Golden Notes in
ENT

List of Videos (QR Codes)

 Access the Videos by Scanning the QR Code Inside

Sl. No	Video title	Chapter number	Page number
1.	Examination of Ear with Otoscope and Aural Speculum	5, 75	47, 441, 442, 443
2	Rinne's Test and Absolute Bone Conduction Test	5	49, 50
3.	Weber's Test	5	50
4.	Fistula Test	5, 10	53, 86
5.	Epiley's and Dix–Hallpike Maneuver	15, 84	112, 116, 542
6.	Ear Syringing	53	368
7.	Anterior Rhinoscopy	20, 75, 84	151, 450, 542
8.	Posterior Rhinoscopy	20, 75, 84	152, 449, 542
9.	Cottle's Test	20, 84	152, 542
10.	Cold Spatula Test	20, 84	152, 542
11.	Indirect Laryngoscopy	30, 75, 84	214, 460, 543
12.	Laryngeal Crepitus	30, 44, 84	215, 300, 543
13.	Pure Tone Audiometry	79	503
14.	Impedence Audiometry	79	505

Golden Notes in ENT

[Previously Known as Exam Preparatory Manual for Undergraduates Otorhinolaryngology (ENT)]

As per the Revised Competency-based Medical Education Curriculum (NMC)

SECOND EDITION

Nilam Uttam Sathe MBBS MS (ENT) FCPS DORL

Associate Professor and Head of Unit
Department of Otorhinolaryngology
Seth GS Medical College (GSMC)
King Edward Memorial (KEM) Hospital
Mumbai, Maharashtra, India

Consultant ENT Surgeon
Fortis Hiranandani Hospital
Navi Mumbai, Maharashtra, India

Wockhardt Hospital
Mumbai, Maharashtra, India

Forewords
D S Grewal
Sanjay N Oak

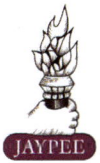

JAYPEE BROTHERS MEDICAL PUBLISHERS
The Health Sciences Publisher
New Delhi | London

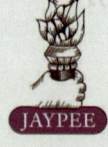

Jaypee Brothers Medical Publishers (P) Ltd

Headquarters
EMCA House
23/23-B, Ansari Road, Daryaganj
New Delhi 110 002, India
Landline: +91-11-23272143, +91-11-23272703
+91-11-23282021, +91-11-23245672
E-mail: jaypee@jaypeebrothers.com

Overseas Office
J.P. Medical Ltd
83 Victoria Street, London
SW1H 0HW (UK)
Phone: +44 20 3170 8910
E-mail: info@jpmedpub.com

Corporate Office
4838/24, Ansari Road, Daryaganj
New Delhi 110 002, India
Phone: +91-11-43574357
Fax: +91-11-43574314
E-mail: jaypee@jaypeebrothers.com

EU GPSR Authorised Representative
Logos Europe, 9 rue Nicolas Poussin
17000, La Rochelle, France
Phone: +33 (0) 6 67 93 73 78
E-mail: contact@logoseurope.eu

Website: www.jaypeebrothers.com
Website: www.jaypeedigital.com

© 2026, Jaypee Brothers Medical Publishers

The views and opinions expressed in this book are solely those of the original contributor(s)/author(s) and do not necessarily represent those of editor(s) and publisher of the book.

All rights reserved. No part of this publication may be reproduced, stored or transmitted in any form or by any means, electronic, mechanical, photocopying, recording or otherwise, without the prior permission in writing of the publishers.

All brand names and product names used in this book are trade names, service marks, trademarks or registered trademarks of their respective owners. The publisher is not associated with any product or vendor mentioned in this book.

Medical knowledge and practice change constantly. This book is designed to provide accurate, authoritative information about the subject matter in question. However, readers are advised to check the most current information available on procedures included and check information from the manufacturer of each product to be administered, to verify the recommended dose, formula, method and duration of administration, adverse effects and contraindications. It is the responsibility of the practitioner to take all appropriate safety precautions. Neither the publisher nor the author(s)/editor(s) assume any liability for any injury and/or damage to persons or property arising from or related to use of material in this book.

This book is sold on the understanding that the publisher is not engaged in providing professional medical services. If such advice or services are required, the services of a competent medical professional should be sought.

Every effort has been made where necessary to contact holders of copyright to obtain permission to reproduce copyright material. If any have been inadvertently overlooked, the publisher will be pleased to make the necessary arrangements at the first opportunity.

Inquiries for bulk sales may be solicited at: jaypee@jaypeebrothers.com

Golden Notes in ENT

First Edition: 2023
   Reprint: 2024
Second Edition: **2026**

ISBN: 978-93-6616-908-8

Printed in India

Foreword

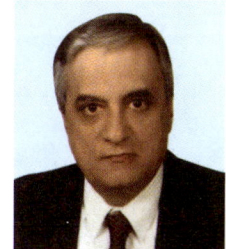

It is a great honour for me to write the foreword of *Exam Preparatory Manual for Undergraduate: Otorhinolaryngology (ENT)*. I have known Dr Nilam Uttam Sathe, one of the most dynamic and versatile ENT surgeons and academician from her postgraduate days. She got the Gold Medal by standing first in the MS (ENT) in Mumbai University. Her astute clinical skills and her passion to teach over a period of years has fully culminated to the publishing of this book, a competency-based medical education (CBME) teaching medium for both, the teachers and the students.

Out of the many salient features of this unique book, a few key ones are:
- All chapters are in question and answer format as per competencies.
- All the chapters are illustrated in tables and flowcharts format, along with relevant clinical photographs.
- Video links for various procedures is a novel feature for better understanding of students which is not seen in most ENT textbooks.
- In practical section, sample long cases and short cases presentation chapters along with frequently asked questions with clinical pictures are added. Also, the chapters of history taking and examination are added with self-explanatory photographs.
- Along with chapters of instruments, radiology, pure tone audiogram and impedance audiometry, and recent advances, a novel chapter on "Specimens" has been added with the markings of the operative specimens and the commonly asked viva voce questions.
- New chapters like objective structured clinical/practical examination (OSCE) and mock question papers have also been added.
- For the very first time, video demonstration of audiology procedures has been added.

Dr Nilam Sathe has provided comprehensive knowledge by the way of question and answers which will help the MBBS students to face the examination with confidence.

It will also help them in their preparations for the NEET PG examinations.

I wish her all the very best in this latest academic endeavor of hers.

D S Grewal MS DLO FACS
Former Professor and Head
Department of ENT
Topiwala National Medical College (TNMC) and BYL Nair Charitable Hospital
President, Association of Otolaryngologists of India (AOI), 2005
Mumbai, Maharashtra, India

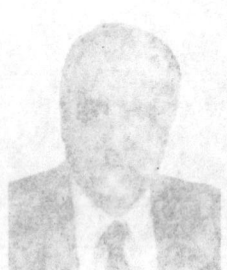

Foreword

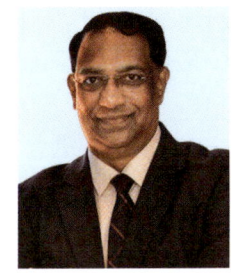

Dear Students, it gives me a great please in writing a foreword for a wonderful effort executed by Dr Nilam Uttam Sathe. I know Nilam for more than two decades now and regard her as a very passionate, persistent and meticulous ENT surgeon who cares for welfare of her undergraduates as well as postgraduate students. She is a teacher in the true sense. I have gone through the contents of the index book *Exam Preparatory Manual for Undergraduate: Otorhinolaryngology (ENT)* and find it extremely practically oriented and student friendly, presentation is lucid and in question-and-answer format. These are the general questions that are asked in examinations either in a case or in a viva voce or even for that matter in a long answer theory question paper. Illustrations in the form of tables, flowcharts, graphics and clinical photographs add to the values of the book. What I liked most was that she has provided video links in the book. Education now has to be hybrid and the students can avail benefit of the live operative procedures through the links quoted in the books. Chapters on history taking and presentation of a case are exemplary. She has covered every aspect of the practical examination by referring to instruments, operations, X-rays, specimens and there is nothing left out. Recent advances are touched upon and students are also oriented to objective structured clinical/practical examination (OSCE) type questions and how to approach them. Overall, I find the book extremely informative and will boost the confidence of an examination undergoing student.

Sanjay N Oak MCH (Paediatric Surgery) MS (General Surgery)
Ex-Vice Chancellor, DY Patil University, Navi Mumbai
Ex-Director, Medical Education and Municipal Hospitals, Municipal Corporation of Greater Mumbai, Mumbai
Ex-Dean, Topiwala National Medical College (TNMC) and BYL Nair Charitable Hospital, Mumbai
Ex-Dean, Seth Gordhandas Sunderdas Medical College (GSMC) and King Edward Memorial (KEM) Hospital, Mumbai
Ex-Professor and Head, Department of Paediatric Surgery, TN Medical College, Mumbai
Ex-CEO, Aga Khan Health Services, India
Task Force In-Charge, COVID-19, Maharashtra
Director Professional Services and Project Management, Kaushalya Hospital, Mumbai, Maharashtra, India

Preface to the Second Edition

It gives me immense pleasure to present the second edition of this unique textbook, now titled *Golden Notes in ENT*, a refined and updated successor to the earlier edition *Exam Preparatory Manual for Undergraduates in ENT*. With evolving academic needs and the implementation of the Competency-based Medical Education (CBME) curriculum by the National Medical Commission (NMC), this edition has been comprehensively revised to meet the current standards and expectations of undergraduate medical education.

This book is structured into seven logically organized sections, thoughtfully structured to integrate both theoretical and practical components. Each chapter is designed in a question-and-answer format, aligning with prescribed competencies, and enriched with visual learning aids for better understanding and retention.

Key Features of this Edition:
- **Competency-aligned content:** All chapters have been structured in a Q&A format following the NMC CBME curriculum, focusing on both theory and practical competencies.
- **Enhanced visual learning:** The content is supported by tables, flowcharts, and clinical photographs that simplify complex concepts and enhance clarity.
- **Integrated video content:** A novel addition to this edition is the inclusion of video links demonstrating key ENT procedures, curated by our team to aid visual learning—a feature rarely found in conventional ENT textbooks.
- **Practical section expansion:** The practical segment now includes sample long and short cases, frequently asked questions, and high-quality clinical images. Detailed chapters on History Taking and Clinical Examination are also included with self-explanatory illustrations.
- **Innovative chapters:** For the first time, chapters on specimens featuring operative samples along with viva questions have been added, alongside content on instruments, radiology, audiology, and recent advances in the field.
- **OSCE and mock exams:** A dedicated section on Objective Structured Clinical Examinations (OSCEs) and mock question papers is included to help students prepare effectively for exams.
- **Audiology video demonstration:** A first-of-its-kind feature—video-based demonstration of audiology procedures—has been added to bridge the gap between theory and practice.

This second edition is the result of a sincere, collaborative effort aimed at equipping students with a comprehensive, clinically oriented, and exam-focused resource. It is designed to serve as a complete companion for undergraduate students in Otorhinolaryngology.

I hope that this updated version will not only help students succeed in examinations but also strengthen their clinical acumen and understanding of ENT. I welcome your valuable feedback and suggestions for continuous improvement.

Nilam Uttam Sathe

Preface to the First Edition

It gives me immense pleasure to bring out and write this unique *Exam Preparatory Manual for Undergraduate: Otorhinolaryngology (ENT)*. As the time changes the method of studies also changes. And now we have the new competency-based medical education (CBME) curriculum of 2019. This book is compliant with NMC CBME curriculum.

This book is divided into four parts. It forms an integral and important part of theory and practical. All the chapters are presented in question-and-answer format with highlighting points as per the competencies.

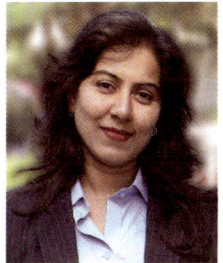

Key points of this book are:
- Theory and practical chapters are in question answer format as per competencies.
- All the chapters are powered by tables, flowcharts format and clinical photographs.
- Video links for various procedures prepared by our team would be novel feature for better understanding of students which would not be seen in many other ENT textbooks.
- In practical section, sample long cases and short cases presentation chapters along with frequently asked questions with clinical pictures are added. Also, the chapters of history taking and examination are added with self-explanatory photographs.
- This is for the first-time chapters on instruments, radiology, pure tone audiogram and impedance audiometry, recent advances and chapter on operative specimens with viva questions are covered.
- New chapters like objective structured clinical/practical examination (OSCE) and mock question papers have also been added to accustom the students with exam patterns.
- First time video demonstration of various procedures and audiology have been added.

It's a sincere attempt of our team so that the expectations of the students are met and the book will help them achieving greater success in writing the exam and improving clinical approaches and understanding otorhinolaryngology.

Theory and practical all available in one textbook. Crisp, complete and comprehensive textbook useful for undergraduates and primer for postgraduates.

Looking forward for your sincere feedback.

Nilam Uttam Sathe

Acknowledgments

My journey in medicine and in this world started with the great efforts and unbelievable support of my parents **Mr Uttam Bansi Sathe, my father, Ms Shanta Uttam Sathe, my mother.** My family members, sisters, Poonam, Varsha, Pallavi especially my brother, Mr Amit Sathe (Advocate), my nephew, Pratham Bhalerao, my niece, Marvika Kedar and my respected teachers. I am extremely thankful to these supporting pillars of my life journey.

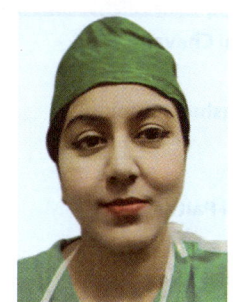

Nilam Uttam Sathe

My journey into medicine and ENT started with excellent teachers. I had an opportunity to learn from the best teachers. I am extremely thankful to my role models and teachers **Dr D S Grewal**, Ex-Head, Department of ENT, Topiwala National Medical College and BYL Nair Charitable Hospital, Mumbai, **Dr Sanjay Oak**, Ex-Vice Chancellor, DY Patil University, Director, Medical Health and Medical Education, Municipal Mumbai Medical Colleges, Ex-Dean BYL Nair Hospital and Topiwala National Medical College and Seth GS Medical College and King Edward Memorial (KEM) Hospital, Mumbai. I am thankful to my PG guide *Late* **Dr Navin L Hiranandani**; My Teachers, Dr Jyoti Dabholkar, Dr Dinaz Namdarian, Dr Ninad Gaikwad, Head, Department of Otorhinlaryngology, HBT Medical College and Dr RN Cooper Municipal Hospital, Mumbai; Dr AG Pusalkar, Ex-Head, Department of ENT, BYL Nair Charitable Hospital and Topiwala National Medical College, Mumbai and DY Patil Medical College; Dr Ajay Shah, Dr KK Ezzy. Padmashree Dr MV Kirtane, Ex-Head, Department of ENT, Seth GS Medical College and KEM Hospital, Mumbai, Consultant ENT Surgeon, Hinduja Hospital, Breach Candy Hospital, Mumbai; Dr Hemant Sheode, Dr Narayanan Janakiram, Royal Pearl Hospital, Trichy, Tamil Nadu. I am thankful to my colleague residents for grooming me in ENT during my residency: Dr Trupti Gadkari, Dr Manoj Bhaskaran, Chennai, Tamil Nadu; Dr Chandrakiran, Mysuru, Karnataka; Dr Anurag

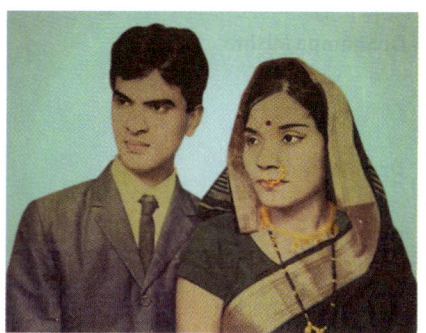

Mr Uttam Bansi Sathe, my father
Ms Shanta Uttam Sathe, my mother

Singhal, Ghaziabad, Uttar Pradesh; Dr Manish Patankar, Dubai; Dr Rohan Walvekar, LSU Hospital, New Orleans, USA; Dr Paresh Tankwal, Bhopal, Madhya Pradesh; Dr Sameer Lambay, Dr Makrand Damle, Dr Amit Sheth, Dr Jayesh Ranawat, Dr Vijay Jagasia, Dr Vikram Khanna, Dr Neha Shah, Dr Meenesh Juvekar.

I am filled with gratitude towards our Seth GS Medical College and KEM Hospital, Mumbai Dean **Dr Sangeeta Ravat** for her blessings and support. I am also thankful to my teacher **Dr Shailesh Mohite**, Head, Department of Forensic Medicine and Dean, HBT Medical College and Dr. RN Cooper Municipal General Hospital, Mumbai.

No publication is complete without the support of publishers. I am thankful to the whole team of M/s Jaypee Brothers Medical Publishers (P) Ltd, New Delhi, India, who helped and guided me, Shri Jitendar P Vij (Group Chairman), Mr Ankit Vij (Managing Director), Mr MS Mani (Group President), Dr Madhu Choudhary (Director-Educational Publishing), Ms Pooja Bhandari [Director-Production (Books and Journals)], Mr Ajay Kumar Sharma [Deputy General Manager (Books and Journals)], Ms Sunita Katla (Executive Assistant to Group Chairman and Publishing Manager), Ms Samina Khan (Executive Assistant to Director–Educational Publishing), Dr Aditya Tayal (Senior Editorial Manager–Content Strategy), Mr Vijay Kumar Bhatia (Manager-Production), Mr Bishan Singh (Production Manager), Ms Seema Dogra (Cover Visualizer), Ms Neha Verma (Graphic Designer-Cover), Mr Dilip Kumar Jha (Quality Analyst), Mr Kulwant Singh (Typesetter), Mr Nitesh Jain (Graphic Designer) and their team members, for all their support to work in this project and make it a success.

Special acknowledgment to:
Marketing heads of all zones (Delhi): Mr Narendra Shekhawat (Vice President—Sales), Mr Sandeep Gupta (RBM—East), Mr CS Gawde (RBM—West), Mr A Maran (RBM—South), Mr Dinesh S Dheek (RBM—North), Mr Rishi Sharma (RBDM—North-East-West)
Branch managers and sales managers from various branches: Mr Sameer S Mulla (Mumbai Branch), Mr Dinesh Waghade (Ahmedabad Branch), Mr Sanjoy Chakraborthy (Kolkata Branch), Mr BS Rawat (Delhi Branch), Mr Rajesh Shrivas (Nagpur Branch), Mr Parimal Guha Neogy (Hyderabad Branch), Mr Gajanan Prabhu (Bengaluru Branch), Mr Dharani Kumar (Chennai Branch), Mr Sujeesh VS (Kochi Branch).

Acknowledgments

A teacher's journey cannot be complete without her students. I am extremely thankful to my one of the pillars, my students Dr Vijay Prakash, Dr Mukesh Kumar, Dr Palak Bhatti, Dr Sonal Sarraiya, USA, Dr Prashant Sharma, Dubai; Dr Sarika Chapne, Dr Sanjana Chirmade, Head, SKN Medical College, Pune; Dr Gaurav Wadkar, Dr Samir Thakre, Dr Manoj Patil, Dr Rameshwar Pawar, Assistant Professor, Government Medical College, Latur, Maharashtra; Dr Sheetal Shelke, Assistant Professor, MIMSR Medical College, Latur; Dr Abhijeet Shirude, Dr Ankur Pareek, Dr Anup Srinivas, Dr Pravin Misal and our audiologist for their unconditional support. Special thanks to:

Name	Designation
Dr Kamini Chavan	Assistant Professor, Seth GS Medical College (GSMC) and King Edward Memorial (KEM) Hospital, Mumbai, Maharashtra, India
Dr Dhanashree Chiplunkar	Ex-Assistant Professor, Seth GS Medical College (GSMC) and King Edward Memorial (KEM) Hospital, Mumbai, Maharashtra, India Consultant DNB Teacher, KB Bhabha Hospital, Mumbai, Maharashtra, India
Dr Pallavi Paithankar	Head, Department of Speech and Audiology, Seth GS Medical College (GSMC) and King Edward Memorial (KEM) Hospital, Mumbai, Maharashtra, India
Dr Swapnal Sawarkar	Ex-Resident, Seth GS Medical College (GSMC) and King Edward Memorial (KEM) Hospital, Mumbai, Maharashtra, India Consultant ENT Surgery, Century Super speciality Hospital and Kamineni Hospital, Hyderabad, Telangana, India
Dr Shampa Mishra	Ex-Resident, Seth GS Medical College (GSMC) and King Edward Memorial (KEM) Hospital, Mumbai, Maharashtra, India Ex-Assistant Professor, Sir JJ Hospital and Grant Medical College, Mumbai, Maharashtra, India
Dr Anjali Taku	Senior Resident, Seth GS Medical College (GSMC) and King Edward Memorial (KEM) Hospital, Mumbai, Maharashtra, India
Dr Muniram Pawra	Senior Resident, Seth GS Medical College (GSMC) and King Edward Memorial (KEM) Hospital, Mumbai, Maharashtra, India
Dr Akshay Jegarkal	Otology Fellow, Seth GS Medical College and King Edward Memorial (KEM) Hospital, Mumbai, Maharashtra, India
Dr Shraddha Bhoyar	Senior Resident, Seth GS Medical College (GSMC) and King Edward Memorial (KEM) Hospital, Mumbai, Maharashtra, India
Dr Manisha Sharma	Senior Resident, Seth GS Medical College (GSMC) and King Edward Memorial (KEM) Hospital, Mumbai, Maharashtra, India
Dr Sivasubramanium Nagrajan	Otology Fellow, Seth GS Medical College (GSMC) and King Edward Memorial (KEM) Hospital, Mumbai, Maharashtra, India
Dr Saad Ahmed	Senior Resident, Seth GS Medical College (GSMC) and King Edward Memorial (KEM) Hospital, Mumbai, Maharashtra, India
Dr Lalpek Thangi	Senior Resident, Seth GS Medical College (GSMC) and King Edward Memorial (KEM) Hospital, Mumbai, Maharashtra, India
Dr Rajat Magdum	Senior Resident, Seth GS Medical College (GSMC) and King Edward Memorial (KEM) Hospital, Mumbai, Maharashtra, India

Contents

Part 1: Diseases of ENT, Head and Neck

Section 1: Basic Sciences

Chapter 1:	Anatomy and Physiology of Ear	3
Chapter 2:	Anatomy and Physiology of Nose and Paranasal Sinuses	15
Chapter 3:	Anatomy and Physiology of Oral Cavity and Pharynx	27
Chapter 4:	Anatomy and Physiology of Larynx and Esophagus	33

Section 2: Otology

Chapter 5:	History Taking and Examination of Ear	41
Chapter 6:	Diseases of the External Ear	55
Chapter 7:	Diseases of Middle Ear	64
Chapter 8:	Eustachian Tube and its Disorders	68
Chapter 9:	Chronic Suppurative Otitis Media	73
Chapter 10:	Complications of Chronic Suppurative Otitis Media	82
Chapter 11:	Otosclerosis	92
Chapter 12:	Meniere's Disease	95
Chapter 13:	Hearing Loss	99
Chapter 14:	Tinnitus	105
Chapter 15:	Assessment and Disorders of Vestibular System	108
Chapter 16:	Deaf Child and Rehabilitation of Hearing Impaired	120
Chapter 17:	Facial Nerve and its Disorders	127
Chapter 18:	Benign Conditions and Malignant Tumors of External Ear and Middle Ear	133
Chapter 19:	Vestibular Schwannoma	143

Section 3: Rhinology

Chapter 20:	History Taking and Examination of Nose and Paranasal Sinuses	147
Chapter 21:	Diseases of External Nose	154
Chapter 22:	Nasal Septum and its Diseases	158
Chapter 23:	Acute and Chronic Rhinitis and Sinusitis and its Complications	163
Chapter 24:	Allergic, Vasomotor Rhinitis and Nonallergic Rhinitis	173
Chapter 25:	Nasal Polyp	177
Chapter 26:	Epistaxis	179
Chapter 27:	Facial Trauma	183
Chapter 28:	Granulomatous Diseases of Nose	192
Chapter 29:	Neoplasms of the Nasal Cavity and Paranasal Sinuses	202

Section 4: Laryngology, Head and Neck

Chapter 30:	History and Examination of Oral Cavity, Throat, Head and Neck	210
Chapter 31:	Disorders and Tumors of Oral Cavity	219
Chapter 32:	Disorders and Tumors of the Salivary Glands	229
Chapter 33:	Acute and Chronic Tonsillitis	237
Chapter 34:	Adenoiditis (Nasopharyngeal Tonsil)	243
Chapter 35:	Acute and Chronic Pharyngitis	246
Chapter 36:	Head and Neck Space Infections	248
Chapter 37:	Tumors of Nasopharynx, Hypopharynx, Oropharynx and Pharyngeal Pouch	256
Chapter 38:	Laryngotracheal Trauma	266
Chapter 39:	Acute and Chronic Inflammation of Larynx	270
Chapter 40:	Congenital Lesions of Larynx	284
Chapter 41:	Laryngeal Paralysis	287
Chapter 42:	Stridor and Stertor	291
Chapter 43:	Benign Tumors of Larynx	295
Chapter 44:	Carcinoma Larynx (Malignant Tumors of Larynx)	299
Chapter 45:	Voice and Speech Disorders	304
Chapter 46:	Snoring and Sleep Apnea	308
Chapter 47:	Foreign Bodies in Air and Food Passages	315
Chapter 48:	Disorders of Esophagus and Dysphagia	320
Chapter 49:	Human Immunodeficiency Virus in Ear, Nose, and Throat	335

Part 2: Operative Procedures

Section 1: Ear

Chapter 50:	Tympanoplasty	357
Chapter 51:	Mastoidectomy	360
Chapter 52:	Myringotomy	364
Chapter 53:	Wax Removal	367

Section 2: Nose

Chapter 54:	Septoplasty and Submucous Resection of Septum	369
Chapter 55:	Polypectomy	373

Chapter 56:	Functional Endoscopic Sinus Surgery	375
Chapter 57:	Endoscopic Septoplasty	379
Chapter 58:	Nasal Packing	381

Section 3: Throat

Chapter 59:	Tonsillectomy	384
Chapter 60:	Adenoidectomy	389
Chapter 61:	Thyroidectomy	391
Chapter 62:	Tracheostomy	394
Chapter 63:	Cricothyroidotomy	404

Section 4: Various Scopy

Chapter 64:	Laryngoscopy	406
Chapter 65:	Microlaryngoscopy	409
Chapter 66:	Esophagoscopy	411
Chapter 67:	Bronchoscopy	413

Section 5: Recent Advances

Chapter 68:	Laser in ENT	417
Chapter 69:	Coblation	420
Chapter 70:	Radiofrequency	423
Chapter 71:	Cryosurgery	425
Chapter 72:	Robotics in ENT	427
Chapter 73:	Chemotherapy in ENT	429
Chapter 74:	Radiotherapy in ENT	434

Part 3: Miscellaneous Topics

Chapter 75:	Instruments in ENT	441
Chapter 76:	Radiology in ENT (X-rays)	473
Chapter 77:	CT Scan and MRI	491
Chapter 78:	Anesthesia in ENT	499
Chapter 79:	Pure Tone Audiogram and Impedance Audiometry	503

Part 4: Questions

Chapter 80:	Objective Structured Clinical/Practical Examination (OSCE)	513
Chapter 81:	Operative Specimens in ENT	520
Chapter 82:	Mock Question Papers	529
Chapter 83:	Multiple Choice Questions (MCQs)	532
Chapter 84:	Case Presentation	538

Index   *553*

Competency Table

Number	Competency The student should be able to	Core (Y/N)	Chapter Number	Page Number
EN1.1	Describe the anatomy and physiology of ear, nose, throat, head and neck	Y	1 2 3 4 33	3 15 27 33 237
EN1.2	Describe the pathophysiology of common diseases in ENT like chronic otitis media, otosclerosis, adenotonsillitis, nasal polyposis	Y	9 11 25 34	73 92 177 243
EN2.1	Elicit document and present an appropriate history in a patient presenting with an ENT complaint	Y	5 20 30	41 147 210
EN2.2	Demonstrate the correct use of conventional methods including head lamp in the examination of ear, nose and throat, the correct technique of examination of the nose and paranasal sinuses including the use of nasal speculum, examination of the throat including the use of a tongue depressor, examination of neck including elicitation of laryngeal crepitus	Y	20 30 75	150 210 441
EN2.3	Demonstrate the correct technique of examination of the ear including Otoscopy and demonstrate the correct technique of performance and interpretation of tuning fork tests	Y	5	46, 49
EN2.4	Describe the correct technique to perform and interpret pure tone audiogram and impedance audiogram	Y	79	503
EN2.5	Demonstrate the correct technique of otoscopy, to hold visualize and assess the mobility of the tympanic membrane, interpret and diagrammatically represent the findings	Y	5	49
EN2.6	Choose correctly and interpret radiological, microbiological and histological investigations relevant to the ENT disorders	Y	76 77	473 491
EN2.7	Identify and describe the use of common instruments used in ENT surgery. Nose: FESS, septoplasty, nasal bone reduction ear tympanoplasty, mastoidectomy, myringotomy Throat: Adenotonsillectomy, foreign body removal from airway and food passage, tracheostomy	Y	47 75	315 441
EN2.8	Enumerate suspect high-risk patients and risk factors associated with and identify by clinical examination malignant and premalignant ENT diseases	Y	31	221
EN2.9	Counsel and administer informed consent to patients and their families in a simulated environment for Ear: Tympanoplasty, mastoidectomy, myringotomy nose: FESS, septoplasty, nasal bone reduction throat: Adenotonsillectomy, foreign body removal from airway and food passage, tracheostomy	Y	47 66 67	315 411 413
EN2.10	Identify, resuscitate and manage ENT emergencies in a simulated environment (including tracheostomy, anterior nasal packing, removal of foreign bodies in ear, nose, throat, upper respiratory tract and food passages)	Y	47 58 62 66 67	315 381 394 411 413
EN2.11	Demonstrate the correct technique to instill topical medications into the ear, nose and throat in a simulated environment	Y	78	499
EN3.2	Observe and describe the indications for and steps involved in the performance of diagnostic nasal endoscopy	N	56	377
EN3.3	Observe and describe the indications for and steps involved in the performance of rigid/flexible laryngoscopy	N	64	406

Competency Table

Number	Competency — The student should be able to	Core (Y/N)	Chapter Number	Page Number
EN4.1	Elicit document and present a correct history, demonstrate and describe the clinical features, choose the correct investigations and describe the principles of management of otalgia	Y	5	43
EN4.2	Elicit document and present a correct history, demonstrate and describe the clinical features, choose the correct investigations and describe the principles of management of diseases of the external ear	Y	6	55
EN4.3	Elicit document and present a correct history, describe the clinical features, choose the correct investigations and describe the principles of management of ASOM	Y	7	64
EN4.4	Elicit document and present a correct history, describe the clinical features, choose the correct investigations and describe the principles of management of OME	Y	7	66
EN4.5	Elicit document and present a correct history, demonstrate and describe the clinical features, choose the correct investigations and describe the principles of management of ear discharge	Y	5, 9	41, 73
EN4.6	Elicit document and present a correct history demonstrate and describe the clinical features, choose the correct investigations and describe the principles of management of mucosal type of CSOM	Y	9	73
EN4.7	Elicit document and present a correct history, demonstrate and describe the clinical features, choose the correct investigations and describe the principles of management of squamosal type of CSOM	Y	9	77
EN4.8	Describe the clinical features, choose the correct investigations and the principles of management of complications of CSOM.	Y	10	82
EN4.9	Demonstrate the correct technique for wax removal from the ear in a simulated environment	Y	53	367
EN4.10	Observe and describe the indications for and steps involved in myringotomy and tympanoplasty	Y	50, 52	357, 364
EN4.11	Observe and describe the indications for and steps involved in mastoidectomy	Y	51	360
EN4.12	Describe the clinical features, investigations and principles of management of acoustic neuroma	Y	19	143
EN4.13	Describe the clinical features, investigations and principles of management of otosclerosis	Y	11	92
EN4.14	Describe the clinical features, investigations, and principles of management of conductive hearing loss and sensorineural hearing loss including sudden sensorineural hearing loss and noise induced hearing loss	Y	13	99
EN4.15	Describe the anatomy of eustachian tube and discuss the clinical features, investigations, and management of eustachian tube disorders	Y	8	68
EN4.16	Describe the clinical features, investigations, and principles of management of facial nerve palsy	Y	17	129
EN4.17	Describe the clinical features, investigations and management of vertigo and assessment of vestibular functions.	Y	15	108
EN4.18	Describe the clinical features, investigations, and principles of management of Meniere's disease	N	12	95
EN4.19	Describe the clinical features, investigations, and management of Tinnitus	Y	14	105
EN4.20	Describe the clinical features, investigations, and management of deaf child	Y	16	120
EN4.21	Elicit document and present a correct history demonstrate and describe the causes, choose the correct investigations and describe the principles of management of nasal obstruction	Y	20	148
EN4.22	Describe the clinical features, investigations and management of DNS and observe and discuss the indications for the steps in septoplasty	Y	22, 54	159, 369
EN4.23	Elicit document and present a correct history, demonstrate and describe the clinical features, choose the correct investigations and describe the principles of management of adenoids	Y	34	243
EN4.24	Elicit document and present a correct history, describe the clinical features, choose the correct investigations and describe the principles of management of allergic rhinitis	Y	24	174
EN4.25	Elicit document and present a correct history, describe the clinical features, choose the correct investigations and describe the principles of management of vasomotor rhinitis	Y	24	173

Competency Table

Number	Competency The student should be able to	Core (Y/N)	Chapter Number	Page Number
EN4.26	Elicit, document and present a correct history, describe the clinical features, choose the correct investigations and describe the principles of management of acute and chronic rhinitis	Y	23	163
EN4.27	Elicit, document and present a correct history, describe the clinical features, choose the correct investigations and describe the principles of management of nasal polyps	Y	25	177
EN4.28	Elicit document and present a correct history, demonstrate and describe the clinical features, choose the correct investigations and describe the principles of management of epistaxis	Y	26	179
EN4.29	Describe the clinical features, choose the correct investigations and describe the principles of management of obstructive sleep apnea	N	46	308
EN4.30	Describe the clinical features, investigations and principles of management of head and neck trauma	N	27 38	183 266
EN4.31	Describe the clinical features, investigations and principles of management of nasopharyngeal angiofibroma	Y	37	256
EN4.32	Elicit document and present a correct history demonstrate and describe the clinical features, choose the correct investigations and describe the principles of management of acute and chronic sinusitis and its complications	Y	23	163
EN4.33	Describe the clinical features, investigations and principles of management of tumors of nose, nasopharynx and para nasal sinus	Y	29 37	202 256
EN4.34	Describe the clinical features, investigation and management of granulomatous diseases of nose	N	28	192
EN4.35	Describe the clinical features, investigations and principles of management of diseases of the salivary glands	N	32	229
EN4.36	Describe the clinical features, investigations and principles of management of deep neck space infection	Y	36	248
EN4.37	Elicit document and present a correct history describe the clinical features, choose the correct investigations and describe the principles of management of dysphagia	Y	48	331
EN4.38	Elicit document and present a correct history, describe the clinical features, choose the correct investigations, complications and describe the principles of management of acute and chronic tonsillitis	Y	33	238
EN4.39	Observe and describe the indications for and steps involved in a tonsillectomy/adenoidectomy and its complications	Y	59 60	384 389
EN4.40	Elicit, document and present a correct history, describe the clinical features, choose the correct investigations and describe the principles of management of hoarseness of voice	Y	45	304
EN4.41	Describe the clinical features, investigations and principles of management of benign lesion of larynx, acute and chronic inflammation of larynx, laryngeal paralysis	Y	39 41 43	270 287 295
EN4.42	Describe the clinical features, investigations and principles of management of malignancy of the larynx and hypopharynx	Y	37 44	263 299
EN4.43	Describe the clinical features, investigations and principles of management of stridor	Y	42	291
EN4.44	Observe and describe the indications for and steps involved in tracheostomy and the care of the patient with a tracheostomy	Y	62	394
EN4.45	Describe the clinical features, investigations and principles of management of diseases of esophagus	N	48	320
EN4.46	Describe the clinical features, investigations and principles of management of HIV manifestations of the ENT	N	49	335

PART 1

Diseases of ENT, Head and Neck

Outline

Section 1: Basic Sciences
1. Anatomy and Physiology of Ear
2. Anatomy and Physiology of Nose and Paranasal Sinuses
3. Anatomy and Physiology of Oral Cavity and Pharynx
4. Anatomy and Physiology of Larynx and Esophagus

Section 2: Otology
5. History Taking and Examination of Ear
6. Diseases of the External Ear
7. Diseases of Middle Ear
8. Eustachian Tube and its Disorders
9. Chronic Suppurative Otitis Media
10. Complications of Chronic Suppurative Otitis Media
11. Otosclerosis
12. Meniere's Disease
13. Hearing Loss
14. Tinnitus
15. Assessment and Disorders of Vestibular System
16. Deaf Child and Rehabilitation of Hearing Impaired
17. Facial Nerve and its Disorders
18. Benign Conditions and Malignant Tumors of External Ear and Middle Ear
19. Vestibular Schwannoma

Section 3: Rhinology
20. History Taking and Examination of Nose and Paranasal Sinuses
21. Diseases of External Nose
22. Nasal Septum and its Diseases
23. Acute and Chronic Rhinitis and Sinusitis and its Complications
24. Allergic, Vasomotor Rhinitis and Nonallergic Rhinitis
25. Nasal Polyp
26. Epistaxis
27. Facial Trauma
28. Granulomatous Diseases of Nose
29. Neoplasms of the Nasal Cavity and Paranasal Sinuses

Section 4: Laryngology, Head and Neck
30. History and Examination of Oral Cavity, Throat, Head and Neck
31. Disorders and Tumors of Oral Cavity
32. Disorders and Tumors of the Salivary Glands
33. Acute and Chronic Tonsillitis
34. Adenoiditis (Nasopharyngeal Tonsil)
35. Acute and Chronic Pharyngitis
36. Head and Neck Space Infections
37. Tumors of Nasopharynx, Hypopharynx, Oropharynx and Pharyngeal Pouch
38. Laryngotracheal Trauma
39. Acute and Chronic Inflammation of Larynx
40. Congenital Lesions of Larynx
41. Laryngeal Paralysis
42. Stridor and Stertor
43. Benign Tumors of Larynx
44. Carcinoma Larynx (Malignant Tumors of Larynx)
45. Voice and Speech Disorders
46. Snoring and Sleep Apnea
47. Foreign Bodies in Air and Food Passages
48. Disorders of Esophagus and Dysphagia
49. Human Immunodeficiency Virus in Ear, Nose, and Throat

PART 1

Diseases of ENT, Head and Neck

Outline

Section 1: Basic Sciences

Chapter 1

Anatomy and Physiology of Ear

EN1.1: Describe the anatomy and physiology of ear, nose, throat, head and neck.

■ ANATOMY OF EAR

Q. Enumerate the structures and parts of the ear.

■ EXTERNAL EAR

Auricle or Pinna

Q. Write a short note on anatomy of auricle/pinna.

- ❖ **Parts:**
  - ➢ Helix
  - ➢ Antihelix
  - ➢ Tragus
  - ➢ Antitragus
  - ➢ Lobule
- ❖ **Pinna** → Single piece of yellow elastic cartilage covered with skin except lobule and outer part of external auditory canal (EAC)
- ❖ **Incisura terminalis:** Area where no cartilage between tragus and crus of the helix
  Various elevations and depressions on the lateral surface of the pinna:
- ❖ Concha
- ❖ Cymba conchae
- ❖ Triangular fossa

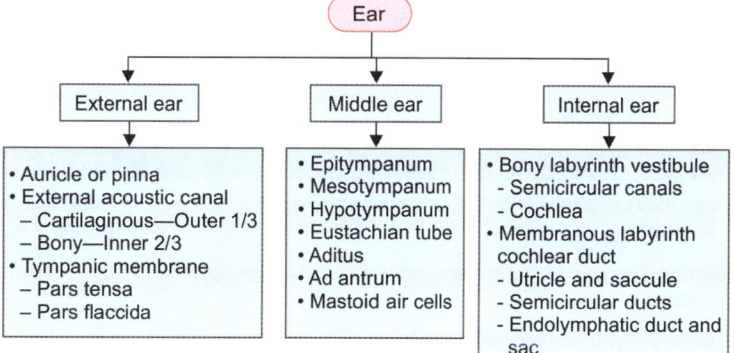

External Acoustic Canal

Q. Write a short note on external acoustic canal.

- ❖ Bottom of concha to tympanic membrane
- ❖ 24 mm along the posterior wall
- ❖ Not a straight tube, outer part directed upwards, backward, and medially and Inner part is directed downwards, forwards, and medially

Note: To see tympanic membrane, pinna is pulled upwards, backward, and laterally so as to bring two parts in alignment.

Cartilaginous Part

- ❖ Forms outer one-third (8 mm) of the canal.
- ❖ It is a continuation of cartilage that forms framework of the pinna.

PART 1: Diseases of ENT, Head and Neck

Q. How ear infections can transmit to parotid?

- **In fissure of Santorini:** Transverse slits in the anterior inferior wall of cartilaginous external auditory canal. Through them spread of infection happens.
- **Skin over the cartilaginous canal:** Thick
- Ceruminous and pilosebaceous glands → wax
- Hair is only confined to outer canal

Note: Therefore, furuncles (staphylococcal infection of hair follicles) are seen only in the outer one-third of the canal.

Bony Part

- Inner two-third (16 mm)
- Skin lining bony canal thin and continuous over the tympanic membrane
- Devoid of hair and ceruminous glands
- **Foramen of Huschke** (anterio inferior part of bony canal, posteromedial to TM joint) establishes a connection between external acoustic canal and mandibular fossa.
- Infections can transmit in children up to 4 years

Tympanic Membrane

Q. Write a short note on tympanic membrane.

- Obliquely set, the posterosuperior part is lateral than anteroinferior part.
- 9–10 mm tall, 8–9 mm wide, and 0.1 mm thick.

Parts

These are divided into two parts:

Pars tensa	Pars flaccida
Annulus tympanicus: Thickened periphery forming a fibrocartilaginous ring	Above lateral process of malleus between the notch of Rivinus and anterior, posterior malleolar folds
Umbo: Central part of pars tensa tented inwards at the tip of malleus	
Cone of light: Anteroinferior quadrant	

Layers of Tympanic Membrane

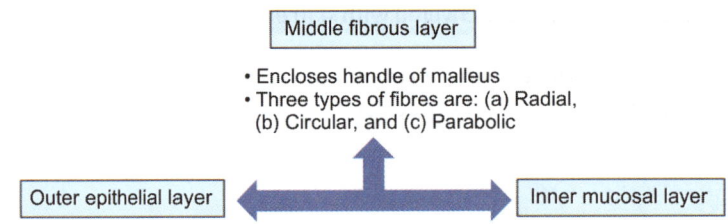

Nerve Supply of External Ear

Q. Write a short note on nerve supply of external ear.

External Auditory Canal

Nerve	Area supplied
Auriculotemporal (V3)	Anterior wall and roof
Auricular branch of vagus (CN X)	Posterior wall and floor
CN VII fibers through auricular branch of the vagus	Posterior wall

Pinna

Nerve	Area supplied
Greater auricular nerve (C2 and C3)	Medial surface of pinna and only posterior part of the lateral surface
Lesser occipital (C2)	Upper part of medial surface
Auriculotemporal (V3)	Tragus, crus of helix, and adjacent part of the helix
Auricular branch of vagus [cranial nerve (CN) X], also called Arnold's nerve	Concha and corresponding eminence on the medial surface
Facial nerve	Concha and retro auricular groove

Tympanic Membrane

Nerve	Area supplied
Auriculotemporal (V3)	Anterior half of lateral surface
Auricular branch of vagus (CN X)	Posterior half of lateral surface

MIDDLE EAR

Q. Write a short note/essay on anatomy of middle ear.

Walls of Middle Ear

Six-sided box

1. Roof
2. Floor
3. Medial
4. Lateral
5. Anterior
6. Posterior wall

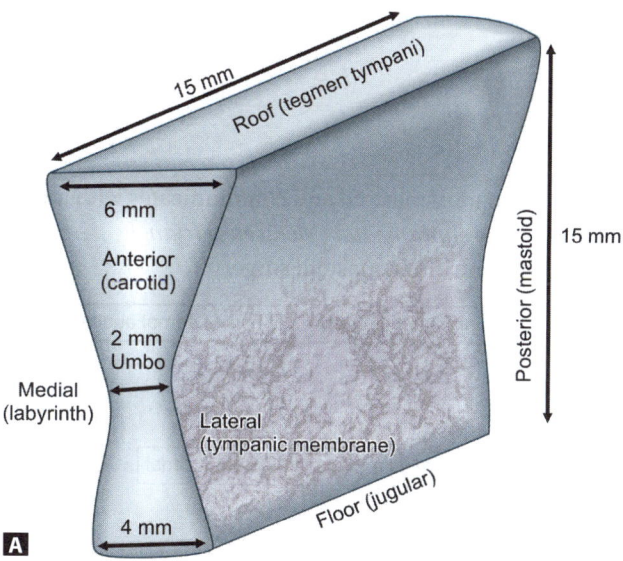

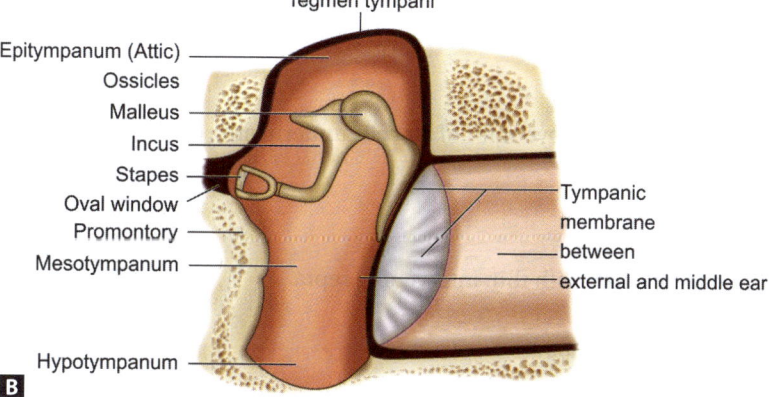

Figs. 1A and B: Middle ear structures.

PART 1: Diseases of ENT, Head and Neck

Structures of Middle Ear

Roof	Thin plate of bone → *tegmen tympani* Separates the tympanic cavity from the middle cranial fossa
Floor	Thin plate of bone separating tympanic cavity from jugular bulb

Posterior wall	❖ **Pyramid:** Bony projection through which appears tendon of stapedius muscle to get an attachment to the neck of stapes
	    Facial nerve runs in posterior wall just behind a pyramid
	 ❖ **Aditus:** Opening through which attic communicates with antrum, lies above pyramid
	 ❖ **Facial recess:** Depression in posterior wall lateral to pyramid
	    Medially: Vertical part of VIIth nerve, laterally: Chorda tympani
	    Above: Fossa incudes

Medial wall	❖ Formed by the labyrinth
	 ❖ **Promontory**—due to basal coil of the cochlea
	 ❖ **Oval window**—into which is fixed stapes footplate
	 ❖ **Round window** is covered by a secondary tympanic membrane.
	 ❖ **Canal for facial nerve**—Above the oval window
	 ❖ Prominence of lateral semicircular canal
	 ❖ **Processus cochleariformis**—hook-like projection anterior to the oval window
	    Importance:
	    Tendon of tensor tympani takes a turn here to get an attachment to the neck of the malleus
	    Level of genu of the facial nerve which is an important landmark for surgery of facial nerve
	 ❖ *Sinus tympani:* Medial to pyramid
	    ➢ Bounded by *subiculum* below *ponticulus* above

Lateral wall	Tympanic membrane Bony outer attic wall → *scutum*

Mastoid Antrum

Q. Write a note on mastoid antrum.

- Large, air-containing space in the upper part of mastoid and communicates with attic through aditus.
- Marked externally on surface of mastoid by *suprameatal (McEwen's) triangle*

Note: Important landmark to locate mastoid antrum in mastoid surgery

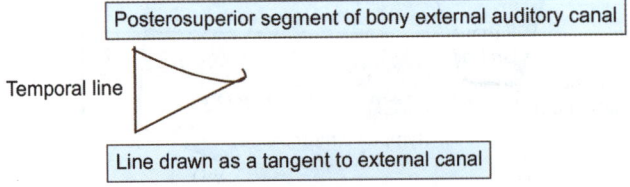

Aditus and Antrum

Aditus is an opening through which the attic communicates with the antrum.

Mastoid and its Air Cell System

Mastoid consists of a bone cortex with a "honeycomb" of air cells underneath.

Types of Mastoid

There are three types of mastoid:
1. **Cellular:** Well-developed mastoid cells with thin intervening septa.
2. **Diploic:** Marrow spaces and few air cells.
3. **Sclerotic:** There are no cells or marrow spaces.

Ossicles of Middle Ear

There are three ossicles in the middle ear—(1) Malleus, (2) Incus, and (3) Stapes.

Ossicles	Parts
Malleus	❖ Head ❖ Neck ❖ Handle (Manubrium) ❖ Lateral process ❖ Anterior process
Incus	❖ Body ❖ Short-process ❖ Long-process
Stapes	❖ Head ❖ Neck ❖ Anterior and posterior crura ❖ Footplate

Footplate is held in oval window by an annular ligament.
- ❖ Ossicles conduct sound energy from the tympanic membrane to the oval window and then to inner ear fluid.

Intratympanic Muscles

Muscles	Action	Nerve supply
Tensor tympani	Tenses tympanic membrane	❖ First arch ❖ Supplied by a branch of the mandibular nerve (V3)
Stapedius	Attaches to neck of stapes and helps to dampen very loud sounds thus preventing noise trauma to inner ear	❖ Second arch muscle ❖ Supplied by a branch of cranial nerve (CN) VII

Nerve Supply of Middle Ear

Tympanic Plexus

- ❖ Lies on a promontory
- ❖ Formed by:
  - ➢ Tympanic branch of the glossopharyngeal
  - ➢ Sympathetic fibers from plexus around the internal carotid artery
- ❖ Supplies innervation to:
  - ➢ Medial surface of tympanic membrane
  - ➢ Tympanic cavity
  - ➢ Mastoid air cells
  - ➢ Bony eustachian tube

Chorda Tympani

- ❖ Branch of facial nerve enters the middle ear through posterior canaliculus, and runs on medial surface of tympanic membrane between the handle of malleus and the long process of incus.
- ❖ **Afferent:** Anterior two-third of the tongue
- ❖ **Efferent:** Secretomotor fibers to submaxillary and sublingual salivary glands.

Blood Supply of Middle Ear

Main	Minor
❖ Anterior tympanic branch of a maxillary artery which supplies tympanic membrane ❖ Stylomastoid branch of the posterior auricular artery which supplies middle ear and mastoid air cells	❖ Petrosal branch of middle meningeal artery ❖ Superior tympanic branch of middle meningeal artery ❖ Branch of artery of pterygoid canal ❖ Tympanic branch of internal carotid

Veins drain into the pterygoid venous plexus and superior petrosal sinus.

INTERNAL EAR

Q. Describe the features of internal ear.

Important organ of hearing and balance.

Bony Labyrinth

It consists of three parts: (1) Vestibule, (2) Semicircular canals, and (3) Cochlea.

Vestibule

Central chamber
- In its lateral wall lies an oval window
- It consists of two recesses:
  - *Spherical recess* → lodges saccule
  - *Elliptical recess* → lodges utricle
- Opening of aqueduct of vestibule through which passes endolymphatic duct.
- Five openings of semicircular canals

Semicircular Canals

- Three in number:

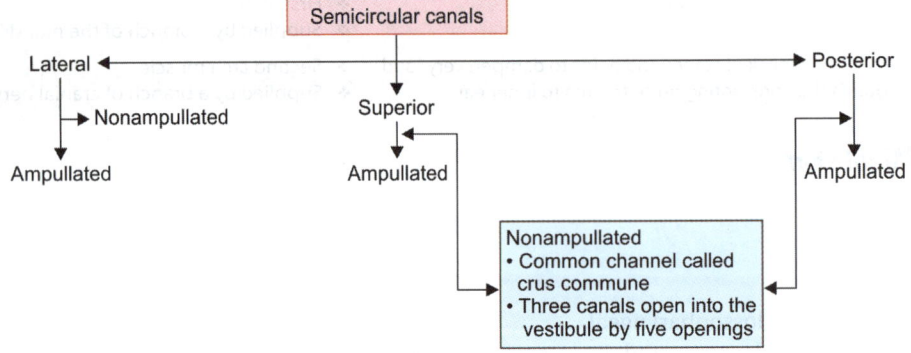

Peripheral Receptors

It consists of two types:

Cristae	Macula
• Located in ampullated ends of three semicircular ducts • Crest-like mound of connective tissues on which sensory epithelial cells are present • Sensory hair cells cilia project into cupula, which is a gelatinous mass extending from surface of crista to ceiling of ampulla and displaced with movements of endolymph • Respond to angular acceleration • Projection of a single hair, kinocilium, and stereocilia	Two parts: • A sensory neuroepithelium, made up of type I, and type II cells, similar to the crista • An otolithic membrane, made up of a gelatinous mass and on top, calcium carbonate crystals are present called otoconia. Linear, gravitational, and head tilt movements displaces otolithic membrane and stimulate hair cells which lie in different planes

Type I hair cell	Type II
• Flask-shaped • Single large cup-like nerve terminal surrounding the base	• Cylindrical • Multiple nerve terminals at the base

CHAPTER 1: Anatomy and Physiology of Ear

Vestibular Nerve

- Vestibular or Scarpa's ganglion is situated in the lateral part of the internal acoustic meatus.
- It contains bipolar cells.
- Distal processes of bipolar cells innervate sensory epithelium of the labyrinth and central processes aggregate to form the vestibular nerve.

Cochlea

Coiled tube making 2.5–2.75 turns around a central pyramid of bone → *modiolus*.
- **Osseous spiral lamina:** Around modiolus, winds spirally like a thread of a screw
- Divides bony cochlea incompletely, and gives attachment to the basilar membrane
- There are three compartments of the cochlea:
    1. Scala vestibuli
    2. Scala tympani
    3. Scala media or membranous cochlea
- **Helicotrema:** Scala vestibuli and scala tympani communicate with each other at the apex of cochlea through an opening
- Scala vestibuli is closed by the footplate of stapes
- Scala tympani is closed by secondary tympanic membrane

Membranous Labyrinth

Cochlear Duct

Also called membranous cochlea or scala media
- Blind coiled tube
    - Basilar membrane → supports the organ of Corti
    - Reissner's membrane → separates it from the scala vestibule
    - Stria vascularis → Contains vascular epithelium and secretes endolymph
- Cochlear duct is connected to saccule by *ductus reunions*
- Length of the basilar membrane increases as we proceed from the basal coil to the apex

Note: Therefore, higher frequencies of sound are heard at the basal coil while lower ones are heard at the apical coil.

Utricle and Saccule

Utricle	Saccule
❖ Lies in posterior part of bony vestibule	❖ Saccule also lies in posterior part of bony vestibule anterior to utricle
❖ Receives five openings of semicircular ducts	❖ Anterior to utricle and opposite stapes footplate
❖ Sensory epithelium is called macula	❖ Sensory epithelium is also called macula
❖ Concerned with linear acceleration and deceleration	❖ It probably also responds to linear acceleration and deceleration
❖ More sensitive to horizontal acceleration	❖ More sensitive to vertical acceleration

Semicircular Ducts

- Three in number
- Correspond to three bony canals
- Opens in utricle
- Ampullated end of each duct contains a thickened ridge of neuroepithelium called *crista ampullaris*.

Endolymphatic Duct and Sac

- Endolymphatic duct is formed by union of the two ducts, one each from the saccule and utricle
- Terminal part is dilated to form an endolymphatic sac

Blood Supply of Labyrinth

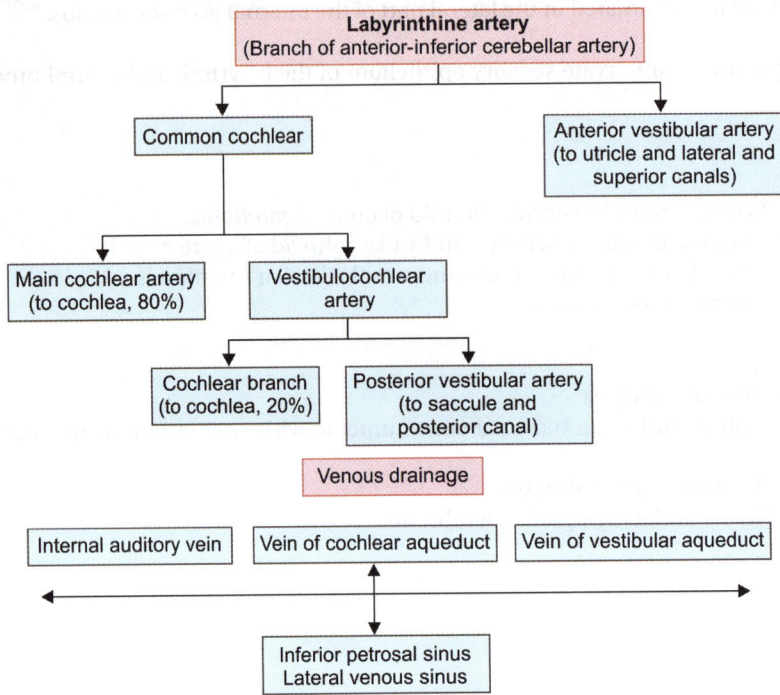

DEVELOPMENT OF EAR

Q. Write a note on development of ear.

Structure	Develops from	Begins	Complete
Pinna	❖ First branchial cleft ❖ **Tragus:** Tubercle of the first arch ❖ **Rest of the pinna:** Remaining five tubercles of second arch	6 weeks	20 weeks
External auditory meatus	First branchial cleft	16 weeks	28 weeks

Middle ear cleft	❖ **Malleus and incus:** Mesoderm of first arch
	❖ **Stapes:** Second arch except footplate, annular ligament—otic capsule
	  ▸ Eustachian tube
	  ▸ Tympanic cavity
	  ▸ Attic
	  ▸ Antrum
	  ▸ Mastoid air cells
	❖ Endoderm of tubotympanic recess arises from first and partly from the second pharyngeal pouch.
		3 weeks	30 weeks

Membranous inner ear	**Otocyst** (anatomy vesicles): part of anatomy placode—from which develops membranous inner ear structures develops (endolymphatic duct and sac, utricle, semicircular canal, saccule, cochlea)	3 weeks	16–20 weeks

PHYSIOLOGY OF EAR

There are two main functions of ear:
1. Hearing
2. Balance

Auditory System

Q. Write a note on auditory system of ear.

❖ Organ of corti
  ▸ Sense organ of hearing
  ▸ Components:

Tunnel of Corti	❖ Formed by inner and outer rods	
	❖ Contains a fluid called cortilymph	
Hair cells	Transduce sound energy into electrical energy	
	Inner hair cells	**Outer hair cells**
	❖ Single row	❖ Three/four rows
	❖ Supplied by afferent cochlear fibers	❖ Receive efferent innervation from olivary complex
	❖ Transmission of auditory impulses	❖ Modulating function of inner hair cells
	❖ More resistant	❖ Damaged by ototoxic drugs and high intensity noise
	❖ Flask-shaped	❖ Cylindrical
Supporting cell	❖ Deiters' cells	
	❖ Hensen cells	
Tectorial membrane	❖ Gelatinous matrix with delicate fibers	
	❖ Overlies organ of Corti	
	❖ Shearing force between hair cells and tectorial membrane produces stimulus to hair cells	

Physiology of Hearing

Q. Write a short note/essay on physiology of hearing/hearing mechanism.

Mechanism of hearing broadly divided into:
❖ Mechanical conduction of sound (conductive apparatus)
❖ Transduction of mechanical energy to electrical impulses
❖ Conduction of electrical impulses to the brain (neural pathways)

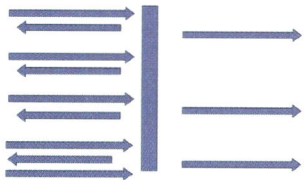

Cochlear fluids
99.9% of the sound energy is reflected away

Conduction of Sound

Impedance Matching Mechanism/Transformer Action

Q. What is impedance matching action of the middle ear?

Sound of greater amplitude but lesser force 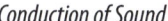 lesser amplitude but greater force.
        (middle ear)

This is accomplished by:

❖ **Lever action of the ossicles**	Handle of malleus is 1.3 times longer than long process of incus, giving a mechanical advantage of 1.3
❖ **Hydraulic action of tympanic membrane**	Out of a total of 90 mm² areas of human tympanic membrane, only 55 mm² is functional and area of stapes footplate is (3.2 mm²), the areal ratio is 17:1 and the total transformer ratio
Total transformer ratio	(17 × 1.3) is 22.1
❖ **Curved membrane effect**	Movements of tympanic membrane are more at the periphery than at the center where malleus handle is attached. This too provides some leverage

Other Factors

Q. Explain acoustic separation of windows. How it is achieved?

Phase differential between oval and round windows/ acoustic separation of windows Phase differential between windows contributes 4 dB in an intact tympanic membrane	When sound waves strike the tympanic membrane, they do not reach oval and round windows simultaneously. Oval window is struck first because of ossicular chain. Thus, when oval window is receiving a wave of compression, the round window is at phase of rarefaction If sound waves strike at both windows simultaneously, they would cancel each others effect with no movement of perilymph and therefore, no hearing Acoustic separation is achieved by: ❖ Intact tympanic membrane ❖ Cushion of air in the middle ear around the round window
Natural resonance of external and middle ear External ear canal: 3,000 Hz Middle ear: 800 Hz	Frequencies transmitted by: Ossicular chain: 500–2,000 Hz Tympanic membrane: 800–1,600 Hz Greatest sensitivity of sound transmission is between 500 and 3,000 Hz which is the most important to a man in day-to-day conversation

Transduction of Mechanical Energy to Electrical Impulses

Traveling wave theory of Von Bekesy:
A sound wave, depending on its frequency, reaches maximum amplitude at a particular place on the basilar membrane and stimulates that segment

Mechanism

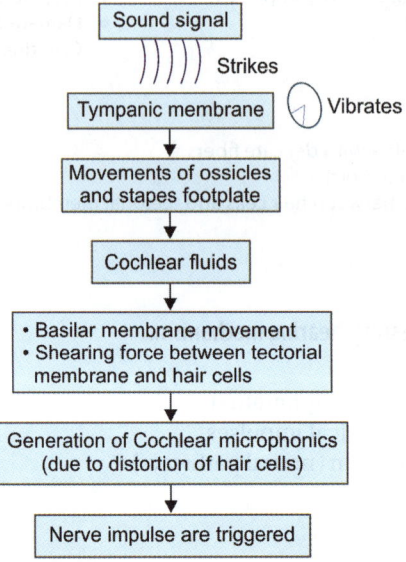

Neural Pathways

Q. Briefly explain auditory nerve transmission pathway.

Auditory neural pathways and their nuclei

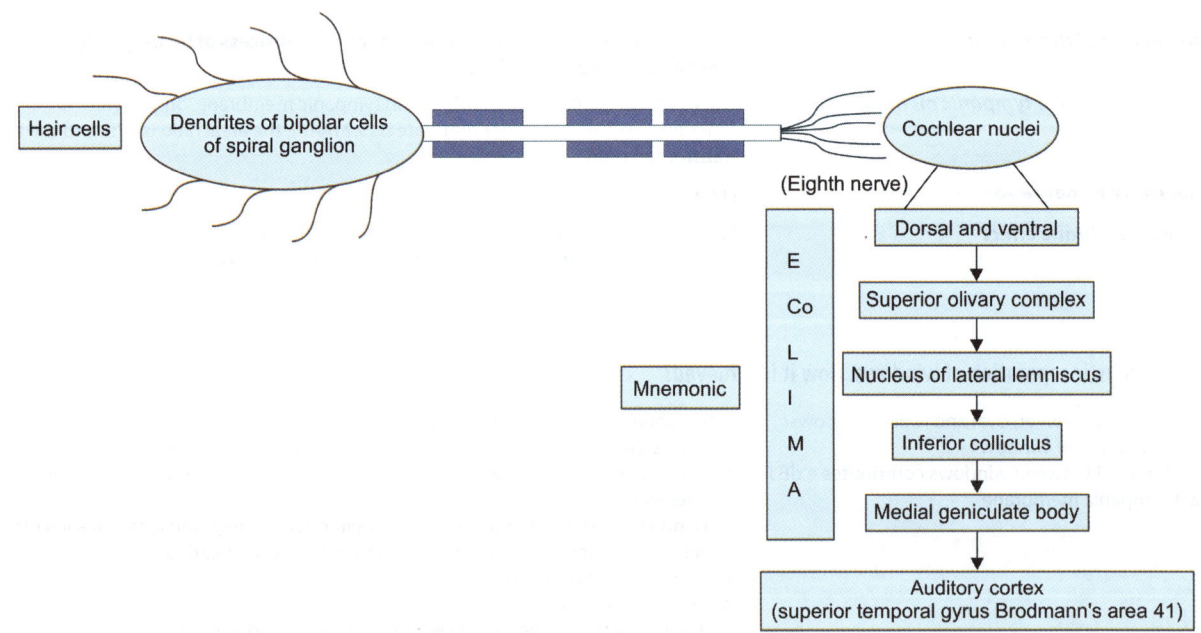

Electrical Potentials of Cochlea and CN VIII

Name	Type	Recorded from	Features
1. Endocochlear potential	Direct current (DC)	Cochlea	❖ Recorded from scala media ❖ +80 mV ❖ Generated from stria vascularis by Na+/K+-ATPase pump ❖ "Battery" to drive current through hair cells when they move in response to the sound stimulus
2. Cochlear microphonic (CM)	Alternating current (AC)	Cochlea	When sound stimulates the basilar membrane, electrical resistance at tips of hair cells changes which allows the flow of K+ through hair cells and produces voltage fluctuations
3. Summating potential (SP)	DC potential	Cochlea	❖ Negative or positive ❖ Used in diagnosis of Ménière's disease ❖ Produced by hair cells
4. Compound action potential		VIIth nerve	All or no response

Vestibular System

Registers changes in:
- Head position
- Linear or angular acceleration, deceleration
- Gravitational effects

Q. Briefly explain the mechanism of vestibular system.

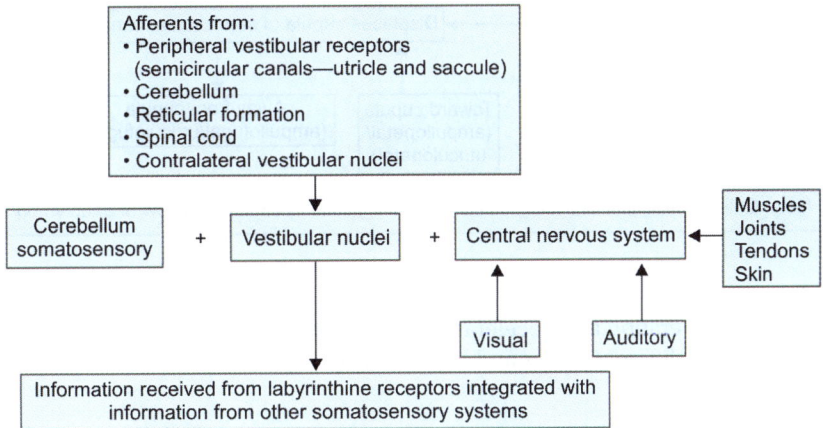

Efferents go to:
- CN III, IV, and VI nuclei via medial longitudinal bundle—vestibulo-ocular reflexes
  - Explains the genesis of nystagmus
- Motor part of spinal cord—vestibulospinal fibers
  - Coordination of movements of the head, neck, and body and maintaining balance
- **Cerebellum:** Vestibulocerebellar fibers
  - Coordinate input information to maintain body balance
- Autonomic nervous system—this explains:
  - It causes nausea, vomiting, palpitation, sweating, and pallor seen in vestibular disorders (e.g., Ménière's disease).
- Vestibular nuclei of the opposite side
- Cerebral cortex (temporal lobe)
  - Responsible for subjective awareness of motion

All this information is integrated and used in the regulation of equilibrium and body posture.

Physiology of Vestibular System

Vestibular system is divided into:

Peripheral	Central
Membranous labyrinth (semicircular ducts—utricle and saccule) Vestibular nerve	Nuclei and fiber tracts in the central nervous system to integrate vestibular impulses with other systems to maintain body balance

Semicircular Canals

Q. Briefly explain the generation of nystagmus.

Respond to angular acceleration and deceleration.

Mechanism

- Three canals lie at right angles to each other
- Due to this arrangement of three canals in three different planes, any change in position of head can be detected

Principle: Canal which lies at the right angles to axis of rotation is the most stimulated.
Stimulation of semicircular canals produces nystagmus and direction of nystagmus is determined by plane of canal being stimulated.

Horizontal canal	Horizontal
Superior canal	Rotatory
Posterior canal	Vertical

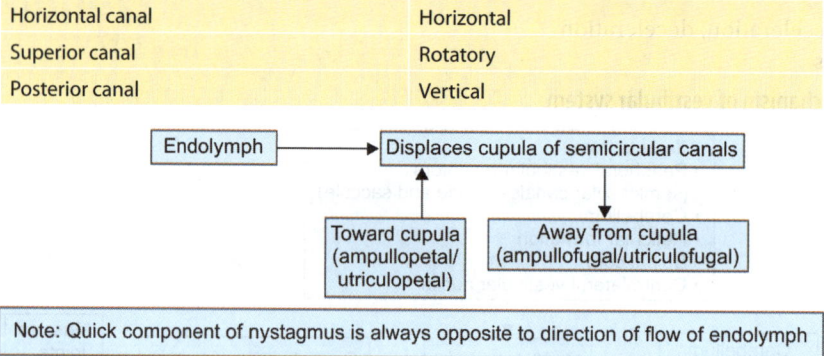

Utricle and Saccule

- Utricle stimulated by linear acceleration and deceleration or gravitational pull during head tilts.
- Sensory hair cells of macula lie in different planes and stimulated by displacement of otolithic membrane during head tilts.

Chapter 2

Anatomy and Physiology of Nose and Paranasal Sinuses

EN1.1: Describe the anatomy and physiology of ear, nose, throat, head and neck.

■ ANATOMY OF NOSE

Q. Briefly explain the anatomy of the nose.

Nasal Skin

- Thin and freely mobile skin over nasal bones and upper lateral cartilages
- Thick and adherent over alar cartilages
- Contains sebaceous glands

APPLIED ANATOMY

Hypertrophy of sebaceous glands gives rise to a lobulated tumor called *rhinophyma*.

Parts of Nose

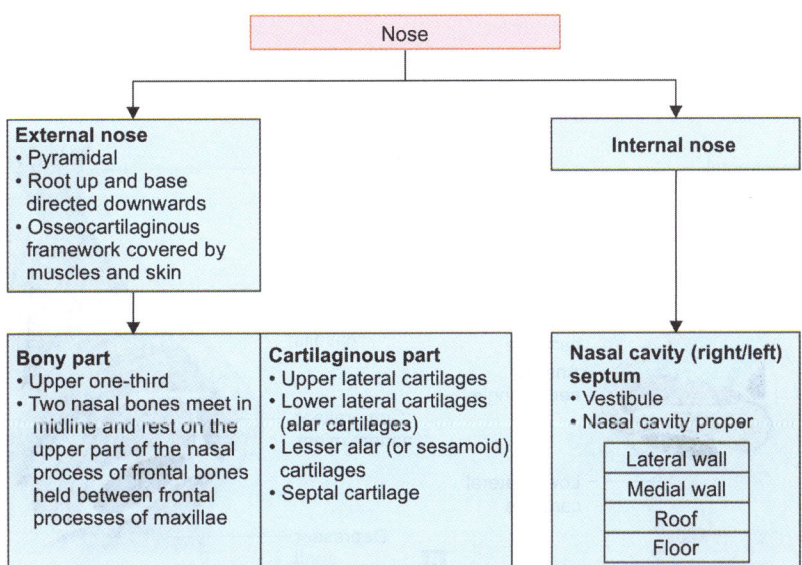

Cartilages (Fig. 1)

Q. Write a short note on nasal cartilages and musculature.

Upper lateral cartilages	❖ Extends from the undersurface of nasal bones above, to the alar cartilages below ❖ Lower free edge of upper lateral cartilage seen intranasally as *limen vestibuli* or *nasal valve* on each side
Lower lateral cartilages	❖ U-shaped ❖ Lateral crus forms ala and medial crus runs in columella ❖ Lateral crus overlaps the lower edge of upper lateral cartilage on each side
Lesser alar cartilages	❖ Two or more ❖ Lie above and lateral to alar cartilages

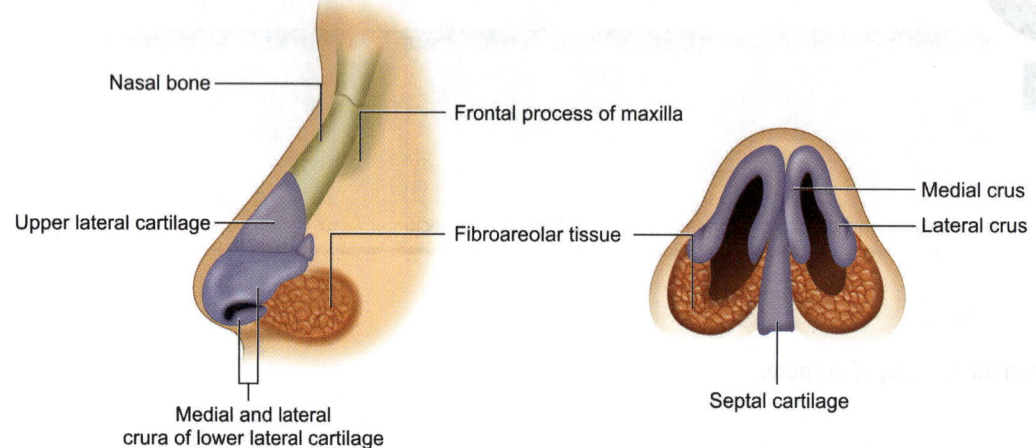

Fig. 1: Nasal cartilages and pyramid.

Nasal Musculature

- ❖ Osseocartilaginous framework of nose covered by muscles
- ❖ Responsible for movements of the nasal tip, ala and overlying skin

Nasal Muscles (Figs. 2A and B)

- ❖ Procerus
- ❖ Nasalis (transverse and alar parts)
- ❖ Levator labii superioris alaeque nasi
- ❖ Anterior and posterior dilator nares
- ❖ Depressor septi

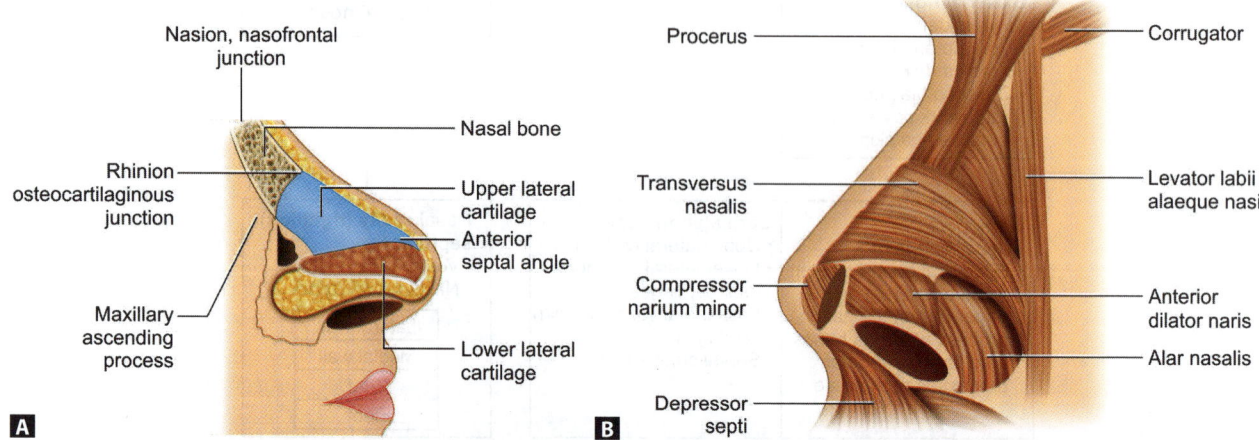

Figs. 2A and B: Nasal muscles.

Internal Nose

Q. Write short note on anatomy of internal nose.

Each nasal cavity communicates with exterior through *naris* or nostril and with nasopharynx through posterior nasal aperture/ *choana*.

Vestibule of Nose

- Anterior and inferior part of nasal cavity
- Lined by skin, contains sebaceous glands, hair follicles, and hair called *vibrissae*.
- Upper limit on the lateral wall formed by limen nasi (also called nasal valve).

1. **Nasal valve:**
   - *Laterally:* Lower border of upper lateral cartilage
     - Fibro fatty tissue
     - Anterior end of inferior turbinate
   - *Medially:* Cartilaginous nasal septum
   - *Caudally:* Floor of pyriform aperture
     - Angle between the nasal septum and lower border of upper lateral cartilage is 30°
2. **Nasal valve area:**
   - Cross-sectional area bounded by structures forming valve.
   - Least cross-sectional area of nose, regulates airflow and resistance on inspiration.

Nasal Cavity Proper

Lateral Nasal Wall (Fig. 3)

Q. Explain various structures of the lateral nasal wall.

Concha

- Three and sometimes four turbinates/conchae present at lateral wall of nose.
- Conchae or turbinates are scroll-like bony projections covered by mucous membrane.
- Spaces below turbinates are called meatuses.

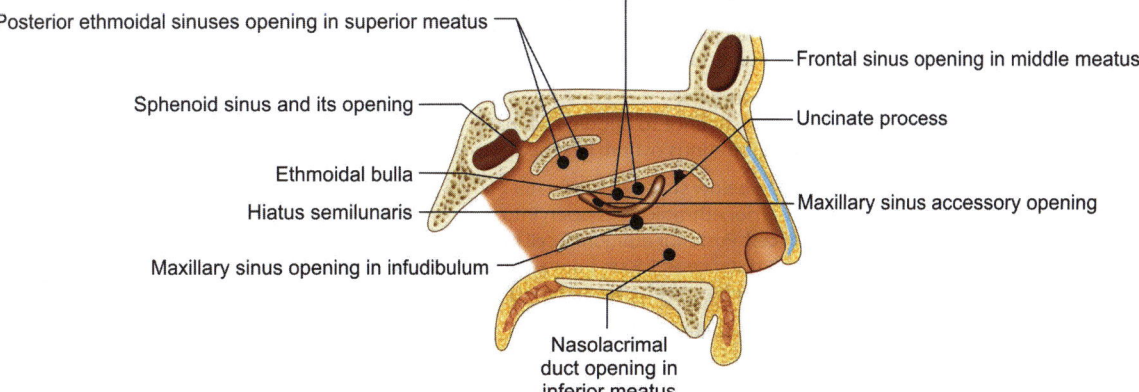

Fig. 3: Lateral nasal wall.

Inferior Turbinate

- Separate bone:
  - Nasolacrimal duct opens into the inferior meatus, guarded by a mucosal valve called ***Hasner's valve***.

Middle Turbinate

- Ethmoturbinal—a part of the ethmoid bone.
- Attached to the lateral wall by a bony lamella called *ground/basal lamella*.
- Pneumatized middle turbinate → *concha bullosa*
- Attachment → S-shaped

Anterior third	Middle third	Posterior third
❖ Sagittal plane	❖ Frontal plane	❖ Horizontally
❖ Attached to lateral edge of cribriform plate	❖ Attached to lamina papyracea	❖ Attached to lamina papyracea and medial wall of maxillary sinus ❖ Forms roof of middle meatus

❖ Ostia of sinuses draining:
  ➢ Anterior to the basal lamella form *anterior group of paranasal sinuses*
  ➢ Posterior and superior to it form *posterior group*

Middle Meatus

Q. Describe structures seen in the middle meatus.

Important structures which are important in endoscopic surgery of sinuses.

Uncinate process	❖ Hook-like structure
	❖ Sharp posterosuperior border, runs parallel to anterior border of bulla ethmoidalis; gap between the two is called *hiatus semilunaris* (inferior)
	❖ It is a two-dimensional space of 1–2 mm in width
	❖ Anteroinferior border attached to the lateral wall
	❖ Posteroinferior end attached to inferior turbinate dividing membranous part of lower-middle meatus into anterior and posterior fontanelle
	❖ Fontanel area consists of a membrane only, when perforated, leads into the maxillary sinus
	❖ Upper attachment variable:
	  ➢ Into lateral nasal wall
	  ➢ Upwards into base of skull
	  ➢ Medially into middle turbinate
	❖ Infundibulum—space bounded by:
	  ➢ **Medially:** Uncinate process, frontal process of maxilla, lacrimal bone
	  ➢ **Laterally:** Lamina papyracea
	❖ Natural ostium of maxillary sinus situated in lower part of the infundibulum
	❖ Accessory ostium sometimes seen in anterior or posterior fontanel

Bulla ethmoidalis	❖ Ethmoidal cell behind uncinate process.
	❖ May be pneumatized or solid.
	❖ May extend superiorly to the skull base and posteriorly to fuse with ground lamella
	❖ When there is a space:
	  ➢ Above bulla: *Suprabullar*
	  ➢ Behind bulla: *Retrobullar recesses*] Sinus lateralis of Grunwald

Atrium	Shallow depression in front of the middle turbinate and above nasal vestibule
Agger nasi	❖ Elevation just anterior to attachment of middle turbinate ❖ If pneumatized → agger nasi cells
Superior turbinate	❖ Ethmoturbinal ❖ Posterosuperior to middle turbinate ❖ Sphenoid sinus ostium lies medial to it
Superior meatus	❖ Space below superior turbinate ❖ Posterior ethmoid cells open into it **Onodi cell:** Posterior ethmoidal cell may grow posteriorly by side of sphenoid sinus or superior to it for as much distance as 1.5 cm from anterior surface of sphenoid ❖ Optic nerve may be related to its lateral wall
Sphenoethmoidal recess	❖ Above superior turbinate ❖ Sphenoid sinus opens into its medial to superior turbinate ❖ Endoscopically about 1 cm above upper margin of posterior choana close to posterior border of septum
Supreme turbinate	Sometimes present above superior turbinate and has a narrow meatus beneath it

Osteomeatal Complex (OMC)

Also known as osteomeatal unit/key area

❖ Common pathway for the drainage and ventilation of maxillary, anterior ethmoidal and frontal sinuses.
❖ Obstruction of this region is a key factor in the development of chronic sinusitis.
❖ It is composed of five structures:
  1. Maxillary ostium
  2. Infundibulum: Common channel that drains the ostia of the maxillary antrum and anterior ethmoid air cells to the hiatus semilunaris.

CHAPTER 2: Anatomy and Physiology of Nose and Paranasal Sinuses

3. Ethmoid bulla
4. Uncinate process
5. Hiatus semilunaris

Medial Wall

Q. Describe nasal septum anatomy.

Nasal septum forms the medial wall (**Fig. 4**).

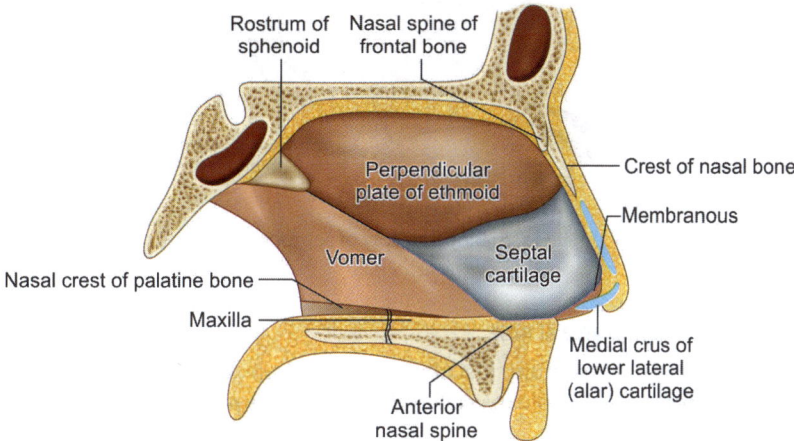

Fig. 4: Nasal septum.

Nasal septum consists of three parts:

Columellar septum	Membranous septum	Septum proper
Formed of columella containing medial crura of alar cartilages united together by fibrous tissue and covered on either side by skin	❖ Double layer of skin ❖ No bony or cartilaginous support ❖ Lies between the columella and caudal border of septal cartilage	❖ Osteocartilaginous framework, covered with mucous membrane ❖ Its components are: ➢ The perpendicular plate of ethmoid ➢ The vomer ➢ Quadrilateral cartilage wedged between above two bones anteriorly **Minor contributions:** ❖ Crest of nasal bones ❖ Nasal spine of frontal bone ❖ Rostrum of sphenoid ❖ Crest of palatine bones and maxilla ❖ Anterior nasal spine of maxilla

Blood Supply of Nasal Septum (Fig. 5)

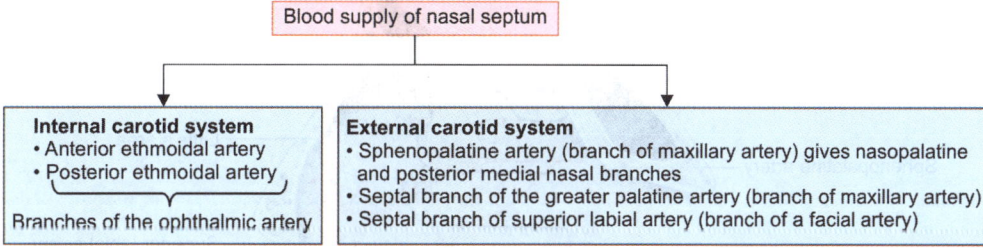

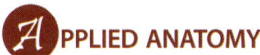

APPLIED ANATOMY

Septal cartilage provides support to the tip and dorsum of cartilaginous part of nose. Its destruction, e.g., in septal abscess, injuries, tuberculosis, or excessive removal during septal surgery, leads to supratip depression.

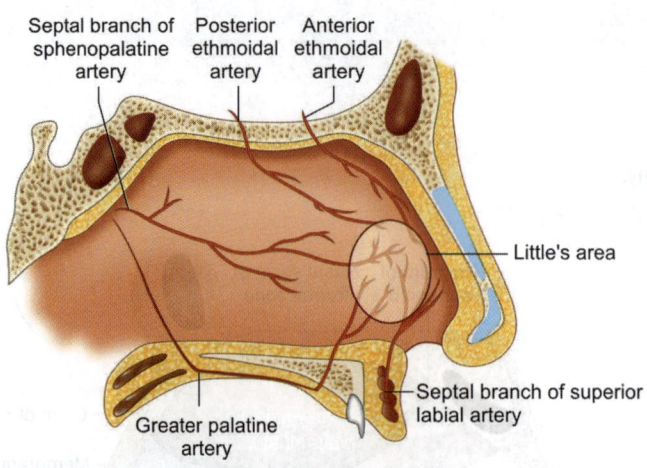

Fig. 5: Blood supply of septum.

Little's Area (Fig. 6)

Q. Write a short note on little's area/dangerous area of nose.

❖ Situated in anterior inferior part of nasal septum, just above the vestibule.
❖ Four arteries anastomose to form a vascular plexus called *"Kiesselbach's plexus"*.

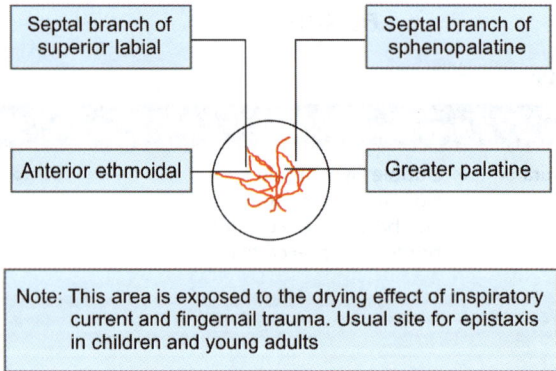

Note: This area is exposed to the drying effect of inspiratory current and fingernail trauma. Usual site for epistaxis in children and young adults

Retrocolumellar vein: Runs vertically downwards just behind columella, crosses floor of nose, and joins venous plexus on the lateral nasal wall.

❖ Common site of venous bleeding in young people.

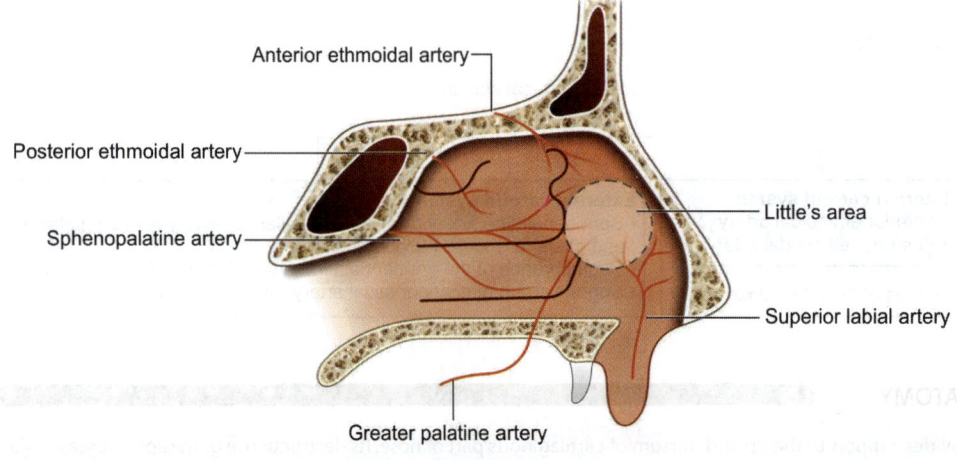

Fig. 6: Little's area.

CHAPTER 2: Anatomy and Physiology of Nose and Paranasal Sinuses

Roof and Floor

Q. What are structures forming the nasal roof and floor?

Roof

Anterior sloping part	Nasal bones
Posterior sloping part	Body of sphenoid
Middle horizontal part	Cribriform plate of ethmoid through which olfactory nerves enter nasal cavity

Floor

- **Anterior three-fourth:** Palatine process of maxilla
- **Posterior one-fourth:** Horizontal part of palatine bone

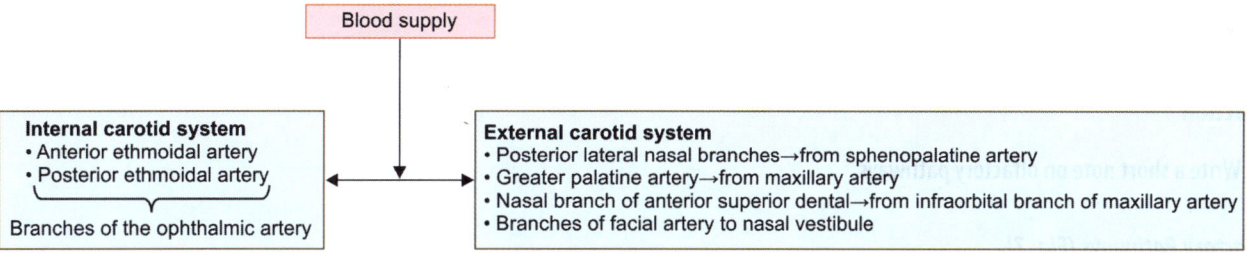

Nerve Supply of Nose

Q. Write as short note on nerve supply of the nose.

Olfactory nerves	Nerves of common sensation		Autonomic nerves	
			Parasympathetic	Sympathetic
Carry a sense of smell and supply olfactory region of nose	❖ Anterior ethmoidal nerve ❖ Branches of sphenopalatine ganglion ❖ Branches of infraorbital nerve	❖ Supply vestibule of nose both on the medial and the lateral side ❖ Posterior two-thirds of nasal cavity (both septum and lateral wall) ❖ Anterior and superior part of nasal cavity (lateral wall and septum)	❖ It comes from the greater superficial petrosal nerve ❖ It supplies the nasal blood vessels and causes vasodilation ❖ Supply nasal glands and control nasal secretion	❖ It comes from the upper two thoracic segments of the spinal cord ❖ Stimulation causes vasoconstriction

Lymphatic Drainage

External nose and anterior part of nasal cavity	Submandibular lymph nodes
Rest of nasal cavity	Upper jugular nodes

PHYSIOLOGY OF NOSE

Q. What are the various functions of the nose?

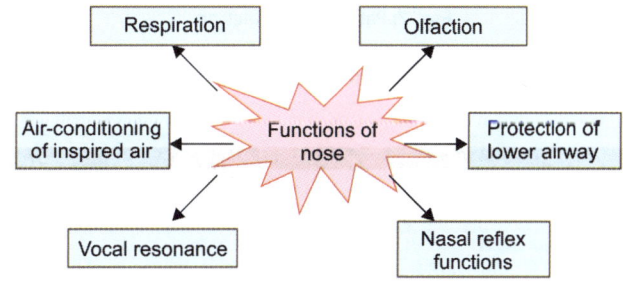

Respiration

Q. What is a nasal cycle?

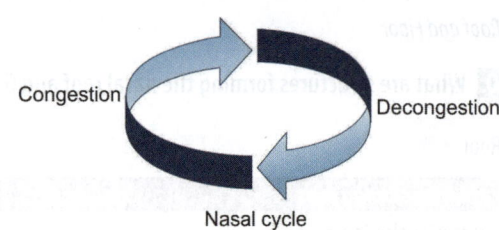

- Varies every 2½–4 hours
- Rhythmic cyclical changes
- When one nasal chamber is working, total nasal respiration, equal to that of both nasal chambers, is carried out by it.

Quiet inspiration	Inspiratory air current passes through middle part of nose between turbinates and nasal septum
Quiet expiration	• Entire air current is not expelled directly through nares • Friction at limen nasi converts it into eddies under cover of inferior and middle turbinates and ventilation of sinuses occurs through ostia • Swelling and shrinkage of anterior end of inferior turbinate regulate the inflow of air

Olfaction

Q. Write a short note on olfactory pathways.

Olfactory Pathways (Fig. 7)

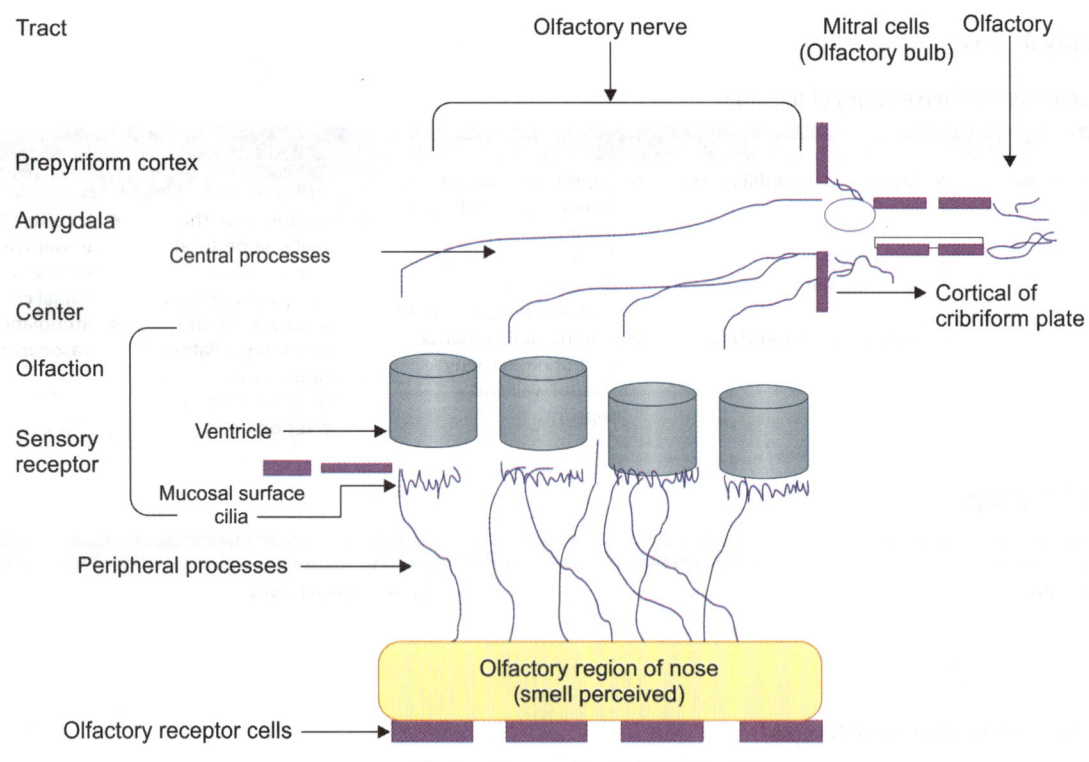

Fig. 7: Pathway of olfaction.

- Also associated with autonomic system at hypothalamic level.

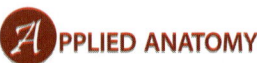 **PPLIED ANATOMY**

- Total loss of sense of smell: *Anosmia*
- Partial loss of sense of smell: *Hyposmia*
- Perversion of smell: *Parosmia*

Air-conditioning of Inspired Air

Q. Briefly explain role of nose in the air conditioning of inspired air. What is a radiator mechanism?

Action	Mechanism
Filtration and purification	❖ Nasal vibrissae at entrance of nose act as filters ❖ Front of nose: Up to 3 µm ❖ Mucus: 0.5–3.0 µm ❖ Spread like a sheet all over surface of mucous membrane
Temperature control of inspired air	❖ Large surface of nasal mucosa ❖ Inspired air heated to near body temperature ❖ "Radiator" mechanism: Mucous membrane, in region of middle and inferior turbinates and adjacent septum, is highly vascular with sinusoids which control blood flow, and increase or decrease turbinate's size
Humidification	Nasal mucous membrane, rich in mucous and serous secreting glands, adjusts relative humidity of inspired air to 75% or more

Protection of Lower Airway

Q. How does nose help in the protection of lower airways?

Mucociliary mechanism	❖ **"Conveyer belt":** Mucous blanket consists of a superficial mucus layer and a deeper serous layer, floating on top of constantly beating cilia towards the nasopharynx ❖ Cilia has a rapid "effective stroke" slow "recovery stroke" ❖ Complete sheet of mucus cleared into pharynx every 10–20 minutes ❖ Inspired bacteria, viruses, and dust particles entrapped on viscous mucous blanket carried to the nasopharynx, and swallowed
Enzymes and immunoglobulins	❖ Nasal secretions contain: ❖ Muramidase → kills bacteria and viruses. ❖ IgA, IgE, interferon → immunity against upper respiratory tract infections
Sneezing	❖ Protective reflex ❖ Foreign particles irritating nasal mucosa expelled by sneezing

Vocal Resonance

❖ Nose forms resonating chamber for (M/N/NG), when sound passes through nasopharyngeal isthmus.
❖ If nose (or nasopharynx) is blocked → denasal speech.

Nasal Reflexes

❖ Nasal function is closely related to pulmonary functions through nasobronchial and nasopulmonary reflexes.
❖ Nasal obstruction leads to increased pulmonary resistance.

ANATOMY AND PHYSIOLOGY OF PARANASAL SINUSES

Q. Write a short note/essay on anatomy of paranasal sinuses.

❖ Air-containing cavities in the skull bones
❖ Four on each side

Two groups:

Anterior group	Posterior group
Maxillary	Posterior ethmoidal → superior meatus
Frontal	Sphenoid sinus
Anterior ethmoidal ↓	↓ Sphenoethmoidal recess

(opens into)
Middle meatus

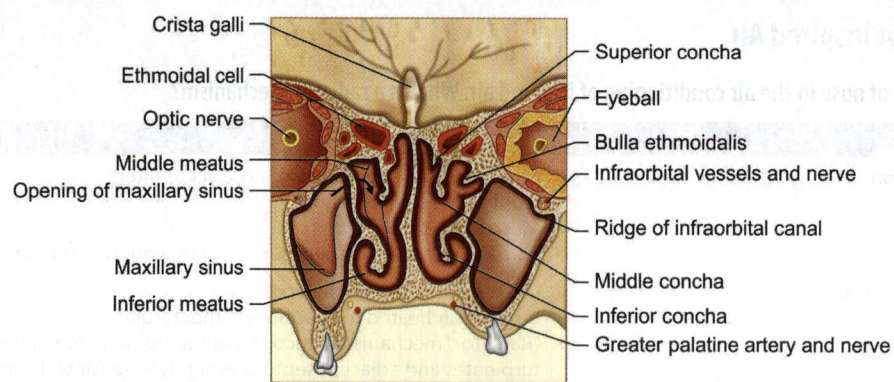

Fig. 8: Sinuses.

Maxillary Sinus (Also Known as "Antrum of Highmore") (Fig. 8)

Q. Write a short note on largest paranasal sinuses/maxillary sinus/antrum of Highmore.

- Largest paranasal sinus
- Present at birth
  - Radiologically earliest evidence: 4–5 months after birth
- Lies in the body of maxilla
- **Shape:** Pyramidal
- **Base:** Lateral wall of nose
- **Apex:** Zygomatic process of maxilla

Relations

Anterior wall	Facial surface of maxilla and soft tissues of cheek
Posterior wall	Infratemporal and pterygopalatine fossae
Medial wall	<ul><li>Middle meatus</li><li>Uncinate process</li><li>Anterior and posterior fontanelle</li><li>Inferior turbinate and meatus</li></ul>
Floor	<ul><li>Alveolar, palatine processes of maxilla</li><li>Roots of second premolar and first molar teeth</li></ul>
Roof	<ul><li>Floor of orbit</li><li>Traversed by infraorbital nerve and vessels</li></ul>

Note: Maxillary sinus ostium is situated high up in the medial wall and opens in posteroinferior part of the ethmoidal infundibulum into middle meatus.

- Location is unfavorable for natural drainage.
- An accessory ostium sometimes (30% of cases) present behind the main ostium.

Frontal Sinus (Fig. 9)

Q. Write short note on frontal sinus.

- Not present at the birth
  - Radiologically earliest evidence: 6 years
- **Location:** Between inner and outer tables of frontal bone, above, and deep to supraorbital margin.
- Loculated by incomplete septa
- Asymmetric with thin intervening bony septum

Relations

Wall	Relations
- Anterior wall	- Skin over forehead
- Posterior wall	- Meninges and frontal lobe of brain
- Inferior wall	- Orbit and its contents

CHAPTER 2: Anatomy and Physiology of Nose and Paranasal Sinuses

Drainage

Drainage: Through its ostium into frontal recess

Frontal Recess

Location: Anterior part of middle meatus
- **Medially:** Middle turbinate
- **Laterally:** Lamina papyracea
- **Anteriorly:** Agger nasi cells
- **Posteriorly:** Bulla ethmoidalis

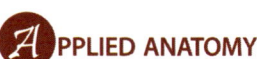

Fig. 9: Frontal sinus, its ostium, and frontal recess form an hourglass structure.

Drainage: Into infundibulum or medial to it, depending on the superior attachment of uncinate process.

Ethmoidal Sinuses (Ethmoid Air Cells)

Q. Write a short note on ethmoid air cells/ethmoid sinus.

- Thin-walled air cavities in the lateral masses of ethmoid bone
- Number varies from 3 to 18
- Present at the birth
  - Radiologically earliest evidence: 1 year
- **Location:** Space between upper third of lateral nasal wall and medial wall of orbit.
- **Roof:** Medial extension of orbital plate of frontal bone, which shows depressions on its undersurface, called fovea ethmoidalis.
- **Lateral wall:** Lamina papyracea.

Groups of Ethmoidal Sinuses

Cells in anterior group
- Agger nasi cells:
  - Ethmoid bulla—forms posterior boundary of hiatus semilunaris
  - Supraorbital cells
  - Frontoethmoid cells—situated in area of frontal recess and may encroach frontal sinus
  - Haller cells—situated in orbital floor

Posterior group
It lies posterior to the basal lamina of middle concha.

Onodi cell: Posterior most cell extends along lamina papyracea, lateral or superior to sphenoid, and may extend 1.5 cm behind the anterior face of sphenoid.

APPLIED ANATOMY

Optic nerve and sometimes carotid artery related to it laterally and are in danger during endoscopic surgery.

Sphenoid Sinus

Q. Write short note on sphenoid sinus.

- Not present at the birth
  - Radiologically earliest evidence: 6 years
  - *Location:* Body of sphenoid
- Two, right and left sinuses, rarely symmetrical
- Separated by a thin bony septum
  - *Ostium:* Situated high up in the anterior wall and opens into sphenoethmoidal recess, medial to superior or supreme turbinate

APPLIED ANATOMY

In adults, the ostium is situated about 1.5 cm from upper border of choana and can be approached endoscopically.

Relations

- ❖ **Lateral wall:**
  - ▸ Optic nerve, carotid artery. Between them-------Carotico-optic recess
  - ▸ Usually covered by a thin bone, sometimes dehiscent, covered only by mucosa.
- ❖ **Floor:** Vidian nerve
- ❖ **Roof:**
  - ▸ *Anterior part:* Related to olfactory tract, optic chiasma, and frontal lobe
  - ▸ *Posterior part:* Related to pituitary gland in sella turcica
- ❖ **Laterally:** Cavernous sinus

Posterior wall of sphenoid forms clivus.

Functions of Paranasal Sinuses

Q. Enumerate functions of paranasal sinuses.

- ❖ Due to a large surface area, inspired air is humidified and warmed thus air conditioning.
- ❖ To provide a certain resonance to voice.
- ❖ Protection of orbital structures and cranium from variations of intranasal temperature and act as buffers against trauma.
- ❖ To provide an extended surface for olfaction, olfactory mucosa is situated in upper part of nasal cavity and over ethmoid.
- ❖ To provide local immunologic defense against microbes.
- ❖ Act as an immunologic barrier against microbes.

Lymphatic Drainage

- ❖ Retropharyngeal
- ❖ Jugulodigastric nodes

Mucous Membrane of Paranasal Sinuses

- ❖ Mucous membrane is continuous with that of nasal cavity through sinuses ostia.
- ❖ Ciliated columnar epithelium with mucus-secreting goblet cells.

Physiology of Paranasal Sinuses

Q. Describe the mechanism of ventilation and mucociliary action of paranasal sinuses.

Ventilation of Sinuses

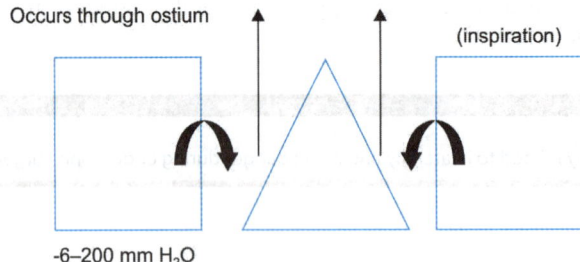

Fig. 10: Schematic diagram showing ventilation of sinuses is paradoxical; they are emptied of air during inspiration and filled with air during expiration because of negative pressure created in the nose during inspiration.

Mucociliary Action

Maxillary sinus	Frontal sinus	Sphenoid sinus	Ethmoid sinuses	
Mucus from all walls of maxillary sinus is transported by cilia to natural ostium and then through it into the middle meatus.	❖ Mucus travels up along interfrontal septum, along the roof of lateral wall, along floor, and then exits through natural ostium ❖ Circulation is anticlockwise in right and clockwise in left frontal sinus	Mucociliary clearance is towards its ostium into sphenoethmoidal recess	Anterior ❖ Mucus joins that from frontal and maxillary sinuses, and travels towards Eustachian tube, passing in front of torus tubarius, into the nasopharynx	Posterior ❖ Mucus drains into superior or supreme meatus and then joins mucus from sphenoid sinus in sphenoethmoidal recess, passes above and behind torus tubarius into nasopharynx

Chapter 3

Anatomy and Physiology of Oral Cavity and Pharynx

EN1.1: Describe the anatomy and physiology of ear, nose, throat, head and neck.

ANATOMY AND PHYSIOLOGY OF ORAL CAVITY (FIG.1)

Q. Write a short note on parts of oral cavity, its lymphatic draige and its functions.

Oral cavity extends from the lips to the oropharyngeal isthmus.

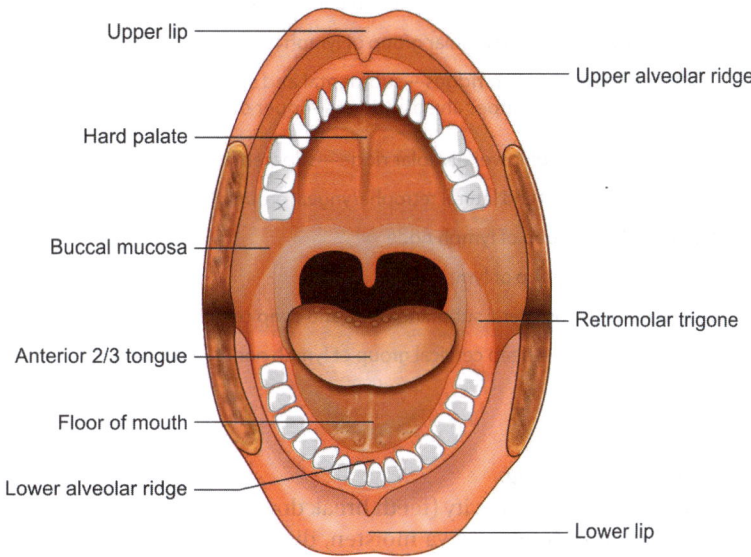

Fig. 1: Anatomy of tongue and oral cavity.

Embryology

- Oral cavity develops from stomatodaeum
- Palate from horizontal process of maxillary and palatine bone

Parts of Oral Cavity

Oral cavity consists of:
- **Lips**—forms the anterior boundary.

- ❖ **Parts**: Two surfaces of lip
  - ➤ Skin
  - ➤ Mucosal membrane
  - ➤ Vermillion border—dry and smooth
  - ➤ Epithelium—nonkeratinized stratified squamous epithelium
- ❖ **Buccal mucosa**—lines cheeks (from lips to pterygomandibular raphe)
  Epithelium—nonkeratinized stratified squamous epithelium
- ❖ **Gums** (gingivae) **and alveoli**—cover upper and lower alveolar ridge
- ❖ **Hard palate**—forms roof of oral cavity
- ❖ **Oral tongue**—anterior two-thirds of tongue (dorsum, tip of tongue, under surface, and lateral border of tongue) separated from posterior one-third of tongue by foramen cecum and circumvallate papillae.
- ❖ **Taste buds are present** in tongue and palate, innervated by facial nerve—anterior two-thirds tongue, glossopharyngeal nerve-posterior one-third, and vagus nerve—vallecula, and epiglottis.
- ❖ **Floor of mouth**—area between gingivae and under surface of tongue (crescent-shaped)
  - ➤ Tongue attached to the floor of the moth by frenulum
  - ➤ Wharton's duct opens on either side of frenulum
- ❖ **Retromolar trigone**—triangular area covering anterior surface of ramus of mandible
  - ➤ Apex is near maxillary tuberosity
  - ➤ Base is behind the lower second molar

Lymphatic Drainage of Oral Cavity

Parts of oral cavity	Draining lymph nodes
Lips	❖ Lower lip—central portion into the submental group of lymph nodes ❖ Lateral portion into the submandibular groups of lymph nodes
	Upper lip—preauricular, infraparotid, submandibular group of lymph nodes
Buccal mucosa	Submental and a submandibular group of lymph nodes
Upper and lower alveolar ridge	❖ Buccal aspect of both ridges—submental and submandibular group of lymph nodes ❖ Lingual aspect of upper alveolar ridge—upper deep cervical and lateral retropharyngeal group of lymph nodes ❖ Lingual aspect of lower alveolar ridge—submental and submandibular group of lymph nodes
Hard palate	Upper deep cervical and lateral retropharyngeal group of lymph nodes
Floor of mouth	Submandibular group of lymph node
Tongue	Tip—submental group of lymph node
	Lateral border—ipsilateral submandibular and deep cervical group of lymph nodes
	Dorsum of tongue—deep cervical group of lymph nodes of both sides

Functions

- ❖ Sensory analysis of material before swallowing.
- ❖ **Mechanical digestion of food**—begins at oral cavity (teeth break down the food particles).
- ❖ **Lubrication and chemical digestion of food**—saliva moisten, dissolve food chemical so they can be tasted, (salivary amylase) start chemical breakdown of starchy food.
- ❖ **Creates bolus so it can travel down to oropharynx** (though action of tongue, palatal surface and teeth).

ANATOMY AND PHYSIOLOGY OF PHARYNX (FIG. 2)

Q. Write a short note/essay on anatomy and physiology of pharynx.

Introduction

- ❖ Fibromuscular tube forms the upper part of the airway and food passages.
- ❖ Extending from the base of the skull to the lower border of the cricoid cartilage there on continuing as the esophagus.

❖ Measuring 3.5 cm at its base, tapering like a cone towards the lower border of the cricoid, forming the narrowest part of the digestive tract—the cricopharyngeal junction (measuring 1.5 cm).

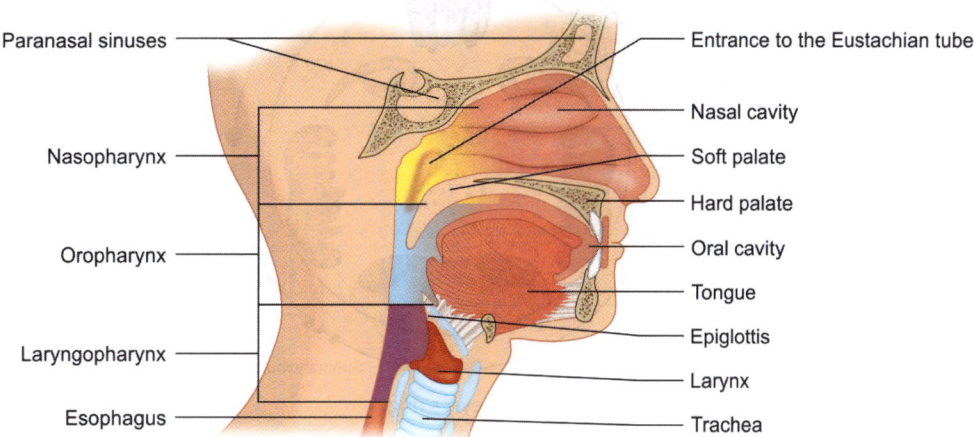

Fig. 2: Pharynx.

Outline Structure of the Pharyngeal Wall

1. **Mucous membrane**: Continuous with the mucous membrane of the Eustachian tube, nasal cavity, esophagus, and larynx.
   ▷ Ciliated columnar in the region of the nasopharynx
   ▷ Stratified squamous in other parts. Contains multiple mucous glands.
2. **Pharyngobasilar fascia** (pharyngeal aponeurosis): Fibrous layer lining the muscular part of the pharynx.
   ▷ More prominent in the region of the base of the skull.
3. **Muscular layer:**
   ▷ *External layer:* Superior, middle, and inferior constrictors
   ▷ *Internal layer:* Stylopharyngeus, salpingopharyngeus, and palatopharyngeus muscles
4. **Buccopharyngeal fascia**: It covers the outer part of the pharyngeal muscles and above the level of the superior constrictor muscle it blends with pharyngeal aponeurosis.

Clinically Important Components of the Pharynx

Killian's Triangle (Fig. 3)

Q. Write a note on Killian's triangle.

❖ Triangular space is created by the two parts of the inferior constrictor muscle—transverse fibers of the cricopharyngeus and oblique fibers of the thyropharyngeus muscle.
❖ Potential area of weakness—the common site for tears during endoscopic procedures (gateway of tear).
❖ Site for herniation of pharyngeal mucosa resulting in pharyngeal pouch.

Waldeyer's Ring (Fig. 4)

Subepithelial collection of scattered lymphoid tissue forming aggregate masses at different sites in the pharynx. It includes:
❖ Adenoids/nasopharyngeal tonsil
❖ Palatine tonsil
❖ Lingual tonsil
❖ Tubal tonsil (contained in fossa of Rosenmuller)
❖ Lateral pharyngeal buds
❖ Nodules in the posterior pharyngeal wall

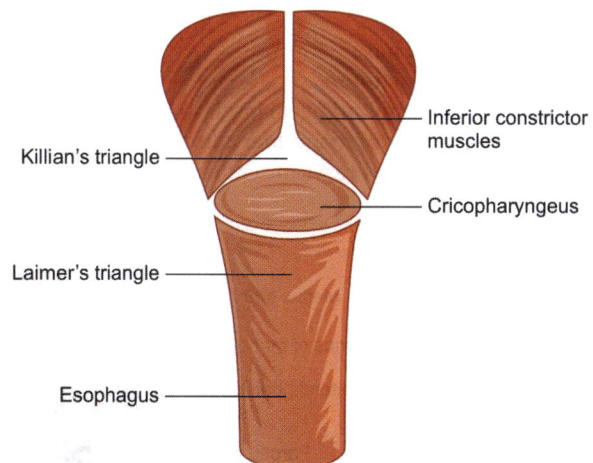

Fig. 3: Killian's triangle.

PART 1: Diseases of ENT, Head and Neck

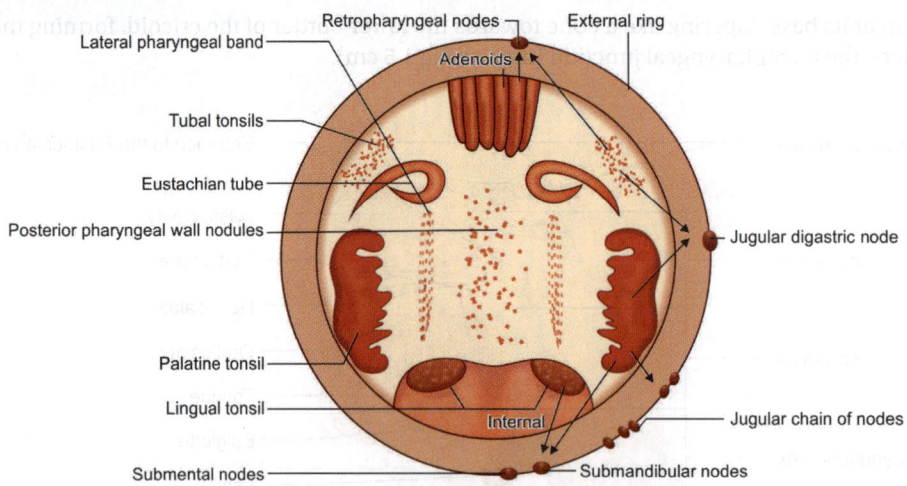

Fig. 4: Waldeyer's ring.

Pharyngeal Spaces (Fig. 5)

Q. Write a note on pharyngeal spaces.

Notorious for abscess formation

Retropharyngeal Space (Gillette's Space)

Potential space behind the pharynx, extending from the base of the skull to the bifurcation of the trachea.

Boundaries

- Anteriorly—buccopharyngeal fascia
- Posteriorly—prevertebral fascia
- Median partition divides space into right and left

Parapharyngeal Spaces

They are located on either side of the pharynx.

Boundaries

- Superior—skull base
- Inferior—mediastinum
- Medially—buccopharyngeal fascia, prevertebral muscles, and fascia
- Laterally—ramus of mandible, parotid gland, sternocleidomastoid containing the carotid vessels, jugular vein, I, X, XI, and XII nerves, and cervical sympathetic chain.

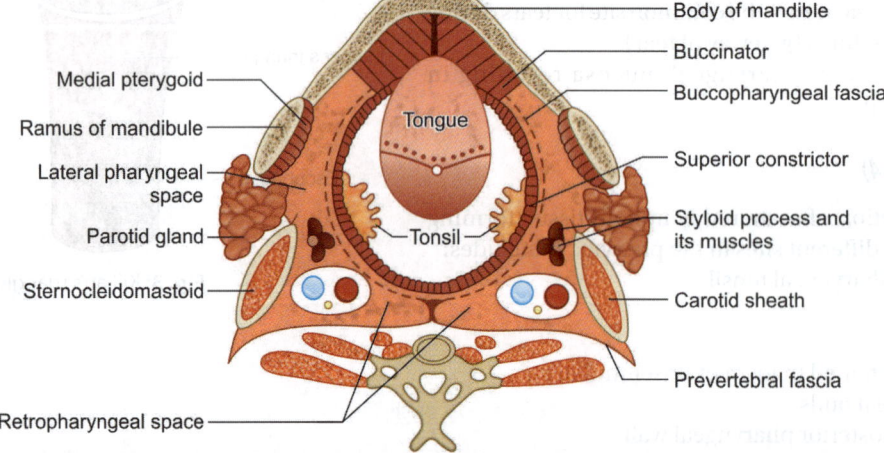

Fig. 5: Pharyngeal spaces.

CHAPTER 3: Anatomy and Physiology of Oral Cavity and Pharynx

Divisions of the Pharynx

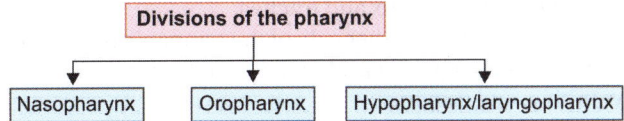

Nasopharynx (Epipharynx)

Q. Write a note on nasopharynx/epipharynx.

The upper most part of the pharynx extends from the base of the skull to the soft palate or level of horizontal plane passing through the hard palate. Lined by pseudostratified ciliated columnar epithelium.

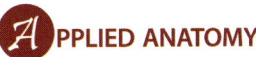 **PPLIED ANATOMY**

- **Roof:** Basisphenoid/basiocciput
- **Posterior wall:** Arch of the atlas vertebrae, covered by the prevertebral muscles and fascia
- **Floor:** Anteriorly formed by the soft palate.
- Posteriorly deficient—(nasopharyngeal isthmus) communication between the nasopharynx and the oropharynx.
- **Anterior wall:** Posterior nasal aperture/choanae
- **Lateral wall:** This contains the pharyngeal opening of the Eustachian tube.
- Bounded behind and above by torus tubarius—an elevation formed by the cartilage of the tube. Above and behind the torus lies a recess called fossa of Rosenmuller—the most common site for origin of carcinoma of the nasopharynx.

Nasopharyngeal Tonsil (Adenoids)
- Subepithelial collection of lymphoid tissue at the junction of the roof and posterior wall
- Increases in size up to 6 years and then gradually atrophies.

Nasopharyngeal Bursa
- Epithelial lined median recess located within the adenoids extending from pharyngeal mucosa to the basiocciput periosteum.
- Represents embryological attachment of notochord to the pharyngeal endoderm.
- Potential site for abscess formation (Tornwaldt's disease).

Ratkhe's Pouch: Hypophyseal Diverticulum
- Represented by dimple above the adenoids (superior out pouching of stomodeal ectoderm to form anterior lobe of pituitary).
- Potential site for formation of craniopharyngioma.

Passavants Ridge
- Mucosal ridge is formed by fibers of the palatopharyngeus muscle, covering the posterior and lateral walls of the nasopharyngeal isthmus.
- During deglutition or speech, it helps cut off communication between the nasopharynx and the oropharynx by making firm contact with the soft palate.

Tubal Tonsil
- Subepithelial lymphoid tissue in the region of the tubal elevation, continuous with the adenoid tissue.
- Its enlargement causes Eustachian tube occlusion.

Sinus of Morgagni
- Space between the base of the skull and the superior free border of the superior constrictor muscle.
- Through it enters the Eustachian tube, levator veli palatini, tensor veli palatini, and ascending palatine artery.

Lymphatic Drainage
- Upper deep cervical lymph nodes
- May also drain into the spinal accessory chain of nodes in the posterior triangle of the neck.
- Can also cross the midline to drain into contralateral lymph nodes.

Functions

- Conduit for passage of air from the nose to the larynx and trachea.
- Ventilate the middle ear and equalize pressure of either side of the tympanic membrane.
- Elevation of the soft palate against the posterior pharyngeal wall to cut off communication between the naso and oropharynx during a speech, deglutition, vomiting, and gagging.
- Resonating chamber for voice production
- Clearing out secretions of the nasal and nasopharyngeal glands.

Oropharynx

Q. Write a short note on oropharynx.

Extends from the plane of the hard palate above to the plane of the hyoid bone below, lying opposite the oral cavity.

Boundaries

- Posterior wall—corresponding to the second and upper part of the third cervical vertebrae
- Anterior wall—it is deficient in its upper part where the oropharynx communicates with the oral cavity. Below it is formed by the base of the tongue, lingual tonsils, and the valleculae.
- Lateral wall—palatine tonsil, anterior pillar (palatoglossal arch), and posterior pillar (palatopharyngeal arch).

Lymphatic Drainage

Jugulodigastric nodes

Functions

- Acts as a conduit for air and food
- Helps in pharyngeal phase of deglutition
- Taste sensation
- Provides a local defense and immunity against harmful pathogens entering air and food passages.

Hypopharynx (Laryngopharynx)

Q. Write a short note on hypopharynx/laryngopharynx.

The lower-most part of the pharynx and lies behind and partly to the sides of the larynx.

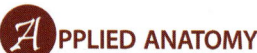
APPLIED ANATOMY

- Superior limit is marked by the horizontal plane passing from body of hyoid to the posterior pharyngeal wall.
- Lower limit is marked by the lower border of the cricoid cartilage where it continues below as the esophagus.
- It is subdivided into three parts—(1) pyriform sinus, (2) postcricoid region, and (3) posterior pharyngeal wall.
- Pyriform sinus: It lies on either side of the larynx extending from the pharyngoepiglottic fold to the upper end of the esophagus.
- It is bounded laterally by the thyroid cartilage and the thyrohyoid membrane. Medially by the aryepiglottic fold, posterolateral surfaces of the arytenoid and cricoid cartilages. The common site for foreign body lodgment.
- Internal laryngeal nerve runs submucosally in the lateral wall of the sinus.

Lymphatic Drainage

- Pyriform sinus is richly supplied by lymphatics and drains into the upper jugular chain.
- Lymphatics from the posterior wall terminate into the parapharyngeal and thereby into the deep cervical nodes.
- Lymphatics from the postcricoid region drain into the parapharyngeal. It can also drain into the supraclavicular and paratracheal chain.

Functions

- A common pathway for air and food.
- Helps in deglutition by properly coordinating pharyngeal muscle contraction and esophageal sphincter relaxation.

Chapter 4

Anatomy and Physiology of Larynx and Esophagus

EN1.1: Describe the anatomy and physiology of ear, nose, throat, head and neck.

ANATOMY OF THE LARYNX

Larynx is also called a voice box which is formed by cartilaginous framework joint by ligaments.
- **Location:** In front of the hypopharynx correspond (level of the third to sixth cervical vertebrae)
  Mucous membrane of the larynx is lined by the ciliated columnar epithelium, except over the vocal cords, and the upper part of the vestibule where it is lined by stratified squamous type.
- **Development:** Ventral midline respiratory diverticulum of foregut (tracheobronchial groove).

Laryngeal Cartilages (Figs. 1A and B)

Q. Write a short note on laryngeal cartilages and its joints.

- Thyroid, cricoid, and most of the arytenoid are hyaline cartilages.
- Epiglottis, cuneiform, corniculate, and tip of arytenoid are elastic fibrocartilage.

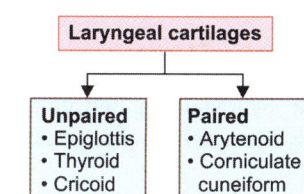

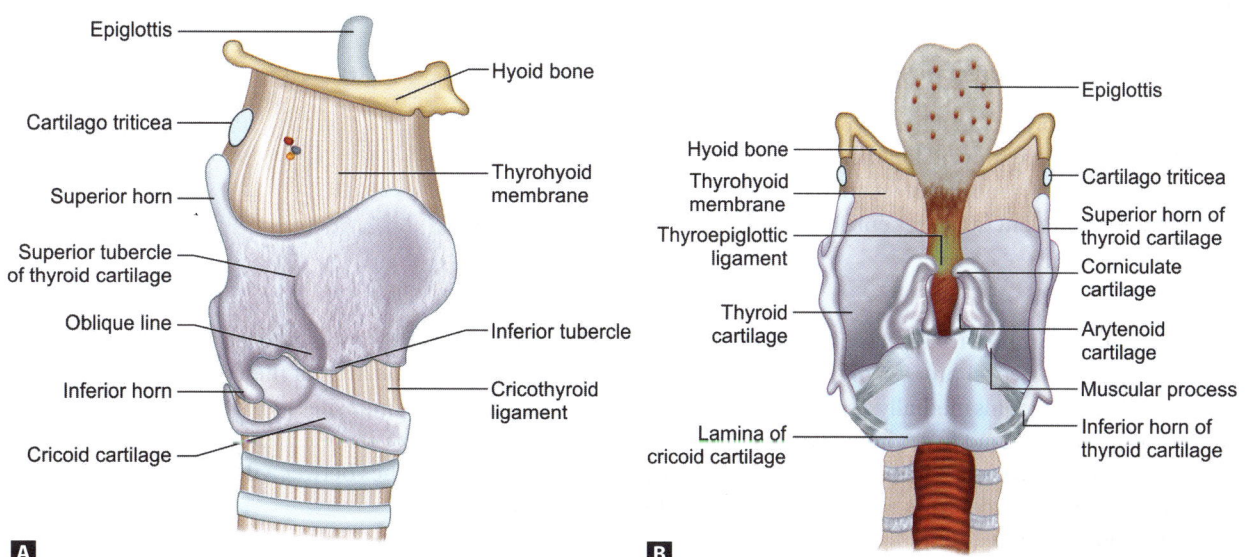

Figs. 1A and B: Laryngeal cartilages.

TABLE 1: Laryngeal cartilages.

Thyroid	<ul><li>Largest of all</li><li>Two alae meet anteriorly forming the thyroid angle—120° in males (Adam's apple), 90° in females</li><li>Vocal cords are attached to the middle of the thyroid angle</li></ul>
Cricoid	<ul><li>Only cartilage to form a complete ring</li><li>Posteriorly it is expanded to form a lamina. Anteriorly, it is narrow forming an arch</li></ul>
Epiglottis	<ul><li>Leaf-like elastic cartilage forms the anterior wall of the laryngeal inlet</li><li>Attached to the body of the hyoid bone by hyoepiglottic ligament</li><li>Attached to the thyroid angle by a stalk-like process called petiole through thyroepiglottic ligament, just above the attachment of the vocal cord</li></ul>
Arytenoid	<ul><li>Paired</li><li>Pyramidal in shape: *Base* that attaches it to the cricoid</li><li>*The lateral muscular process* that gives attachment to the internal laryngeal muscles</li><li>*Vocal process* is directed anteriorly that gives attachment to the vocal cord, *apex* that supports the corniculate cartilage</li></ul>
Corniculate	<ul><li>Paired</li><li>Attaches to the apex of the arytenoid cartilages forming a horn</li></ul>
Cuneiform	<ul><li>Paired and rod-shaped</li><li>Situated in the aryepiglottic fold in front of the corniculate cartilage</li></ul>

Laryngeal Joints

Cricoarytenoid Joint

- Synovial joint formed between base of arytenoid and a facet in the upper border of the cricoid lamina.
- **Two movements:** Rotatory movement—arytenoid moves around its vertical axis thus abducting and adducting the vocal cord. Gliding movement—where one cartilage glides towards and away from its counterpart thus opening or closing the posterior part of the glottis.

Cricothyroid Joint

- Synovial joint between the inferior cornua of the thyroid cartilage and a facet on the cricoid cartilage.
- Rotatory movement along a transverse axis.

Laryngeal Membranes and Ligaments

Q. Write short note on membranes of larynx and ligaments.

Extrinsic Membrane (Joins Larynx to Hyoid Bone and Trachea)

- Thyrohyoid membrane (attaches thyroid to hyoid)
- Medial and lateral thyrohyoid ligament
- Cricotracheal membrane (connect cricoid to the trachea)
- Hyoepiglottic ligament (attaches epiglottis to hyoid)

Intrinsic Membranes

- **Cricovocal membrane**—triangular fibroelastic membrane. Upper border is free and stretches from the middle of the thyroid angle to the vocal process of the arytenoid. Lower border attaches to the arch of the cricoid cartilage. From its lower attachment, it folds medially and upwards and joins its counterpart on the opposite side to form the conus elasticus, where foreign bodies tend to get impacted.
- **Quadrangular membrane**—lies deep in the mucosa of the aryepiglottis. It stretches between the epiglottis and arytenoid cartilages. Its lower border from the vocal ligament within the false vocal cord.
- **Cricothyroid ligament**
- **Thyroepiglottic ligament**—it attaches the epiglottis to the thyroid cartilage.

CHAPTER 4: Anatomy and Physiology of Larynx and Esophagus

Laryngeal Muscles (Figs. 2A and B)

Q. Write a short note on laryngeal muscles and its nerve supply and blood supply with actions of muscles.

Intrinsic Muscles

Acting on the vocal cords or laryngeal inlet.

Acting on the Vocal Cords

- **Abductors**: Posterior cricoarytenoid
- **Adductors**: Lateral cricoarytenoids, interarytenoid, and thyroarytenoid (external part) cricothyroid
- **Tensors**: Vocalis (internal part of the thyroarytenoid)

Acting on Laryngeal Inlet

- **Openers of the laryngeal inlet**: Thyroepiglottic (part of the thyroarytenoid)
- **Closers of the laryngeal inlet**: Interarytenoid and aryepiglottic (oblique part of inter arytenoid)

Extrinsic Muscles

They are connecting the larynx to the neighboring structures.

Elevators

- **Primary elevators**: They are directly attached to the thyroid cartilage—stylopharyngeus, salpingopharyngeus, palatopharyngeus, and thyrohyoid
- **Secondary elevators**: They act indirectly as they are attached to the hyoid bone—mylohyoid, digastric, stylohyoid, and geniohyoid.

Depressors

- Sternothyroid
- Sternohyoid
- Omohyoid

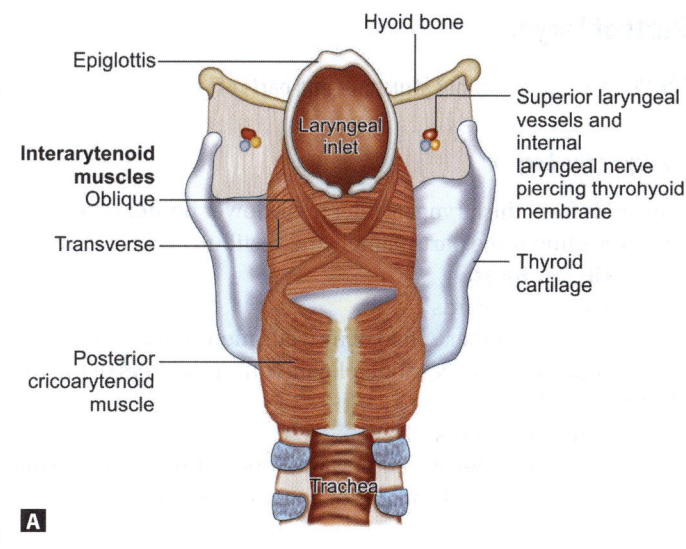
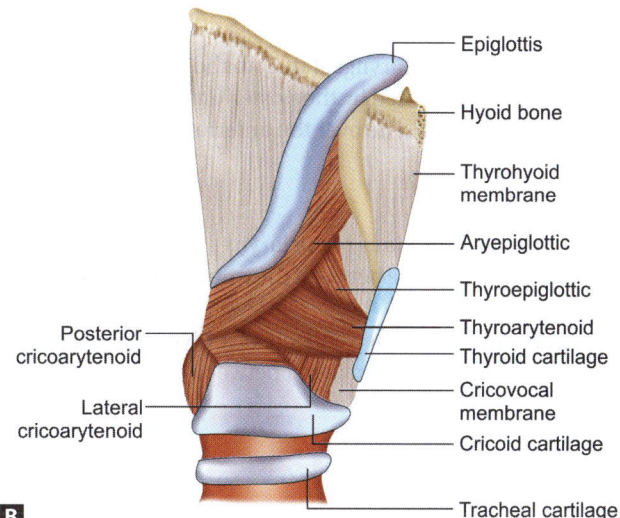

Figs. 2A and B: Laryngeal muscles.

TABLE 2: Origin, insertion, and action of the intrinsic muscles of the larynx.

Muscle	Origin	Insertion	Action
Posterior cricoarytenoid	Posterior surface of the cricoid lamina	Muscular process of arytenoid	Abducts vocal folds
Lateral cricoarytenoids	Upper border of the cricoid arch	Muscular process of arytenoid	Adducts vocal folds
Transverse interarytenoid	Back of one arytenoid and its muscular process	Back of on other arytenoid and its muscular process	Anterolateral
Thyroarytenoid (external part)	Lower half of the thyroid angle	Anterolateral Arytenoid surface	Anterolateral
Cricothyroid	Anterolateral surface of the cricoid arch	Lower border and inferior cornu of thyroid	Lengthens vocal folds (tensor)
Thyroarytenoid (internal part) vocalis	Lower half of the thyroid angle	Lateral surface arytenoid vocal process	Shortens vocal folds and thickens them
Thyroepiglottic (part of thyroarytenoid)	Lower half of the thyroid angle	Back of arytenoid muscular process	Opens laryngeal inlet
Oblique part of interarytenoid	Back of arytenoid muscular process	Apex of opposite arytenoid	Closes laryngeal inlet
Aryepiglottic (prolongation of oblique interarytenoid)	Back of arytenoid muscular process	Back of arytenoid muscular process	Closes laryngeal inlet

Parts of Larynx

Q. Write a note on various structures and parts of larynx.

Cavity of the Larynx

It extends from the laryngeal inlet to the lower border of the cricoid cartilage. Two pairs of folds—vocal and vestibular divide the larynx into three parts namely the vestibule, ventricle, and subglottic space.

- ❖ **Vestibular folds:**
  - ▸ False vocal cords
  - ▸ Two in number. A fold of mucous membrane extending anteroposteriorly across the laryngeal cavity.
  - ▸ It contains the vestibular ligament, a few fibers of the thyroarytenoids muscle, and mucous glands.
- ❖ **Vocal folds:**
  - ▸ True vocal cords
  - ▸ Two in number. Extending anteroposteriorly from the middle of the thyroid angle to the vocal process of the arytenoid.
  - ▸ Each vocal cord consists of a vocal ligament which is the true upper edge of the cricovocal membrane.

Vestibule

- ❖ It extends from the laryngeal inlet to the vestibular folds.
- ❖ Anterior wall is formed by the posterior surface of the epiglottis, sides by the aryepiglottic folds, and the posterior wall by the mucous membrane over the anterior surface of the arytenoids.

Ventricle

- ❖ It is also called the sinus of the larynx
- ❖ It is an elliptical space between the true and false cords and also extends a short distance above and lateral to the vestibular folds.
- ❖ The saccule part of the ventricle is a diverticulum of mucous membrane that originates from the anterior part of the ventricle and extends upwards between the vestibular folds and the thyroid cartilage. Site for laryngocele and saccular retention cyst formation

Glottis (Rima Glottidis)

- ❖ The space between the vocal cords anteriorly and the vocal processes posteriorly.
- ❖ Anteroposteriorly it is 24 mm in men and 16 mm in women.
- ❖ The narrowest part of the larynx.
- ❖ Anterior two-third is called phonatory glottis as it is concerned with phonation, posterior one-third is called respiratory glottis.

Subglottic Space

It extends from the vocal cords to the lower border of the cricoid cartilage.

Lymphatic Drainage of Larynx

- ❖ Supraglottic region drains into the upper deep cervical lymph nodes.
- ❖ Infraglottic larynx drains into prelaryngeal and pretracheal lymph nodes and thus into the lower deep cervical lymph nodes.

Nerve Supply of Larynx (Fig. 3)

- ❖ All muscles that move the vocal cord (abductors, adductors, and tensors) are supplied by the recurrent laryngeal nerve except the cricothyroid muscle.
- ❖ Cricothyroid receives its innervation from the external laryngeal nerve (branch of the superior laryngeal nerve).
- ❖ Sensory supply above the vocal cord larynx is supplied by the internal laryngeal nerve (branch of the superior laryngeal nerve) and below the vocal cord, it is supplied by the recurrent laryngeal nerve.

CHAPTER 4: Anatomy and Physiology of Larynx and Esophagus

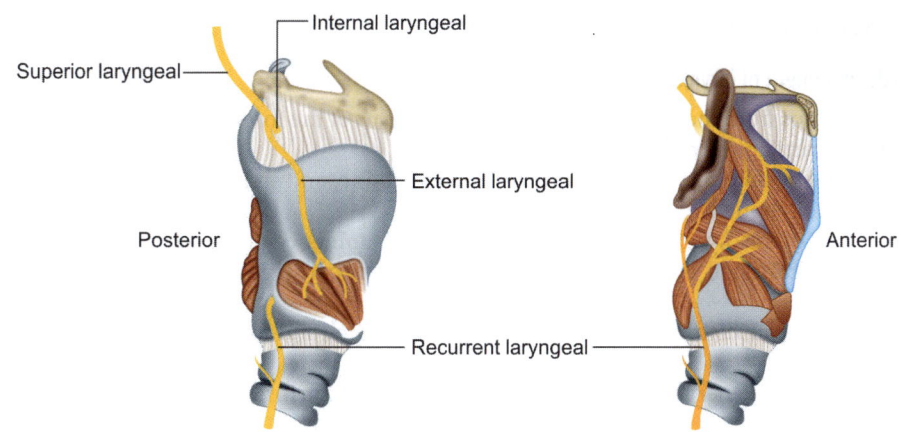

Fig. 3: Laryngeal nerve supply.

Spaces of the Larynx

Q. Write short note in spaces of the larynx.

- **Pre-epiglottic space of Boyer**: it is bounded by upper part of thyroid cartilage and thyrohyoid membrane in front, hyoepiglottic ligament above, and infrahyoid epiglottis and quadrangular membrane behind.
- **Paraglottic space**: Bounded by the thyroid cartilage laterally, conus elasticus inferomedially, the ventricle and quadrangular membrane medially, and mucosa of the pyriform fossa posteriorly.
- **Reinke's space**: A potential space under the epithelium of the vocal cords. It is bounded above and below by the arcuate lines, in front by the anterior commissure, and behind by the vocal process of the arytenoids. Edema of this space causes swelling of the membranous cords (Reinke's edema).

■ PHYSIOLOGY OF THE LARYNX

Functions

Q. Write short note on functions of larynx.

Protection of Lower Airways

- When food is swallowed, its entry is prevented into the air passage by the closure of three successive sphincters—(1) laryngeal inlet, (2) false cords, and (3) true cords.
- Respiration temporarily ceases when food comes in contact with the posterior pharyngeal wall/base of the tongue. This reflex is mediated through afferent fibers of the ninth nerve.
- The cough is an important mechanism to dislodge and expel foreign particles when it comes into contact with the respiratory mucosa.

Phonation and Speech

- Vocal cords are kept adducted. Infraglottic air pressure is increased by the air exhaled from the lungs.
- The air forces open the vocal cord and are released as small puffs that vibrate the vocal cord to produce a sound which is amplified by the nose mouth pharynx and chest.
- Sound is converted into speech by modulatory action of lips tongue palate teeth and pharynx.

Respiration

Regulates air flow into the lungs. Vocal cord adducts during expiration and abducts during inspiration.

Fixation of the Chest

When the larynx is closed the chest wall gets fixed thus facilitating various actions like digging, climbing, pulling, etc.

EMBRYOLOGY OF THE LARYNX

Q. Write short note on development of larynx.

- Laryngeal mucosa develops from the endoderm of the cephalic part of the foregut
- Laryngeal muscles and cartilage develop from the mesenchyme
- Upper part of body of the hyoid bone, lesser cornua of the hyoid bone, and stylohyoid ligament—2nd arch
- Lower part of body of hyoid bone and greater cornua—3rd arch
- Epiglottis and upper part of the thyroid cartilage—hypobranchial eminence of the 4th arch
- Lower part of the thyroid cartilage, cuneiform cartilage, corniculate cartilage, and intrinsic muscles of the larynx—6th arch
- Superior laryngeal nerve branch of the vagus nerve—nerve of the 4th arch and supplies cricothyroid muscle and constrictors of the pharynx
- Recurrent laryngeal nerve is the nerve of the 6th arch and supplies all intrinsic muscles of the larynx.

PEDIATRIC LARYNX

The larynx of an infant differs significantly from that of the adult and is very important clinically.

- It is positioned higher up in the larynx (C3 or C4). During swallowing it reaches the C1 or C2 level. Epiglottis meets the soft palate and creates a nasopharyngeal channel for nasal breathing during swallowing. Thus allowing breathing and feeding to go on simultaneously in an infant.
- Funnel in shape (cylindrical in adult)
- Subglottis is the narrowest part (rima glittidis in adults).
- Epiglottis shorter, floppy omega-shaped, angled more over the glottis.
- Vocal cords are slanted—anterior commissure more inferiorly placed.
- Vocal process constitutes 50% of anteroposterior length of glottis.
- Thyroid cartilage is flat and overlaps the cricoid cartilage, hyoid bone overlaps thyroid cartilage. Thus the cricothyroid and the thyrohyoid spaces are narrow, hence landmarks are not well-defined.
- Mucosal and submucosal tissue of the infant's larynx are comparatively loose and friable, thus easily subjected to mucosal edema following trauma or inflammation leading to obstruction.
- Infant's larynx shows two growth spurts—first in the primary 3 years of life and thus obviating the need for any airway surgery in certain congenital anomalies. The second growth spurt occurs during adolescence.
- With the growth of the neck, the larynx gradually descends to its normal adult level; vocal cords lies at the level of C5.

ANATOMY AND PHYSIOLOGY OF THE ESOPHAGUS

Q. Briefly discuss applied anatomy of esophagus.

APPLIED ANATOMY

- **Fibromuscular tube**: 25 cm in length extending from the lower end of the pharynx (C6) to the cardiac end of the stomach (T11).
- **It has 3 curves**
  - One in the sagittal plane—follows cervical vertebral column (concave forward)
- Two in the coronal plane—leftward from the origin of esophagus to T5 level and again from T7 level bending to left up to lower-end esophagus joining the stomach.
- **It harbors three normal constrictions** at the following site
  - At cricopharynx (C6)—15 cm from the upper incisors.
  - At crossing of arch of aorta (T4)—25 cm from the upper incisors
  - At crossing of left main bronchus—27 cm from upper incisors.
  - Where it pierces the diaphragm (T10)—40 cm from upper incisors.
- Foreign bodies can get lodged at these sites (the most common site—at the cricopharyngeal constrictor)
- Wall of the esophagus consists of four layers from within outwards
  1. Mucosa—lined by stratified squamous epithelium
  2. Submucosa
  3. Muscular layer—inner circular and outer longitudinal muscle fibers
  4. Fibrous layer

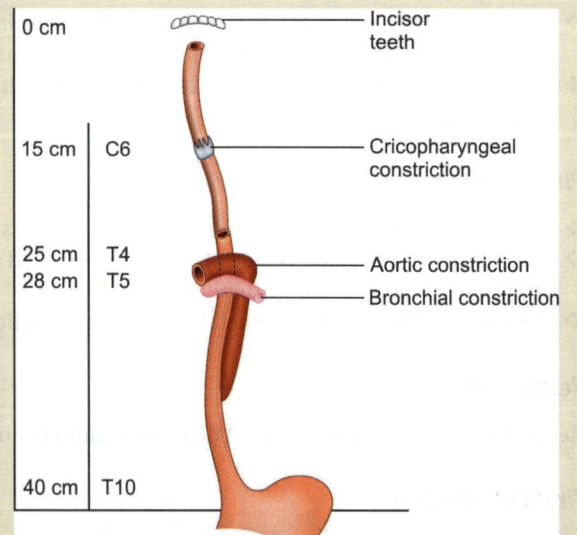

Fig. 4: Constrictor of esophagus with distance of constrictor from upper incisor teeth.

Blood Supply, Nerve Supply and Lymphatic Drainage

Q. Write a note on blood supply, nerve supply and lymphatic drainage of oesophagus.

Arterial

- **Cervical part:** Inferior thyroid artery
- **Thoracic part:** Branches from descending thoracic aorta
- **Abdominal part:** Left gastric artery

Venous Drainage

- **Cervical part:** Inferior thyroid vein
- **Thoracic part:** Azygos vein
- **Abdominal part:** Left gastric vein

Nerve Supply

Parasympathetic nerve supply comes from the vagus nerve and sympathetic supply comes from the sympathetic trunk.

Lymphatic Drainage

Cervical, thoracic, and abdominal parts of the esophagus drain into deep cervical, posterior mediastinal, and gastric nodes respectively.

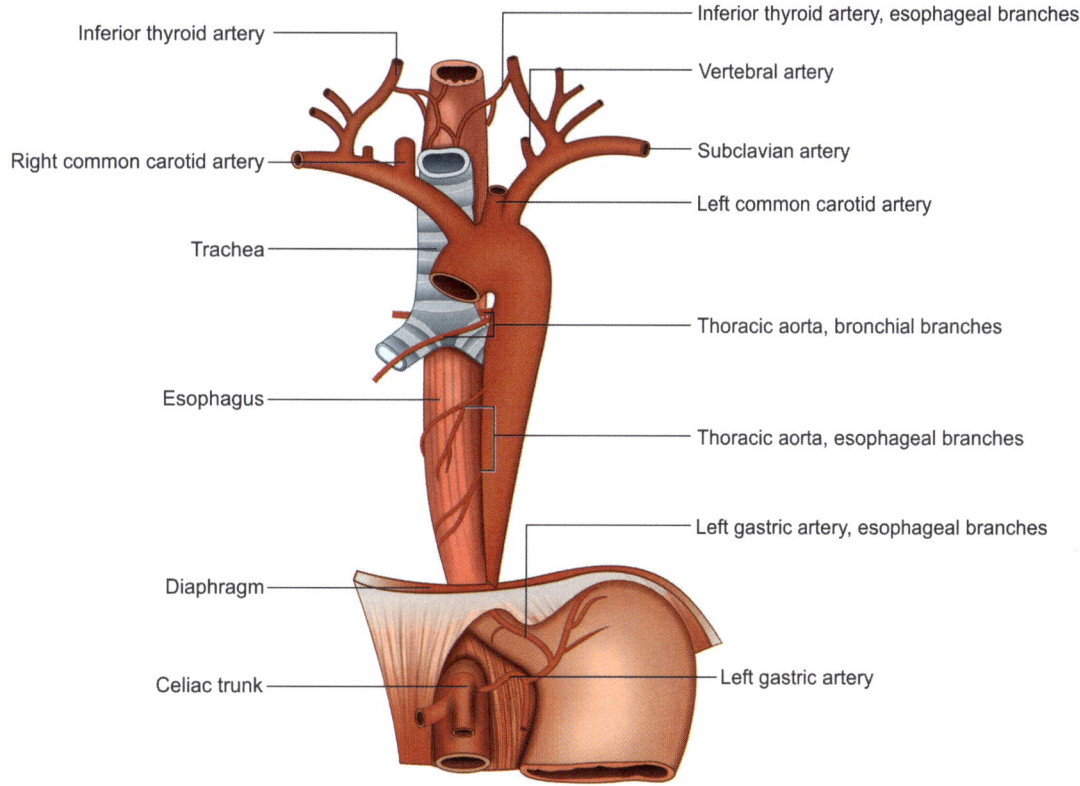

Fig. 5: Esophagus and its relation.

Applied Physiology

- Manometric studies have shown two high pressure zones in the esophagus which form the physiologic sphincters.
- Upper esophageal sphincter is present at the upper border of the esophagus is about 3–5 cm in length and plays an important role in the act of swallowing.
- Lower esophageal sphincter lies at the lower end of the esophagus and also measures about 3–5 cm in length and prevents esophageal reflux.

PHYSIOLOGY OF SWALLOWING

Q. Write a short note on physiology of swallowing.

Act of swallowing can be divided into three phases:
1. **Oral/buccal phase:** The food which is placed in the mouth is chewed and lubricated with saliva and converted into a bolus and then propelled into the pharynx by elevation of the tongue against the palate.
2. **Pharyngeal phase**: Initiated when the food bolus comes into contact with the pharyngeal mucosa. A series of coordinated reflex actions take place culminating into the passage of the food bolus past the oro- and laryngopharynx into the esophagus, while the communications into the nasal cavity, oral cavity, and the larynx are cut off.
    - *Closure of the nasopharynx:* A soft palate contracts against the Passavant's ridge on the posterior pharyngeal wall and completely cuts off the nasopharynx from the oropharynx.
    - *Closure of the oropharyngeal isthmus:* A contraction of the tongue against the palate and contraction of the palatoglossal muscle blocks the entry of the bolus back into the oral cavity.
    - *Closure of the larynx:* A communication of the food bolus into the larynx is prevented by temporary cessation of respiration, closure of the laryngeal inlet by contraction of the aryepiglottic folds, closure of false and true vocal cords, and rising of the larynx under the tongue.
    - Contraction of the pharyngeal muscles and relaxation of the cricopharyngeus.
3. **Esophageal phase**: After the bolus enters the esophagus, the upper esophageal sphincter relaxes and the bolus is pushed down to the stomach by the peristaltic movements of the esophagus. The lower esophageal sphincter relaxes well before the peristaltic wave reaches the lower end. After the bolus reaches the stomach the lower esophageal sphincter closes. Regurgitation back into the esophagus from the stomach is prevented by:
    - Tone of the lower esophageal sphincter
    - Negative intrathoracic pressure
    - Pinch-cock effect of the diaphragm
    - Mucosal folds
    - Esophagogastric angle
    - Slightly positive intrabdominal pressure

Section 2: Otology

Chapter 5

History Taking and Examination of Ear

EN2.1: Elicit document and present an appropriate history in a patient presenting with an ENT complaint.

DEMOGRAPHICS

- **Age:** Certain diseases are common in particular age group. Tonsillitis is seen in childhood. Nasopharyngeal angiofibroma is seen in teenagers.
- **Sex:** Certain diseases are common in particular sex. Nasopharyngeal angiofibroma is commonly seen in males while otosclerosis is more common in females.
- **Residence:** Allergic rhinitis is seen in areas where pollens, dusts, molds, animal dander, etc., are most common. Residence also gives rough idea about socioeconomic status of patients like chronic suppurative otitis media (CSOM) is more likely seen in low socioeconomic group.
- **Occupation:** Allergic rhinitis is seen in patients working in air-conditioned room for longer time. Noise-induced hearing loss is seen in saw mills, crushers, printing, etc.

HISTORY

- Chief complaints
- Presenting illness
- Negative complaints
- History of etiology
- History of complications
- Past history
- Personal history
- Family history

Chief Complaints

- Ear discharge (**otorrhea**)
- Decreased hearing (**deafness**)
- Earache (**otalgia**)
- **Tinnitus**
- **Vertigo**

History of Presenting Illness

EN4.5: Elicit document and present a correct history, demonstrate and describe the clinical features, choose the correct investigations and describe the principles of management of discharging ear.

Ear Discharge (Otorrhea)

Q. Write a short note on ear discharge/discharging ear/otorrhea.

- ❖ **Site**: Right/left/bilateral
- ❖ **Onset**: Acute/chronic
- ❖ **Duration**
- ❖ **Consistency of ear discharge** can be mucoid, mucopurulent, purulent, hemorrhagic, serous, and watery.

Mucoid	Mucopurulent	Purulent

Mucoid discharge indicates discharge is from middle ear as goblet cells are seen in the lining mucosa of middle ear cavity. It is seen most commonly in mucosal chronic otitis media (COM)	Seen in:
	❖ Mucosal CSOM
	❖ Marginal perforations with discharge
	❖ Grade V pars tensa retraction with discharge
		❖ Otitis externa
		❖ Otomycosis
		❖ Granular myringitis
		❖ Squamous CSOM
		❖ Most common organism:
		  ➤ Streptococcus pneumoniae
		  ➤ H. influenzae
		  ➤ Moraxella

Hemorrhagic	Serous	Watery
❖ Trauma to ear ❖ Foreign body ❖ Granulations, polyps ❖ In acute otitis media (AOM) in stage of suppuration when drum ruptures (blood-tinged discharge) ❖ Squamosal CSOM ❖ Vascular tumors like glomus jugulare, arteriovenous (AV) malformations, etc. ❖ Malignancy	Atopic/eczematous otitis externa	Cerebrospinal fluid (CSF) otorrhea (spontaneous/traumatic) Diagnostic test is serum $\beta 2$ transferrin test. $\beta 2$ transferrin is found in CSF, perilymph of cochlea, aqueous, and vitreous humor of eye

- ❖ **Smell**: Foul smelling/nonfoul smelling

Foul smelling ear discharge	Nonfoul smelling ear discharge

❖ Squamous CSOM
❖ Malignant otitis externa
❖ Otomycosis
❖ Forgotten ear foreign body
❖ Malignancy
❖ Causative organism in cholesteatoma:
  ➤ Proteus
  ➤ Pseudomonas
  ➤ Klebsiella
Reason: Proteus releases mercaptans causing the fishy odors while anaerobic infection with osteitis and bony erosions also causes foul smelling discharge.
	❖ Mucosal CSOM
	❖ Acute suppurative otitis media (ASOM)

- ❖ Blood stained/nonblood stained
- ❖ **History of upper respiratory tract infection (URTI):** It is usually preceding complaint seen in AOM and mucosal CSOM.
- ❖ **History of ear drops reaching throat/air bubbles in ear discharge:** It suggests perforation in the tympanic membrane with anatomically patent Eustachian tube. It is seen mostly in mucosal CSOM.

Mucosal/tubotympanic/safe CSOM	Squamous/atticoantral/unsafe CSOM
❖ Mucoid/mucopurulent ❖ Not foul smelling ❖ Not blood stained ❖ Profuse ❖ Associated with URTI ❖ History of ear drops reaching throat	❖ Purulent/mucopurulent ❖ Foul smelling ❖ May be bloodstained ❖ Scanty ❖ +/−URTI ❖ No history of ear drops reaching throat

Decreased Hearing

❖ Unilateral/bilateral

Unilateral hearing loss	Bilateral hearing loss
Wax, foreign body, otitis externa, malignant otitis externa, otomycosis, ruptured tympanic membrane, CSOM, AOM, SOM, sudden sensorineural hearing loss, CP angle tumors, glomus tumors, malignancy	Congenital causes: Mondini's, incomplete partition, cochlear nerve aplasia, etc. Bilateral CSOM, SOM, Eustachian tube dysfunction, otosclerosis, Meniere's disease, presbycusis, barotrauma, noise-induced hearing loss, bilateral acoustic neuromas

❖ **Gradual/sudden onset:** Sudden onset hearing loss is seen in severe noise trauma seen in bomb blast, fire cracker injuries, sudden sensorineural hearing loss (idiopathic), and acute Eustachian tube dysfunction.
❖ Progressive/nonprogressive
❖ Fluctuant/nonfluctuant
❖ **Associated symptoms:** Fluctuant hearing loss associated with vertigo and tinnitus seen in Meniere's disease.

> **EN4.1:** Elicit document and present a correct history, demonstrate and describe the clinical features, choose the correct investigations and describe the principles of management of otalgia.

Earache (Otalgia)

Q. Write short note on otalgia/earache.

❖ **Site:** Patients should be asked to point the area of maximum tenderness with one finger. Causes of earache differ as per areas like preauricular region, tragus, pinna, external auditory canal (EAC), postauricular region or mastoid tip.
❖ Intensity
❖ **Aggravating factors:** Otalgia due to tympanomandibular joint dysfunction aggravates on jaw movement while it increases in AOM due to Eustachian tube dysfunction secondary to URTI.
❖ **Relieving factors:** Pain reduces when tympanic membrane ruptures in suppurative stage of acute otitis media.
❖ **Referred otalgia:** Earache occurs due to the cause at distant region and due to common innervation. It occurs due to either involvement of mandibular division of CN V (temporomandibular joint disorders), CN IX (tonsils, base of tongue, pharynx) or CN X (larynx, pyriform fossa) disorders.

Tinnitus

❖ Unilateral/bilateral
❖ Continuous/intermittent
❖ **Type:** Ringing/hissing/humming, etc.
❖ Whether affecting daily routine?
❖ **Associated with other symptoms:** Hearing loss/vertigo/earache/ear discharge

Vertigo

❖ Whether it is sense of dizziness/rotatory giddiness/blackout/imbalance
❖ Continuous/intermittent
❖ Positional/not associated with position change
❖ **Duration of each episodes:** Vertigo in benign paroxysmal positional vertigo (BPPV) last for few seconds to minutes while vertigo in labyrinthitis or vestibular neuronitis last for few hours to days
❖ Associated with autonomous symptoms like nausea, vomiting, sweating, etc.
❖ Associated with other conditions like anemia, pregnancy, cervical spondylosis, etc.

History of Etiology

❖ Unilateral/bilateral nasal blockage, rhinitis, sneezing [to rule out deviated nasal septum (DNS), sinusitis or allergic rhinitis]
❖ Recurrent sore throat, odynophagia, mouth breathing (to rule out chronic tonsillitis or adenoiditis)
❖ History of trauma
❖ History of use of ototoxic drugs (drugs used in TB, malaria, diabetes, etc.)

History of Complications

- History of fever, headache, projectile vomiting, imbalance, loss of consciousness: To rule out intracranial complications of CSOM like meningitis, encephalitis, brain abscesses.
- History of facial weakness (facial palsy), giddiness (labyrinthine fistula), postaural or neck swelling (mastoid abscesses), retro-orbital pain (Gradenigo's syndrome): To rule out extracranial complications of CSOM.

Past History

- History of medication or surgery of ear in past. In case same ear has been operated in past, we must look for causes of failure of surgery.
- History of diabetes, hypertension, bronchial asthma:
  - Diabetes can be the cause of recurrent infections. It is also the main factor in malignant otitis externa.
  - History of asthma is needed for association of allergic rhinitis.
  - All those diseases are important in preoperative anesthesia evaluation in case of surgery is treatment of choice.
- History of Kochs or Koch's contact:
  - Tuberculous otitis media has distinctive features like multiple perforations (Fig. 1), pale granulations, and sensorineural hearing loss. Patient has more signs than symptoms.
- History of exanthematous fever:
  - Acute necrotizing otitis media is seen following exanthematous fever like measles, mumps, etc.
  - In acute necrotizing otitis media, there is rapid destruction of tympanic membrane, ossicles along with annulus which can lead to secondary cholesteatoma.

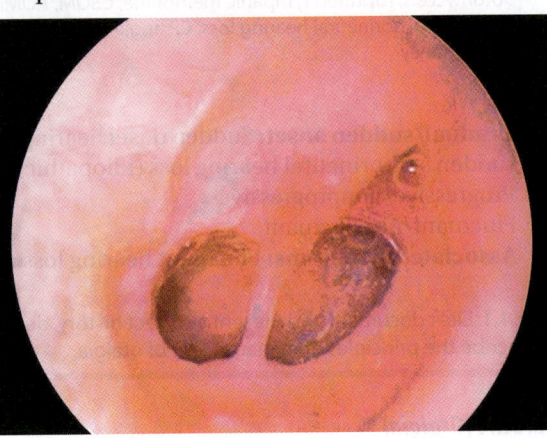

Fig. 1: Multiple perforations of tympanic membrane (TM).

Personal History

It is important to know the history of addiction. Smoking can irritate Eustachian tube as well as middle ear mucosa. Nicotine and alcohol addiction can cause tinnitus, vertigo as well as ototoxicity.

Family History

Allergy can run in family as genetic factors and also common environment. Familial otosclerosis is autosomal dominant disease.

EXAMINATION

Local Examination

Local examination is to be done for each ear differently.

Preauricular Region

Look for any visible swelling (Fig. 2A), sinus (Fig. 2B), cyst, discharge, pulsations, tag (Fig. 2C) and scar of surgery. Palpate for any tenderness.

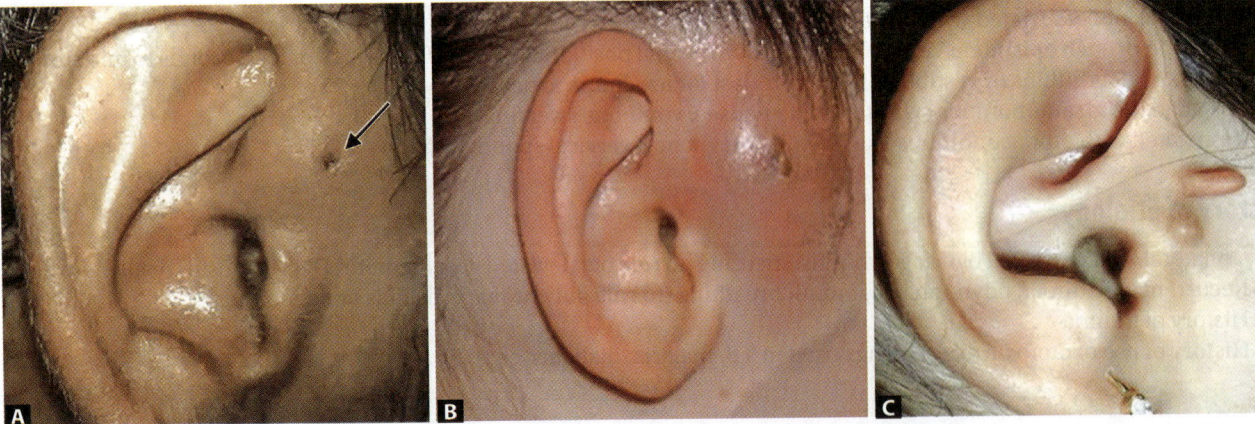

Figs. 2A to C: (A) Preauricular sinus; (B) Preauricular cyst; (C) Preauricular tags.

Pinna

Look for position of pinna. It should be in the mid-third of face. Note any low-lying pinna or other congenital malformation of pinna-like malformed pinna tag **(Fig. 3A)**. Note if it is pushed forward as in mastoiditis tag **(Fig. 5A)**. Note any sinus, scar, and vascular malformations. Look for normal cartilaginous framework of pinna. Look for anomalies like bat ear/lop ear tag **(Fig. 3B)**, Stahl ear **(Fig. 4B)**, cup ear **(Fig. 4A)**, cauliflower ear **(Fig. 5B)**, and swimmer's ear **(Fig. 5C)**, etc.

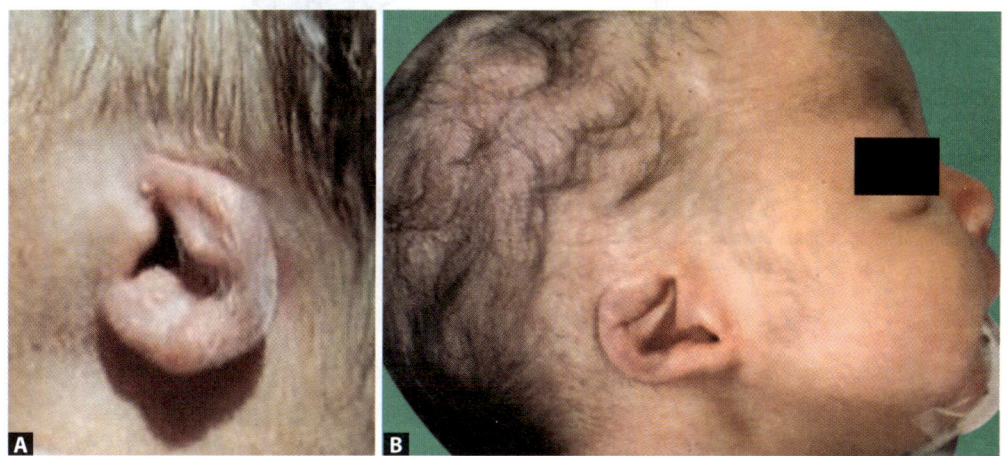

Figs. 3A and B: (A) Malformed pinna; (B) Low set and lop ear.

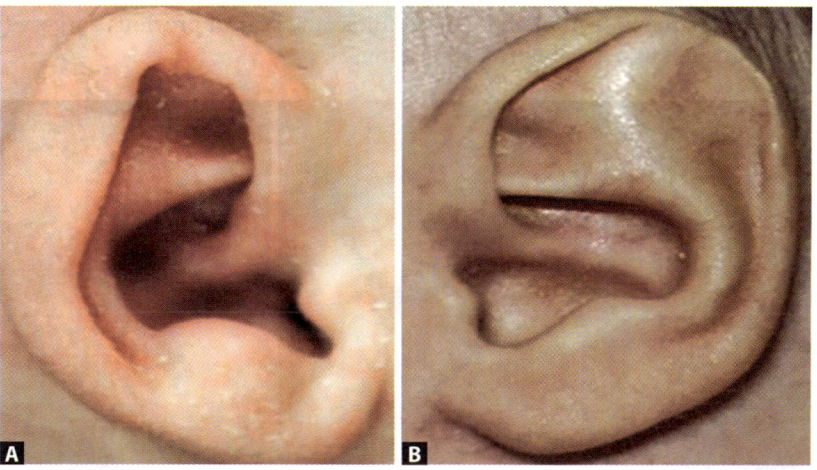

Figs. 4A and B: (A) Cup ear; (B) Stahl's ear.

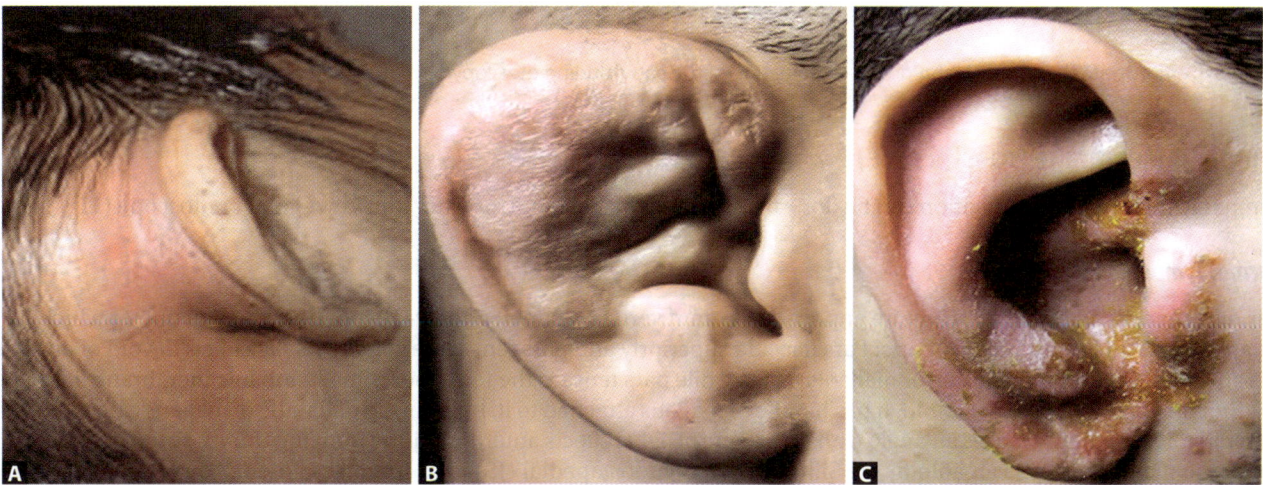

Figs. 5A to C: (A) Mastoiditis. (B) Cauliflower ear. (C) Swimmer's ear.

External Auditory Canal

It is 24 mm in size with outer one-third cartilaginous and inner two-third bony. It is **"S" shaped**, directed laterally, downward, and forward. Color of canal is same as skin with few hairs in outer cartilaginous area. Look for any narrowing, partial or complete atresia **(Fig. 6)**, wax, discharge, and foreign body.

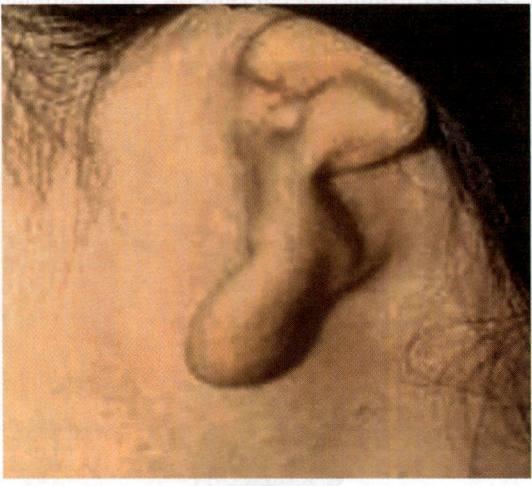

Fig. 6: Aural atresia.

Postauricular Region

Look for obliteration of postaural groove seen in acute mastoiditis, any scar of previous surgery **(Figs. 7A and B)**, sinus, swelling, and cyst. Palpate for any tenderness, abnormal pulsations.

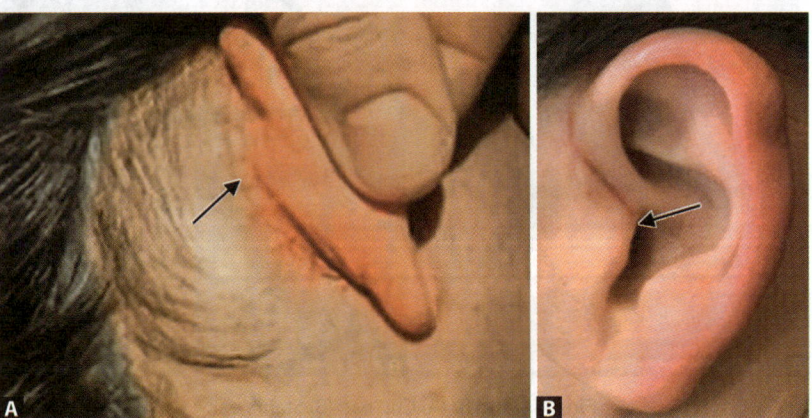

Figs. 7A and B: (A) William Wilde's incision scar; (B) Lempert's incision scar.

EN2.3: Demonstrate the correct technique of examination of the ear including otoscopy.

Tympanic Membrane (scan QR code)

Tympanic membrane examination can be done using headlight, head mirror with Bull's eye-lamp or otoscope **(Fig. 8)**.

Normal Tympanic Membrane (Fig. 9)

It is oval shaped, pearly white structure approx. 11–12 mm vertical diameter and 9–10 mm horizontal diameter which lie at an angle of 55° to EAC. It has two parts: Pars flaccida superiorly and pars tensa inferiorly. Pars flaccida is devoid of annulus, lies above the anterior and posterior malleolar folds while pars tensa is the tense portion of tympanic membrane lies below anterior and posterior malleolar fold. It has handle of malleus attached to it, bulbous tip of handle of malleus called "Umbo." As tympanic membrane makes an angle with EAC, cone of light reflects anteroinferiorly from the Umbo. Through the normal tympanic membrane, we can able to see Silhouette of incudostapedial (IS) joint in posteroinferior quadrants. Tympanic membrane moves with Valsalva maneuver.

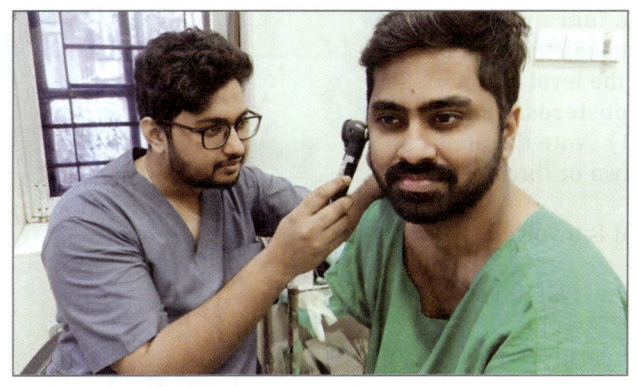

Fig. 8: Ear examination using otoscope.

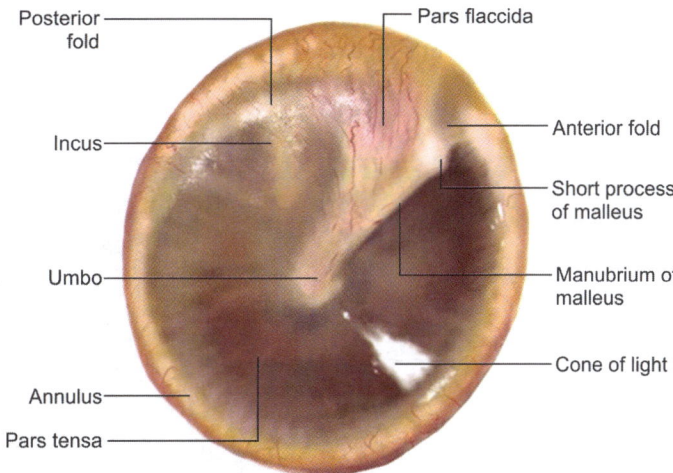

Fig. 9: Tympanic membrane.

Perforation

Q. Write short note on tympanic membrane perforations.

❖ Tympanic membrane perforations are of three types:
  1. *Central perforation:* It lies in pars tensa and surrounded by annulus and remnant of drum.
  2. *Marginal perforation:* It lies in pars tensa but some of perforation is devoid of annulus. This is the dangerous type of perforation and should be treated as unsafe ear **(Fig. 10A)**.
  3. *Attic perforation:* It lies in pars flaccida and commonly seen in unsafe CSOM **(Fig. 10B)**.

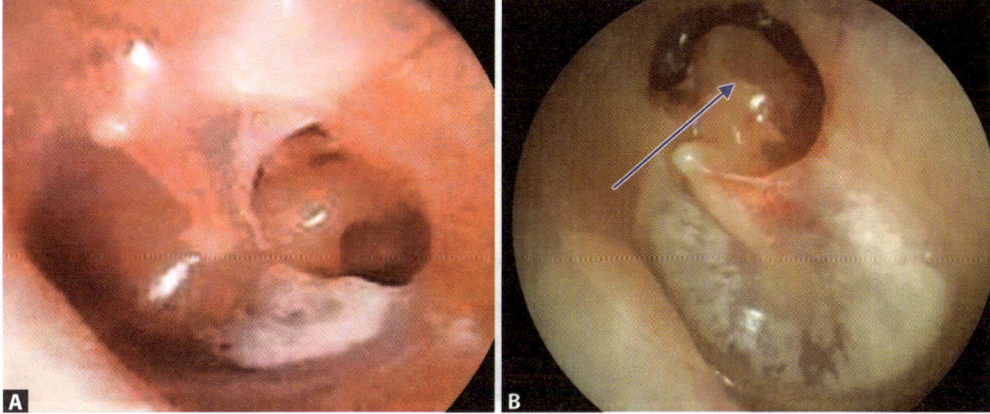

Figs. 10A and B: (A) TM marginal perforation; (B) TM attic perforation.

❖ **Site and size:** Pars tensa is divided into **four quadrants by** line drawn vertical passing through handle of malleus and other perpendicular to first line at the level of umbo into **anterosuperior, anteroinferior, posterosuperior, and posteroinferior quadrant (Fig. 11)**. Note the areas involving perforation. It can be one or two or three or all quadrant involved.
  ➢ *Small perforation:* Only one quadrant is involved **(Fig. 12A)**.
  ➢ *Medium perforation:* Any two quadrants are involved **(Fig. 12B)**.
  ➢ *Large perforation:* Any three quadrants are involved **(Fig. 12C)**.
  ➢ *Subtotal perforation:* All four quadrants are involved but thin rim of drum and annulus present **(Fig. 13A)**.
  ➢ *Total perforation:* Entire pars tensa along with annulus absent. It can be seen in acute necrotizing otitis media **(Fig. 13B)**.

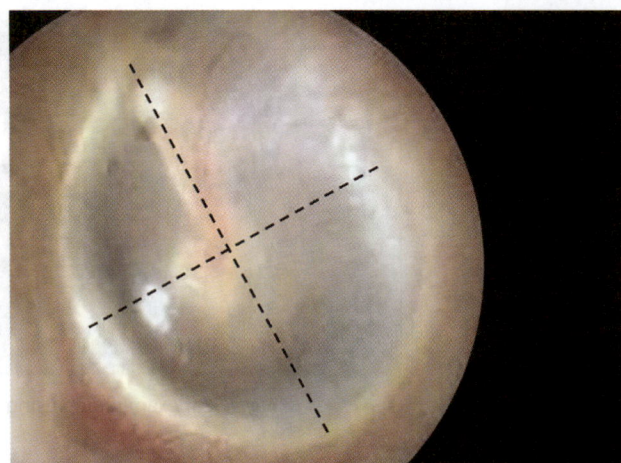

Fig. 11: Normal right tympanic membrane divided into four quadrants.

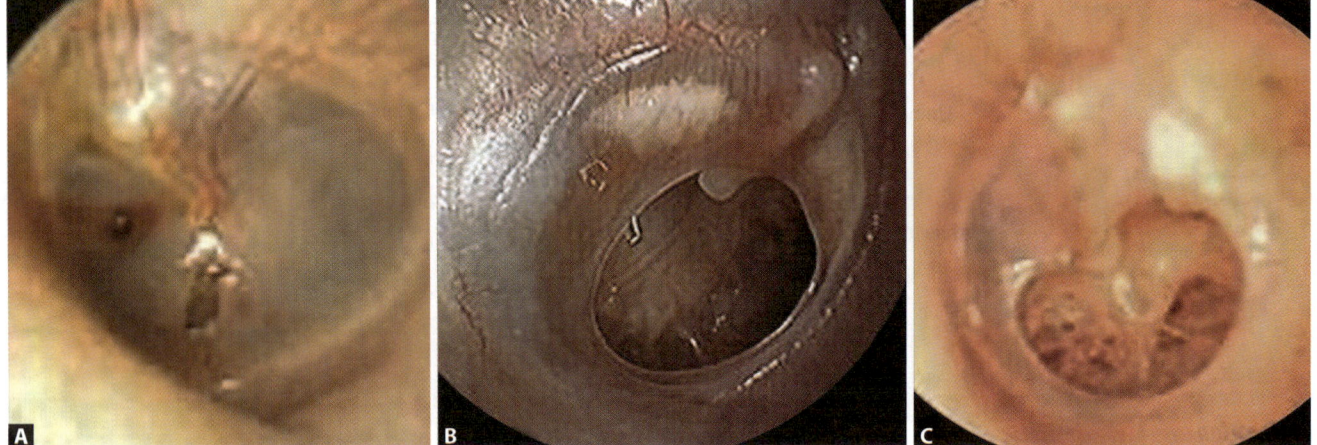

Figs. 12A to C: (A) TM small central perforation; (B) TM medium sized perforation; (C) TM large sized perforation.

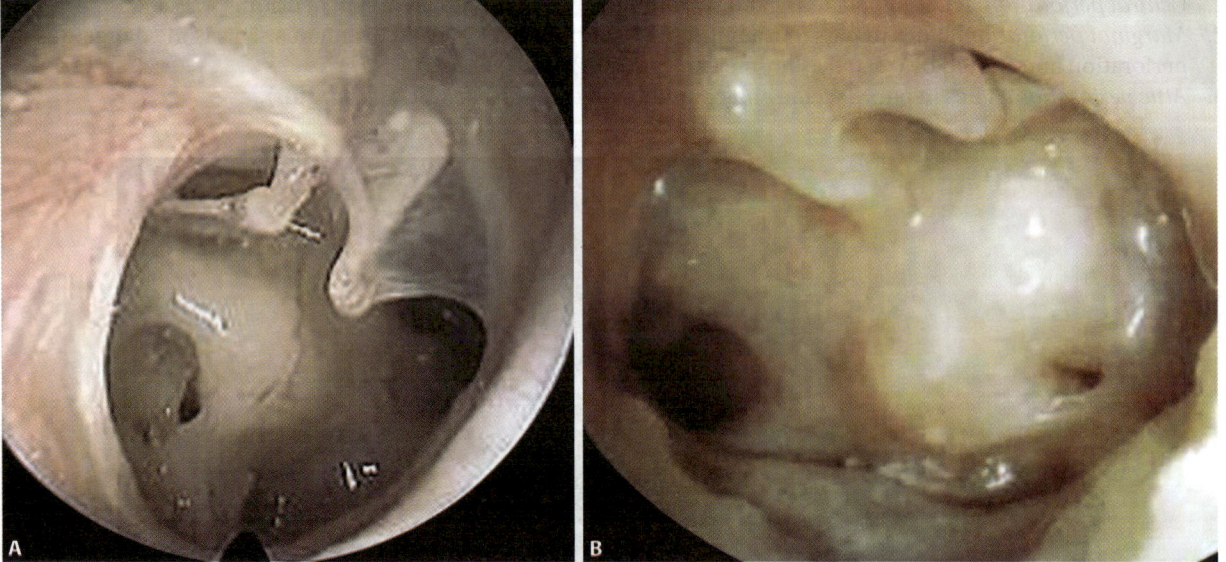

Figs. 13A and B: (A) TM subtotal perforation; (B) TM total perforation.

- ❖ **Margins:** Regular and irregular. Irregular margin is seen in traumatic perforation **(Fig. 14)**.
- ❖ **Edges:** Thick, thin.
- ❖ **Condition of middle ear mucosa**:
  - ➢ Pink seen in normal ear
  - ➢ Reddish, velvety—acute infections
  - ➢ Pale granular—TB
  - ➢ Pale—anemia
- ❖ **Structure seen through perforation:**
  - ➢ If perforation involves posterosuperior quadrant, we can able to see incus, stapes, IS joint, chorda tympani, and facial canal in most of the cases.
  - ➢ If perforation involves posteroinferior quadrant, round window niche, and hypotympanic air cells can be visible.
  - ➢ If perforation involves anterosuperior quadrant, Eustachian tube opening can be seen.
  - ➢ If perforation involves anteroinferior quadrant, hypotympanic air cells are seen.

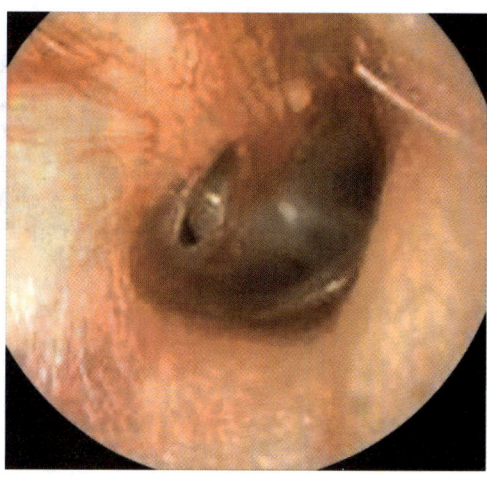

Fig. 14: Right TM traumatic perforation in posterior quadrant. Look the irregular margin with peripheral prominent blood vessels.

EN2.5: Demonstrate the correct technique of otoscopy, to hold visualize and assess the mobility of the tympanic membrane and its mobility and interpret and diagrammatically represent the findings.

Mobility of intact tympanic membrane:
- ❖ Ask the patient to do **Valsalva maneuver** while looking at tympanic membrane through otoscope or ear speculum and look for mobility of pars tensa.
- ❖ It is not appreciated in perforated drum.
- ❖ Mobility is restricted in serous otitis media, Eustachian tube dysfunction, and adhesive drum.
- ❖ Mobility is increased in hypermobile tympanic membrane.

EN2.3: Demonstrate the correct technique of performance and interpretation of tuning fork tests.

Tuning Fork Tests

Q. Discuss briefly various tuning fork tests.

Rinne's Test (scan QR code)

Q. Write short on Rinne's tuning fork test.

A tuning fork is stroke on hard surface or rubber pad at the junction of anterior one-third and posterior two-third and kept over nonhairy part of mastoid region **(Fig. 15)**, once the patient stops hearing the sound, tuning fork is then transferred in front of ear, 1 inch parallel to the EAC and ask the patient if he still hears the sound **(Fig. 16)**.
- ❖ If patient still hears the sound, then air conduction is better than bone conduction, **it is seen in normal ear or sensorineural hearing loss (Rinne's positive).**
- ❖ If patient hears bone conduction better than air conduction, he has **conductive deafness (Rinne's negative).**
- ❖ When air conduction is equivalent to bone conduction, it is called Rinne's equivocal.
- ❖ This test can be done vice-versa also or you can just compare the loudness of sound in front of EAC and mastoid region.

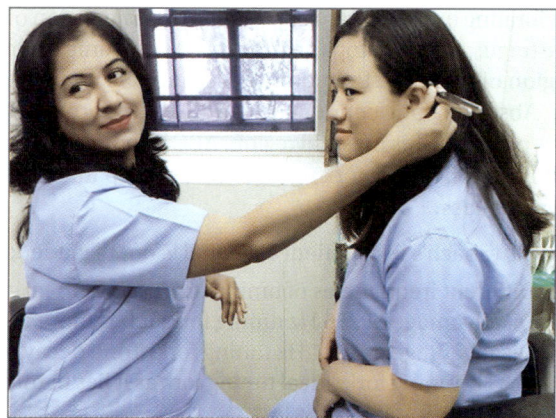

Fig. 15: Rinne's test, bone conduction being checked.

Almost 15 dB of hearing loss is needed for Rinne's to become negative. So roughly if only 256 Hz tuning fork is negative, ≈15 dB of hearing loss (mild), for 256 Hz and 512 Hz tuning forks negative ≈25–30 dB of hearing loss (moderate), and all three tuning fork negative 9 **(256, 512, 1024 Hz),** ≈40–45 dB of hearing loss (severe) is expected.

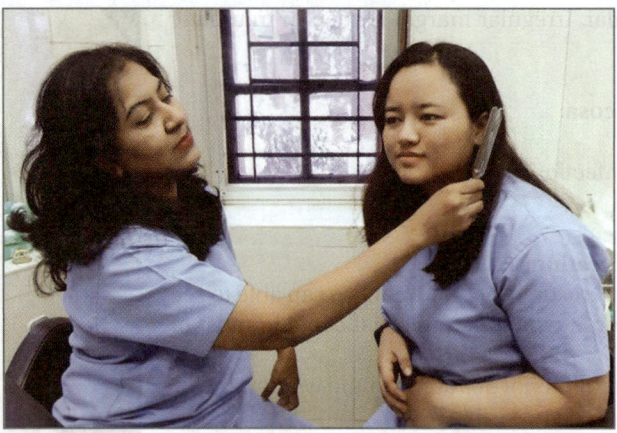

Fig. 16: Rinne's test, air conduction being checked.

Weber's Test (scan QR code)

Q. Write short note on Weber's tuning fork test

A vibrating tuning fork is kept over the bony prominence of midline, i.e., over glabella, midline parietal region, bony dorsum, teeth or chin and patient is asked in which ear he hears the sound best.

- In normal patient, he can hear sound equally in both ears, i.e., Weber is central.
- In conductive hearing loss, Weber is lateralized to worst ear **(Fig. 17)**.
- In sensorineural hearing loss, it is lateralized to better ear.

There is minimum 5 dB hearing loss difference is required for Weber to get lateralized to one ear.

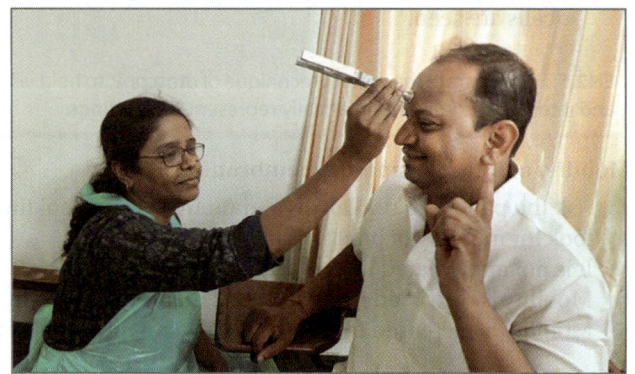

Fig. 17: Weber's test using 512 Hz tuning fork.

Absolute Bone Conduction Test/Modified Schwabach's Test (scan QR code)

Q. Write short note on ABC tuning fork test/Modified Schwabach's tuning fork test.

A vibrating tuning fork is kept over the mastoid region of patient after occluding his ear canal by pressing the tragus, once he stops hearing the sound, same tuning fork is then transferred to examiner's mastoid region of same ear. Prerequisite is examiner should have normal hearing.

Absolute bone conduction (ABC) test is normal when examiner also do not hear sound of tuning fork placed on his mastoid region. ABC is reduced as compared to examiner when examiner still hears sound when tuning fork is transferred from patient to his mastoid region. **It is seen in sensorineural hearing loss.**

In Schwabach's test, patient ear canal is not occluded; rest of the procedure is same.

- Different frequencies of tuning fork used for hearing test: 256 Hz, 512 Hz, 1024 Hz
- Disadvantage of 256 Hz tuning fork: It has more of vibratory sensation than sound.
- Disadvantage of 1024 Hz tuning fork: Tone decay is more.
- 512 Hz tuning fork: Ideal tuning fork as it lies in midspeech frequency. Sensations are better heard than felt. Tone decay is less.
- At the end of tuning fork test, we can actually guess the type (conductive/sensorineural/mixed hearing loss) and intensity (mild/moderate/severe) hearing loss.

Mastoid Tenderness

Mastoid tenderness can be elicited by pressing over cymba concha, mastoid tip, MacEwan's triangle, and root of zygoma. It is positive in acute mastoiditis and mastoid abscesses.

Three Fingers Test

Three fingers namely middle finger over cymba concha, index finger over mastoid area behind the pinna, and thumb are placed over mastoid tip and alternatively pressed gently to elicit mastoid tenderness.

If the tenderness is elicited over cymba concha, it is due to mastoiditis, if it is over mastoid area, it is due to thrombophlebitis of mastoid emissary vein and tenderness over mastoid tip is due to mastoid abscess. Out of these three sites, tenderness over cymba concha is an important indicator of mastoiditis.

Tragal Tenderness

It is elicited by gently pressing tragus or pulling the pinna gently. Patient will have pain in otitis externa, EAC boils, or abscess.

Nystagmus

Q. Write short note on nystagmus.

Finger is kept at the level of patient's eyes in center at the distance of 1 ft and moves till the angle of 30° each side of midline and check for any oscillatory movements in patient's eye **(Fig. 18)**. Note that finger should not go beyond 30° to avoid physiological nystagmus.

Alexander's Law for Grading of Nystagmus

- Only present while looking toward the fast component of nystagmus (irritative nystagmus)
- Also present on looking straight
- Present on looking toward slow component also (paralytic nystagmus)

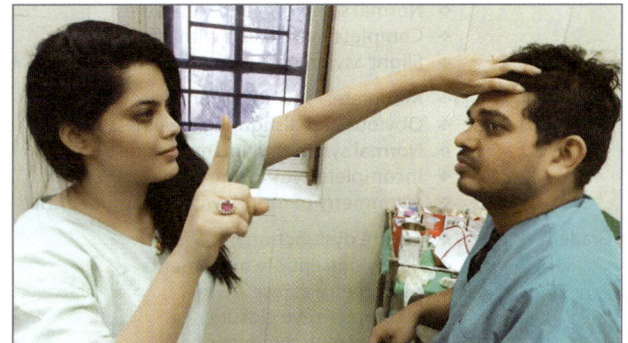

Fig. 18: Checking for nystagmus.

Peripheral Causes of Nystagmus

- BPPV
- Meniere's disease
- Vestibular neuronitis
- Labyrinthitis
- Labyrinthine or promontory fistula
- Superior semicircular
- Canal dehiscence
- Trauma
- Ototoxicity
- Can be seen in immediate postoperative of stapedotomy patient

Causes of Central Nystagmus

- Vascular lesions
- Tumors (benign or malignant)
- Trauma
- Demyelinating disorders
- Multiple sclerosis
- Toxins like anticonvulsant drugs, aspirin, alcohol, etc.
- Stroke

Central nystagmus	Peripheral nystagmus
- Horizontal, vertical, or rotatory - It can change the direction with change in gaze - It does not disappear with fixation of gaze - Nonfatigable - Mostly associated with other neurological symptoms like diplopia, cranial nerve, neuropathies, etc.	- Usually, rotatory - Unidirectional - It disappears with fixation of gaze - Fatigable - Not associated with other neurological symptoms

Facial Palsy

It is important to differentiate between upper motor neuron and lower motor neuron (LMN) facial palsy. Look for any visible asymmetry and check movement of each group of facial muscles individually and look for any weakness like:
- Ask the patient to look up to the ceiling without moving his head and look for symmetrical wrinkling over forehead
- Tight closure of eyes

❖ Nasolabial fold
❖ Ask patient to blow the balloon or hold the air in mouth or clench the teeth.

House Brackmann's Grading of LMN Facial Palsy

Grade I	❖ Normal facial function
Grade II (Fig. 19A)	❖ Mild dysfunction ❖ Slight weakness noticeable on close inspection ❖ Slight synkinesis ❖ Normal symmetry and tone at rest ❖ Complete eye closure with minimum efforts ❖ Slight asymmetry of mouth
Grade III	❖ Moderate dysfunction ❖ Obvious but not disfiguring weakness ❖ Noticeable synkinesis and/or hemifacial spasms ❖ Normal symmetry and tone at rest ❖ Complete eye closure with efforts ❖ Slight asymmetry of mouth with maximum efforts
Grade IV (Fig. 19B)	❖ Moderately severe dysfunction ❖ Obvious and disfiguring weakness ❖ Normal symmetry and tone at rest ❖ Incomplete eye closure ❖ Asymmetry of mouth with maximum efforts
Grade V	❖ Severe dysfunction ❖ Barely perceptible movements ❖ Asymmetry at rest ❖ Incomplete eye closure ❖ Slight mouth movement
Grade VI	❖ Total paralysis ❖ No facial movement

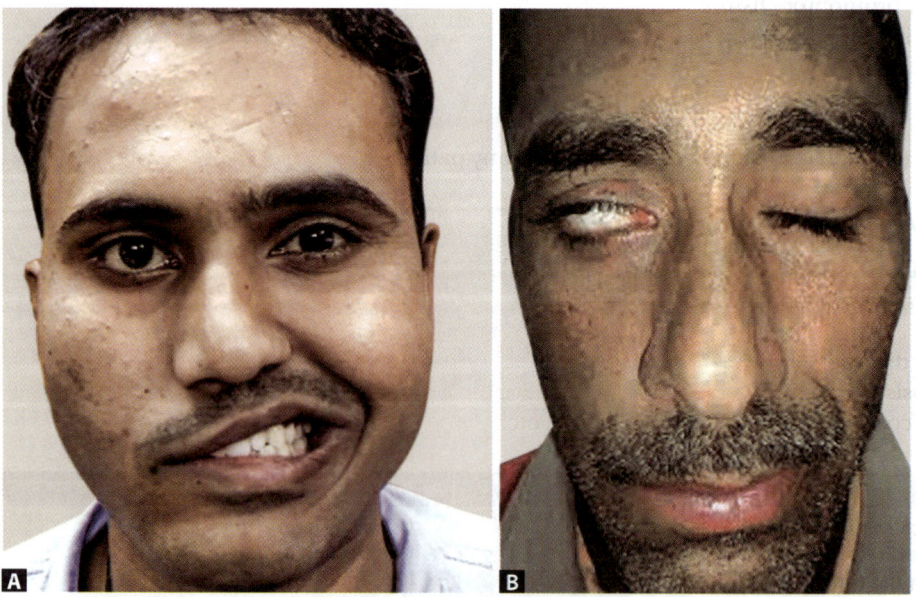

Figs. 19A and B: (A) Grade 2 LMN facial palsy; (B) Grade 4 LMN facial palsy.

Causes of LMN Facial Palsy

❖ **Trauma:** Road traffic accidents (RTA), fracture temporal bone
❖ Iatrogenic trauma during mastoidectomy, labyrinthectomy, etc.
❖ Complicated unsafe CSOM
❖ Facial neuroma or cerebellopontine (CP) angle tumors
❖ Congenital facial canal dehiscence with ASOM
❖ Parotid malignancy

Fistula Test (scan QR code)

Q. Write short note on fistula test.

Fistula test is performed either by pressing tragus alternatively or by Siegel speculum to alternatively increase pressure in ear canal and looking for signs of nystagmus or vertigo.

Fistula test is positive in:
- In cholesteatoma due to horizontal semicircular canal (SCC)/labyrinthine/promontory fistula
- Poststapedotomy
- Fenestration surgery
- Round window membrane rupture

False positive fistula test is seen (fistula is absent but test is positive).
- Congenital syphilis (Hennebert's sign) due to hypermobile or membranous stapes footplate.
- Meniere's disease due to stapes is connected to utricle by fibrous band.

False negative fistula test is seen (fistula is present but test is negative).
- Dead labyrinth
- Improper technique of fistula test

Cerebellar Sign

It is important to perform cerebellar test to rule out complication of cholesteatoma.

Test to be performed:
- Gait
- Romberg's test
- Dysdiadochokinesis
- Finger-nose test
- Finger-finger test

Examination of Nose and Paranasal Sinuses and Throat (*refer* chapter 20 and 30)

■ DIAGNOSIS

At the end of history and examination, student should able to give diagnosis in following headings:

My patient XYZ, age/sex is suffering from unilateral/bilateral, acute/chronic, mucosal/squamous, CSOM, active/inactive with intensity (mild/moderate/severe) and type (conductive/sensorineural/mixed) hearing loss, with/without any complication (intracranial /extracranial), with/without any etiological factors (DNS/tonsilloadenoiditis/trauma/allergy, etc.).

■ MANAGEMENT

Q. Discuss management of CSOM.

Investigation

Ear Microscopy
- To confirm findings of CSOM
- To remove wax, discharge, or debris and look for underlying structure if not seen during examination.

Swab for Culture And Sensitivity

Only in active discharging ear.

Pure Tone Audiometry
- To confirm the degree and type of hearing loss
- To compare preoperative audiogram with postoperative improvement
- For medicolegal purpose

Imaging

X-ray Mastoid Schuller's View

- ❖ To check of cellularity of mastoid air cells—sclerosed or pneumatic
- ❖ To check for low lying dura or forward lying sigmoid sinus to prevent complication during mastoid surgery
- ❖ Lucency in mastoid area can be cholesteatoma sac or postoperative mastoid cavity.

High-resolution Computed Tomography Temporal Bone

- ❖ It is the preferred imaging modality over X-ray mastoid Schuller's view.
- ❖ It gives precise bony details of temporal bone, thus helps in the deciding the approach for surgery.
- ❖ It is the must investigation in suspected complications of disease.

Preoperative Investigation for Anesthesia Fitness

Routine investigations like complete blood count (CBC), bleeding time (BT), clotting time (CT), fasting blood sugar test (FBS), postprandial blood sugar (PPBS), renal function test, serum electrolytes, chest X-ray posteroanterior (CXR–PA), electrocardiogram (ECG), etc.

Treatment

Medical Management

- ❖ **Oral antibiotics:** In patients with active mucopurulent or purulent ear discharge or nasal discharge.
- ❖ Aural toilet
- ❖ Antihistaminics
- ❖ **Ear drops:** Antibiotic ± steroid combination ear drops
- ❖ **Nasal drops or nasal spray:** In patients with ear discharge associated with sinusitis or allergic rhinitis.

Surgical Management

- ❖ Written informed consent is necessary. You should able to explain the procedure, alternative management if any and probable complications to patient in the language which he understands the best.
- ❖ Surgical correction of etiological factors (if any) is must before actual management of mucosal CSOM patient like septoplasty in DNS and tonsilloadenoidectomy in chronic tonsilloadenoiditis patient (But in squamous CSOM, mastoidectomy should be performed as early as possible to prevent the complications).
- ❖ Surgery of choice is tympanoplasty (repair of tympanic membrane with inspection of middle ear and possible ossicular chain reconstruction).
- ❖ Myringoplasty (repair of tympanic membrane without inspecting middle ear) can be performed with mild hearing loss.
- ❖ Incisions:
  - ➢ Postaural: WilliamWilde's incision
  - ➢ Endaural: Lempert's incision
  - ➢ Endomeatal: Rosen's incision
- ❖ Preferred graft material is temporalis fascia.
  - ➢ It is available in abundant in operative site through same incision.
  - ➢ It has same thickness as that of tympanic membrane.
  - ➢ It has low metabolic rate.
- ❖ **Other graft materials:** Cartilage, perichondrium, vein graft, tensor fascia lata, skin, etc.
- ❖ **Graft material for ossiculoplasty:** Autologous incus or malleus, cartilage, allografts, total ossicular replacement prosthesis (TORP), partial ossicular replacement prosthesis (PORP), gold or hydroxyapatite prosthesis.
- ❖ **Complications of tympanoplasty:**
  - ➢ Infections
  - ➢ Bleeding
  - ➢ Medialization or lateralization of graft
  - ➢ Residual perforation
  - ➢ Discharging ear
  - ➢ Granular myringitis

Chapter 6

Diseases of the External Ear

EN4.2: Elicit document and present a correct history, demonstrate and describe the clinical features, choose the correct investigations and describe the principles of management of diseases of the external ear.

■ DISEASES OF THE PINNA

Q. Enumerate different diseases of pinna and discuss congenital anomalies of it.

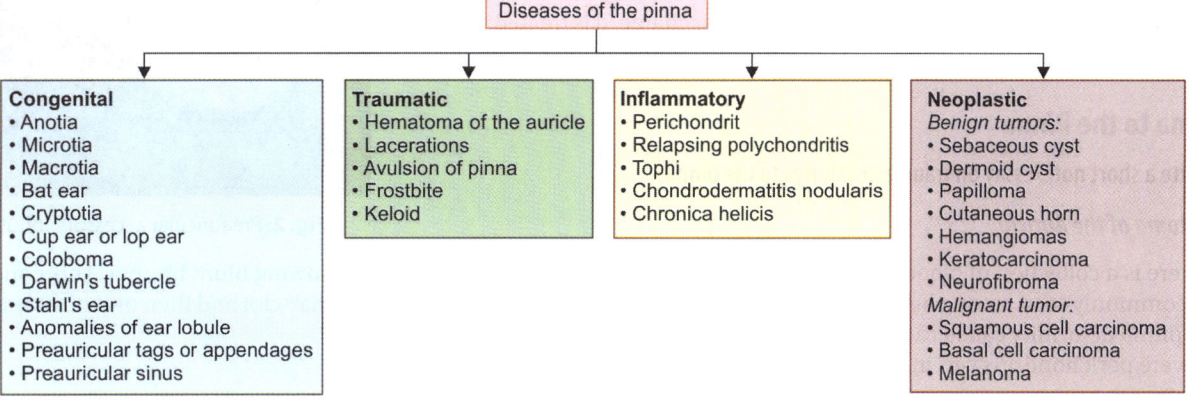

Congenital Disorders

Anotia

Forms part of the first arch syndrome. There is a complete absence of the pinna and lobule (**Fig. 1**).

Microtia

It is a small-sized pinna, and it is frequently associated with anomalies of the external auditory canal (EAC), middle ear, and internal ear. The degree of microtia varies and may be unilateral or bilateral. It is usually associated with hearing loss.

Macrotia

Excessively large pinna.

Bat Ear

Abnormal protrusion of the pinna outwards. It is characterized by large concha with poorly developed antihelix and scapha.

Cup Ear or Lop Ear

Upper portion of the helix or pinna is cupped due to hypoplasia of the upper third of the auricle.

Cryptotia

Upper third of the auricle is embedded under the scalp skin.

Coloboma

It is characterized by a transverse cleft in the pinna.

Darwin's Tubercle

A pointed tubercle present on the upper part of the helix.

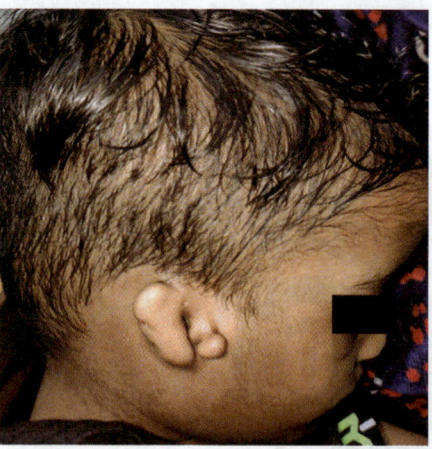

Fig. 1: Anotia and preauricular lobule.

Stahl's Ear

The helix which is normally folded is flat. The upper crust of the antihelix is duplicated and reaches the rim of the helix.

Anomalies of Ear Lobule (Figs. 1 and 2)

- The ear lobule may be absent, excessively large, bifid, or fixed lobule.
- They are skin-covered tags that appear on a line drawn from the tragus to the angle of the mouth.

Preauricular Sinus

- It is an epithelial tract formed due to incomplete fusion of the tubercles.
- It may be recurrently infected causing purulent discharge. It is treated with oral antibiotics and excision of the tract once the infection subsided.

Trauma to the Pinna

Q. Write a short note/essay on traumatic injuries to the pinna.

Hematoma of the Auricle

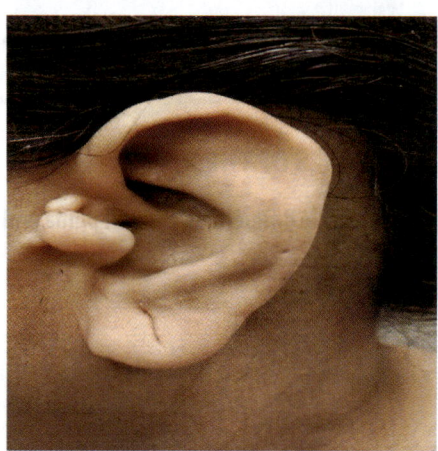

Fig. 2: Preauricular accessory lobule.

- There is a collection of blood between the perichondrium and cartilage, usually following blunt trauma. This condition is commonly seen among boxers, wrestlers, and rugby players. The collected blood may clot and then organize, resulting in pinna deformity called cauliflower ear.
- Severe perichondritis sets in if the hematoma gets infected.

Treatment

- Aspiration of hematoma under strict aseptic precautions with a pressure dressing.
- Incision and drainage are done if aspiration failed.
- Prophylactic antibiotics are given in all cases.

Lacerations

They should be repaired as soon as possible and broad-spectrum antibiotics should be given. Precautions should be taken to prevent stripping of perichondrium from cartilage as there is a risk of avascular necrosis.

Avulsion of Pinna

- Primary reattachment should be considered when pinna is attached to the head by a small pedicle of skin.
- Reimplantation is done in cases of complete avulsion.

Frostbite

It is characterized by initial erythema and edema, followed by bullae formation, necrosis of skin, and subcutaneous tissue, and finally complete necrosis with loss of the affected part.

Treatment

- ❖ Rapid tissue warming via circulating warm water or warmed moistened dressings.
- ❖ Aseptic dressing of the pinna using 1% silver sulfadiazine cream.
- ❖ Antibiotics are given to prevent and treat a secondary infection.
- ❖ The use of radiant heat is contraindicated as it may worsen the injury.

Keloid

They are benign hypertrophic, fibrous lesions that develop following trauma or surgery, usually located at the helix and lobule.

Treatment

- ❖ Intralesional triamcinolone injections.
- ❖ Surgical excision.
  Despite combined excision and intralesional corticosteroid therapy, recurrence is quite high (50%).

Inflammatory Disorders

Q. Write short note/essay on inflammatory disorders affecting pinna.

Perichondritis

- ❖ It is the infection and inflammation of the perichondrium and cartilage of the pinna.
- ❖ It results from infection secondary to lacerations, hematoma, or surgical procedures.
- ❖ The pinna appears red and swollen. There is severe pain and may be associated with headache, fever, and malaise. An abscess may be informed.
- ❖ Treatment consists of systemic antibiotics, aural toilets, and debridement. Incision and drainage are done if an abscess is present.
- ❖ Ciprofloxacin is the drug of choice.

Relapsing Polychondritis

- ❖ This is a rare autoimmune disorder involving cartilage of the ear. The entire auricle except the lobule becomes inflamed and tender; the external ear canal is stenosed.
- ❖ Treatment consists of a high dose of systemic steroids.

Tophi

This is characterized by urate crystal deposits in the helix, seen in gout. There is a salmon pink nodule on the helix. When compressed, tophi exude a whitish, chalky substance. Treatment consists of the correction of the underlying abnormality in uric acid metabolism.

Chondrodermatitis Nodularis Chronica Helicis

This is seen most commonly in males about the age of 50 years. It is characterized by small painful nodules on the free border of the helix. It is treated by excision of the nodules.

Neoplastic

Q. Discuss:
a. Benign tumors affecting pinna.
b. Malignant tumors affecting pinna.

Benign Tumors

Sebaceous Cyst

- ❖ Common site is the postauricular sulcus or below and behind the ear lobule.
- ❖ *Treatment*: Excision.

Dermoid Cyst

Usually presents as a rounded mass over the upper part of the mastoid behind the pinna.

Hemangiomas

Congenital tumors are often seen in childhood. It may be capillary, cavernous, or vascular malformations.

Papilloma

It is viral in origin and presents as a tufted growth or flat grey plague. Treatment consists of surgical excision or curettage with cauterization of base of the papillomatous swelling.

Cutaneous Horn

It is a form of papilloma, commonly seen at the rim of the helix in elderly people. It is treated by surgical excision.

Keratoacanthoma

It presents as a rapidly growing nodule with a central crater. Treatment is excision biopsy.

Neurofibroma

It presents as a nontender, firm swelling. It may be associated with von Recklinghausen disease. Treatment is surgical excision.

Malignant Tumors

Squamous Cell Carcinoma

- It presents as a nodule or an ulcer with everted edges and indurated base. It has a predilection for the helix and is more common among males who are in their 5th decade of life and is associated with exposure to sunlight.
- Metastasis to lymph nodes occurs at a late stage.
- Treatment consists of excision of the lesion with 1 cm of the healthy area around it. If the lesion comes within 1 cm of the external auditory canal or has metastasized to lymph nodes, total removal of the pinna along with en bloc removal of the parotid gland and cervical lymph nodes is required.

Basal Cell Carcinoma

- It presents as a nodule with a central crust, commonly at the helix and tragus. It is more common in men above 50 years of age.
- It tends to extend circumferentially into the skin. It may also involve the underlying cartilage or bone **(Fig. 3)**.

Treatment

- Superficial lesions without cartilage involvement can be irradiated.
- If the cartilage is involved, surgical excision is required.

Melanoma

It is more common in men and may occur anywhere over the auricle.

Treatment

Lesion >1 cm, situated over the helix—wedge resection and primary closure. Lesion <1 cm, infiltrative, situated in posterior auricular surface or concha, recurrent—resection of the pinna along with parotidectomy with radical neck dissection.

DISEASES OF THE EXTERNAL AUDITORY CANAL

Q. List different diseases affecting external auditory canal.

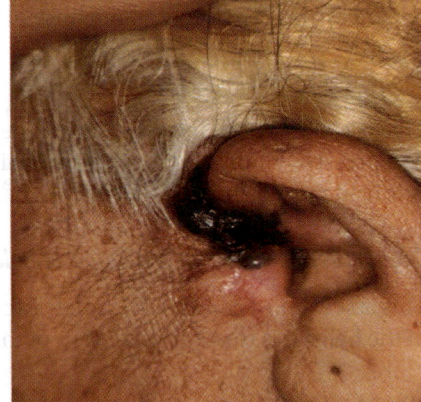

Fig. 3: Basal cell carcinoma of the ear.

Congenital	Inflammations	Neoplastic	Miscellaneous
❖ Atresia of the external canal ❖ Collaural fistula	❖ Furuncle ❖ Bacterial and fungal otitis externa ❖ Otitis externa hemorrhagica ❖ Herpes zoster oticus ❖ Aural polyps ❖ Malignant otitis externa/skull base osteomyelitis ❖ Primary cholesteatoma of the external auditory canal	*Benign tumors:* ❖ Osteoma ❖ Exostoses ❖ Ceruminoma ❖ Sebaceous adenoma *Malignant tumors:* ❖ Squamous cell carcinoma ❖ Basal cell and adenocarcinomas ❖ Malignant ceruminoma	❖ Impacted wax or cerumen ❖ Foreign bodies of the ear ❖ Keratosis obturans ❖ Acquired atresia and stenosis of the meatus

Congenital Disorder

Q. Write short note on congenital disorders of external auditory canal.

Atresia of the External Canal

This is due to failure of canalization of the ectodermal core of the first branchial cleft. The outer meatus is obliterated with fibrous tissue or bone while the inner meatus and the tympanic membrane are normal. Atresia of the meatus may occur alone or along with microtia. It may also be associated with abnormalities of the middle ear, and internal ear.

Collaural Fistula

This is also an abnormality of the first branchial cleft. The fistula has two openings—one situated in the neck just below and behind the angle of the mandible and the other in the external canal or the middle ear.

Infections and Inflammations of the Ear Canal

Furuncle

Q. Write a short note on Furuncle.

- It is a bacterial of the hair follicle by *Staphylococcus*. Hair follicles present up to the cartilaginous part of the meatus, hence furuncle is seen only in this part.
- Patients present with severe pain and tenderness. There is pain in moving the pinna and the jaw.
- On examination, there is edema over the mastoid with obliteration of the retroauricular groove. Periauricular lymph nodes may also be enlarged and tender.
- Treatment consists of oral antibiotics, analgesics, and an ear pack with 10% glycerine ichthammol. Glycerine ichthammol is hygroscopic in nature and helps to reduce edema; it is mildly antiseptic as well.
- Diabetes mellitus should be ruled out in a case of recurrent furunculosis. Also, the patient's vestibule may harbor staphylococci and the infection transferred by the patient's fingers.

Bacterial and Fungal Otitis Externa

Q. Write a short note/essay on Otitis externa.

- Acute diffuse otitis externa is a bacterial infection and inflammation of meatal skin and may spread to involve the pinna and epidermal layer of the tympanic membrane.
- It is commonly seen in a hot and humid climate and in swimmers (swimmer's ear).
- There is usually a history of trauma to the ear canal with Q tips or matchsticks, vigorous cleaning of the ear canal or following foreign body removal.
- There is itching, pain, and tenderness of the pinna with associated hearing loss.
- On examination, there is erythema and edema of the external canal skin and sometimes the concha and lobule.
- Otomycosis is an acute fungal infection of the ear canal. *Candida* and *Aspergillus* are the most common causative fungal species.
- There is intense pruritus with an earache.
- Examination reveals erythematous canal skin. The presence of fungal debris is critical for the diagnosis.

Treatment

- Thorough removal of all purulent or fungal elements to allow penetration of antimicrobial therapy.
- When edema is severe, a medicated wick is inserted in the ear canal which is replaced every 2–3 days.
- Ototopical preparations containing acidifying agents and antibiotics against *Pseudomonas aeruginosa* and *Staphylococcus aureus* are used.
- Oral antibiotics are used when the infection involves preauricular soft tissue.
- Otomycosis is treated with appropriate topical antifungal medications.
- Analgesics are used for the relief of pain.

Otitis Externa Hemorrhagica

- This is thought to be viral in origin. There is a hemorrhagic bulla on the tympanic membrane and the ear canal.
- There is severe earache and blood-stained discharge.
- Treatment consists of analgesics and antibiotics to prevent secondary infection.

Herpes Zoster Oticus

There are vesicles on the tympanic membrane, meatal skin concha, and postauricular groove.

Aural Polyps

Q. Write a short note on aural polyps.

- They are well-circumscribed, soft, and fleshy masses.
- They may arise from middle ear mucosa and protrude into the external meatus through a tympanic membrane perforation or tube.
- They are frequently seen in patients with otorrhea and hearing loss.
- It is frequently seen in pediatric patients as a result of a foreign body reaction to a pressure equalization tube.
- They may also be a manifestation of myringitis, malignant otitis externa, temporal bone malignancy or other neoplastic, or inflammatory lesions.

Treatment

- Gentle aural cleansing and antibiotic and steroid-containing ear drops.
- A thorough examination of the ear is done once the polyp is reduced in size.
- Cauterization with silver nitrate may be helpful in initial therapy.
- Aggressive debridement/avulsion should be avoided.
- Biopsy and histologic analysis should be done to rule out malignancy and to diagnose the underlying cause.

Malignant Otitis Externa/Skull Base Osteomyelitis

Q. Write short note on malignant otitis externa/skull base osteomyelitis.

- It is a bacterial infection, seen among diabetics or low immunity status.
- **Pseudomonas** is the causative organism.

Clinical Features

- Excruciating pain resembling diffuse otitis externa.
- Granulation in the ear canal.
- Facial asymmetry.
- Infection spreads to the skull base and invades the jugular foramen causing multiple cranial nerve palsies.
- Computed tomography (CT) scan may show bony erosion.
- Gallium 67 is the investigation of choice and is useful for follow-up.
- Technetium 99 bone scan can be used to detect infection. But it cannot be used to monitor the disease.

Treatment

- Strict control of diabetes.
- Aural toilet to remove discharge, granulations, and debris.
- Antibiotic treatment:
    - It requires prolonged antibiotic treatment for at least 6–8 weeks
    - Intravenous third generation cephalosporins combined with aminoglycosides.
    - Quinolones can be given orally.

Primary Cholesteatoma of the External Auditory Canal

- It is characterized by invasion of the bony canal by squamous epithelium.
- It is usually posttraumatic or postsurgery.
- Clinical features include purulent ear discharge with the intact tympanic membrane.

CHAPTER 6: Diseases of the External Ear

Neoplastic

Benign Tumors

Q. Discuss various benign tumors affecting external auditory canal.

Osteoma

- Originate from cancellous bone, most commonly arising from the posterior wall of the bony canal.
- It is a single, smooth, bony, hard, and pedunculated tumor.

Treatment

Surgical removal.

Exostoses

- They are often seen in those exposed to cold water in the meatus such as swimmers and divers.
- They are multiple, bilateral, smooth sessile, and bony swellings that arise from the deeper part of the ear canal, in close proximity to the tympanic membrane.
- Sometimes they may extend deeply and lie in close relation to the facial nerve.
- Males are affected three times more than females.

Treatment

- For asymptomatic and small tumors, no active treatment is required.
- Tumors causing decreased hearing, retention of wax, and debris are removed using high-speed drill.

Ceruminoma

- It is a tumor of modified sweat glands that secrete cerumen. It presents as a smooth, firm, skin-covered polypoid swelling in the outer part of the meatus.
- It leads to retention of wax and debris due to obstruction of the meatus.

Treatment

Wide local excision with regular follow-up as it has the tendency to recur.

Sebaceous Adenoma

- It arises from the sebaceous glands of the meatus and presents as a smooth, skin-covered swelling in the outer meatus.
- It is treated surgically.

Malignant Tumors

Q. Write a short note on malignant tumors affecting external auditory canal.

Squamous Cell Carcinoma

- It may arise from the meatus itself or maybe as an extension of the middle ear carcinoma.
- It is most often seen in cases of long-standing ear discharges.
- It is characterized by blood-stained ear discharge associated with a severe earache.

Clinical Features

- It may present as ulceration or a bleeding polypoidal mass or granulations.
- Facial asymmetry is seen in cases of local extension through the posterior meatal wall or due to the middle ear extension.

Treatment

En bloc-wide surgical excision with postoperative radiation.

Basal Cell and Adenocarcinomas

They are rare conditions and present with similar features to that of squamous cell tumors.

Treatment

It includes wide surgical excision and postoperative radiation.

Malignant Ceruminoma

- This is more common than benign type.
- Clinical features are similar to that of benign type.

Treatment

It includes surgical excision and postoperative radiotherapy.

Miscellaneous Conditions

Impacted Wax or Cerumen

Q. Write a short note on Cerumen/impacted wax.

- Wax has a protective function of lubricating the ear canal. It is acidic, bacteriostatic, and fungistatic. It entraps any foreign materials that enter the ear canal.
- Wax secreted is small in quantity and is expelled from the ear canal by the movement of the jaw.
- Impacted wax may be due to excessive secretion or other factors such as narrow and tortuous ear canal, stiff hair, or obstructive lesion of the canal like exostosis.

Clinical Features

- Patients often complain of aural fullness and decreased hearing. It may present as an earache.
- Tinnitus and giddiness may present due to impaction against the tympanic membrane.

Treatment

- Removal by syringing or instrumentation.
- Hard wax may require prior softening with wax solvents.

Foreign Bodies of the Ear

Q. Write a short note on living and nonliving foreign bodies in ear and its management.

Nonliving Foreign Bodies

- Common among children
- Common foreign bodies—a piece of paper or sponge, grains of seeds, slate pencil, and piece of chalk or metallic ball bearings.
- Adults may present with a broken end of a matchstick used for scratching the ear or a cotton swab.
- Vegetable foreign bodies swell up and get impacted in the ear canal.

Treatment

- *Forceps removal*: For soft and irregular foreign bodies such as a piece of paper, swab, and sponge.
- *Syringing*: It should not be done for vegetables as it will cause swelling of the foreign body and get impacted.
- Suction using ear suction tips.
- Impacted foreign bodies are removed using a microscope under general anesthesia.

Living Foreign Bodies

- Crawling or flying insects such as mosquitoes, beetles, cockroaches, and an ant may enter, and they are the common foreign bodies.
- Cause intense irritation and pain.

Treatment

The insect should be killed by instilling oil, spirit, or chloroform. Then the insect can be removed by forceps, syringing, or suction.

Keratosis Obturans

Q. Write a short note on keratosis obturans.

There is a collection of pearly white mas of desquamated epithelial cells in the deep meatus due to failure of migration of epithelium onto the posterior meatal wall. It may cause a pressure effect leading to absorption of bone leading to widening of the meatus and facial nerve may be exposed and paralyzed.
- It is commonly seen between 5 and 20 years and presents as earache, hearing loss, tinnitus, and ear discharge.
- On examination, the ear canal is filled with a pearly white mass of keratin material. It may be associated with ulceration and granuloma formation.
- Treatment includes removal of keratotic mass by syringing or instrumentation. Patient should follow-up periodically for recurrence.

Acquired Atresia and Stenosis of Meatus

It can result from the following:
- Infections like chronic otitis externa.
- Trauma such as lacerations, fracture of the tympanic plate, and surgeries.
- Burns

Treatment

Meatoplasty

DISEASES OF TYMPANIC MEMBRANE

Q. Write a short note on diseases of tympanic membrane.
- **Retracted tympanic membrane:** it is due to negative intratympanic pressure due to Eustachian tube dysfunction.
  On examination: Tympanic membrane appears dull with a distorted or absent cone of light. The handle of malleus becomes prominent, and anterior and posterior malleal folds become sickle-shaped.
- **Myringitis bullosa:** It is characterized by formation of hemorrhagic blebs on the tympanic membrane and deep meatus. It is thought to be a viral cause.
- **Herpes zoster oticus:** It is a viral infection by herpes zoster involving geniculate ganglion of facial nerve, characterized by the formation of vesicles on the tympanic membrane, concha, and retroauricular sulcus. The 7th and 8th cranial nerves may be involved.
- **Myringitis granulosa**: There is a formation of nonspecific granulations on the outer surface of the tympanic membrane. It may be associated with impacted wax, long-standing foreign body or external ear infection.
- **Traumatic rupture**: It may be due to the following:
  - Trauma due to a hairpin, matchstick, or unskilled attempts to remove a foreign body.
  - Sudden change in air pressure, e.g., a slap on the ear or a sudden blast.
  - Pressure by a fluid column such as diving, water sports, and forceful syringing.
  - Fracture of the temporal bone.

  Treatment
  - In maximum cases, there is a spontaneous healing of the tympanic membrane.
  - Exploration may be required if there is associated facial paralysis, vertigo, nystagmus, or sensorineural hearing loss.
- **Atrophic tympanic membrane:** Serous otitis media causes absorption of the middle fibrous layer of the tympanic membrane. It is also seen when perforation heals by epithelial and mucosal layers without intervening fibrous layer.
- **Retraction pockets and atelectasis**: When the tympanic membrane is thin and atrophic, a segment of it or the entire membrane may collapse inwards due to eustachian tube insufficiency. It may form a retraction pocket or get plastered onto the promontory or may be wrapped around the ossicles. Keratin debris may accumulate in the retraction pocket and form a cholesteatoma.
- **Tympanosclerosis**:
  - It is characterized by hyalinization and calcification in the fibrous layer of tympanic membrane. It appears as chalky white plaque.
  - It is frequently seen in cases of serous otitis media. It commonly affects tympanic membrane. Joints of ossicles, muscle tendons, and submucosal layer of middle ear cleft may also be involved.

Chapter 7

Diseases of Middle Ear

EN4.3: Elicit document and present a correct history, demonstrate, and describe the clinical features, choose the correct investigations and describe the principles of management of acute suppurative otitis media (ASOM).

ACUTE SUPPURATIVE OTITIS MEDIA

Q. Write a short note/essay on acute suppurative otitis media.

It is an acute infection of the mucosa of the middle ear cleft by pyogenic organisms.

Causative Organisms

- *Streptococcus pneumoniae*
- *Haemophilus influenzae*
- *Staphylococcus aureus*
- *Pneumococcus*
- *Moraxella catarrhalis*
- *Pseudomonas aeruginosa*

Etiology

- **Age:** More common in infants and children as the Eustachian tube is shorter, wider, and more horizontal.
- Commonly bilateral
- **Sex:** No gender predilection
- Recurrent attacks of upper respiratory tract infections and exanthematous fevers such as measles, diphtheria, or whooping cough.
- Infections of tonsils and adenoids
- Obstruction of the Eustachian tube by nasopharyngeal tumors
- Swimming
- Cleft palate
- **Iatrogenic:** Scarring of the Eustachian tube orifice during surgical procedures like adenoidectomy can damage the Eustachian tube.

Stages

Stage of Tubal Occlusion

There is edema and inflammation of the Eustachian tube causing a tubal obstruction which causes absorption of air in the middle ear cleft and negative intratympanic pressure. There is irritation of the middle ear mucosa and the tympanic membrane is retracted due to the negative pressure.

Patient complains of aural fullness and pain in the ear (otalgia).

On examination, the tympanic membrane is congested "cartwheel appearance." There is a loss of cone of light, the drum looks dull and is retracted.

Stage of Exudation

If occlusion persists, there is an exudation from capillaries in the middle ear due to congestion **(Fig. 1)**. There is a collection of seromucinous exudate in the middle ear causing the tympanic membrane to bulge.

There is a marked throbbing type of earache with deafness and tinnitus. There is a high-grade fever and malaise.

The tympanic membrane is congested and bulged. A pressure point may be seen as a yellow nipple at one spot on the drum.

Stage of Suppuration

The middle ear cavity is invaded by pyogenic organisms causing pus formation. Tension in the middle ear increases and ultimately leads to tympanic membrane perforation.

There is a mucopurulent otorrhea. Pain and fever reduce while deafness and tinnitus persist.

Tympanic membrane shows perforation usually in the anteroinferior quadrant with a pulsatile discharge "lighthouse sign".

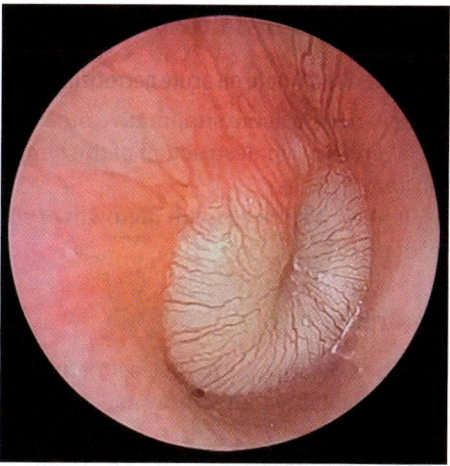

Fig. 1: Bulging and congested tympanic membrane in exudation stage.

Stage of Resolution

The infection resolves with the release of pus and subsidence of symptoms. It depends on the immunity of the host, virulence of organisms, and efficacy of antibiotics.

This stage can begin after any stage. Earache, fever, and malaise are relieved. If it occurs after suppuration, there may be a small perforation in the anteroinferior quadrant of the drum or may heal completely with a small scar formation or tympanosclerosis.

Stage of Complications

If the infection remained untreated or virulence of the organism is high or the immunity of the patient is low, the disease spreads beyond the middle ear cleft. It may lead to acute mastoiditis, subperiosteal postaural abscess, zygomatic abscess, Luc's abscess, Citelli's abscess, Bezold's abscess, facial paralysis, labyrinthitis, petrositis, extradural abscess, meningitis, brain abscess, or lateral sinus thrombophlebitis.

Investigations

- Tuning fork tests (Rinne's and Weber's tests) show a conductive hearing loss.
- **Tympanometry/impedance audiometry:** "C" type of curve in tubal occlusion/Eustachian catarrh stage
- Pus for culture and antibiotic sensitivity is done.
- **X-ray mastoid Schuller's view and high resolution computed tomography (HRCT) temporal bone:** Usually is normal. In cases of coalescent mastoiditis, there is a ground-glass appearance.
- **Pure tone audiogram:** It is not possible to perfume in the initial stage of the disease due to severe pain.
- It reveals conductive hearing loss. In cases of labyrinthitis due to complications, there is sensorineural hearing loss.

Treatment

Conservative Management

It consists of:
- **Systemic antibiotics:** Broad-spectrum antibiotics, mostly ampicillin and amoxicillin are given. Those allergic to penicillin may be given cefaclor, cotrimoxazole, or erythromycin.
- Anti-inflammatory analgesics to decrease inflammation and pain.
- Nasal decongestants to decrease Eustachian tube edema and promote ventilation of the middle ear.
- Antihistaminics
- Local antibiotics ear drops if there is perforation of the tympanic membrane.

Surgical Management

Myringotomy: An incision is made on the tympanic membrane to evacuate pus and to improve the middle ear cleft.

ACUTE NECROTIZING OTITIS MEDIA

Q. Write a short note on acute necrotizing otitis media.

It is a variety of acute suppurative otitis media, caused by β-hemolytic **Streptococcus**.

There is rapid destruction of the tympanic membrane with its annulus, mucosa of the promontory, ossicular chain, and mastoid air cells.

It heals by fibrosis with ingrowth of squamous epithelium into the middle ear cleft leading to secondary cholesteatoma formation.

Treatment

Antibacterial therapy for at least 7–10 days.

Cortical mastoidectomy may be indicated if medical treatment fails or there is acute mastoiditis.

> **EN4.4**: Elicit document and present a correct history, demonstrate, and describe the clinical features, choose the correct investigations and describe the principles of management of otitis media with effusion.

OTITIS MEDIA WITH EFFUSION

Q. Write a short note on otitis media with effusion.

Also known as:
Serous otitis media, Secretory otitis media, Mucoid otitis media, Glue ear, Catarrhal otitis media.

It is characterized by nonpurulent effusion in the middle ear. The effusion is often thick and viscid but may be thin and serous.

Etiology

- **Age:** It is commonly seen in children, especially those below the age of 10 years.
- **Climate:** It is common in winter.
- **Eustachian tube obstruction:** Adenoid hypertrophy, nasopharyngeal tumors, scarring due to surgical procedure, chemoradiation.
- **Eustachian tube dysfunction:** Chronic rhinitis and sinusitis, patulous Eustachian tube.
- **Allergy:** It causes Eustachian tube obstruction along with the increased secretory activity of middle ear mucosa.
- **Viral infections:** Viral organisms of the upper respiratory tract may invade middle ear mucosa and stimulate it to increase secretory activity.
- **Barotrauma:** Sudden change in atmospheric pressure leads to negative intratympanic pressure and leads to serous effusion in the middle ear.
- Cleft palate, palatal paralysis.
- Impaired mucociliary clearance such as Young's syndrome and Kartagener's syndrome.
- Inadequate treatment of acute suppurative otitis media.

Clinical Features

Symptoms

- **Decreased hearing:** This is the most common presenting symptom. It is insidious in onset and usually bilateral.
- **Tinnitus:** It may present as a bubbling or whistling type.
- **Delayed and defective speech:** Due to hearing loss, there may be delayed or defective speech development.

Clinical Examination (Signs) and Investigations

- **Tympanic membrane:** Intact, dull, and maybe bulging **(Fig. 2)**. A cone of light is absent and sometimes fluid level or air bubbles may be seen behind an intact eardrum.
- Tuning fork test reveals conductive hearing loss.

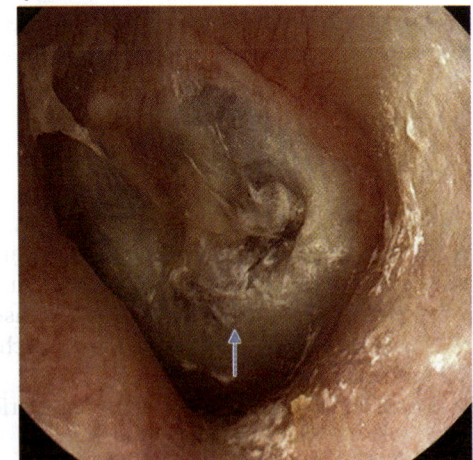

Fig. 2: Bulging and dull tympanic (arrow) membrane.

- Pure tone audiometry reveals a conductive hearing loss of 20–40 dB. Sometimes a sensorineural component of hearing loss may be present.
- **Impedance audiometry**: It shows a flat "type B" curve.
- **X-ray mastoid Schuller's view:** Clouding of air cells due to fluid.

Treatment

Medical

- Nasal decongestants to decrease Eustachian tube edema.
- Antihistaminics to decrease allergic rhinitis.
- Antibiotics are helpful in cases of upper respiratory tract infections or unresolved acute suppurative otitis media.
- Valsalva maneuver, politzerization, or Eustachian tube catheterization to improve middle ear ventilation.

Surgical

- **Myringotomy and aspiration of fluid:** An incision is made in the tympanic membrane to drain the effusion. Radial incision is made in the anterosuperior quadrant of pars tensa.
- **Grommet insertion:** A grommet can be inserted through a myringotomy incision to provide prolonged aeration of the middle ear.
- **Tympanotomy or cortical mastoidectomy:** It is indicated in cases of recurrence or the presence of sequelae.
- **Surgical management of causative factor:** In children, adenoid hypertrophy is the most common cause of secretory otitis media (SOM), so **adenoidectomy is useful in most cases.**

Prophylaxis

- All children who seem inattentive should be investigated for middle ear effusion.
- Prompt treatment of rhinitis and upper respiratory infection.
- Proper treatment of acute suppurative otitis media.

Sequelae of Chronic Secretory Otitis Media

Q. What is the sequelae of chronic secretory otitis media?

- **Atelectasis**: It is characterized by medial retraction of the pars tensa **(Fig. 3)**. Due to prolonged effusions, the tympanic membrane becomes thin, atrophic, and retracts into the middle ear.
- **Tympanosclerosis:** It is characterized by chalky calcareous plaques in the subepithelial layer of the tympanic membrane **(Fig. 4).** There is hyaline degeneration of the fibrous layer with calcifications in the tympanic membrane or around the ossicular chain.
- **Ossicular necrosis**: A long process of incus is most commonly necrosed. If ossicular necrosis is present, the conductive hearing loss is >45 dB.

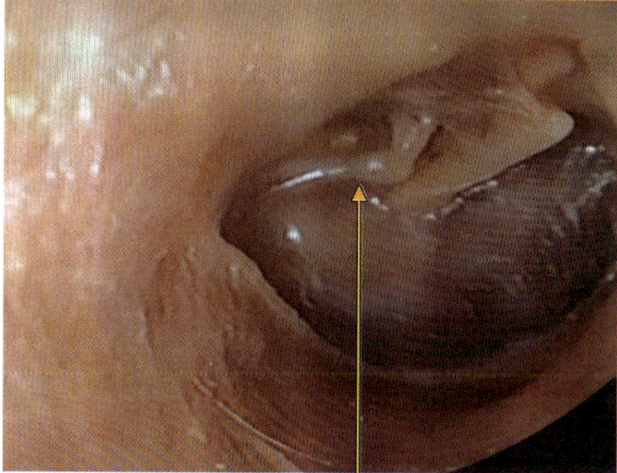

Fig. 3: Atelectasis (adhesive otitis media).
Draping of tympanic membrane over incudostapedial joint and prominent anterior and posterior malleolar folds

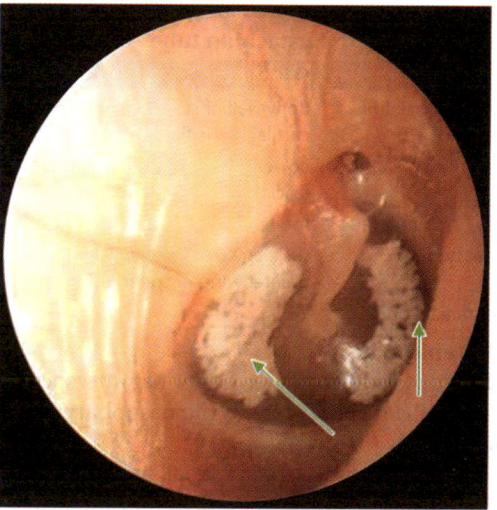

Fig. 4: Tympanic membrane with tympanosclerosis (arrows).

Chapter 8

Eustachian Tube and its Disorders

EN4.15: Describe the anatomy of eustachian tube and discuss the clinical features, investigations, and management of Eustachian tube disorders.

■ ANATOMY OF EUSTACHIAN TUBE

Q. Describe the anatomy of the Eustachian tube.

- A narrow osteocartilaginous channel connecting the tympanic cavity to the nasopharynx.
- Also called the pharyngotympanic tube or the auditory tube
- Develops from the endoderm of first pharyngeal pouch from the proximal portion of the tubotympanic recess
- Directed anteriorly, inferiorly, and medially from anterior wall of the middle ear. Forms 45° angle with the horizontal
- Enters nasopharynx 1.25 cm behind posterior end of the inferior turbinate.
- Adult length—36 mm. Two parts:
  a. Posterior third—bony—12 mm (one-third)
  b. Anterior two-third—cartilaginous—24 mm (two-third)
  Note: Junction between two parts: Narrowest part of Eustachian tube—called isthmus
- Tympanic end-bony lies just above the floor of the middle ear:
  - Just below the opening of the canal for tensor tympani
- Pharyngeal end—opens 1.25 cm behind posterior end of inferior turbinate:
  - Forms tubal elevation/torus tubarius
  - Lymphoid tissue around torus—Gerlach's tubal tonsil
  - Posterosuperior to torus tubarius—fossa of Rosenmuller
- **Muscles related to Eustachian tube**

Muscles	Attachment	Action	Nerve supply
Tensor veli palatini	Bony wall of scaphoid and whole length of short cartilaginous flange	Opens the tubal lumen actively	Mandibular branch of trigeminal
Levator veli palatini	Lower surface of petrous bone and cartilage and fascia of upper carotid sheath	Assists in opening the tube passively	Pharyngeal plexus (cranial part of CN XI through vagus)
Salpingopharyngeus	Inferior part of cartilage near its pharyngeal end		Pharyngeal plexus
Tensor tympani	Cartilage of ET, surrounding bony canal, and greater wing of sphenoid		

(CN: cranial nerve)

- **Lining epithelium**
  - Pseudostratified ciliated columnar interspersed with mucus-secreting goblet cells
  - With cilia beating towards the nasopharynx.
- **Blood supply**
  - *Arterial:* Ascending pharyngeal, middle meningeal arteries
  - *Venous:* Pharyngeal and pterygoid venous plexus
- **Lymphatic drainage:** Retropharyngeal node
- **Nerve supply:** Tubal mucosa—the tympanic branch of cranial nerve IX

PHYSIOLOGY OF EUSTACHIAN TUBE

Q. Describe the physiology of the Eustachian tube.
- Bony part—always open, cartilaginous part—closed at rest
- Opens on:
  - Swallowing
  - Sneezing
  - Yawning
  - Forceful inflation
- Opens—actively by contraction of tensor veli palatini
- Passively by contraction of levator veli palatini
- Closes—elastic recoil of elastin hinge + deforming force of Ostmann's fat pad

Q. What is Ostmann's pad of fat?

Fatty mass over lateral end of the cartilaginous Eustachian tube which helps to close the tube—protections from reflux of nasopharyngeal secretions.

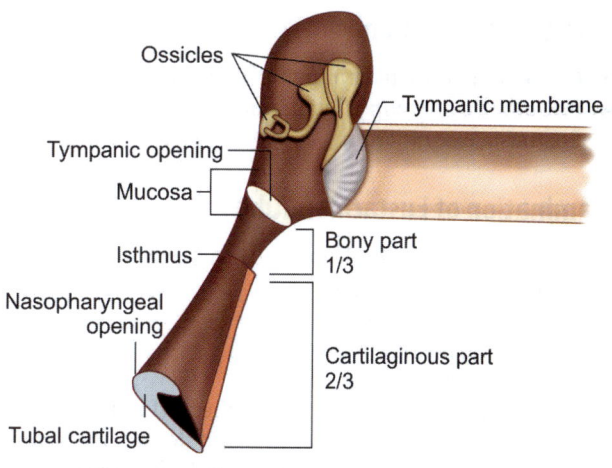

Fig. 1: Eustachian tube in relation to middle ear.

Q. What are the functions of Eustachian tube?

Three main functions are as follows:
- Ventilation of middle ear:
  - Equalization of middle ear pressure with the ambient pressure thus maintaining same pressure on either side of the tympanic membrane—essential for optimum hearing
- Protection of middle ear:
  - From sound pressure transmission via nasopharynx—thus preventing interference with normal hearing From reflux of nasopharyngeal secretions into the middle ear
- Clearance of middle ear secretions:
  - Cilia in the Eustachian tube direct the secretions toward nasopharynx

Q. What is the difference between infant and adult Eustachian tubes?

	Infant	Adult
Length	13–18 mm	36 mm
Angle with horizontal	10° (more horizontal) Normalizes at 7 years of age	45°
Angulation at isthmus	None	Angulated
Cartilaginous portion	Flaccid	Rigid (protection from reflux)
Elastic recoil	Not efficient, as less elastin density	Present, as dense elastin
Ostmann's fat	Less volume	More in volume

CLINICAL EVALUATION

Q. Describe the evaluation to assess Eustachian tube function.

History

Symptoms of Eustachian tube dysfunction:
- Fullness of ears
- Pain and discomfort
- Hearing loss
- Tinnitus
- Dizziness

Symptoms of nasopharyngeal or nasal pathology:
- Nasal obstruction
- Mouth breathing
- Nasal twang to speech
- Nasal discharge

Physical Examination

- **Otoscopy:** Retracted tympanic membrane (TM)/middle ear effusion
- **Pneumatic otoscopy:** Tympanic membrane mobility
- Postnasal examination

Examination of Eustachian Tube

- Pharyngeal end (to rule out extrinsic obstruction):
  - Posterior rhinoscopy
  - Rigid nasal endoscopy
  - Flexible nasopharyngoscope
- Tympanic end:
  - Microscope/endoscope—via the perforated tympanic membrane
  - Eustachian tube endoscopy/middle ear endoscopy by fine flexible endoscopy

Note: Various causes of Eustachian tube dysfunction—assessed by—nasal endoscopy/allergy tests/CT scan of temporal bone/magnetic resonance imagining (MRI) for patulous Eustachian tube in multiple sclerosis.

■ EUSTACHIAN TUBE FUNCTION TESTS

Q. Enumerate the tests used for Eustachian tube function.

- Valsalva test
- Politzer test
- Catheterization
- Toynbee's test
- Tympanometry
- Radiological test
- Saccharin or methylene blue test
- Sonotubometry

Valsalva Test

Q. Describe the Valsalva test—procedure, inference, and contraindications.

- Principle—increase air pressure in nasopharynx to let air enter the Eustachian tube
- Procedure—patient is asked to take a deep breath, pinch his nose to close it completely, and close the mouth, followed by an attempt to blow air into the ears

Note: Successfully performed only in 65% of persons

- Inference on otoscopy:
  - Reveals outward movement of tympanic membrane during the increase in pressure
  - Hissing sound—in perforated tympanic membrane
  - Crackling sound—in ear discharge
- Contraindications:
  - Atrophic scar on the tympanic membrane—to avoid rupture
  - Infections of nose and nasopharynx—to avoid spread to middle ear

Note:
Politzer test works on same principle as Valsalva. It is done in patients who are not able to perform Valsalva. Air is introduced via olive tip of a Politzer bag into the nostril on the side to be tested and patient is asked to swallow simultaneously. A hissing sound from patients ear heard by introducing auscultation tube, confirms patency of Eustachian tube.

Catheterization test: A Eustachian tube catheter is inserted in the nose so that it lies against the Eustachian tubal opening, to insufflate the air which confirms patency using auscultation tube. Has disadvantage of risk of injury to the tubal opening or pressure trauma to tympanic membrane, and risk of introduction of infection through the tube.

Toynbee's Test

- It is reverse of Valsalva test.
- Patient is asked to close his nose and mouth, and swallow—causes middle ear air to escape into nasopharynx—causing retraction of the tympanic membrane confirmed otoscopically.

Tympanometry for Eustachian Tube Testing

- It can be done in both perforated and intact tympanic membrane patients

CHAPTER 8: Eustachian Tube and its Disorders

- ❖ A probe is fit in the external auditory canal (EAC) that creates positive and negative pressures, with patient asked to swallow repeatedly.
- ❖ Ability to equalize middle ear pressure with ambient pressure indicates normal function

Saccharin/Methylene Blue Tests for Eustachian Tube

- ❖ Saccharin/methylene blue is inserted in middle ear through pre-existing perforation and time taken by it to reach the pharynx is noted, which indicates drainage/clearance tubal function
- ❖ Saccharin gives sweet taste while methylene blue can be visualized as stained pharyngeal secretions
- ❖ This principle can be elicited while taking history—ear drops instilled in ear with perforated tympanic membrane causing bitter taste indicates drainage function of tube

Sonotubometry

- ❖ It is a newer noninvasive technique.
- ❖ A tone is delivered into the nose and recorded through the ear.
- ❖ It is heard louder in case of patulous tube. Also measures the time for which tube is open.

■ EUSTACHIAN TUBE DISORDERS

Q. Describe the disorders of Eustachian tube.

- ❖ Tubal blockage:
  - ➢ Functional obstruction—mucosal inflammation due to laryngopharyngeal reflux, allergies—edema—obstruction
  - ➢ Dynamic obstruction—muscular abnormality. Infants, cleft palate, Down's syndrome
  - ➢ Anatomical obstruction—adenoids, unilateral dysfunction—nasopharyngeal or infratemporal fossa tumors should be ruled out
- ❖ Barotrauma–scuba diving, flying in an airplane (avoid by using decongestants, Valsalva maneuver or pressure equalizing ear plugs)
- ❖ Patulous Eustachian tube

Q. What are effects of acute and prolonged tubal blockage?

Tubal blockage → absorption of middle ear gases → negative middle ear pressure → tympanic membrane retraction → transudate in middle ear → otitis media with effusion (OME) → prolonged blockade atelectasis/TM perforation/retraction pocket

Q. Elaborate the relation between blocked Eustachian tube and the retraction pockets.

- ❖ Pathway of ventilation of middle ear cleft = Eustachian tube > mesotympanum > attic > aditus > antrum > mastoid air cell system.
- ❖ Blockage in this pathway—retraction/atelectasis > thin atrophic tympanic membrane > cholesteatoma > ossicular necrosis/tympanosclerosis
- ❖ **Treatment:**
  - ➢ Correction of pathologic process
  - ➢ Ensure ventilation

Obstruction level	Sequelae
Eustachian tube	Atelectatic tympanic membrane
Middle ear	Posterior retraction pocket
Isthmi	Attic retraction pocket
Aditus	Cholesterol granuloma/mucoid collection in mastoid

Eustachian Tube Obstruction

Q. Enumerate the causes of Eustachian tube obstruction.

- ❖ Allergy causing nasal congestion
- ❖ Sinus infections
- ❖ Cold (upper respiratory tract infection—viral/bacterial)
- ❖ Narrow Eustachian tube
- ❖ Deviated nasal septum
- ❖ Polyps
- ❖ Tumors (in adults)
- ❖ Adenoids (in children)
- ❖ Activities with large, rapid altitude changes—flying in an airplane/scuba divings
- ❖ Cleft palate
- ❖ Down's syndrome

Patulous Eustachian Tube vs Eustachian Tube Blockage

Q. How will you differentiate patulous Eustachian tube from Eustachian tube blockage?

	Patulous Eustachian tube	*Eustachian tube blockage*
Definition	Abnormal patency	Obstruction of tube
Causes	❖ Idiopathic ❖ Rapid weight loss ❖ Pregnancy ❖ Multiple sclerosis	❖ Infection ❖ Allergy ❖ Nasopharyngeal mass ❖ Sudden change in altitude
Symptoms	Autophony (hearing his own voice/even breath sounds)	❖ Aural fullness/block sensation ❖ Earache—mild to severe ❖ Hearing loss ❖ Ringing sensation ❖ Dizziness ❖ Symptoms cannot be relieved by swallowing/yawning/chewing
Signs (on otoscopy)	Tympanic membrane moves with inspiration and expiration	❖ Retracted tympanic membrane ❖ Congestion along handle of malleus and pars tensa ❖ Transudate behind intact tympanic membrane ❖ In barotrauma—marked as tympanic retraction with hemorrhage in subepithelial layer or sometimes perforation
Medical treatment	❖ Acute episode—self-limiting (no treatment required) ❖ Weight gain ❖ Oral potassium iodide	❖ Intranasal steroids sprays ❖ Oral steroids ❖ Decongestants ❖ Nasal/oral antihistaminics ❖ Leukotriene antagonists ❖ Proton pump inhibitors in laryngopharyngeal reflux
Surgical treatment	In long standing cases—cauterization (laser vaporization) of tubes or insertion of a grommet	❖ Adenoidectomy ❖ Treatment of tumors ❖ Myringotomy ❖ Pressure equalization tubes ❖ Balloon dilation of Eustachian tube ❖ Eustachian tuboplasty—using laser/microdebrider

Note: Surgery in nasopharynx has risks of bleeding, scarring.

Chapter 9

Chronic Suppurative Otitis Media

EN4.5: Elicit document and present a correct history, demonstrate and describe the clinical features, choose the correct investigations and describe the principles of management of discharging ear.
EN4.6: Elicit document and present a correct history, demonstrate and describe the clinical features, choose the correct investigations and describe the principles of management of mucosal type of CSOM.

■ DEFINITION

Q. What are types of CSOM? Enumerate differences between tubotympanic and atticoantral type of CSOM.

Chronic suppurative otitis media (CSOM) is a chronic infection of middle ear mucosa lining the middle ear cleft.

Duration of infection should be >3 months characterized by ear discharge and a permanent perforation (edges of perforation are covered by squamous epithelium).

■ EPIDEMIOLOGY

Higher incidence seen in developing countries due to poor economic status, poor nutrition, lack of health education.

■ TYPES

a. Tubotympanic CSOM.
b. Atticoantral CSOM.

	Tubotympanic CSOM	Atticoantral CSOM
Type	Safe/benign type	Unsafe/dangerous type
Site of involvement	Anteroinferior part of middle ear cleft (i.e., mesotympanum, Eustachian tube associated with central perforation)	Posterosuperior part of the middle ear cleft (i.e., attic, antrum, mastoid associated with attic, marginal, or total perforation)
Discharge	Profuse, mucoid, nonblood stain, nonfoul-smelling	Scanty, purulent, blood-stained, foul-smelling
Granulations	Uncommon	Common
Bone erosion	Uncommon	Common
Polyp	Pale	Red fleshy
Cholesteatoma	Absent	Present
Complication	Rare	Common
Hearing loss	Conductive hearing loss (CHL)	Conductive or mixed hearing loss

Tubotympanic CSOM

Q. Write a short note/essay on tubotympanic CSOM.

Etiology of CSOM

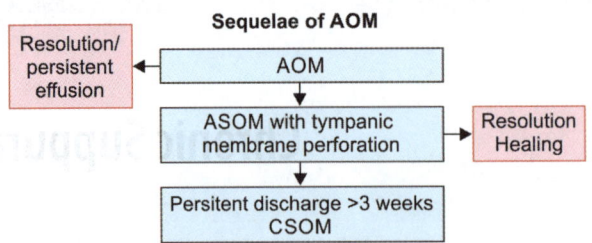

(AOM: acute otitis media; CSOM: chronic suppurative otitis media)

Causes of Persistent Perforation (Fails to Heal Spontaneously)

1. Large central perforation	❖ ASOM in exanthematous fever (measles, chicken pox) results in acute necrotizing otitis media ❖ Large perforation following trauma
2. Inadequately treated ASOM	❖ Persistent foci on infection at tonsil, adenoid, sinus ❖ Resulted in recurrent ascending infection via the Eustachian tube
3. Persistent mucoid discharge	❖ Allergic rhinitis ❖ Foreign body in middle ear ❖ GERD

(ASOM: acute suppurative otitis media; GERD: gastroesophageal reflux disease)

Bacteriology

- Culture shows both aerobic and anaerobic organisms
- Common aerobic organisms are:
  - *Pseudomonas aeruginosa*
  - *Escherichia colli*
  - *Proteus*
  - *Staphylococcus aureus*
  - *Klebsiella*
- Common anaerobic organisms are:
  - *Bacteroides fragilis*
  - Anaerobic streptococci
  - *Propionibacterium*

Pathological Changes in CSOM

Q. Describe pathological changes of CSOM.

Eardrum
Central perforation (varies in size and location).

Middle Ear Mucosa
- Inactive stage (quiescent) normal mucosa seen
- Active stage (inflammation) velvety edematous congested mucosa seen

Polyp
- Benign fleshy growth of edematous inflamed mucosa protruded through perforation found in external auditory canal
- In tubotympanic CSOM—pale edematous
- In atticoantral CSOM—pink-red fleshy

Ossicles
- Mostly intact and mobile
- Partial necrosis of bone may be seen (a long process of incus most common site)
- Destruction of bone is due to hyperemic decalcification

Tympanosclerosis

Reparative response is secondary to middle ear inflammation caused by hyalinization and subsequent calcification of subepithelial connective tissue of tympanic membrane and middle ear cleft.

Brittle chalk-like plaque seen on:
- Tympanic membrane
- Promontory
- Ossicle joints
- Tendons
- Oval window
- Round window
- Tympanosclerosis restricts the mobility of tympanic membrane (TM) and ossicle resulting in conductive hearing loss (CHL)
- Tympanosclerosis of cochlea that leads to sensorineural hearing loss (SNHL)

Fibrosis and Adhesions

Further decreases the mobility of ossicles, which may cause Eustachian tube obstruction.

Tympanic Membrane Perforation

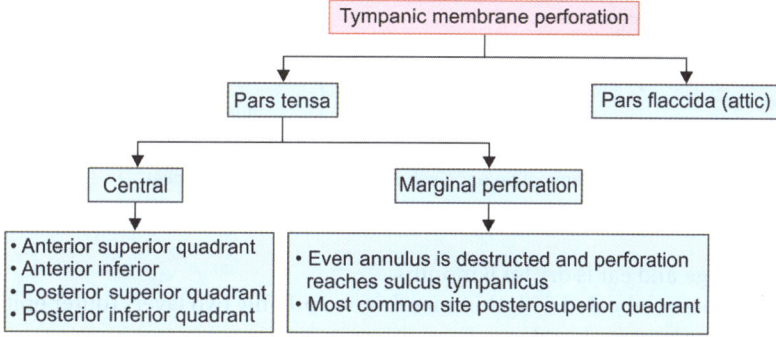

Types Depending upon Size of CP (Figs. 1 to 4)

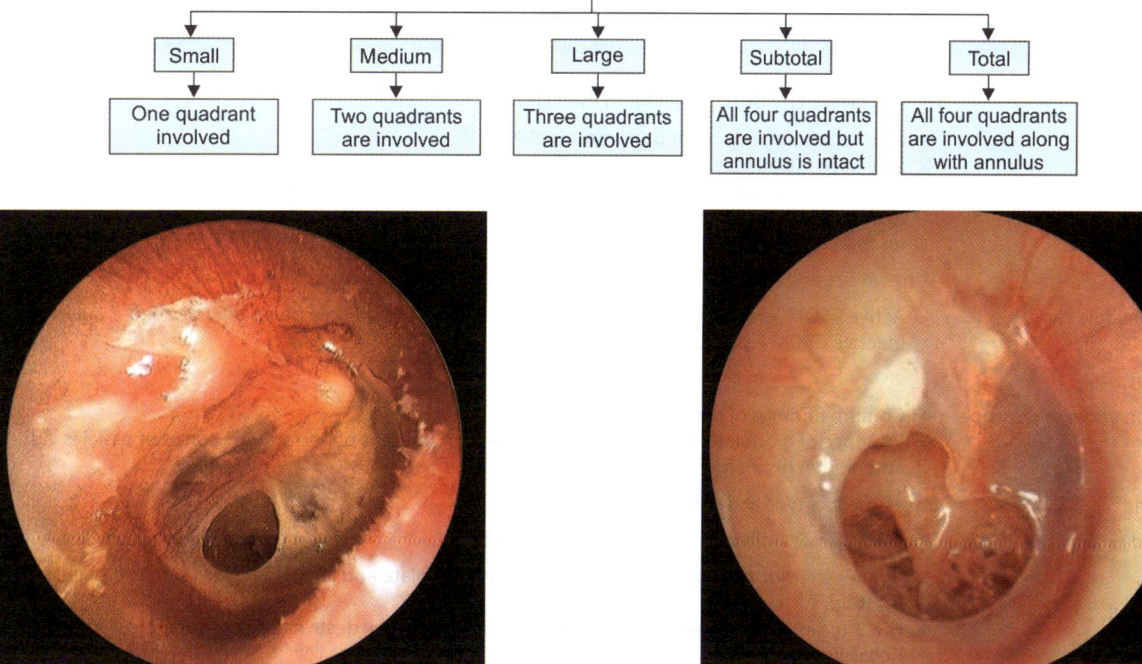

Fig. 1: Small perforation in pars tensa of the tympanic membrane (TM).

Fig. 2: Medium perforation in pars tensa of the tympanic membrane (TM).

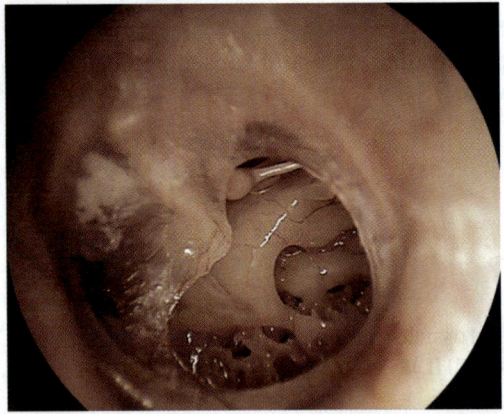

Fig. 3: Large perforation in pars tensa.

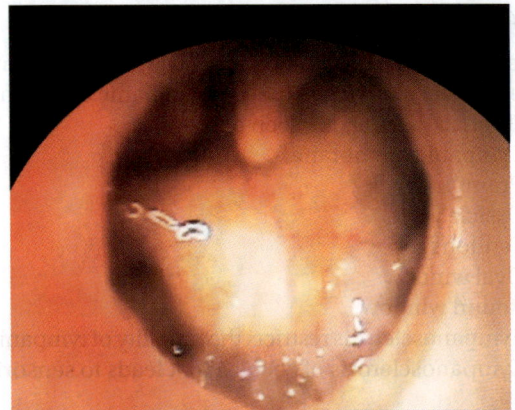

Fig. 4: Total perforation in pars tensa.

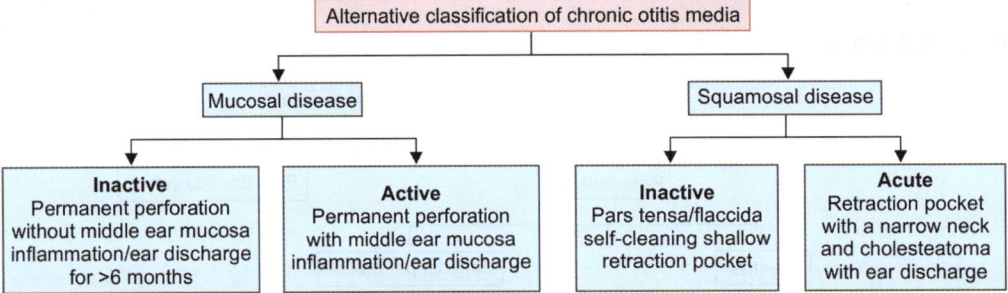

Note:
- ❖ **Quiescent stage:** No discharge and ear is dry for 6 months.
- ❖ **Healed CSOM:** Central perforation healed with thin membrane and only two layers (outer epithelial and inner mucosal layers present). Middle fibrous layer is absent.

Mucosal Type CSOM

Q. Describe clinical features, assessment and treatment of the mucosal type of CSOM and management.

	Clinical features
Ear discharge	❖ Mucopurulent, nonfoul-smelling, nonblood-stained, profuse ❖ Aggravated by URTI, relieving on medications
Hearing loss	❖ CHL depending on size of perforation, <50 dB ❖ May have mixed HL due to cochlear damage by absorption of toxins through oval and round windows. ❖ **Round window shielding effect:** Patients hear better during active ear discharge than dry ear, in the dry ear sound waves strike both oval window and round window thus cancelling each other's effect, in discharging ear phase difference get maintained
Perforation	Varies in size and location (*refer* tympanic membrane perforation chart)
Mucosa of middle ear	❖ Active CSOM—red, edematous, velvety, inflamed mucosa, a pale polyp may be seen ❖ Inactive CSOM—pale pink mucosa
Assessment	
Examination under microscope	❖ Confirm findings of otoscopic examination ❖ Presence of granulations, epithelial ingrowth from margins of perforation, status of ossicles, adhesions, and hidden discharge
Audiogram	Assessment of type and degree of hearing loss
Culture and sensitivity	To select proper antibiotics (reduces drug-resistance)
Imaging	❖ X-ray—sclerotic type of mastoid (look for low dural plate and forwardly place sigmoid plate, contracted mastoid) ❖ HRCT temporal bone—soft tissue in middle ear cleft, bony destruction, ossicular erosion (hyperemic decalcification)

Contd...

Contd...

Treatment	
Aural toilet	❖ Clearing all discharge/debris ❖ By dry mopping with a cotton swab, ear suctioning ❖ Irrigation of ear with body temperature normal saline
Ear drops	❖ Antibiotic ear drops: Neomycin, polymyxin, Chloromycetin ❖ Combined with steroids (hydrocortisone, betamethasone) for anti-inflammatory action ❖ 1.5% acetic acid drops used for *Pseudomonas* infection ❖ In case of polyp: Polypectomy is done by cutting polyp, which permits ear drops to reach effectively (avulsion of polyp is contraindicated as polyp can arise from ossicles or facial nerve, avulsion leads to ossicular discontinuity or facial palsy)
Systemic antibiotics	Useful in active CSOM
Treatment of foci of infection	Treatment of acute tonsillitis, adenitis, rhinosinusitis, and nasal allergy
Precaution	❖ Keep ear dry while bathing, use ear plugs for swimming ❖ Avoid nose blowing
Surgical treatment	❖ Once ear is dry, TM repair is done ❖ Myringoplasty—repair of TM perforation without ossicular reconstruction ❖ Tympanoplasty—repair of TM perforation with ossicular reconstruction

(CHL: conductive hearing loss; CSOM: chronic suppurative otitis media; HL: hearing loss; URTI: upper respiratory tract infection; TM: tympanic membrane)

EN4.7: Elicit document and present a correct history, demonstrate, and describe the clinical features, choose the correct investigations and describe the principles of management of the squamosal type of CSOM.

Atticoantral CSOM (Unsafe/Dangerous CSOM)

Q. Write short note/essay on atticoantral type of CSOM or cholesteatoma.

Posterosuperior part of middle ear cleft is involved and associated with cholesteatoma.
    Cholesteatoma is a misnomer—neither contains cholesterol crystal nor it is a tumor to merit suffix "oma"

Normal lining of middle ear
- Ciliated columnar in anterior and inferior middle ear cleft
- Cuboidal in mesotympanum area
- Pavement like in attic

Presence of squamous epithelium (which is the lining epithelium of external ear) in the middle ear results in cholesteatoma (skin in the wrong place).

Definition

It is squamous epithelium-lined sac in middle ear cleft which contains desquamated debris (keratin).

Consists of:
- **Matrix:** Keratinizing squamous epithelium resting on thin fibrous stroma
- **Keratin debris:** Central white mass containing desquamated debris produced by matrix
- **PriMatrix:** Granulation tissue lining bone secretes multiple proteolytic enzymes resulting in bone destruction

Classification

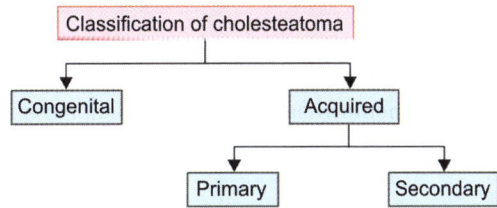

Congenital cholesteatoma	❖ White mass behind the intact eardrum ❖ Normal pars tensa and flaccida ❖ No prior history of perforation/ear discharge ❖ No prior history of ontological procedure Common site: Anterosuperior quadrant, petrous apex, cerebellopontine angle Theories: ❖ **Teed's epithelial cell rest theory**—presence of squamous cell rest in temporal bone results in formation of congenital cholesteatoma ❖ **Friedberg's implantation theory**—viable squamous cell in amniotic fluid present in middle ear of neonates ❖ **Michael's epidermoid formation theory**—nest of squamous epithelium in lateral wall of tympanic cavity, which usually involute, failure of involution result in cholesteatoma
Primary acquired	No history of previous otitis media, pre-existing perforation: ❖ **Toss theory**—persistent negative pressure in middle ear results in a retraction pocket in attic or pars tensa, this retraction pocket is later filled with desquamated squamous epithelium and results in cholesteatoma ❖ **Wittmaack's theory** ❖ **Squamous metaplasia theory**—normal pavement epithelium of attic undergoes squamous metaplasia due to subclinical infection ❖ **Basal cell hyperplasia**—proliferation of basal cell of pars flaccida induced by a subclinical childhood infection

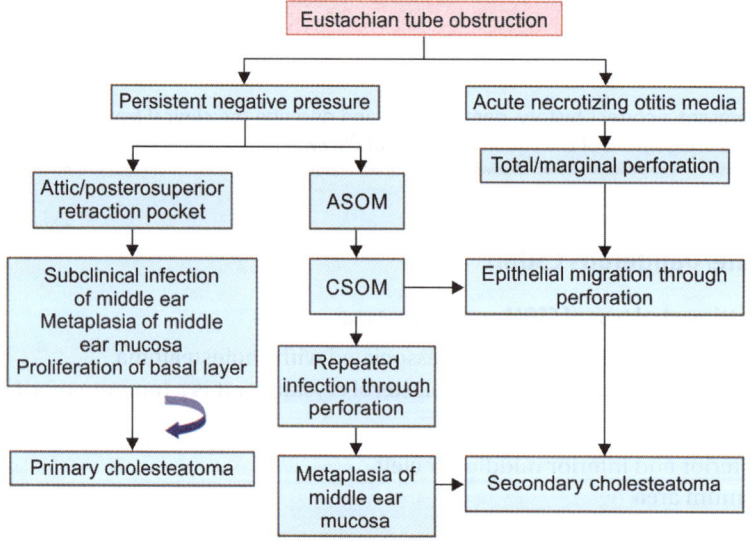

Pathology

❖ **Destruction of bone:**
  ▸ PeriMatrix of cholesteatoma (granulation tissue, mononuclear inflammatory cell) secrets enzymes (collagenase, acid phosphatase, proteolytic enzyme) results in bone destruction (tegmen plate, sinus plat, ossicles, bony labyrinth, facial canal)
  ▸ Ossicular necrosis—long process of incus commonly get affected, may involve the entire ossicular chain
  ▸ Cholesteatoma hearer—cholesteatoma bridges gap of ossicular destruction (sound conducted through cholesteatoma) resulting in hearing loss not apparent to the patient
❖ **Osteitis and granulation:** In response to inflammation bone surrounding cholesteatoma show osteitis, and granulation tissue surrounds affected bone, attic, and antrum.
❖ **Cholesterol granuloma:**
  ▸ It may or may not be associated with cholesteatoma
  ▸ On long standing retention of secretion or hemorrhage mass of granulation tissue with foreign body giant cells surround cholesterol crystals

Clinical Features

Symptoms	
Ear discharge	❖ Scanty, purulent (due to mucus-secreting goblet cells destructed), foul-smelling (fishy odor) ❖ Due to osteolysis and anaerobic infection ❖ Blood-stained due to granulation
Hearing loss	❖ CHL—due to bone erosion ❖ SNHL or MHL—toxins enter the labyrinth through round and oval window ❖ Normal hearing—cholesteatoma hearer
Signs	
Perforation	On ear examination—attic perforation/marginal perforation or total perforation
Retraction pocket	❖ Retraction of pars tensa (posterosuperiorly more common) ❖ Early stage—retraction pocket is shallow and self-cleansing ❖ Later stage—pocket becomes deep with a narrow neck and results in accumulation of keratin mass ❖ Stages of retraction pocket ➢ **Grade I:** Mild retracted TM, loss of cone of light, retraction does not contact incus ➢ **Grade II:** Retracted deep, drape over incus ➢ **Grade III:** Drape over promontory and ossicles (middle ear atelectasis) loss of middle ear space completely or partially, mucosa lining middle ear present, TM can be lifted by Valsalva, suctioning (changes are reversible with ventilating tube) ➢ **Grade IV:** TM drape over promontory, mucosa lining of middle ear is absent, TM cannot be lifted by Valsalva or by suction. Deep retraction pocket plug with keratin debris forms cholesteatoma, erosion of long process of incus, stapes suprastructure is common
Cholesteatoma	Pearly white flakes are seen on otoscopic examination and on examination under microscope
Assessment	
Examination under microscope	❖ Confirmation of findings ❖ Grade of TM retraction ❖ Site and extent of cholesteatoma ❖ Bony and ossicular destruction ❖ Granulation, polyp
Hearing assessment	❖ Tuning fork test ❖ Audiometry ❖ Type and severity of hearing loss assessed
X-ray mastoid HRCT temporal bone	❖ Ct gives more detailed information over X-ray mastoid ❖ Anteposed sigmoid sinus, low-lying dura ❖ Bone destruction, labyrinthine fistula, dehiscent facial, facial erosion ❖ Degree of pneumatization, sclerosis
Culture sensitivity of ear discharge	For proper selection of antibiotics

(CHL: conductive hearing loss; HRCT: high-resolution computed tomography; MHL: mixed hearing loss; SNHL: sensorineural hearing loss; TM: tympanic membrane)

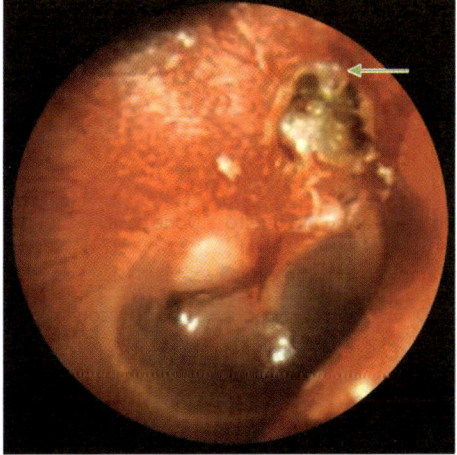

Fig. 5: Pars flaccida perforation and white cholesteatoma matrix (arrow).

Complications of CSOM

Q. Enumerate clinical features of complications of CSOM.

- Pain—seen in mastoid, extradural, perisinus, and brain abscess, otitis externa due to discharge
- Vertigo—lateral semicircular canal fistula leads to labyrinthitis, meningitis (fistula test will be +ve)
- Ataxia—cerebellar abscess, labyrinthitis
- Persistent headache, neck rigidity, projectile vomiting—in raised intracranial temperature (ICT), meningitis, and brain abscess
- Facial weakness lower motor neuron (LMN)—facial erosion
- Deep-seated retro-orbital pain, lateral rectus (LR) palsy, persistent ear discharge (Gradenigo syndrome)—seen in petrositis
- Listless child, refusing feed, lethargic—extradural abscess

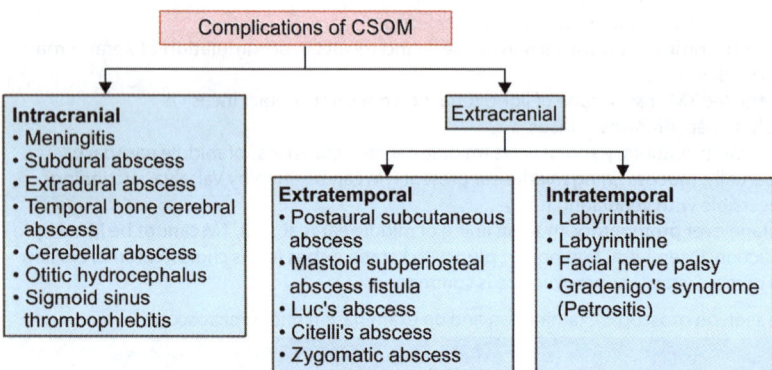

- Luc's abscess: In posterosuperior EAC bulge
- Citelli's abscess: Along posterior belly of digastric muscle
- Luc's abscess: Along sternocleidomastoid muscle
- Zygomatic abscess: Along the root of zygoma bone

Treatment of Atticoantral Type CSOM

Surgery is mainstay of treatment
- **Primary aim**—remove all disease
- **Secondary aim**—preserve hearing, reconstruct hearing (never at cost of primary aim)

Two types of surgical procedures are done—canal wall down mastoidectomy

	Canal wall down mastoidectomy	Canal wall up mastoidectomy
Procedure	• Making mastoid cavity open into EAC • Disease area fully exteriorized • Posterior bony meatal wall removed	• Disease is removed by a combined approach • Through meatus and mastoid • Posterior bony wall kept intact
Recurrence/residual disease	Low rate of recurrence/residual	High rate
Second look surgery	Not required	Since a high rate of residual/recurrence requires second-look surgery
Meatus	Wide meatus (due to meatoplasty)	Normal looking
Cavity problems	• 5 D of cavity problem • Discharging cavity • Doctor dependency—cleaning Disability—of swimming • Deafness—due to shallow middle ear CHL • Dizziness	No cavity problems
Hearing rehabilitation	• Difficulty in fitting hearing aid due to the wide meatus • Difficult to wear in discharging ear	Done easily
Reconstructive procedure	Not be done in CWD	Hearing reconstruction (ossiculoplasty) can be done to restore hearing

(CHL: conductive hearing loss; CWD: canal wall down; EAC: external auditory canal)

Conservative Treatment

- It plays a limited role in management of unsafe ear.
- Reserve for old age patient >65 years did not fit for surgical procedure.
- It includes repeated periodic suction clearance of debris under the microscope.

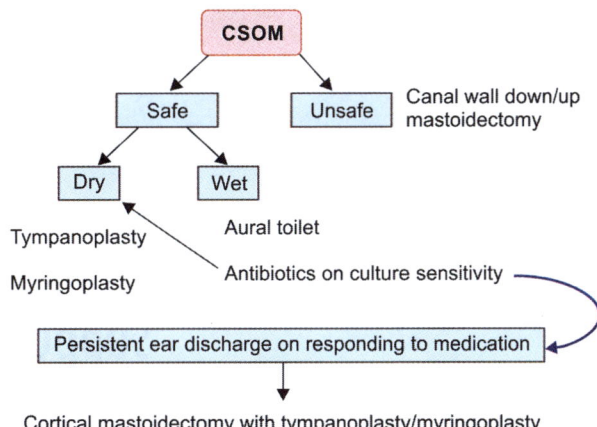

Tubercular Otitis Media

Q. Describe etiology, pathology, clinical features, and management of tubercular otitis media.

Etiology

- It is caused by mycobacterium tuberculosis, secondary to pulmonary tuberculosis (TB)
- Port of entry-Eustachian tube
- Blood-born from lung, tonsil, spine, cervical, mediastinal lymph node

Pathology

It is a gradual process of tubercle formation in submucosal layer of middle ear cleft with caseation.

Signs Out of Proportion to Symptoms

- **Ear discharge:** Painless, foul-smelling (ossicular erosion)
- **Tympanic membrane (TM) perforation:** Painless necrosis of PT, multiple TM perforation coalesce to form large perforation, double perforation
- **Mastoid/middle ear:** Pale pouty granulations +ve
- Ossicle, **mastoid bone erosion**, labyrinthine fistula, mastoiditis, postauricular fistula, osteitis with bony sequestra formation
- **Hearing loss:**
  - Sever CHL due to ossicular erosion
  - SNHL—due to labyrinth involvement
- **Facial palsy:** Presenting complaint in children, most common complication

Investigations

- Chest X-ray, sputum test, fine needle aspiration cytology (FNAC) for cervical lymphadenopathy.
- Ear discharge—acid-fast bacillus (AFB), culture, deoxyribonucleic acid (DNA) probe, polymerase chain reaction (PCR)

Treatment

- Anti Koch's treatment (AKT) to control primary disease
- Aural toilet to control secondary pyogenic infection
- Surgery—mastoid surgery with reconstruction delayed till completion of AKT (anti Koch's treatment)

Chapter 10

Complications of Chronic Suppurative Otitis Media

EN4.8: Describe the clinical features, choose the correct investigations and the principles of management of complications of CSOM.

FACTORS AFFECTING DEVELOPMENT OF COMPLICATIONS

Q. Discuss various factors affecting complications of chronic suppurative otitis media (CSOM) and its spread of infection.

Complications occur when an infection spreads beyond the mucoperiosteal lining of the middle ear cleft.
- **Age**: It is more commonly seen in children and elderly people, low immunity in both the groups make them vulnerable.
- **Socioeconomic status:** Low socioeconomic group are commonly affected.
- Poor nutrition, poor immunity, overcrowding, lack of personal hygiene, and lack of health education and health facility, are several factors that makes them more vulnerable for complications.
- **Virulence of organism:**
  - Inadequate dose for inadequate periods results in drug-resistance, poor control of infection results in chronicity and complication, e.g., *Haemophilus influenza* is developing resistance to β-lactam antibiotics and chloramphenicol.
  - *Pseudomonas aeruginosa* methicillin-resistant *Staphylococcus aureus*.
- **Immune compromised host**: Acquired immunodeficiency syndrome (AIDS), uncontrolled diabetes, transplant patient on an immunosuppressive dose, and cancer patients on chemotherapy are more prone to develop complications.
- **Preformed pathway**:
  - Congenital—congenital dehiscent facial, dehiscent middle ear floor
  - Patent suture line—petrosquamous suture
  - Fracture temporal bone—fracture site heals by fibrosis, scar permit infections
  - Surgical defect—stapedectomy, fenestration with mastoidectomy, iatrogenic dural/sigmoid sinus plate defect
  - Oval window, round window
  - Into brain tissue along with the periarteriolar space of Virchow-Robin
  - Infection from labyrinth spread to IAC, aqueduct of vestibule and cochlear aqueduct to meninges leads to easy spread of infection beyond middle ear cleft through this preformed pathway
- **Cholesteatoma-bony destruction** facilitates the spread of infection deeper

SPREAD OF INFECTION

- **Direct bone erosion:** In acute infection—hyperemic decalcification, in cholesteatoma—bony destruction by osteitis, granulation
- **Venous thrombophlebitis:** Infection from the mastoid bone can cause thrombophlebitis of venous sinuses and even cortical vein thrombosis (veins of Haversian canals are connected with dural venous sinuses and superficial veins of the brain through dural veins)
- **Preformed pathway: Same as above**

CHAPTER 10: Complications of Chronic Suppurative Otitis Media

■ CLASSIFICATION OF COMPLICATIONS CHRONIC SUPPURATIVE OTITIS MEDIA

Q. Classify complications following chronic suppurative otitis media.

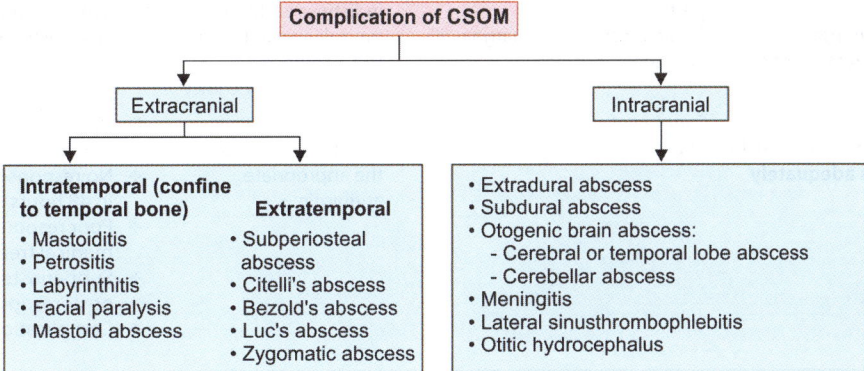

■ ACUTE COALESCENT MASTOIDITIS

Q. Write short note/essay on acute coalescent mastoiditis.

When infection spread from the mucosal lining of mastoid air cells to the bony walls of the mastoid air cell system.

Etiology

It follows acute suppurative otitis media (ASOM) (the following are determining factors):
- Virulence of organism
- Resistance of patient

Pathology

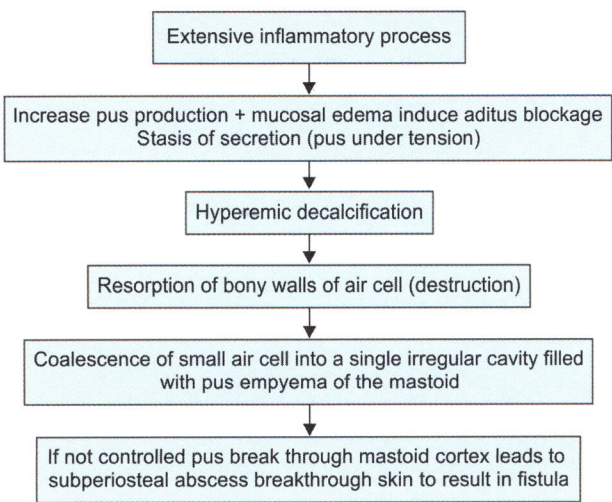

Clinical Features and Management

Symptoms	Sign	Investigation	Management
Pain behind ear	Pinna—pushed forward and downward	CBC—raised leukocyte counts and ESR	Hospitalization of patient and starting broad-spectrum IV antibiotic till sensitivity report awaited, analgesic
Persistent earache >2 weeks	Obliteration of postauricular groove		
Recurrence within 3 weeks or increase in intensity	Swelling over the mastoid imparts smooth "ironed out" feel		

Contd...

Contd...

Symptoms	Sign	Investigation	Management
Ear discharge Persistent profuse ear discharge >3 weeks If an obstruction in drainage discharge ceases with worsening of pain	Light house effect—pulsatile ear discharge coming from central perforation Reservoir sign—discharge refills EAC after cleaning	X-ray mastoid—the clouding of air cells with indistinct partition Irregular walled cavity HRCT temporal—investigation of choice	Early cases of mastoiditis treated with antibiotics alone or in combination with myringotomy (pus under tension is relived with myringotomy)
Fever Persistent/recurrence of fever in AOM treated with antibiotics adequately indicates mastoiditis	Sagging of posterosuperior wall of EAC	Pus culture and sensitivity—to select the appropriate antibiotic	Cortical mastoidectomy is indicated in: ❖ +ve reservoir sign ❖ No response to medical treatment in 48 hours ❖ Poor response to 2 weeks of medical treatment ❖ Subperiosteal abscess, sagging of posterosuperior wall of EAC ❖ Complication of mastoiditis

Differential diagnosis of mastoiditis		
Suppurative mastoid lymph node	**Furunculosis of EAC**	**Infected sebaceous cyst due to scalp infection**
❖ No history of ear discharge	❖ No history of preceding AOM	❖ No history of ear discharge
❖ No history of decreased hearing	❖ No history of decreased ❖ Swelling over the bony cartilaginous, junction of EAC, normal TM	❖ No history of decreased hearing
❖ No sagging of meatal wall	❖ No sagging of meatal wall ❖ No obliteration retroauricular groove ❖ Serous/purulent ear discharge ❖ Pre and postauricular lymph node enlargement	❖ No obliteration retroauricular groove
❖ X-ray mastoid normal	❖ X-ray mastoid normal tragal tenderness +ve	❖ X-ray mastoid normal

(AOM: acute otitis media; CBC: complete blood count; EAC: external auditory canal; ESR: erythrocyte sedimentation rate; HRCT: high resolution computed tomography; TM: tympanic membrane)

Aim of cortical mastoidectomy is to exenterate all pus-filled mastoid air cells. Postoperative antibiotics to be continued minimum for 5 days.

Complications of Mastoiditis

❖ Subperiosteal abscess
❖ Labyrinthitis
❖ Facial paralysis
❖ Petrositis
❖ Extradural abscess
❖ Subdural abscess
❖ Meningitis
❖ Brain abscess
❖ Lateral sinus thrombophlebitis
❖ Otitic hydrocephalus.

■ VARIOUS MASTOID ABSCESSES

Q. Describe abscesses in relation to mastoid infection.

Postauricular subperiosteal mastoid abscess	❖ Most common abscess ❖ Most common site—MacEwen's triangle ❖ Course—direct cortex erosion/through vessels of lamina cribrosa ❖ Occur in 50% of acute coalescent mastoiditis
Zygomatic abscess	❖ Posterior root of zygoma (zygomatic air cell) involvement ❖ Swelling in front of pinna +ve ❖ Edema of upper eyelid +ve ❖ Pus collected either superficial or deep to the temporalis muscle

Contd...

Contd...

Bezold's abscess
• Acute coalescent mastoiditis
• Pus break through thin medial side of the mastoid tip
• Selling present at upper part of neck
  ➤ Push sternocleidomastoid muscle outwards
  ➤ Follow post belly digastric (swelling between mastoid tip and angle of mandible)
  ➤ Reaches supper part of posterior triangle
  ➤ Parapharyngeal space
  ➤ Track down along carotid vessel
	• **Clinical features**—sudden onset of pain, fever with neck swelling, torticollis with a history of otorrhea
	• **Differential diagnosis:** Upper jugular lymphadenitis
	  ➤ Jugular vein thrombosis
	  ➤ Tail of parotid mass
	  ➤ Parapharyngeal abscess
	  ➤ Infected branchial cyst
	• **Specific investigation**—HRCT temporal bone with neck
	• **Treatment:**
	  ➤ **Hospital admission**, under IV antibiotic coverage post for cortical mastoidectomy with the exploration of mastoid tip (fistulous opening in soft tissue)
	  ➤ **Drainage of neck abscess** with a separate incision in neck and keeping drain
	  ➤ Continue appropriate IV antibiotic (culture sensitivity of pus)

Luc's abscess (meatal abscess)	• From antrum pus breaks through the bony wall between antrum and EAC • **Present as swelling in deep part of meatus**
Citelli's abscess	Abscess **along posterior belly of digastric muscle**
Parapharyngeal abscess • B-masked (latent mastoiditis) slow destruction of mastoid air cells without signs and symptoms • Due to inadequate antibiotics are given in terms of dose duration frequency • Acute stage of infection gets controlled but infective foci persist, and continue to destruct mastoid	Due to involvement of peritubal cells **Clinical features:** • Most commonly seen in a child, not entirely feeling well • Mild earache with persistent hearing loss after treatment • TM—thick, loss of translucency • Mild mastoid tenderness • PTA—CHL, X-ray-clouding of air cell with the indistinct outline of cell • **Treatment—cortical mastoidectomy with IV antibiotics**

(CHL: conductive hearing loss; EAC: external auditory canal; HRCT: high resolution computed tomography; IV: intravenous; PTA: pure tone audiometry; TM: tympanic membrane)

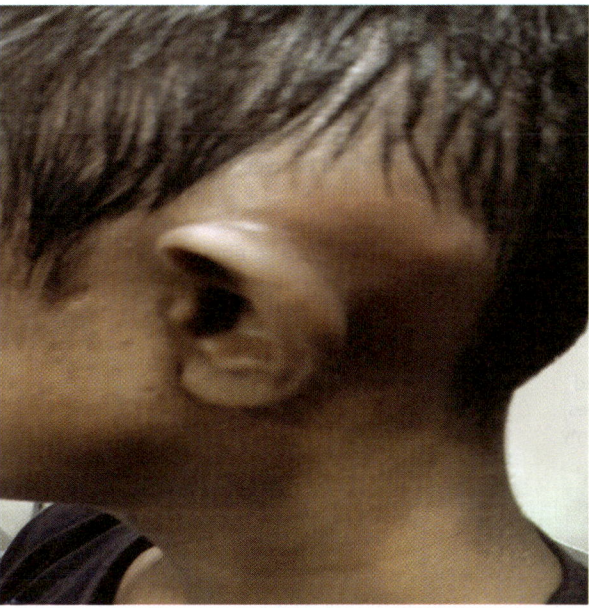

Fig. 1: Postaural mastoid abscess with forward downward displacement of the pinna.

PETROSITIS

Q. Write a short note/essay on petrositis.

Involvement of petrous apex air cell (pneumatized in 30% cases)

Pathology	Clinical features	Management

Petrous bone have variation in air cell of bone similar to mastoid
Infection spread via following cell track to reach petrous apex:
❖ Posterosuperior track—from mastoid run above and behind labyrinth, some through the arc of superior semicircular canal
❖ Anteroinferior track—from hypotympanum near eustachian tube run around cochlea to reach a petrous apex:
  ➢ Epidural abscess is formed
Involves IV nerve and trigeminal ganglion
	Gradenigo syndrome (triad of):
	❖ **Lateral rectus palsy (IV nerve involvement)**
	❖ **Deep-seated retro-orbital pain** (V nerve involvement)
	❖ Persistent ear discharge
	Persistent ear discharge (with/without deep-seated pain) after cortical mastoidectomy/MRM points to petrositis:
	➢ Fever, headache, and neck rigidity may be present
	➢ Facial nerve involvement—facial palsy
	➢ Vestibular nerve involvement—vertigo
		❖ **Specific investigation**—HRCT temporal-bony details of petrous apex
		❖ **Treatment**:
		  ➢ **Medical**—hospitalization IV antibiotic, anti-inflammatory
		  ➢ **Surgical**—(cortical/MRM/radical mastoidectomy) clearance of fistulous track
		❖ **Without residual hearing**:
		  ➢ Translabyrinthine route—posterior cell
		  ➢ Transcochlear route—anterior cell
		❖ **With residual hearing**:
		  ➢ Retrolabyrinthine/subarcuate route (Trautmann's triangle)—posterior cells
		  ➢ Infracochlear/subtemporal route—anterior cell

(HRCT: high resolution computed tomography; MRM: modified radical mastoidectomy)

■ LABYRINTHITIS (THREE TYPES)

Q. Write short note/essay on Labyrinthitis and its types.

Etiology	Clinical features	Management

❖ **Circumscribed labyrinthitis**
Thinning/erosion of bony labyrinth (lateral semicircular canal most common site) caused by:
  ➢ CSOM with cholesteatoma (most common)
  ➢ Neoplasm of middle ear (carcinoma, glomus)
  ➢ Trauma-accidental, surgical
	Membranous labyrinth is exposed and makes sensitive to pressure changes (vertigo on pressing tragus, performing Valsalva):
	❖ **Fistula test**—intermittent inward pressure applied to tragus, positive pressure stimulates labyrinth (ampullopetal displacement of cupula) induces nystagmus with a fast component towards test ear
	❖ Siegel's speculum—on test ear + pressure applied (ampullopetal flow)
	❖ On –ve pressure ampullofugal displacement of cupula, induces nystagmus with a fast component towards nontest ear (vertigo last for few seconds to minutes)
		❖ **Specific Investigation:** HRCT temporal—erosion of bony capsule of labyrinth
		❖ **Definitive treatment:** Tympanomastoidectomy CWU/CWD, with repair of labyrinthine fistula
		
		In CWU—keep cholesteatoma matrix intact over fistula, do second stage surgery—matrix turn into small cyst which can be easily removed at second stage/remove matrix in initial stage with repair of fistula
		
		In CWD—keep matrix in intact/remove with fistula repair

❖ **Diffuse serous labyrinthitis**
Diffuse inflammation of membranous labyrinth without pus formation. caused by:
  ➢ Circumscribed labyrinthitis associated with CSOM or cholesteatoma
  ➢ Spread of infection through round widow, annular ligament of stapes Fenestration surgery/stapedectomy
	❖ Mild cases—vertigo
	❖ Severe case—severe vertigo, vomiting, spontaneous nystagmus (fast component towards affected ear)
	❖ Some degree of SNHL (but no total hearing loss) which is reversible
		❖ **Medical management:**
		  ➢ Hospitalization, bed rest, head immobilization
		  ➢ IV antibiotics
		  ➢ Vestibular sedative-prochlorperazine, cinnarizine, betahistine
		  ➢ Myringotomy for labyrinthitis in AOM with bulging TM
		❖ **Surgical:**
		  ➢ For acute mastoiditis—cortical mastoidectomy
		  ➢ For CSOM with cholesteatoma—modified radical mastoidectomy (MRM)

❖ **Diffuse suppurative labyrinthitis** – diffuse pyogenic infection of labyrinth with permanent loss of vestibular and cochlear function: ➢ Follows serous labyrinthitis if not treated adequately progress to suppurative labyrinthitis	❖ Patient is toxic ❖ Acute vestibular failure ❖ Severe vertigo, vomiting nystagmus fast component towards healthy side ❖ Total hearing loss ❖ Vertigo last for 4–6 weeks till adaptation	Same as serous labyrinthitis

(AOM: acute otitis media; CSOM: chronic suppurative otitis media; CWD: canal wall down; CWU: canal wall up; HRCT: high resolution computed tomography; SNHL: sensorineural hearing loss; TM: tympanic membrane)

CHAPTER 10: Complications of Chronic Suppurative Otitis Media

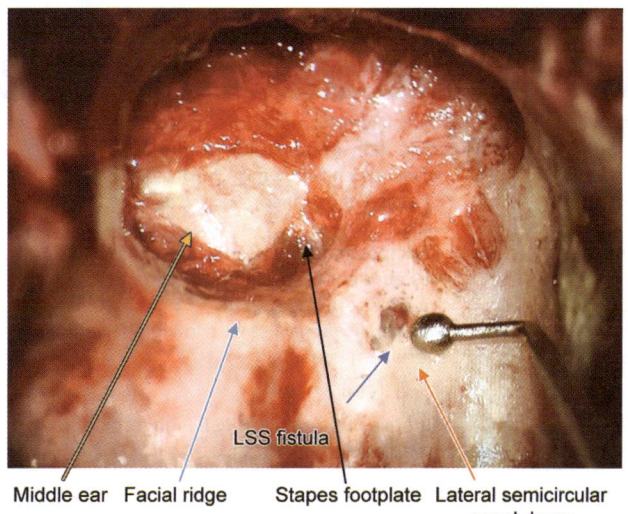

Fig. 2: Intraoperative photograph of canal wall up (CWD) mastoidectomy showing lateral semicircular canal fistula.

FACIAL PARALYSIS

Q. Write a short note on facial paralysis following otitis media.

It occurs in both ASOM and CSOM.

ASOM	CSOM
Result of—congenital dehiscence of facial nerve: ❖ Edema within fallopian canal induced by ASOM ❖ Hyperemic decalcification of fallopian canal Inflammation of epi, perineurium leads to facial palsy	Result of—cholesteatoma erodes fallopian canal causes pressure on nerve: ❖ Osteitis ❖ Granulations Facial palsy insidious in onset, slowly progressive
Investigation: HRCT temporal bone **Treatment:** ❖ Paralysis of facial is reversible with control of ASOM with antibiotic ❖ Myringotomy—ASOM with bulging TM relieves pressure over dehiscent facial ❖ Cortical mastoidectomy may be required	**Investigation:** Same **Treatment:** ❖ Under antibiotic coverage urgent facial nerve exploration and decompression ❖ CWD mastoidectomy and nerve exploration from first genu to stylomastoid foramen ❖ Granulation invading bony canal uncapped, if involving nerve sheath left in place ❖ Granulation destroying nerve segment—resection of nerve end to end anastomosis, grafting

(ASOM: acute suppurative otitis media; CWD: canal wall down; epi: epineurium; HRCT: high resolution computed tomography; TM: tympanic membrane)

INTRACRANIAL COMPLICATION

Q. Write short note/essay on.

❖ Extradural abscess
❖ Meningitidis
❖ Subdural abscess
❖ Otogenic brain abscess
❖ Lateral sinus thrombophlebitis
❖ Otic hydrocephalus

PART 1: Diseases of ENT, Head and Neck

Extra Dural Abscess (Collection of Pus between the Skull Bone and Dura)

Pathology	Clinical features	Management
❖ In ASOM—bone over dura is destroyed by hyperemic decalcification ❖ In CSOM—bone destroyed by cholesteatoma, pus directly comes in contact with dura ❖ By venous thrombophlebitis (bone over dura is intact) ❖ Affected dura covered by granulations ❖ Location—dura of middle or posterior cranial fossa, at dura of lateral venous sinus (perisinus abscess)	❖ Mostly asymptomatic (discovered accidentally on mastoidectomy) ❖ Suspected on following symptoms: ➤ Persistent headache on side of affected ear ➤ Disappearance of headache with free flow of purulent ear discharge (spontaneous abscess drainage) ➤ Generalized malaise with low-grade fever ❖ Severe pain in ear	❖ Investigation—contrast enhance HRCT temporal/MRI ❖ Treatment—cortical/MRM with evacuation of extradural abscess by removing overlying bone till the limits of healthy dura is reached ❖ IV antibiotic to be given minute for 5 days

(ASOM: acute suppurative otitis media; CSOM: chronic suppurative otitis media; HRCT: high resolution computed tomography; IV: intravenous; MRI: magnetic resonance imaging; MRM: modified radical mastoidectomy)

Meningitidis

Pathology	Clinical features	Management
Inflammation of leptomeninges (pia and arachnoid) by bacterial invasion of CSF in subarachnoid space Most common intracranial complication of otitis media: ❖ In adult—due to CSOM ❖ In children—due to ASOM Mode of spread: ❖ In infant and children—bloodborne ❖ In adults—follows CSOM (bone erosion, venous thrombophlebitis), which may be associated with extradural abscess	Presentation is due to inflammation, raise ICT, meningeal irritation ❖ High-grade fever with chills and rigors ❖ Nausea, vomiting (projectile) ❖ Headache, neck rigidity, irritability ❖ Tachypnea, tachycardia ❖ Sleeplessness ❖ Photophobia ❖ Seizures ❖ Altered mental status (confusion) **Signs-positive Kernig's sign**—extension of leg with flexion of thigh on abdomen causes pain **Positive Brudzinski sign**—neck flexion causes hip and knee flexion: ❖ Exaggerated tendon reflex ❖ Papilledema	**Investigation**: ❖ CT/MRI with contrast (also reveal associate intracranial lesion) ❖ Diagnosis—lumbar puncture and CSF study ❖ Raise pressure ❖ Raised cell counts >1,000/mL (polymorph cells) ❖ Elevate CSF protein level ❖ Lower CSF: Blood sugar ratio ❖ CSF culture sensitivity **Management:** ❖ **Hospitalization**, head high 30° ❖ IV antibiotic covering both aerobic and anaerobic till culture sensitivity report available ❖ Corticosteroids **Surgical**—once patients general condition improves on medical treatment, otogenic foci of infection is surgically removed **ASOM—cortical mastoidectomy** **CSOM—radical/MRM** Partial improvement on medical line of management requires urgent mastoid surgery

(ASOM: acute suppurative otitis media; CSF: cerebrospinal fluid; CSOM: chronic suppurative otitis media; CT: computed tomography; ICT: intracranial temperature; MRI: magnetic resonance imaging; MRM: modified radical mastoidectomy)

Subdural Abscess

Pathology	Clinical features	Management
❖ Pus collected between dura and arachnoid ❖ By erosion of bone or dura/venous thrombophlebitis ❖ Rapidly spread over in subdural space compressing cerebral hemisphere it lies against the cerebral hemisphere	❖ **Meningeal irritation**—fever, headache, neck rigidity, positive Kernig's and Brudzinski sign ❖ **Raise ICT:** Papilledema, dilated pupil, ptosis (third nerve involvement) ❖ **Cortical venous thrombophlebitis**—thrombophlebitis of vein over cerebral hemisphere may present as hemiplegia, hemianopia, aphasia, Jacksonian type epilepsy	Lumbar puncture (LP) contraindicated—LP may causes herniation of cerebellar tonsil: ❖ Drainage of subdural abscess by burr hole/craniotomy ❖ IV antibiotic—to control the infection ❖ Once patients general condition improves, otogenic foci of infection is removed by mastoidectomy

Otogenic Brain Abscess

- Accounts for 50% of brain abscess in adults and 25% in children
- Aerobic organisms—staphylococci, streptococci (*pneumoniae, haemolyticus*), Escherichia coli (*E. coli*)
- Anaerobic—peptostreptococci, *Bacteroides fragilis*

Pathology	Clinical features	Management
In adult—CSOM (cholesteatoma) In children- ASOM Incidence of cerebral (temporal) to cerebellar is 2:1 Route of spread Direct erosion of tegmen (cerebral)/ Trautmann's triangle (cerebellar) **Venous thrombophlebitis** Usually associated with other complications—subdural, extradural abscess, sigmoid sinus thrombophlebitis Stages of abscess formation: ❖ Invasion (encephalitis): Mild symptoms of low-grade fever, headache, malaise ❖ Localization (quiescent abscess): Capsule formation, asymptomatic stage last for several weeks ❖ Enlargement (manifest abscess): Edema appears around abscess resulting in raised ICT and focal cerebral/cerebellar dysfunction due to lesion ❖ Rupture of abscess—into ventricle and subarachnoid space result in fatal meningitis	Clinical features overlapped due to presence of other complications: ❖ **Raised intracranial tention (ICT)**: Severe headache, nausea, projectile vomiting ➢ Lethargy progressing to drowsiness, coma ➢ Papilledema (if raised ICT persists for >2 weeks) ❖ Localizing symptoms for: ➢ Temporal abscess ♦ **Nominal aphasia** (dominant hemisphere) patient unable to name common objects but can demonstrate their use. ♦ **Homonymous hemianopia:** (compression on optic radiation, visual field of opposite side of lesion is lost) examined by confrontation/perimetry test ♦ Contralateral motor paralysis upward spread of abscess (face followed by arm then leg involve) downward spread toward internal capsule (leg then arm followed by face involves) ♦ Epileptic fits (uncinate gyrus involvement causes smell, test hallucination, generalized fits oculomotor palsy) (transtentorial herniation) ➢ Cerebellar abscess ♦ Suboccipital headache ♦ Spontaneous irregular **nystagmus towards side of lesion** ♦ Ipsilateral ataxia, hypotonia, weakness ♦ **Past-pointing and intension tremors** ♦ **Dysdiadochokinesia**	**Investigation:** ❖ X-ray skull (replaced by CT) ❖ Midline shift of brain, gas in abscess cavity revealed **CT with contrast** (brain with temporal bone)—hypodense area with a surrounding area of edema (**ring sign**) seen Size, site, associated other complication, presence of ear disease noted Lumbar puncture (contraindicated due to risk of coning) **Treatment:** ❖ **Medical** ➢ IV antibiotics combination to cover aerobes and anaerobes ➢ Dexamethasone 10 mg 6 hourly for 4 days ➢ Hypertonic mannitol 20% in dose of (0.25–0.5 mg/kg) ❖ **Neurosurgical approaches to drain abscess:** ➢ Burr hole and aspiration ➢ Excision of abscess ➢ Open incision of abscess and evacuation of pus Burr hole and aspiration abscess followed by repeat CT, if no decrease in size/expanding abscess requires excision of abscess **Otological surgery**: To be considered only after abscess is controlled: ❖ For ASOM: Cortical mastoidectomy ❖ CSOM—modified radical mastoidectomy

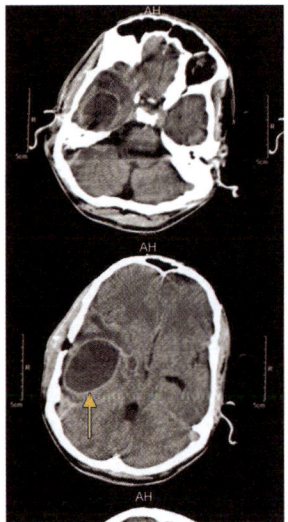

Fig. 3: High resolution computed tomography (HRCT) showing temporal lobe abscess.

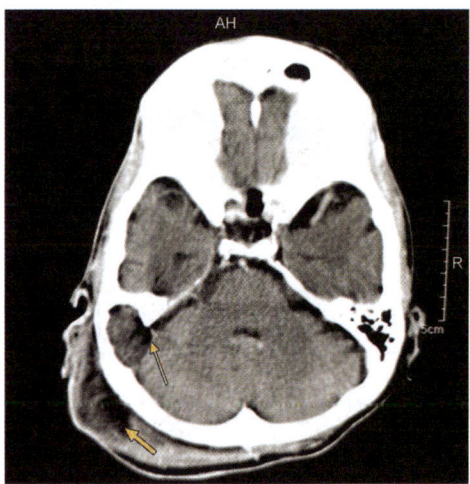

Fig. 4: High resolution computed tomography (HRCT) showing temporoparietal (cerebral abscess) abscess with mastoiditis and destruction of complete sinus plate.

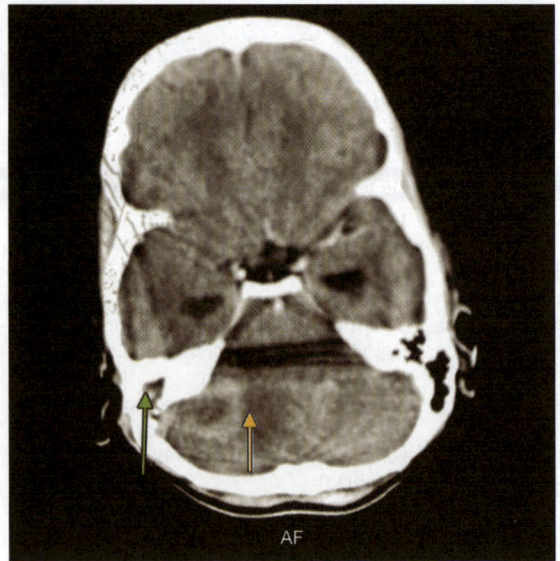

Fig. 5: High resolution computed tomography (HRCT) sinus plate erosion with cerebellar abscess.

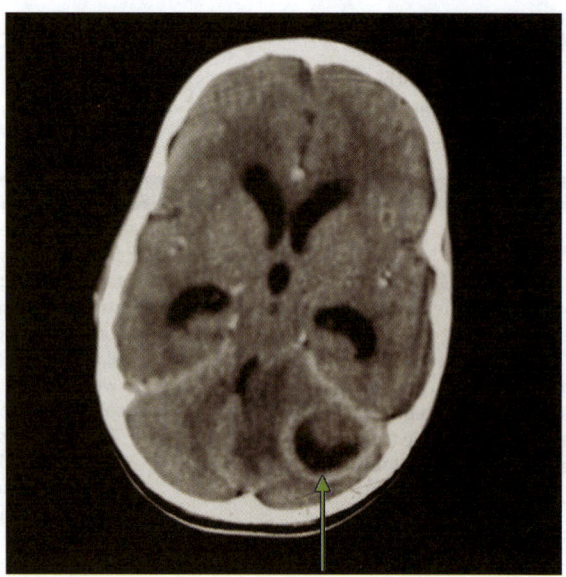

Fig. 6: High resolution computed tomography (HRCT) temporal bone showing cerebellar abscess.

Lateral Sinus Thrombophlebitis (Sigmoid Sinus + Transverse Thrombosis)

Characterized by inflammation of inner wall of lateral sinus and mural thrombus formation

Etiology

ASOM, CSOM, and cholesteatoma

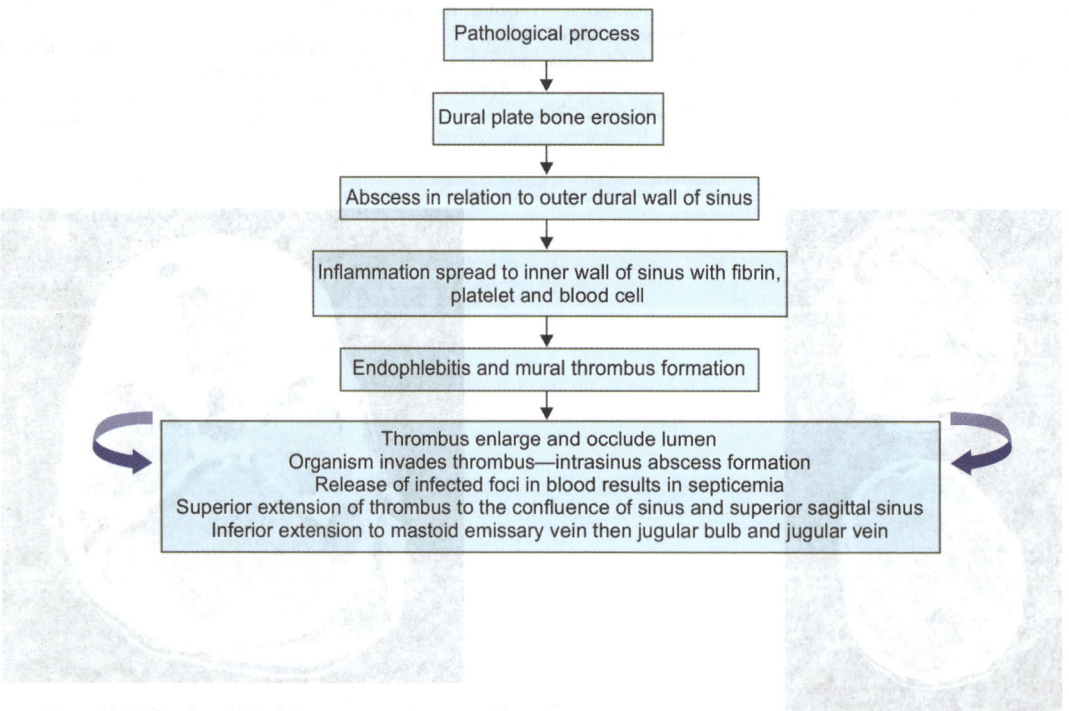

Clinical features	Management

❖ Hectic picket fence type of fever with rigors
Fever coincide with a release of septic emboli into blood characterized by irregular one or more peak of fever with rigor and chills, following profuse sweating fever subsides (resemble malaria which has regular fever spikes)
❖ **Headache:** Initially stage of perisinus abscess it is mild nature progressed to severe due to venous thrombosis induced raised ICT
 	
Signs
❖ **Griesinger's sign:** Edema over mastoid due to thrombosis of mastoid emissary vein
❖ **Papilledema:** Due to raised ICT, retinal hemorrhages/dilated vein
❖ **Tobey–Ayer test:**
  ➢ Recording of CSF pressure by manometer with compression of one or both jugular vein
  ➢ Compression of the thrombosed site—no change in pressure, very slow rise of pressure 10–20 mm Hg
  ➢ Compression of normal site—rapid increase in pressure (2–3 times greater than normal pressure)
❖ Crowe–Beck test—compression of normal jugular vein caused engorgement of retinal vein examined by ophthalmoscope, which subsides on releasing pressure
❖ Tenderness of jugular vein—due to thrombophlebitis of vein, associated with enlarged inflamed jugular lymph node, torticollis
	❖ **Investigations:**
	  ➢ Rule out malaria by blood smear
	  ➢ Blood culture and sensitivity—blood to be collected at time of chills which coincides with septic emboli entering blood stream
	  ➢ CSF study—excludes meningitis, high pressure normal study
	  ➢ CT with contrast brain-filling defect in sinus, delta sign due to sinus thrombosis (inflammatory enhancement of sinus wall but not content of sinus)
	  ➢ Digital subtraction angiography—site and extent of obstruction
	Complications:
	  ➢ Septicemia, pyogenic abscess of lung, bone, and other organs
	  ➢ Meningitis, cerebellar abscess
	  ➢ Cavernous sinus thrombosis
	  ➢ Otic hydrocephalus due to extension to sagittal sinus
	
	Treatment:
	❖ IV antibiotics—broad spectrum (4–6 weeks) covering both aerobic and anaerobic organisms
	❖ Anticoagulant—low molecular weight heparin/warfarin
	❖ **Otological surgery:**
	  ➢ For ASOM—cortical mastoidectomy
	  ➢ CSOM—modified radical mastoidectomy:
	    ♦ Ligation of internal jugular vein (IJV) rarely required in antibiotic era (infection/thrombosis of IJV)

(ASOM: acute suppurative otitis media; CSF: cerebrospinal fluid; CSOM: chronic suppurative otitis media; CT: computed tomography; ICT: intracranial temperature)

Otic Hydrocephalus

Raised intracranial temperature (ICT) with normal CSF finding due to failure of arachnoid villi to absorbed CSF.
CF—headache, nausea, vomiting, VI nerve palsy (diplopia), CSF pressure >300 mm Hg with normal sugar, protein, and bacteriological sterile.

Treatment—aim is to reduce CSF pressure:

- ❖ Acetazolamide
- ❖ Corticosteroids
- ❖ Repeated lumbar puncture

Lumboperitoneal drain:

- ❖ IV antibiotics for sinus thrombosis
- ❖ Once raise ICT controlled—ear disease removed by mastoidectomy

Chapter 11

Otosclerosis

EN4.13: Describe the clinical features, investigations, and principles of management of otosclerosis.

■ DEFINITION AND ETIOPATHOGENESIS

Q. Write short note/essay on otosclerosis.

Definition
It is a disease of altered bone mechanism in which remodeled bone bridges the stapediovestibular joint and fixates it. It usually affects bilateral ears.

Pathology
- It is a disease of abnormal bone remodeling that occurs in the endochondral layer of the temporal bone. It may affect the bony walls of the cochlea as well.
- **Blue mantle:** It is the first histological sign of otosclerosis. It is an extracellular staining pattern due to an unstable matrix that begins to remodel giving rise to an otosclerotic focus.
- Immature bone continues to remodel with prominent osteoblastic involvement called otospongiosis. An immature bone matures into a sclerotic, dense, irregularly woven, and poorly vascularized bone.

Etiology
- **Age:** Most common in the second or third decade of life.
- **Sex:** Females are more commonly affected than males (1.4–2 times common among females)
- **Hereditary:** It is inherited in an autosomal dominant pattern. Monozygotic twins have a nearly 100% concordance rate of otosclerosis.
- **Race:** It is more common in white races.
- **Hormonal factors:** Hormones may have an influence on otosclerosis as it is more prevalent in women, especially during pregnancy.
- **Metabolic theory:** It is thought that disturbances of calcium metabolism may be responsible for abnormal bone remodeling.
- **Van der Hoeve syndrome:** A generalized osseous disease in which patients have otosclerosis along with blue sclera and osteogenesis imperfecta.

Foci of Otosclerosis
Otosclerosis can occur in any part of the otic capsule.
The location and extent of the disease determine the clinical presentation, extent of conductive hearing loss, and presence or absence of sensorineural hearing loss.
- **Anterior to stapes footplate:**
  - The most common type is seen in 96% of the cases.
  - The lesion starts on the anterior footplate, also known as "fistula ante fenestram."

CHAPTER 11: Otosclerosis

- ❖ **Round window niche:**
  - ▷ It is seen in 30% of the cases.
  - ▷ Causes conductive hearing loss irrespective of the state of stapes.
- ❖ **Cochlear apex:**
  - ▷ It is seen in 12% of the cases.
  - ▷ It involves a region of round windows or other areas in the otic capsule.
  - ▷ Causes sensorineural hearing loss.

■ CLINICAL FEATURES

Symptoms

- ❖ Hearing loss—bilateral hearing loss, mostly seen in young females which worsens time and increases during pregnancy. Patients tend to speak in a low voice.
  Paracusis Willisii—patient hears better in noisy environment. Patient's speech discrimination becomes better as people tend to raise their voices in a noisy environment.
- ❖ Vestibular symptoms may present as—benign paroxysmal positional vertigo, dizziness, or unsteadiness.
- ❖ Tinnitus: It is frequently the presenting symptom.
- ❖ Positive family history is seen in 50% of the cases.

Signs

- ❖ Normal/intact tympanic membrane
- ❖ Schwartze's sign: It is a vascular blush on the promontory, indicating the active process of the disease.
- ❖ Other ears, nose, and throat (ENT) examinations are normal.

■ INVESTIGATIONS

Tuning Fork Tests

- ❖ 512 Hz and 1,024 Hz are used to assess hearing.
- ❖ It reveals bilateral symmetrical hearing loss which may be conductive, sensorineural, or mixed.

Pure Tone Audiometry

- ❖ Complete audiometry including air and bone thresholds, speech discrimination, and acoustic reflexes is essential.
- ❖ It confirms the findings of tuning fork tests.
- ❖ The maximal conductive loss is approximately 55–60 dB.
- ❖ **Carhart's notch:** It is a common audiometric finding but not pathognomonic of otosclerosis. It is a depression of bone conduction (5 dB) thresholds at 2,000 Hz. It is a pseudo-loss; may be due to the increase in the mass of the stapes footplate.

Role of Radioimaging in Otosclerosis

It may be helpful in excluding other causes of conductive hearing loss and hence confirming the diagnosis of otosclerosis.

■ DIFFERENTIAL DIAGNOSIS

- ❖ Ossicular discontinuity
- ❖ Tympanosclerosis
- ❖ Congenital fixation or malformations of the ossicles
- ❖ A third mobile window such as superior semicircular canal dehiscence
- ❖ Serous otitis media
- ❖ Stapes suprastructure fracture
- ❖ Fracture or dislocation of the ossicles
- ❖ Congenital absence of the round or oval window.
- ❖ Van der Hoeve's syndrome
- ❖ Paget's disease

■ TREATMENT

Conservative Management

- ❖ **Medical management:** Primarily directed at maturing the involved bone and decreasing osteoclastic activity:
  - ▷ Sodium fluoride and bisphosphonates have been introduced for medical management. However, no medical management is recommended on a consistent basis.

❖ **Hearing aids:** They offer effective means of nonsurgical management of hearing loss in otosclerosis for those who do not benefit from surgery or who are not willing for surgery or where surgery is contraindicated.

Surgical Management

Stapedotomy is the treatment of choice.

Contraindications for Surgery

❖ Infected middle ear or external ear
❖ Perforation of the drum
❖ Only hearing ear
❖ Relatively contraindicated if the other ear has a disease that may threaten to hear in the future.
❖ Meniere's syndrome should be ruled out in patients with vestibular symptoms.
❖ If an intact vestibular system is required for occupational activity, the potential intact of surgery should be considered.
❖ Advanced age is not a contraindication for surgery.

Steps of Stapedotomy Surgery (Figs.1 to 3)

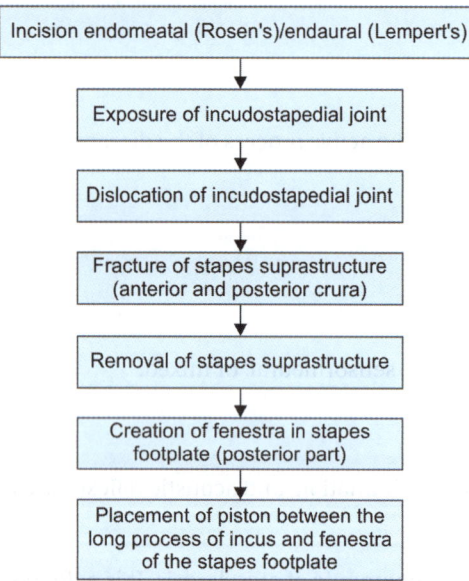

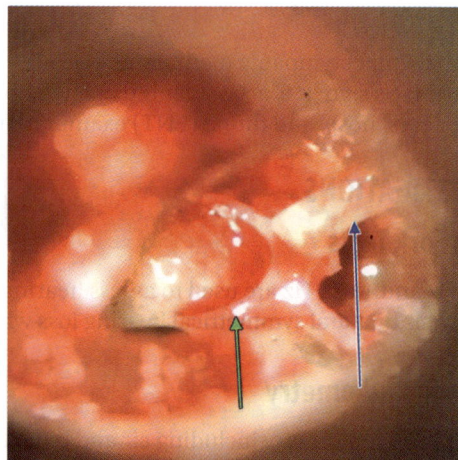

Fig. 1: Fractures stapes suprastructure and separated incus.

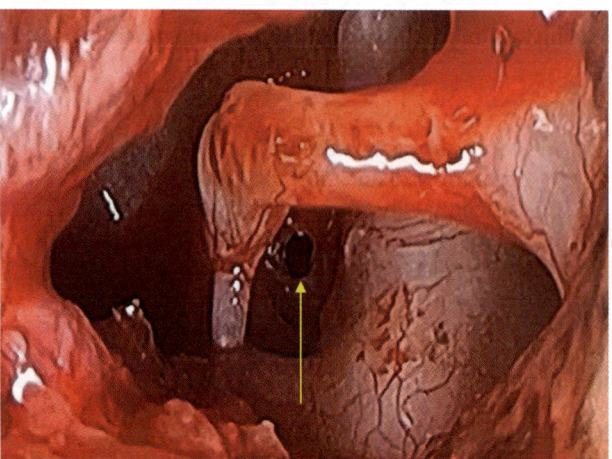

Fig. 2: Fenestra in stapes footplate.

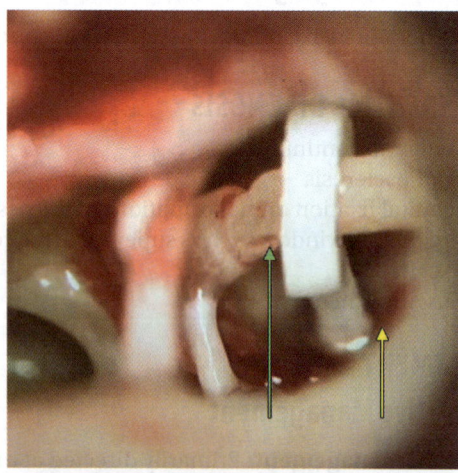

Fig. 3: Teflon piston placed between the incus and stapes footplate.

Chapter 12

Meniere's Disease

EN4.18: Describe the clinical features, investigations and principles of management of Meniere's disease.

■ DEFINITION

Q. Write short note/essay on Meniere's disease.

It is a disorder of the inner ear, characterized by (i) vertigo, (ii) sensorineural hearing loss, (iii) tinnitus, and (iv) aural fullness. It is also known as endolymphatic hydrops. The endolymphatic system is distended with endolymph. The endolymph is normally produced by stria vascularis which fills both the membranous labyrinth and is absorbed through the endolymphatic sac.

It is one of the most common causes of otogenic vertigo.

■ ETIOLOGY

- **Age:** Commonly seen after the third decade of life
- **Sex:** More common among men.
- **Allergy:** The inner ear acts as the "shock organ" producing excess of endolymph. Nearly 50% of patients with Meniere's disease are found to have concomitant inhalant and/or food allergies.
- **Sodium and water retention:** Excessive retention leads to endolymphatic hydrops.
- **Hypothyroidism:** About 3% of cases of Meniere's disease are due to hypothyroidism and are found to benefit from thyroid replacement therapy.
- **Hypoadrenalism and hypopituitarism** are found to be responsible in about 6% of the cases.
- **Syphilis and cochlear otosclerosis** can also produce endolymphatic hydrops.
- **Autoimmune and viral etiologies** have been suggested on the basis of experimental, laboratory, and clinical observations.

■ PATHOPHYSIOLOGY

Distension of the endolymphatic system due to increased volume of endolymph is the main pathology.

The increased volume of endolymph may be due to increased production, impaired absorption, or both.

However, the exact cause of the disease is not yet identified:

- **Impaired absorption by lymphatic sac:** Impaired absorption by the sac may be responsible for raised endolymph pressure. There are experiments that show hydrops when the endolymphatic and its duct is blocked. Ischemia of the sac leads to poor absorption and hence increased volume of endolymph and eventually leading to distension of the sac.
- **Vasomotor disturbance:** Sympathetic overactivity due to vasomotor imbalance leads to spasms of the internal auditory artery and/its branches. This causes deafness and vertigo as this interferes with the functions of the cochlear or vestibular sensory neuroepithelium.

Also, there is increased production of endolymphatic sac due to transudation of fluid as a result of anoxia of capillaries of stria vascularis.

CLINICAL FEATURES

Symptoms

- The cardinal symptoms of Meniere's disease are—(i) episodic vertigo, (ii) fluctuating hearing loss, (iii) tinnitus, and (iv) aural fullness.
- It is commonly seen in the age group of 35–60 years of age. Males are affected more than females.
- This disease is usually unilateral but becomes bilateral later on.

Vertigo

- It is characterized by a feeling of rotation of the patient himself or his surroundings. It is sudden in onset and may be accompanied by nausea and vomiting with ataxia and nystagmus. In severe cases, it may be accompanied by other symptoms of vagal disturbances such as abdominal cramps, diarrhea, cold sweats, pallors, and bradycardia.
- **Tullio phenomenon:** It is a condition that arises due to the distended saccule lying against the stapes footplate where patients develop vertigo due to loud sounds or noise. This is also seen when there are three functioning windows in the ear, e.g., a fenestration of horizontal canal in the presence of mobile stapes.

Hearing Loss

It is a **sensorineural type of hearing loss** and may precede or accompany vertigo. It **improves after the attack** and is normal during the periods of remission. **This fluctuating hearing loss is quite characteristic of the disease.** The recovery of hearing during remission may not be completed with recurrent attacks, leading to slow and progressive hearing loss which is permanent.

Tinnitus

It is characterized by a low-pitched roaring type and disappears after the attack in the initial stage of the disease, however, it becomes continuous with repeated attacks.
- Aural fullness is fluctuating in nature and may precede or accompany the attack.
- Patients are often anxious and stressed due to apprehension of the repetition of attacks.

VARIANTS OF MENIERE'S DISEASE

Cochlear hydrops	Vestibular hydrops	Drop attacks	Lermoyez syndrome
Only cochlear signs and symptoms are present	Cochlear function is normal	Cochlear function is normal	Symptoms occurred in reverse order.
Vertigo is absent	Typical attacks of episodic vertigo	Vertigo is absent	Characterized by progressive deterioration of hearing followed by vertigo
Characterized by increased endolymph pressure due to block at ductus reuniens	• Exact pathology could not be demonstrated. • Often termed as "recurrent vestibulopathy"	• Characterized by sudden drop attack without loss of consciousness. • Also known as "Tumarkin's otolithic crisis"	

STAGING OF MENIERE'S DISEASE

It is based on the average of pure tone thresholds at 0.5, 1, 2, and 3 kHz of the worst audiogram during a period of 6 months before treatment.

Stage	Pure tone average in dB in previous 6 months
1	≤25
2	26–40
3	41–70
4	>70

INVESTIGATIONS

- Otoscopic examination of the tympanic membranes reveals no significant abnormality.
- **Nystagmus:** This is seen only during an acute attack. The quick component of nystagmus is towards the unaffected ear.

- **Tuning fork test:** The test is suggestive of sensorineural hearing loss. Rinne test is positive, absolute bone conduction is reduced in the affected ear and Weber is lateralized to the better ear.
- **Speech audiometry:** Discrimination score is usually good (55-85%) during attacks but much impaired during and immediately following an attack.
- **Special audiometry test:** These tests help to distinguish it from retrocochlear diseases.
  - Recruitment test is positive for the affected ear.
  - *Short increment sensitivity test (SISI):* The normal score is 15%. In two-thirds of the patients, it is better than 70%.
  - Tone decay test
- **Electrocochleography:** It is a diagnostic of Meniere's disease. The normal ratio of summating potential (SP) to action potential (AP) is 30%. In Meniere's disease, this ratio is >30%.
- **Caloric test:** It shows reduced response on the affected side in 75% of cases. It often reveals canal paresthesias on the affected side.
- **Glycerol test:**
  - It shows improvement in hearing. Glycerol is a dehydrating agent and thus decreases the endolymphatic pressure.
  - Patient is given glycerol (1.5 mL/kg). Audiogram and speech discrimination scores are recorded before and 1-2 hours after ingestion of glycerol.

DIFFERENTIAL DIAGNOSIS

- Labyrinthitis
- Acoustic neuroma
- Ototoxicity
- Perilymph fistula

TREATMENT

- Conservative management
- Surgical management

Conservative Management

In-between Attacks/General Measures

- Reassurance of the patient and relatives by explaining the nature of the disease. This helps to alleviate the anxiety and emotional stress.
- **Cessation of smoking:** Smoking should be completely stopped as nicotine causes vasospasm.
- **Low salt diet:** Salt intake should not be >1.5-2.0 g/day. No extra salt should be permitted.
- Avoid excessive intake of water.
- Avoid over-indulgence in coffee, tea, and alcohol.
- **Avoid stress:** Mental relaxation exercises and yoga are helpful to decrease stress.
- Avoid activities requiring good body balance, flying, swimming, or working at great heights as the attack of Meniere's disease is abrupt and almost impossible to predict.

During Acute Attacks

- Reassurance and comfort of the patient.
- Bed rest with head supported on pillows to decrease head movements.
- Labyrinthine sedatives to relieve vertigo. Drugs commonly used are dimenhydrinate, promethazine, or prochlorperazine
- Intravenous fluids and electrolyte administration
- **Vasodilators:** Carbogen (5% CO_2 with 95% O_2) inhalation helps to improve labyrinthine circulation.
- Tranquillizers are given to relieve anxiety and functional overlay.

Management of Chronic Phase

- **Vestibular sedatives:** Oral prochlorperazine (Stemetil) 10 mg three times a day (TID) for 2 months and then reduced to 5 mg TID for 1 month.
- **Vasodilators:** Betahistine is considered to be the most effective vasodilator and helps in rapid endolymph absorption.
- Diuretics like furosemide are given every alternate day with potassium supplements.
- Avoidance of allergens.
- Hormonal cause if present, should be treated accordingly.

Labyrinthine Exercises

- ❖ Cooksey–Cawthorne's vestibular exercises help in labyrinthine adaptation.
- ❖ **Intratympanic gentamicin injection:** Gentamycin is vestibulotoxic and causes destruction of the vestibular labyrinth. It is given weekly or biweekly. It is absorbed through the round window.
- ❖ **Intermittent low-pressure pulse therapy:** Using an instrument called the Meniett device, intermittent positive low pressure is delivered to the inner ear.

Surgical Management

Surgical management is indicated only if medical treatments fail:
- ❖ Conservative procedures:
  - ▻ Stellate ganglion block
  - ▻ Endolymphatic shunt operation
  - ▻ Decompression of endolymphatic sac
  - ▻ Sacculotomy
  - ▻ Selective section of vestibular nerve section
  - ▻ Ultrasonic destruction of the vestibular labyrinth
- ❖ Destructive procedures:
  - ▻ Labyrinthectomy

Chapter 13

Hearing Loss

EN4.14: Describe the clinical features, investigations, and principles of management of conductive hearing loss and sensorineural hearing loss including sudden sensorineural hearing loss and noise induced hearing loss.

■ DEAFNESS

Definition

Q. What is deafness? Classify types of deafness.

Deafness is defined as the impairment of hearing.

Classification

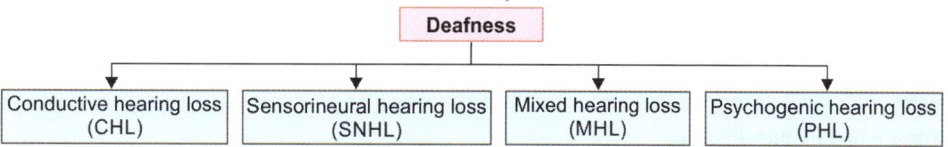

CHL—pathology in the conducting mechanism of the ear, i.e., the external or middle ear
SNHL—pathology in the inner ear, VIIIth cranial nerve, or central connections
MHL—conductive as well as sensorineural deafness components
Psychogenic—no organic cause for hearing loss, it is due to malingering or hysteria

Etiology

Conductive Hearing Loss

Q. Write the etiology for conductive hearing loss (CHL).

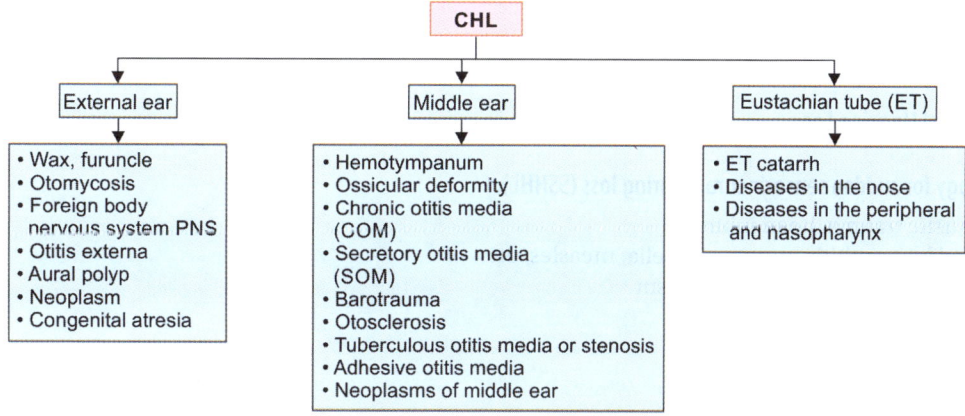

Congenital Causes

- ❖ Congenital cholesteatoma—presenting with white mass behind an intact tympanic membrane
- ❖ Fixation of stapes footplate
- ❖ External auditory canal atresia
- ❖ Ossicular discontinuity

Sensorineural Hearing Loss

Q. Write the etiology for sensorineural hearing loss (SNHL).

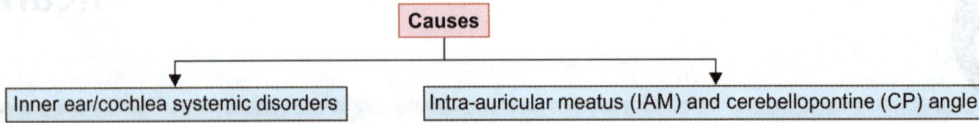

- ❖ Inner ear/cochlea:
  - ➤ Congenital—malformations of inner ear structures
  - ➤ Infective—labyrinthitis—viral, bacterial, syphilitic
  - ➤ Traumatic—fractures due to head injury/iatrogenic
  - ➤ Meniere's disease
  - ➤ Ototoxicity—streptomycin, gentamicin, furosemide, etc.
  - ➤ Tumors—e.g., acoustic neuroma
  - ➤ Presbycusis (age-related hearing loss)
  - ➤ Acoustic trauma (noise-induced)
- ❖ Systemic disorders:
  - ➤ Metabolic disorder—diabetes mellitus
  - ➤ Hypertension
  - ➤ Hypothyroidism
  - ➤ Vitamin deficiency, i.e., vitamin B1, B6 deficiency
  - ➤ Smoking and alcoholism
  - ➤ Cerebrovascular accident (CVA), multiple sclerosis
  - ➤ Atherosclerosis, blood dyscrasias
- ❖ Internal auditory meatus and CP angle:
  - ➤ Acoustic neuroma
  - ➤ Meningioma
  - ➤ Cholesteatoma—unsafe ear disease
  - ➤ Arachnoid cyst

Mixed Deafness

Q. Write the etiology for mixed deafness.

- ❖ Chronic otitis media—cholesteatoma resulting in damage to ossicles or inner ear
- ❖ Advanced otosclerosis
- ❖ Senile deafness
- ❖ Trauma—Acoustic trauma:
  - ➤ Blast injury
  - ➤ Head injury

Sudden Sensorineural Hearing Loss

Q. Write the etiology for sudden sensorineural hearing loss (SSNHL).

- ❖ Trauma—acoustic trauma, head injury
- ❖ Infection—viral labyrinthitis, mumps, rubella, measles, etc.
- ❖ Vascular—spasm, hemorrhage, or embolism
- ❖ Ototoxicity
- ❖ Meningitis
- ❖ Tumors—acoustic neuroma
- ❖ Functional

Diagnosis of Hearing Loss

Q. How will you work up a case of hearing loss?

Examination and Investigations

- Full clinical examination of ears—otomicroscopy, pneumatic otoscopy
- Hearing tests—tuning fork tests and pure tone audiometry (PTA) speech
- Audiometry—speech reception threshold (SRT) and speech discrimination score (SDS)
- Fistula test and caloric test
- Brainstem evoked response audiometry (BERA) to rule out congenital hearing loss
- Complete hemogram with coagulation profile
- Blood sugar, blood pressure monitoring
- X-ray and high resolution computed tomography (HRCT) scan of the temporal bone and CP angle
- Magnetic resonance imaging (MRI) brain (gadolinium contrast) with special mention of VIIth and VIIIth cranial nerves with CP angle.
- Neurological examination

Management

Q. How will you treat a case of hearing loss?

Conductive Deafness

- Treat the underlying cause, i.e., if COM is secondary to tuberculosis or syphilis then treat the underlying cause first, i.e., tuberculosis (TB) or syphilis
- Definitive surgical management:
    - Myringotomy with or without grommet insertion in a case of glue ear.
    - Exploratory tympanotomy for removal of mass (tumors) from middle ear or to check the status of ossicular chain.
    - Myringoplasty/tympanoplasty for repair of tympanic membrane perforation. Ossiculoplasty for repair of the ossicular chain in case of COM
    - Mastoidectomy for mastoiditis in a case of COM
    - Stapedectomy for fixed stapes footplate presenting with conductive hearing loss/mixed hearing loss with intact tympanic membrane
- Hearing aid

Sensorineural Deafness

- Treat the cause—syphilis, diabetes, etc.
- Vasodilators for sudden SNHL—IV nicotinic acid, pentoxifylline
- Intratympanic dexamethasone—5 to 6 sittings. Low salt diet and diuretics
- Oral or IV steroids—some prefer these in place of intratympanic steroids
- Multivitamins with antioxidants—vitamin B complex group with A, C, and E
- Labyrinthine sedatives, i.e., cinnarizine
- Hearing aids/cochlear implant/bone-anchored hearing aid (BAHA)
- Auditory training

Drug Related Hearing Loss

Q. Classify ototoxic drugs causing hearing loss.

- **Aminoglycosides:** It causes vestibulotoxicity and cochleotoxicity
    - *Vestibulotoxic* drugs—*Streptomycin, gentamycin, and tobramycin*
    - *Cochleotoxic* drugs—*Kanamycin, amikacin, neomycin, sisomicin, and* dihydrostreptomycin

    Mechanism of action: Vestibulotoxic drugs destroy type 1 hair cells of the crista ampullaris. Cochleotoxic drugs damage type 2 hair cells
- **Diuretics:** *Furosemide, bumetanide, and ethacrynic acid* which cause bilateral symmetrical hearing loss which is reversible.
    - *Mechanism of action:* It causes edema, inflammation, and cystic changes in the stria vascularis of the vascular duct

- ❖ **Analgesics:** *Salicylates, indomethacin, phenylbutazone, ibuprofen*
  - ▷ Salicylates—It causes tinnitus and bilateral SNHL affecting higher frequencies which is reversible.
  - ▷ Mechanism of action: It interferes at the enzymatic level.
- ❖ **Antimalarials:** *Quinine, chloroquine, and hydroxychloroquine*
  Quinine cause tinnitus and SNHL which is reversible, but higher doses may cause permanent hearing loss
  - ▷ *Mechanism of action of quinine:* Vasoconstriction of the small vessels of the cochlea and stria vascularis.
  - ▷ Chloroquine and hydroxychloroquine cause reversible hearing loss
- ❖ **Cytotoxic drugs:** *Nitrogen mustard, cisplatin, and carboplatin*
  - ▷ Mechanism of action—affects the outer hair cells of the cochlea
- ❖ **Topical ear drops:** *Polymyxin B, neomycin, framycetin, gentamicin propylene glycol, antifungal ear drops,* etc.
- ❖ **Deferoxamine:** It causes high-frequency SNHL which can be sudden onset or delayed onset
- ❖ **Miscellaneous:** Erythromycin, ampicillin, propranolol, propylthiouracil, chloramphenicol tetanus antitoxin
- ❖ **Chemicals**: Alcohol, tobacco, marijuana, carbon monoxide, etc.

■ NONORGANIC HEARING LOSS

Q. Write a short note/essay on nonorganic hearing loss and its diagnosis.

Recruitment

Recruitment is the abnormal growth in the perception of loudness by an individual with a hearing loss.

Nonorganic Hearing Loss

It is a type of hearing loss, where there is no organic lesion. It is either due to malingering or of psychogenic origin.

Diagnosis of Malingering or Nonorganic Hearing Loss

- ❖ Inconsistent results on PTA and speech audiometry
- ❖ Inconsistent results on PTA and speech reception threshold (SRT)
- ❖ Stenger test
- ❖ Chimani–Moos test
- ❖ Lombard test
- ❖ Acoustic reflex threshold
- ❖ BERA

Q. How to calculate the degree of handicap for a person who complains of being hard of hearing and wants to apply for a disability certificate?

- ❖ Do an audiogram first and then calculate the average of the three speech frequencies, i.e., 500, 1,000, 2,000 kHz say = X
- ❖ Deduct 25 from it, i.e., X – 25
- ❖ Multiply it by 1.5, i.e., (X – 25) × 1.5
  This is the percentage of hearing impairment for that ear.
- ❖ Similarly calculate hearing impairment for another ear
- ❖ Total percentage handicap of an individual given by formula = [(better ear% × 5) + worse ear %]/6

■ NOISE-INDUCED HEARING LOSS

Q. Write a short note/essay on noise-induced hearing loss (NIHL).

Types of NIHL

- ❖ **Temporary threshold shift:** Hearing is impaired immediately after exposure to noise but recovers after an interval of few minutes to a few hours which can even extend up to 14 days.
- ❖ **Permanent threshold shift:** The hearing loss is permanent and does not recover at all.

Safe Limits of Noise

- ❖ Maximum safe limit for noise pollution (recommended by the Ministry of labour, Government of India)
  - ▷ A noise of 90 dB (A) SPL, 8 hours a day for 5 days a week

Audiogram Findings

Audiogram shows a typical notch, at 4 kHz for both air and bone conduction.

Clinical Features

- High-pitched tinnitus and difficulty in hearing in noisy surroundings but no difficulty in day-to-day hearing.
- After repeated noise exposure, lower and higher frequencies are involved and the notch at 4 kHz may deepen.
- Hearing loss is evident when speech frequencies are involved.

Pathogenesis

Noise-induced hearing loss causes damage to hair cells starting at the basal turn of the cochlea. Outer hair cells are affected first and then followed by inner chair cells.

Diagnosis and Treatment

Investigations

- Pure tone audiometry to document hearing loss and tympanometry to confirm normal middle ear function. In malingering individuals, cortical evoked response audiometry (CERA) is done.
- Loudness discomfort levels (LDL) are done to document hyperacusis.

Diagnosis

History of prolonged history of unprotected exposure to excessive noise where there is no history of organic ear pathology.

Management

- **Prevention:** Avoiding excessive exposure to noise by use of earmuffs or earplugs.
- **Personal hearing protection:** Earplugs/earmuffs/active noise—electronic method of noise reduction by providing sound in a set of earmuffs.
- **Nonspecific management:** Reduction of background noise as far as possible. In severe hearing loss—psychological counseling, infrared headphones use with TV, telephones.
- **Specific management:** Sound therapy in the form of a binaural hearing aid/white noise generator.

■ SUDDEN SENSORINEURAL HEARING LOSS

Q. Write a short note/essay on sudden sensorineural hearing loss.

Definition

Sudden SNHL is defined as 30 dB of SNHL over at least three contiguous frequencies occurring within 72 hours or less.

Presbycusis

Presbycusis is defined as the sensorineural hearing loss associated with the physiological aging process in the ear.

Six types of presbycusis have been described:
- Sensory
- Neural
- Strial/metabolic
- Cochlear conductive
- Intermediate
- Mixed

Sensory

- Degeneration of organ of corti affecting basal turn of cochlea first followed by apex later.
- Higher frequencies are affected but the speech discrimination score is good.

Neural

This is the most common type:
- ❖ Degeneration of the cells of the spiral ganglion starts at the basal turn of the cochlea and then progresses to apex. Higher frequencies are affected but speech discrimination is poor.
- ❖ Hearing loss is out of proportion to the pure tone loss.

Strial

- ❖ Atrophy of stria vascularis affecting all the turns of the cochlea.
- ❖ An audiogram is flat but speech discrimination is good.

Cochlear Conductive

Stiffening of the basilar membrane affecting its movements. An audiogram is a sloping type.

Intermediate

Changes in the characteristics of the cochlear duct that are not evident on the light microscopy. Following changes have been described in this category:
- ❖ Changes in the intracellular organelles involved in cell metabolism
- ❖ Decrease in synapse numbers
- ❖ Changes in endolymph composition

Mixed

Involving a combination of the above five.

Clinical Features

- ❖ Patients have difficulty hearing in the presence of background noise but they hear well in quiet surroundings.
- ❖ They can hear the speech but cannot understand the speech.
- ❖ Tinnitus is also a common complaint
- ❖ Recruitment is positive, i.e., all the sounds suddenly become intolerant when the volume is raised.

Diagnosis and Management

Investigations

Pure tone audiogram—if hearing loss between two ears is asymmetrical then MRI with gadolinium contrast is done to rule out vestibular schwannoma.

Management

Three broad areas are considered:
- ❖ Psychological (nonspecific)
- ❖ Practical (nonspecific)
- ❖ Sensory (specific)

Nonspecific Management

- ❖ Reduction of background sound (noise) as far as possible.
- ❖ Face-to-face conversation to minimize the nonverbal communication cues.
- ❖ Explanation of the problem to allow legitimization of patient's hearing loss.

Specific Management

- ❖ Binaural hearing aids
- ❖ Managing accompanying tinnitus with cognitive, directive counseling, tinnitus retraining therapy, and sound therapy which includes hearing aids and/or white noise generators

Chapter 14

Tinnitus

EN4.19: Describe the clinical features, investigations and principles of management of tinnitus.

■ DEFINITION

Q. Define tinnitus. What are its types?

- ❖ A sensation of noise in the ear, described variably by the patients as ringing, whistling, booming, blowing, roaring, hissing, sizzling, etc.
- ❖ Characteristics:
  - ➢ Originates inside the patient
  - ➢ Unilateral >bilateral
  - ➢ Quiet surrounding (e.g., at night) → ambient noise absent → masking effect lost → louder perception of tinnitus

Classification

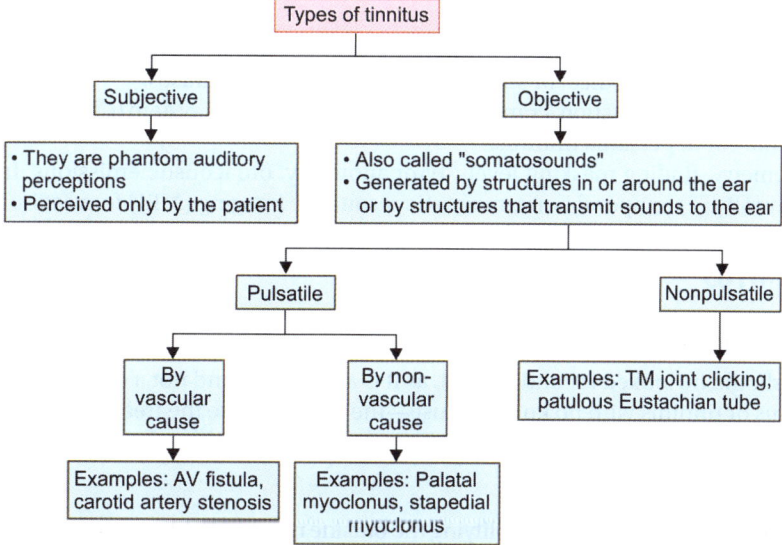

(AV: arteriovenous; TM: tympanic membrane)

CAUSES

Q. What are the causes and pathophysiology of tinnitus?

Causes of Subjective Tinnitus

- ❖ **Local causes** (ear-related): Impacted wax, otitis media (acute/chronic/serous), ototoxicity, noise-induced hearing loss, sudden sensorineural hearing loss (SNHL), presbycusis, Meniere's disease, and acoustic neuroma
- ❖ **Systemic causes**:
  - ▸ *Neurologic causes:* Head injury, fracture temporal bone, brain ischemia, brain hemorrhage, and multiple sclerosis.
  - ▸ *Cardiovascular:* Anemia, hypertension, hypotension, cardiac arrhythmias, and arteriosclerosis.
  - ▸ *Metabolic:* Obesity, hyperlipidemia, and hyper/hypothyroidism.
  - ▸ *Other:* Anxiety and depression.

Causes of Objective Tinnitus

- ❖ **Vascular causes:**
  - ▸ *Arteriovenous (AV) shunt:* Congenital AV malformations, and glomus tumor.
  - ▸ *Arterial:* Carotid stenosis, carotid aneurysm, arteriosclerosis, and persistent stapedial artery.
  - ▸ *Venous:* Dehiscent jugular bulb.
- ❖ **Nonvascular causes**:
  - ▸ Patulous Eustachian tube
  - ▸ Palatal myoclonus
  - ▸ Stapedial myoclonus
  - ▸ Tympanic membrane (TM) joint click

PATHOPHYSIOLOGY

- ❖ It originates from damage/alteration of the inner hair cells or peripheral or central nervous pathway.
- ❖ **Mechanism:** Abnormal afferent excitation at cochlea or efferent dysfunction.
- ❖ Imbalance caused between the damaged outer hair cells and the relatively better inner hair cells.

EVALUATION OF TINNITUS

Q. How will you evaluate a case of tinnitus?

- ❖ **Thorough history:** Nature of tinnitus, continuous/intermittent, impact on sleep/daily life. History of ear disorders or drug intake (ototoxicity). Past history of medical or surgical illness, psychogenic causes.
- ❖ **Examination:** Otomicroscopic examination, cranial nerve and central nervous system (CNS) examination, and auscultation of the neck or around the ear in pulsatile tinnitus.
- ❖ **Investigations:** Audiometry, finding masking levels, tympanometry, otoacoustic emissions. Imaging—high-resolution computed tomography (HRCT) temporal bone, magnetic resonance imaging (MRI) for vestibular schwannoma.

MANAGEMENT OF TINITUS

Q. Write a note on treatment options of tinnitus.

- ❖ The cause of tinnitus should be looked for and treated, as it is a symptom and not a disease
- ❖ For unresolving tinnitus or tinnitus with no known cause—the following are the treatment options:

Hearing Aid and Masking Therapy

- ❖ **Principle:** Tinnitus perception is reduced by amplifying the outside noise with a hearing aid or by applying masking sound designed to match various sounds to a person's tinnitus.
- ❖ **Maskers:** Wearable device—behind the ear or in the ear—low-level sound generators to provide constant neural auditory signals. Should be used for 6–8 hours a day.

Tinnitus Retraining Therapy

- ❖ **Aim:** Habituation of tinnitus by habituation of reaction evoked by tinnitus.
- ❖ **Principle:** Attenuation of the abnormal conditioned reflex arc, between the tinnitus signals within the auditory pathway and emotional and physiological responses involving the limbic and sympathetic system part of the autonomic nervous system.
- ❖ Based on—Jastreboff's neurophysiological model of tinnitus
- ❖ **Requires long-term therapy:** 18–24 months, but gives a significant improvement in 80% of patients.
- ❖ **Components:**
  - ▹ *Counseling:* Educating the patient about the origin, mechanism of generation, and perception at cortical and subcortical levels of tinnitus. About the generation of negative reactions to tinnitus, both emotional and autonomic.
  - ▹ *Sound therapy:* Avoiding silent environment. Continuous low-level broadband noise is generated for 8 hours a day to produce habituation.

Psychological Treatment

Counseling

Pharmacotherapy

- ❖ No proven medications for tinnitus
- ❖ Antidepressants—for coexisting depression and anxiety
  Benzodiazepines—for the suffering associated with tinnitus. Causes recurrence on discontinuation and causes dependence.
- ❖ Other supplementary medicines—*Ginkgo biloba*, antioxidants, vitamins, and minerals
- ❖ Transtympanic therapy—anesthetic/ototoxic drug/corticosteroids/neuroactive antioxidants

Surgical Treatment

- ❖ **Cochlear implantation**—when tinnitus is associated with hearing loss
- ❖ Cochlear nerve section—not recommended

Others

Transcutaneous electrical stimulation.

Chapter 15

Assessment and Disorders of Vestibular System

EN4.17: Describe the clinical features, investigations, and principles of management of vertigo.

■ VERTIGO

Q. What is vertigo? Classify types of vertigo. Write a note on its management.

- ❖ Defined as an illusion of rotation of the surroundings or oneself
- ❖ Ill-defined subjective sense of imbalance
- ❖ Symptom and not a disease

Classification

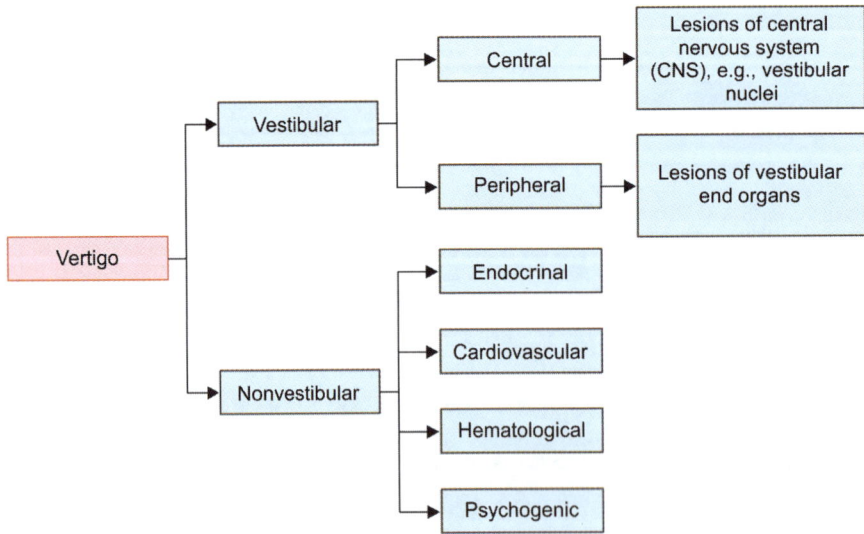

Peripheral and Central Vertigo

Q. State the differences between peripheral and central vertigo.

	Peripheral vertigo	*Central vertigo*
Direction of nystagmus	Fixed	Variable
Torsion component	Present with vertical/horizontal	May or may not
Visual fixation	Inhibits nystagmus	No inhibition
Habituation	Yes	None
Latency of nystagmus	3–40 seconds	No latency
Fatigability	Fatigable	No
Severity of vertigo	Often marked	Mild
Reproducibility	No	Yes

Management

- ❖ **Pharmacological treatment:**
  - ▸ It aims to suppress the symptoms of acute vestibular attacks.
  - ▸ To treat specifically the underlying conditions.
- ❖ **Vestibular rehabilitation**: It is based on the concept of the capacity of the vestibular system for adaptation and recalibration of vestibular reflexes by substitution of sensory input, motor responses, and strategies in order to achieve symptomatic recovery for a vestibular lesion.
- ❖ **Exercise, repositioning maneuvers** for treatment of benign paroxysmal positional vertigo.
- ❖ **Adjunctive treatment**: This may include psychological or psychiatric intervention.

ASSESSMENT OF VESTIBULAR SYSTEM DISORDERS

Q. Describe the evaluation/assessment of vestibular system disorders.

- ❖ **History**
  - ▸ To find the underlying cause—a history of viral infection, systemic illness, surgery, and drugs should be ruled out.
  - ▸ Presenting features of vertigo:
    - ◆ Number of episodes:
      - ◊ Single
      - ◊ Multiple
    - ◆ Spontaneous or provoked
    - ◆ Associated hearing loss
    - ◆ Episodic vertigo:
      - ◊ Positional—benign paroxysmal positional vertigo (BPPV)
      - ◊ Paroxysmal—vestibular paroxysm
      - ◊ Migraine—vestibular migraine
      - ◊ Hearing loss—Meniere's disease and labyrinthitis
  - ▸ Triggering factors:
    - ◆ Lying down or turning in bed—BPPV
    - ◆ Standing up—orthostatic hypotension
    - ◆ Neck movement—any vestibular disorder
    - ◆ Pressure changes—third window/fistula
    - ◆ A loud sound (**Tullio phenomenon**)—Meniere's disease and third window
    - ◆ Alcohol and exercise—episodic ataxia
- ❖ **Examination of a patient with vertigo**
  - ▸ Ear nose and throat examination
  - ▸ **Neurological examination:** Cranial nerve examination

- Cerebellar lesion signs:
  - Nystagmus
  - Dysdiadochokinesia
  - Finger nose test
  - Finger to finger test
  - Heel knee test
  - Gait test
  - Tremors
- Vestibular evaluation:
  - Nystagmus—spontaneous nystagmus
  - Fistula test
  - Positional tests
  - Vestibulo-ocular reflex
    - Romberg's test
    - Sharpened Romberg's test
    - Gait test
    - Unterberger's test

❖ **Laboratory tests for evaluation of vertigo**
- Caloric tests
- Electronystagmography
- Optokinetic test
- Rotation test
- Galvanic test
- Posturography

Fistula Test

Q. Write a short note on fistula test.

❖ The pressure changes induced in the external auditory canal (EAC) are transmitted to the labyrinth, causes its stimulation leading to nystagmus and vertigo.

❖ **Principle**:

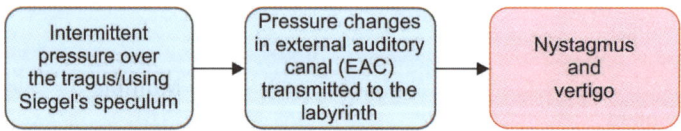

Test results	Fistula	Fistula sign	Conditions

Positive	Present	Positive	❖ Erosion of horizontal semicircular canal
			  ➤ Cholesteatoma
			  ➤ Fenestration operation
			❖ Oval window—poststapedectomy fistula
			❖ Round window—rupture of round window membrane

False positive	Absent	Positive	❖ Congenital syphilis—hypermobile footplate ❖ Meniere's disease—fibrous bands from utricular macula to stapes footplate (Hennebert's sign)
False negative	Present	Negative	❖ Dead labyrinth ❖ Cholesteatoma covering the fistula
Negative	Absent	Negative	Normal ear

Spontaneous Nystagmus

Q. Describe how do you check for spontaneous nystagmus?

❖ Definition—involuntary, rhythmical, oscillatory movements of eyes
❖ Can be horizontal vertical or rotatory
❖ Vestibular nystagmus has a fast and slow component
❖ Direction of nystagmus—indicated by **fast components**
❖ Intensity—described by its degree (**Alexander's laws**)

Degree of nystagmus	Direction of nystagmus
1	Present when the patient looks in direction of fast component (weak)
2	Present when the patient looks straight ahead (strong)
3	Present when the patient looks in direction of slow component (stronger)

❖ **Method to examine:**
  ➤ The patient is advised to be seated in front of the examiner and the examiner keeps moving his fingers 45 cm from the patient's eye to the right-left up and down taking care not to be move the fingers >30° from the central position (to avoid gaze-evoked nystagmus).
  ➤ Watch for nystagmus.
  ➤ Spontaneous nystagmus is seen when there is a static imbalance in tonic levels of activity mediating the semicircular canal. It indicates an organic lesion.
  ➤ Nystagmus can be central or peripheral:

Nystagmus	Peripheral	Central
Origin	Labyrinth or CN VIII	Central vestibular pathway: Vestibular nuclei, brainstem, cerebellum
Duration	<1 minute	>1–2 minutes
Direction of nystagmus	Fixed	Changing
Latency	2–20 seconds	None
Fatigability	Present	Absent
Associated vertigo	Present	None
Optic fixation	❖ Suppressed by looking at a fixed point. ❖ Enhanced in darkness/by use of Frenzel glasses (eliminates optic fixation)	Not suppressed

❖ **Direction of nystagmus depending on the nature of pathology:**
  ➤ Irritative lesions—nystagmus on the side of the lesion, e.g., **serous labyrinthitis**
  ➤ Paretic lesions—nystagmus to the opposite side of the lesion, e.g., purulent labyrinthitis, trauma, lesion of CN VIII
❖ **Types of central nystagmus:**
  ➤ Purely torsional—lesion of the brainstem/vestibular nuclei—syringomyelia
  ➤ Vertical downbeating—lesion of the craniocervical region (Arnold–Chiari malformation/cerebellar degenerative lesion)
  ➤ Vertical upbeating nystagmus—lesion at the junction of pons and medulla or pons and midbrain
  ➤ Pendular nystagmus—multiple sclerosis. Can be disconjugate (vertical in one eye and horizontal in the other)
❖ **Ewald's laws for nystagmus:**
  ➤ The axis of nystagmus parallels the axis of the semicircular canal that generated it.
  ➤ Ampullopetal flow of the endolymph causes more stimulation in the horizontal semicircular canal than ampullofugal flow.
  ➤ Ampullopetal flow of the endolymph is inhibitory and ampullofugal flow excitatory in the vertical canals, i.e., superior and posterior semicircular canals.

Vestibulo-ocular Reflexes

Q. Describe the tests for vestibulo-ocular reflexes.

❖ **Romberg's test:**
  ➤ To assess the patient's ability to stand, feet together arms by the side with eyes opened and with eyes closed.
  ➤ Interpretation:
    ♦ Uncompensated, unilateral, peripheral vestibular lesion—patient sways to the side of the lesion.
    ♦ Central pathology patient shows instability.
❖ **Sharpened Romberg's test:**
  ➤ It is done when a patient performs Romberg's test without swaying.
  ➤ A patient stands with one heel in front of his toes and arms folded across the chest.
  ➤ Inability to maintain balance in peripheral vestibular involvement.
❖ **Gait test:**
  ➤ Patient is asked to walk in a straight line at a fixed point—with eyes open and then with closed.
  ➤ With eyes closed, the patient deviates to the affected side—in the uncompensated lesion of the peripheral vestibular system.

- **Unterberger's test:**
  - It is performed by asking the patient to walk up and down on the spot, with eyes closed and arm outstretched in front, with the hand closed together.
  - Body rotation of >30° or backward or forward displacement of >1 m are regarded as indicative of peripheral vestibular dysfunction.

Dix–Hallpike Maneuver

Q. Describe in detail Dix–Hallpike maneuver.

- **Dix–Hallpike maneuver** is a positional test done in patients complaining of vertigo with change in head positions.
- It also helps to differentiate peripheral from central vertigo.
- **Method (scan QR code):**
  - The patient sits on the couch.
  - Examiner holds the patient's head, and turns it 45° to the right
  - Then places the patient in a supine position so that his head hangs 30° below the horizontal.
  - Patient's eyes are observed for nystagmus.
  - The test is repeated with the head turned to the left and then again in a straight head hanging position.
- **Four parameters are observed:**
  1. Latency
  2. Duration
  3. Direction
  4. Fatigability
- **Interpretation:**
  - In BPPV—nystagmus has a latency (2–20 seconds), lasts 1 minute, is always in one direction (towards the undermost ear—geotropic) and is fatigable on repeating the maneuver for a few times. With patient complained of vertigo when in a critical position.
  - In central lesions—nystagmus is produced immediately, and lasts until the head is in a critical position with no fatigability. The direction of nystagmus changes each time.

Q. How do you differentiate the cerebellar signs based on site of the cerebellar lesion?

Cerebellar hemisphere lesions	Midline disease of cerebellum lesions
❖ Asynergia abnormal finger-nose test) ❖ Dysmetria (inability to control range of motion) ❖ Adiadochokinesia (inability to perform rapid alternating movements) ❖ Rebound phenomenon (inability to control movement of extremity when opposing forceful restraint is suddenly released)	❖ Wide base gait ❖ Falling in any direction ❖ Inability to make sudden turns while walking ❖ Truncal ataxia

Caloric Test

Q. Describe caloric tests with their types.

Principle

To induce nystagmus by thermal stimulation of the vestibular system.

Advantages

- Each labyrinth can be tested separately.
- It also checks for labyrinthine origin of vertigo—indicated by qualitatively the same type experienced by the patient during the vertigo episode.

Types

- **Modified Kobrak test:**
  - A quick office procedure.

- Method:
  - Patient is seated with a head tilted 60° backward to place the horizontal canal in a vertical position.
  - Irrigate with ice water for 60 seconds
    - First with 5 mL
    - If no response—10 mL, 20 mL, and 40 mL
  - Nystagmus to opposite side with 5 mL—normal
  - Nystagmus with >5–40 mL—hypoactive labyrinth
  - No response with 40 mL—dead labyrinth
- **Fitzgerald–Hallpike test (bithermal caloric test) (Fig. 1):**
  - Method:
    - Supine position, head tilt: 30° forward (horizontal canal is vertical)
    - Ear irrigated for 40 seconds alternately with water at 30° and 44°, 5 minutes gap between 2 ears.
    - Observe for nystagmus.
    - If no nystagmus, the test is repeated with water at 20° for 4 minutes before labeling it as a dead labyrinth.
    - Time is noted from the start of the irrigation to the endpoint of nystagmus and it is plotted on a graph.
  - Interpretation:
    - Direction of nystagmus: Cold opposite, warm same (COWS)
      - With cold water—nystagmus is seen directed to opposite side
      - With warm water—nystagmus is seen directed to same side as the ear irrigated
    - Normal—responses from both labyrinths are almost the same, cold water usually has s stronger stimulus than the hot water.
    - Canal paresis—response elicited from one side is less than that from the opposite side.
    - Directional preponderance—25–30% more nystagmus than the other side indicates preponderance on that side.
  - Conditions associated:
    - Canal paresis indicates a depressed function of the ipsilateral side—Meniere's disease, acoustic neuroma, vestibular neurectomy, postlabyrinthectomy.
    - Directional preponderance—occurs to the side of central lesion, away from the side in peripheral lesion.
    - Meniere's disease on one side—shows canal paresis on same side and directional preponderance to the other side. In acoustic neuroma—canal paresis and directional preponderance to the ipsilateral side.
- **Cold air caloric test (Fig. 1):**
  - Done in tympanic membrane (TM) perforation (as irrigating with water is contraindicated).
  - A coiled copper tube wrapped in cloth called Dundas–Grant tube is used.
  - Air inside the tube is cooled by using ethyl chloride and then blown into the ear.

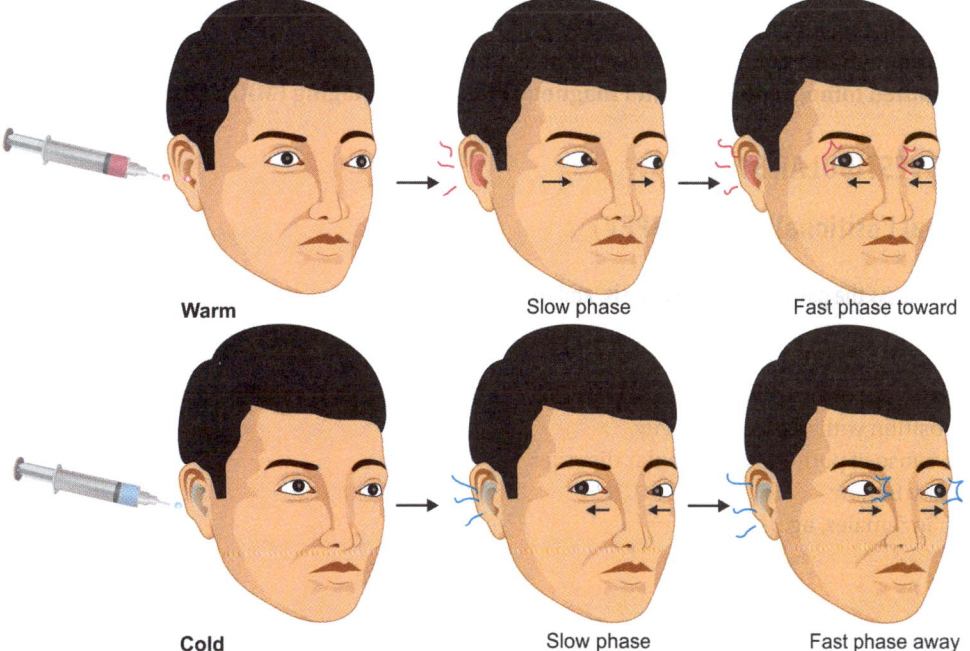

Fig. 1: Caloric reflex test.

Electronystagmography

- Detects both spontaneous and induced nystagmus (by caloric, positional, rotational optokinetic stimulus)
- Depends on the presence of corneo-retinal potentials—recorded using electrodes placed around the eyes
- Useful to detect nystagmus not seen by the naked eyes.
- Also helps in the permanent recording of the nystagmus.

Optokinetic Test

- Useful to diagnose the central lesion—brainstem and cerebral hemispheres
- Patient is asked to follow a series of vertical stripes on a drum from right to left followed by left to right.
- Normally it produces nystagmus with a slow component in the direction of stripes.

Rotational Test

- Patient sits in a Barany's revolving chair with head tilted forward 30° with rotation of chair (10 turns in 20 seconds).
- Chair is stopped abruptly—nystagmus observed
- Normally: 25–40 seconds of nystagmus.
- Useful in congenital anomalies with atresia of ear canal (caloric test cannot be performed)
- Disadvantage—stimulation of both the labyrinths simultaneously during the rotation.
- Now the advanced form of test—with electronystagmography and computer analysis of nystagmus recorded.

Galvanic Test

- It is the only test that differentiates an end-organ lesion from the vestibular nerve.
- A patient stands with the feet together, eyes closed and arms outstretched.
- A current of 1 mA is passed to one ear and body swaying is studied.

Posturography

Evaluates vestibular function by measuring postural stability.

Other Investigations

- **Audiometry test**: Distinguishing peripheral causes.
- **Brainstem evoked audiometry:** 90–95% sense for detecting **acoustic neuroma**.
- **Imaging—computed tomography (CT) and magnetic resonance imaging (MRI)**: Distinguishing central cause.

■ DISORDERS OF VESTIBULAR SYSTEM

Benign Paroxysmal Positional Vertigo (BPPV)

Q. Describe BPPV—discuss the pathogenesis, diagnosis, and treatment.

Definition

It is a peripheral vestibular disorder characterized by brief attack of vertigo with associated nystagmus, precipitated by certain changes in head position with respect to gravity.

- Most common cause of peripheral vestibular disorder
- First described by Bárány
- More common in females, age: 40–50 years

Pathology

Otoconia: Crystals of calcium carbonate, normally found embedded in the gelatinous otolithic membrane of utricle and saccule.

Etiology

- ❖ Idiopathic
- ❖ Head trauma
- ❖ Vestibular neuritis
- ❖ Meniere's syndrome

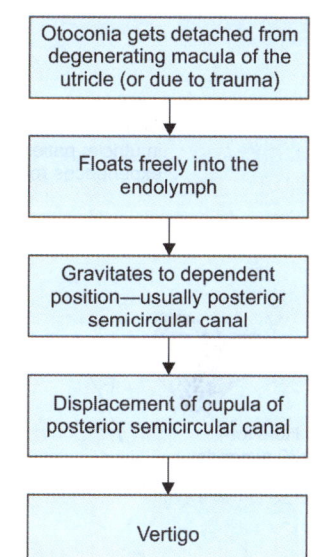

Clinical Features

- ❖ **Symptoms:**
  - ▷ Vertigo:
    - ♦ With a change in head position, rolling over or getting out of the bed
    - ♦ It is side-specific
    - ♦ Sudden onset, lasting for less than a minute
    - ♦ Have few asymptomatic periods in between
- ❖ **Sign:**
  - ▷ Nystagmus: Elicited on Dix–Hallpike maneuver
  - ▷ Caloric test: Normal or hypofunctional
  - ▷ Neurological examination: Normal

Management

- ❖ **Diagnosis:**
  - ▷ Typical history
  - ▷ **Dix–Hallpike maneuver**—the patient is guided through a series of movements known to elicit nystagmus in a BPPV patient.
- ❖ **Treatment:**
  - ▷ Supportive—as most patients have spontaneous resolution of the symptoms
    - ♦ Vestibulosuppressant medication
  - ▷ Persistent symptoms: First line of treatment is—canalith repositioning maneuver (Epley's maneuver)
    - ♦ Principle—attempting to reposition the free-floating canalith particles from semicircular canals to utricle using gravity
    - ♦ Maneuvers are 90% effective
  - ▷ **Epley's maneuver (Fig. 2):**

Q. Write a short note on Epley's repositioning maneuver.

- ❖ Patient is made to sit on the table with legs extended and the doctor stands behind the patient
- ❖ Affected side is identified using Dix–Hallpike maneuver, latency, and duration of nystagmus were noted.
- ❖ Patient is sitting with a head turned 45° to the affected side.
- ❖ Step 1: Patient is brought down and head extended over the edge of the table—vertigo and nystagmus noted—wait till symptoms subside.
- ❖ Step 2: Then turn the head 90° to the opposite side (i.e., affected ear up)
- ❖ Step 3: Rotate head and body 90° away from the affected ear, facing downward (135° from supine position)
- ❖ Step 4: Patient is brought to sitting position and head turned downward 20°
- ❖ Each position to be maintained for 30 seconds or until symptoms subside
- ❖ After completion of maneuver—upright position for 48 hours, and avoid shaking the head.
- ❖ Most patients (80%) recover with a single maneuver, it can be repeated if required.
  - ▷ **Brandt–Daroff positional exercises (Fig. 3):**
    - ♦ Self-treatment exercise
    - ♦ Rapid sequence of head and body tilt
    - ♦ Starting from the sitting position
    - ♦ Lying on the affected side (nose 45° up) and remaining in this position for at least 30 seconds, or until vertigo subsides.
    - ♦ Complete relief from BPPV within 3–14 days in 98% of treated patients.

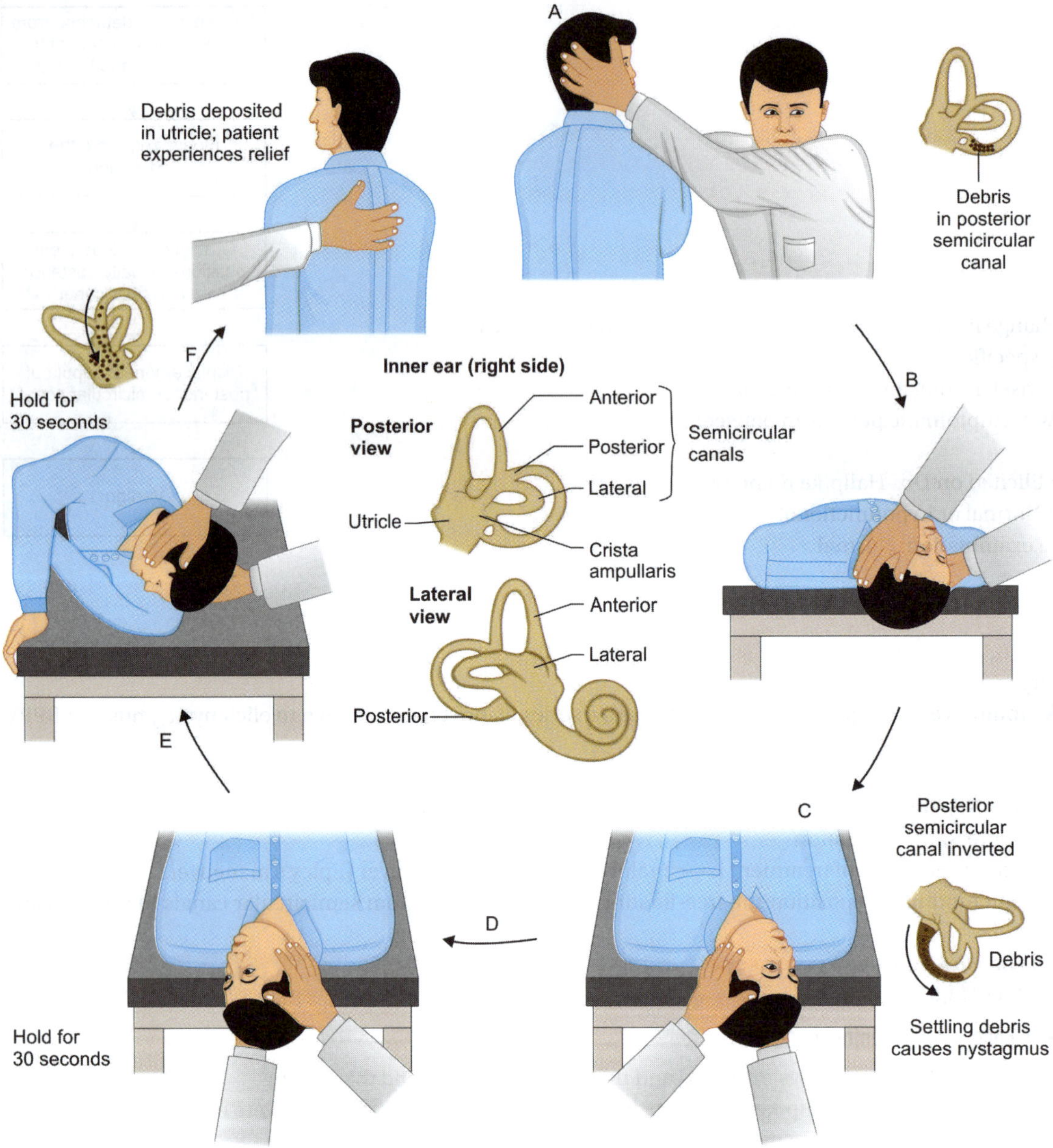

116   **PART 1:** Diseases of ENT, Head and Neck

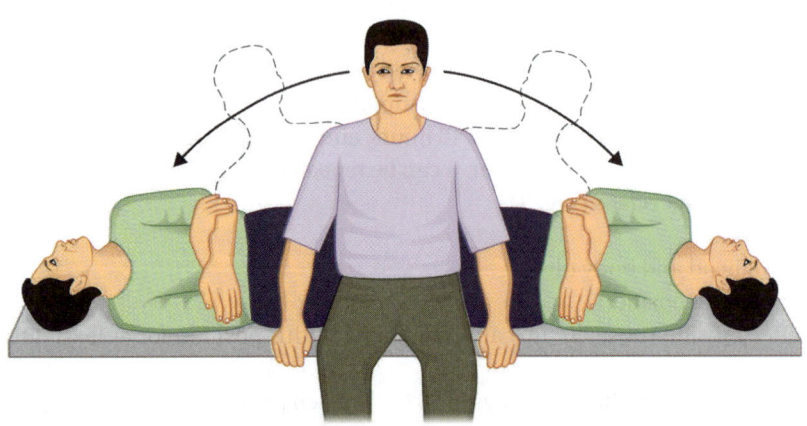

Fig. 2: Epley's repositioning maneuver (scan QR code).

Fig. 3: Brandt–Daroff exercises.

CHAPTER 15: Assessment and Disorders of Vestibular System

Cawthorne–Cooksey Exercises (Fig. 4)

Another set of self-treatment exercises used in BPPV

Exercises in bed

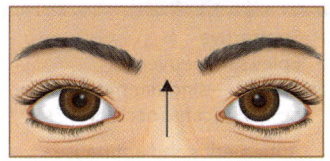
- Looking up and then down

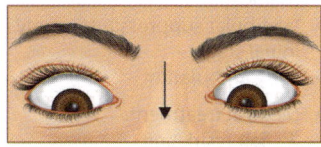
- Looking alternatively left and right

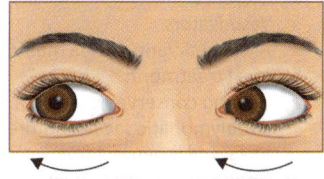

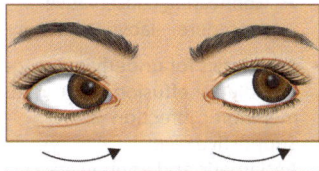
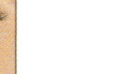
- Convergence exercises

Exercises in sitting position

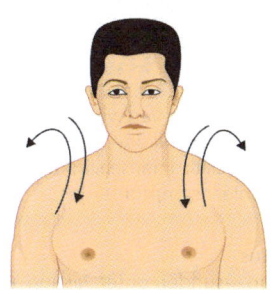
- Shrugging and rotating shoulders

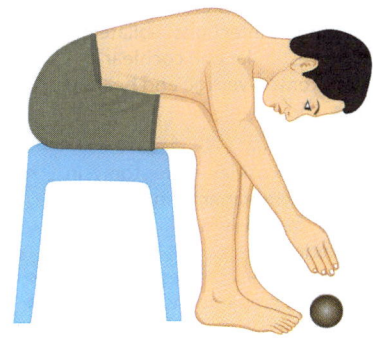
- Bending forward and picking up objects

Head movements

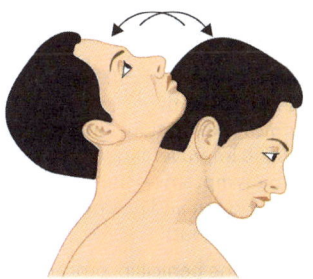
- Bending alternately forward and backward

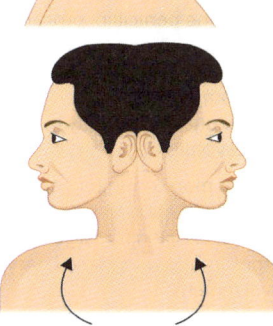
- Turning alternately to left and then right

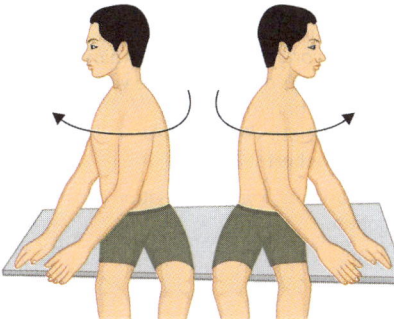
- Turning head and trunk alternately to the left and right

Fig. 4: Cawthorne–Cooksey exercises.

- ❖ **Surgical treatment:**
  - ➢ For patient's refractory to repositioning maneuvers
  - ➢ Surgical procedures—singular neurectomy
  - ➢ Posterior semicircular canal occlusion

Peripheral Vestibular Disorders

Q. Discuss/write an essay on various peripheral vestibular disorder.

	Disorder	Clinical features	Diagnosis	Treatment
1.	BPPV (most common cause of peripheral vestibular disorder)	Positional vertigo nystagmus	Dix–Hallpike maneuver	❖ Supportive ❖ Epley's maneuver ❖ Surgery—singular neurectomy, posterior canal occlusion
2.	Vestibular neuronitis (second most common cause)	❖ Sudden onset severe vertigo lasting for several days ❖ With associated nausea, vomiting ❖ No cochlear symptoms	Audiometry electronystagmography	❖ Antiemetics and antinausea medications ❖ Vestibular suppressants—only in the initial stage ❖ Early ambulation
3.	Meniere's disease	❖ Tinnitus ❖ Vertigo—sudden onset, lasting a few minutes to 24 hours ❖ SNHL—fluctuating ❖ Aural fullness	Audiometry	❖ Medical treatment: ➢ Salt restriction ➢ Diuretics ➢ Vasodilators ➢ Antiemetic/antinausea medications ❖ Surgical treatment: ➢ Hearing conservative—endolymphatic sac decompression, a vestibular neurectomy ➢ Nonhearing conservative procedure—labyrinthectomy
4.	Labyrinthitis	❖ Otogenic—due to ear infection—unilateral ❖ Meningitic infections—bilateral ❖ Both vestibular and cochlear symptoms—vertigo and hearing loss	❖ Audiometry—SNHL/mixed hearing loss ❖ Electronystagmography	❖ Antibiotics for underlying otogenic, (middle ear effusion/mastoiditis) or meningitic infection ❖ Supportive care ❖ Antiemetic and antinausea medications
5.	Vestibulotoxic drugs (damage to hair cells)	Causes: ❖ Aminoglycosides—streptomycin, gentamicin, kanamycin ❖ Antihypertensives ❖ Diuretics ❖ Labyrinthine sedatives ❖ Estrogen preparations ❖ Antimalarials	❖ Audiometry—high frequency—before, during, and after the treatment ❖ Electronystagmography ❖ Posturography	❖ Prevention—dose of the drug should be titrated according to weight, duration of treatment limited ❖ Otoprotective agents: ➢ Antioxidants ➢ Iron chelators for aminoglycoside toxicity
6.	Perilymph fistula	❖ Both vestibular and cochlear symptoms ❖ Tullio's phenomenon ❖ Fistula test positive	❖ Serial audiograms ❖ Fraser test—improvement in audiogram after lying in Trendelenburg position for 30 minutes	❖ Conservative: Bedrest, head elevation, laxatives ❖ Surgical exploration—in patients with no improvement or worsening of the symptoms—the fistula should be found out and patched with a graft (fascia/fat)
7.	Syphilis ❖ Congenital ❖ Acquired	❖ Dizziness, SNHL ❖ Late congenital syphilis—mimics Meniere's diseases (acute vertigo, SNHL, tinnitus) ❖ False-positive fistula test—Hennebert's sign	❖ VDRL test ❖ FTA-ABS ❖ TPHA test	❖ Benzathine penicillin, procaine penicillin ❖ Tetracycline ❖ Erythromycin ❖ Ceftriaxone—especially in neurosyphilis
8.	Acoustic neuroma	Unsteadiness, a vague sensation of motion	❖ Contrast-enhanced MRI ❖ CT temporal bone	❖ Regular monitoring for very small tumors ❖ Surgical excision for large symptomatic with cranial nerves involvement
9.	Head trauma	❖ Mechanism—concussion of labyrinth, perilymph fistula, damage to vestibular end organ ❖ Vertigo	HRCT temporal bone—to rule out fractures	❖ Symptomatic treatment

(BPPV: benign paroxysmal positional vertigo; CT: computerized tomography; EEG: electroencephalogram; FTA-ABS: fluorescent treponemal antibody absorption; HRCT: high-resolution computed tomography; MRI: magnetic resonance imaging; SNHL: sensorineural hearing loss; TPHA: *Treponema pallidum* hemagglutination; VDRL: venereal disease research laboratory)

Central Vestibular Disorders

Q. Discuss/write an essay on various central vestibular disorders.

Disorder	Cause	Vestibular symptoms	Other symptoms
1. Vertebrobasilar ischemic stroke			
2. Vertebrobasilar insufficiency (transient decrease in cerebral blood flow)	❖ Common cause of vertebrobasilar insufficiency in age >50 years ❖ Atherosclerosis ❖ Aggravated by—cervical osteophytes pressing on vertebral arteries or hypotension	❖ Vertigo ❖ Dizziness, nausea and vomiting (symptoms mainly on lateral rotation and extension of head)	Neurological—visual disturbances, diplopia, drop attacks, hemianopia, dysphagia, and hemiparesis
3. Vestibular migraine			
4. Wallenberg syndrome	Thrombosis of the posteroinferior cerebellar artery—cuts off supply to lateral medullary area	❖ Violent vertigo ❖ Horizontal or rotatory nystagmus to side of lesion	❖ Diplopia ❖ Dysphagia ❖ Hoarseness of voice ❖ Horner's syndrome ❖ Sensory loss—on ipsilateral face and contralateral side of body ❖ Ataxia
5. Basilar migraine	❖ Vascular syndrome ❖ Common in adolescent girls and strong menstrual relationship ❖ Positive family history	Vertigo—abrupt onset, lasting 5–60 minutes	❖ Recurrent headache—unilateral, throbbing ❖ Occipital headache—in basilar artery migraine ❖ Visual disturbance ❖ Diplopia
6. Cerebellar disease	❖ Hemorrhage—hypertension ❖ Infarction ❖ Infection ❖ Slow growing tumors	❖ Severe vertigo ❖ Ataxia ❖ Vomiting	❖ Incoordination ❖ Past-pointing ❖ Adiadochokinesia ❖ Rebound phenomenon ❖ Wide-based gait
7. Multiple sclerosis	❖ Demyelinating disease ❖ Young adults	❖ Vertigo ❖ Dizziness ❖ Spontaneous nystagmus ❖ Nystagmus—acquired pendular, dissociated, upbeating vertical (important features)	❖ Blurring/loss of vision ❖ Diplopia ❖ Dysarthria ❖ Paresthesia ❖ Ataxia
8. Tumors of fourth ventricle and brainstem	❖ Midbrain—gliomas, astrocytomas ❖ Fourth ventricle floor—medulloblastoma, ependymoma, epidermoid cyst, teratoma	❖ Vertigo ❖ Dizziness	❖ Neurological symptoms ❖ CT scan and MRI
9. Epilepsy	❖ Vertigo as an aura of epilepsy ❖ Unconsciousness, seizure following aura	Vertigo	❖ EEG abnormal
10. Cervical vertigo	❖ Neck injury (7–10 days back) ❖ Disturbed vertebrobasilar circulation ❖ Sympathetic cervical plexus involvement ❖ Alteration of tonic neck reflexes	Vertigo on moving the neck to the side of injury	❖ Tenderness of neck ❖ Spasms of cervical muscles ❖ Restricted neck movements ❖ X-ray shows loss of cervical lordosis

(CT: computerized tomography; EEG: electroencephalogram; MRI: magnetic resonance imaging)

- ❖ **Other causes of vertigo**
  - ➤ **Endocrine causes:** Hypoglycemia, adrenal failure, and pheochromocytoma
  - ➤ **Cardiovascular causes:** Vasovagal syncope, orthostatic hypotension, and arrhythmias
  - ➤ **Ocular vertigo:** Acute extraocular muscle paresis or high errors of refraction
  - ➤ **Psychogenic vertigo:**
    - ♦ Panic attack, emotional tension and anxiety, and phobias.
    - ♦ It is often described as light headedness.
    - ♦ Other associated symptoms such as palpitation, breathlessness, fatigue, insomnia, profuse sweating, and tremors with no hearing loss or tinnitus. Caloric test shows exaggerated response.

Chapter 16

Deaf Child and Rehabilitation of Hearing Impaired

EN4.20: Describe the clinical features, investigations, and management of Deaf child.

■ INTRODUCTION

Q. Write short note/essay on etiology and signs of hearing loss in a deaf-mute child.

- Hearing loss >90 is profound hearing loss or total deafness
- Deafness is a common childhood problem (seen in 1 in 1,000 births)
- Children born with total deafness fail to develop speech hence termed deaf-mute (speech center is normal, the main defect is deafness)
- Speech and language development occur in the first 5 years of age, and normal hearing plays a crucial role in speech development.
- Early identification, assessment, and rehabilitation (before 6 months of age) play a major role for better vocabulary and comprehensive language skill development

■ ETIOLOGY

- In the developed world—genetic causes
- In the developing world—infectious causes

Prenatal causes	<ul><li>Infant factors: Inner ear anomalies due to genetic or nongenetic factors</li><li>It may affect membranous labyrinth of the inner ear or bony labyrinth or both components are malformed.</li><li>Maternal factors:<ul><li>Infections during pregnancy: TO: Toxoplasmosis R: Rubella C: *Cytomegalovirus* HE: Herpes type 1, type 2 S: Syphilis</li><li>Medication during pregnancy crosses the placental barrier and affects the developing fetus's ear— gentamicin, streptomycin, amikacin, chloroquine</li><li>Radiation during pregnancy, diabetes, hypothyroidism, and maternal alcoholism</li></ul></li></ul>
Perinatal causes	<ul><li>Premature baby with low birth weight (<1,500 g)</li><li>Fetal anoxia—due to prolonged labor, meconium aspiration, cord around neck cord prolapse, anoxia of brain causes damage to cochlear nucleus</li><li>Birth related trauma—forceps delivery resulting in intracranial hemorrhage</li><li>Kernicterus</li><li>Ototoxic drug used—for meningitis, septicemia</li></ul>
Postnatal causes	<ul><li>Post-traumatic hearing loss</li><li>Following infection—measles, mumps, influenza</li><li>Secretory otitis media</li><li>Noise-induced deafness</li><li>Ototoxic drugs use</li></ul>

CLASSIFICATION OF CONGENITAL MALFORMATION OF INNER EAR

Q. Classify congenital malformations of inner ear resulting in deaf-mute child.

- **Malformation limited to membranous labyrinth:**
  - **Siebenmann–Bing:** Complete membranous labyrinthine dysplasia
  - Limited membranous labyrinthine
  - Cochleosaccular dysplasia (Scheibe)
  - Cochlear basal turn dysplasia (Alexander)
- **Malformation of both osseous and membranous labyrinth:**
  - Michel-complete labyrinthine aplasia
  - Cochlear anomalies
  - Cochlear hypoplasia
  - Mondini—incomplete partition
  - Common cavity
- **Labyrinthine anomalies:**
  - Semicircular canal dysplasia
  - Semicircular canal aplasia
- **Aqueductal anomalies:**
  - Enlarged vestibular aqueduct
  - Enlarged cochlear aqueduct
- **Internal auditory canal anomalies:**
  - Narrow internal auditory canal

SYNDROMES ASSOCIATED WITH HEARING LOSS

Waardenburg syndrome (AD) SNHL	❖ Retinitis pigmentosa ❖ White forelock ❖ Heterochromia iridis ❖ Vitiligo ❖ Dystopia canthorum
Usher syndrome (AR) SNHL	❖ Retinitis pigmentosa ❖ Night blindness
Jervell and Lange–Nielsen syndrome (AR) SNHL	❖ Syncopal attacks ❖ Prolonged Q interval in ECG
Pendred syndrome (AR) SNHL	❖ Defective iodine transport ❖ Goiter
Alport syndrome (AD) SNHL	❖ Hereditary progressive glomerulonephritis ❖ Corneal dystrophy
Treacher Collins syndrome (AD) **Mandibulofacial dysostosis** CHL	❖ Antimongoloid palpebral fissure ❖ Coloboma of lower lid ❖ Mandibular, malar bone hypoplasia ❖ Malformation of malleus and incus
Crouzon syndrome (AD) **Conductive/mixed hearing loss**	❖ Frog eyes ❖ Hypertelorism ❖ Parrot beak nose ❖ Mandibular prognathism ❖ Mental retardation with premature closure of cranial sutures
Apert (AD) stapes fixation **Conductive hearing loss**	❖ Syndactyly ❖ With all features of Crouzon syndrome
Branchiootorenal syndrome (AD conductive/mixed hearing loss)	❖ Branchial fistula/cyst ❖ Deformity of pinna, preauricular pits/sinus ❖ Renal abnormalities
Van der Hoeve syndrome (AD) SNHL	❖ Osteogenesis imperfecta with a history of bone fractures ❖ Blue sclera ❖ Hearing loss
Stickler syndrome (AD) SNHL	❖ Small jaw ❖ Cleft plat ❖ Myopia, retinal detachment

Contd...

PART 1: Diseases of ENT, Head and Neck

Contd...

Pierre Robbin sequence (AD) SNHL	❖ Cataract ❖ Juvenile onset arthritis ❖ Micrognathia ❖ Glossoptosis ❖ Cleft palate ❖ Part of stickler syndrome
Goldenhar's syndrome **Facio-auriculo-vertebral dysplasia (AD)** **Conductive/mixed hearing loss**	❖ Facial asymmetry ❖ Low set ear, atretic ear canal ❖ Preauricular tag ❖ Hemivertibrae of cervical region ❖ Coloboma of upper lid
Down's syndrome (trisomy 21) **Conductive hearing loss**	❖ Microcephaly ❖ Mental retardation ❖ Short stature ❖ Epicanthal fold ❖ Stenosis of ear canal ❖ Atlantoaxial instability
Klippel–Feil syndrome (AR) SNHL	❖ Short neck ❖ Fused cervical vertebrae ❖ Spina bifida ❖ Atretic ear canal

(AD: autosomal dominant; AR: autosomal recessive; CHL: conductive hearing loss; ECG: electrocardiogram; SNHL: sensorineural hearing loss)

■ POSSIBLE SIGNS MAY SUGGEST A CHILD IS HAVING HEARING LOSS

❖ Fail to startle to loud noise.
❖ Child sleep through loud noise unperturbed.
❖ Failure to development of speech at 1 year of age.
❖ Child does not respond appropriately unless looking directly at you.
❖ Child's vocabulary is less than other children of his age.
❖ Childs speech is unclear and difficult to understand.
❖ Difficulty in school/poor academic performance.

■ ASSESSMENT OF HEARING IN INFANTS AND CHILDREN

Q. How will you assess the loss of hearing in infants and children?

Neonatal Screening Procedure

❖ **Arousal test**—high-frequency narrow-band noise presented to infants for 2 seconds, a normal infant can be aroused twice in three such stimuli.
❖ **Auditory response cradle**—(newborn) baby is placed in the cradle to monitor his behavior (trunk, limb movement, respiration, and head jerk) by a transducer in response to auditory stimuli.
❖ Auditory brainstem response (ABR)/otoacoustic emissions (OAE).

Behavior Observation Audiometry (0–6 months)

❖ **Moro's reflex**—in a normal infant on exposure to 80–90 dB auditory stimuli will have a startled look (sudden movement of limbs and extension of head), the absence of Moro's reflex is abnormal.
❖ **Cochleopalpebral reflex**—child responds by blinking to aloud sound.
❖ **Cessation reflex**—infant stops activity or start crying in response to a sound of 90 dB.

Distraction Technique (age 6–18 months)

❖ Child is seated on his parent's lap being distracted by the assistant while the examiner produces sound from behind or from side to see if child can locate sound.
❖ Distractor should not look at the tester at any time.

Conditioning Techniques

Visual Reinforcement Audiometry (6–36 months)
- Child on parent's lap.
- One examiner distracts the child, and sound stimuli were given, each time child hears a sound and locates sound he is rewarded by seeing a motivational toy (moving clown/illuminating toy).
- Test is to reduce the habituation to sound (seen in children over the age of 1 year) and reinforces the localization of sound stimulus.

Conditioned Play Audiometry (2–5 years)
- Teach the child to complete a motor act.
- Each time child hears a sound, the child is conditioned to place an object in a box or a ring on a stack.

Tangible Reinforcement Operant Conditioning Audiometry
Child is taught to push a button when a sound is heard, reinforced with chocolate.

Objective Test
- **Electrocochleography:**
  - Invasive procedure requires placement of electrode through the tympanic membrane, it measures auditory sensitivity within 20 dB.
- **Auditory brainstem response:**
  - Noninvasive technique to find the integrity of central auditory pathway (refer to hearing test)
- **Otoacoustic emission test:**
  - Screening test but not for confirmation.
  - Takes only a few minutes to perform.
  - A normal functioning cochlea will produce an echo or emission that suggests that the hair cells in cochlea are functioning.
- **Pure tone audiometry (3 years onwards)**
- **Impedance audiometry**

Imaging
- CT scan [high-resolution computed tomography (HRCT) temporal bone]—to see cochlear dysplasia, cochlear hypoplasia, and small internal auditory canal
- MRI scan—to detect central nervous system (CNS) abnormality

> **3–6 screening goal**
> - Screen all babies = ES for hearing loss by 1 month of age
> - Evaluate or assess by audiologist by 3 months of age
> - Intervene by 6 months of age

MANAGEMENT AND REHABILITATION

Q. Write a short note/essay on management and rehabilitation of deaf-mute child.

Q. Write a note on cochlear implants.

Assessment of type and degree of hearing loss, other handicaps such as developmental delay and mental retardation, whether deafness is prelingual or postlingual.

Aim of Habilitation
- Development of speech and language
- Adjustment in society
- Useful employment in vocation

Parental Guidance
- Deal with sympathetically
- Explain disability of child
- Counseling of parent regarding deaf child rehabilitation requires lots of effort from parents for frequent follow-up visit, home education, and periodic change of hearing aid or ear module

Hearing Aid

In deaf child residual hearing (small but useful) amplified with use of hearing aid as early as possible which is also helpful for learning lip reading

Cochlear Implant

- ❖ **Selection of candidates:**
    - ➢ Bilateral profound sensorineural hearing loss
    - ➢ Age group >12 months
    - ➢ No appreciable benefit from hearing aid us (3–6 months)
    - ➢ Normal neurological, mental development
    - ➢ Normal morphological development of cochlea
    - ➢ Motivational parents
- ❖ **Cochlear implant surgery:** In this case a cochlear implant **(Fig. 7)** might be best option. Cochlear implant bypass the inner ear to directly stimulate the inner ear to directly stimulate the hearing nerve to provide the child with clarity of sound and speech they need to help them understand what is being said.
- ❖ **Steps of cochlear implant surgery**
    - ➢ Postaural incision taken **(Fig. 1)**
    - ➢ Cortical mastoidectomy done
    - ➢ Well created for placement of implant in postaural area **(Fig. 2)**
    - ➢ Implant placed in the well **(Figs. 3 and 5)**
    - ➢ Electrode placed in round window through posterior tympanotomy approach **(Figs. 4 and 6)**
    - ➢ Postaural suturing done
    - ➢ Postoperative X-rays done to confirm placement of implant **(Fig. 8)**
    - ➢ Neural response telemetry (NRT) is done for capturing the action potential of the distal portion of the auditory nerve in cochlear implant users, using the CI itself to elicit and record the answers.
- ❖ **Contraindications:**
    - ➢ Cochlear malformation
    - ➢ Disorder of central auditory pathway
    - ➢ Active middle ear infection

Development of Speech and Language

- ❖ Auditory—oral communication (used by normal person)
- ❖ Hearing aid augments auditory perceptions in moderate-to-severe hearing loss/postlingual deaf along with training of lip reading, face, hand, and body gesture.

Manual Communication

- ❖ Sign language
- ❖ Finger spelling method

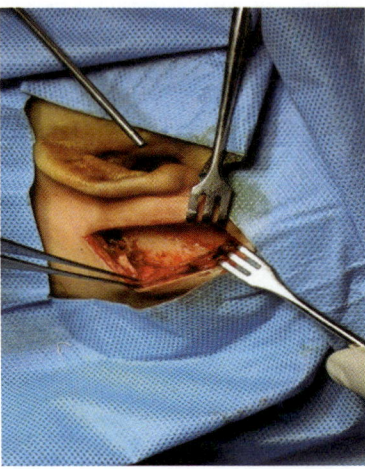

Fig. 1: Postaural incision for cochlear implant surgery.

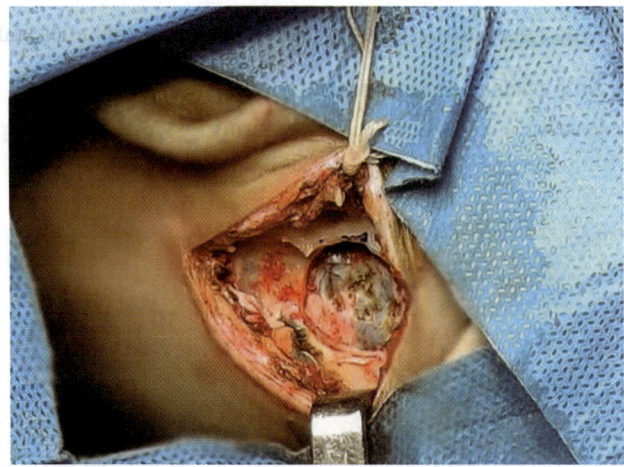

Fig. 2: Well created in postaural area for cochlear implant fitting.

CHAPTER 16: Deaf Child and Rehabilitation of Hearing Impaired

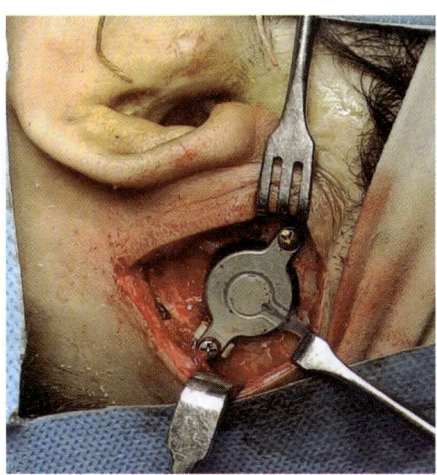

Fig. 3: Cochlear implant device placed.

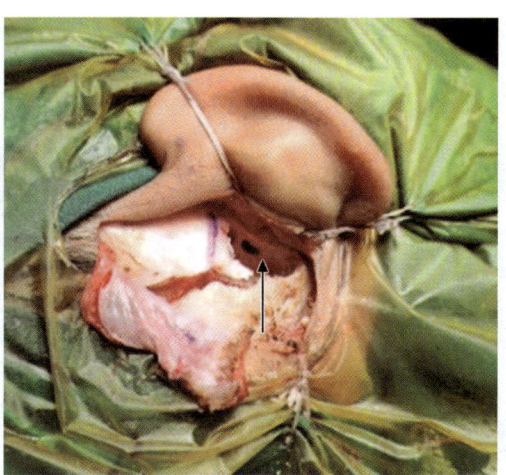

Fig. 4: Posterior tympanotomy done for cochlear implant electrode (arrow).

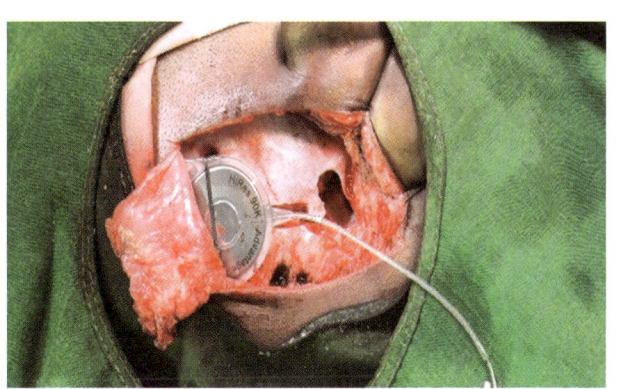

Fig. 5: Cochlear implant device with electrode being placed postaurally.

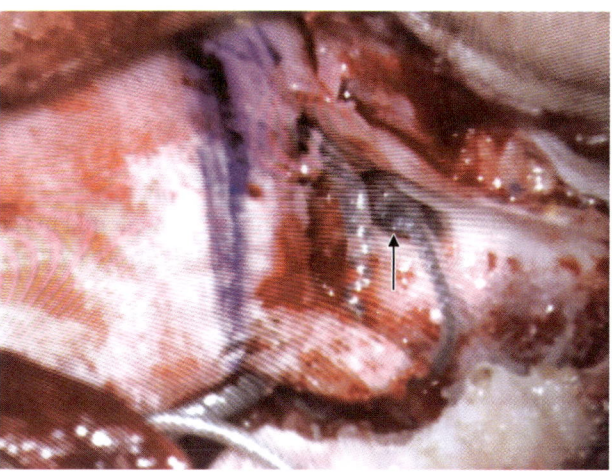

Fig. 6: Cochlear implant electrode being placed in round window (arrow).

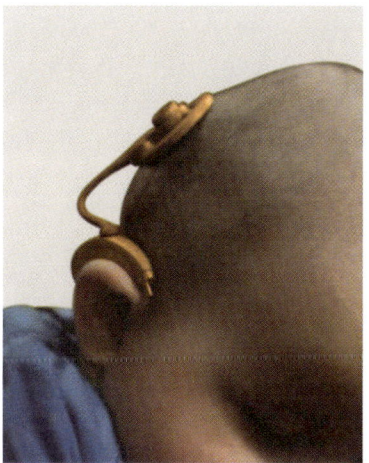

Fig. 7: Cochlear implant.

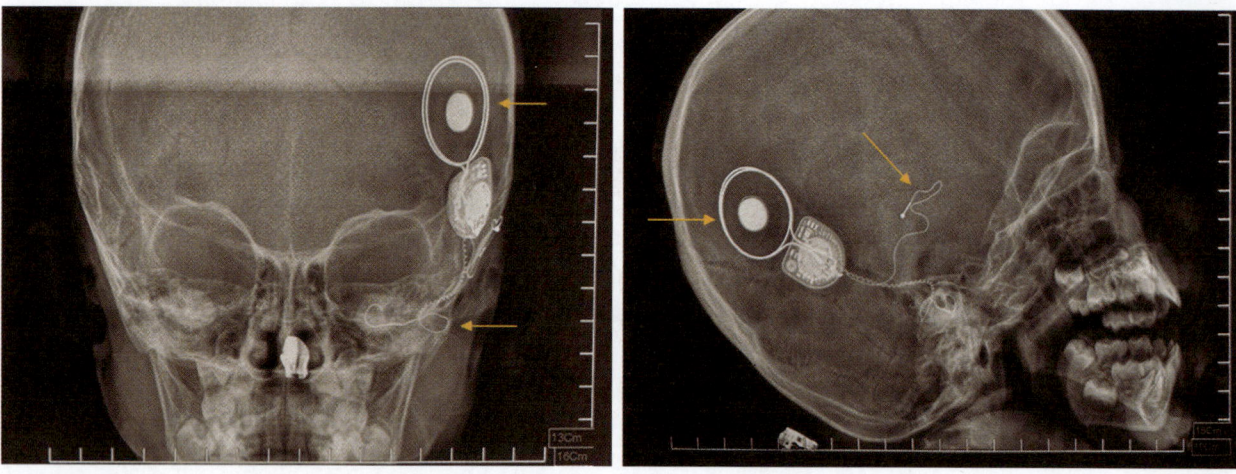

Fig. 8: Postoperative X-rays showing cochlear implant inserted.

Total Communication

- **Using all modalities of sensory input:** Auditory, visual, tactile kinesthetic to teach oral speech, lip reading, sign language for prelingual profound deafness
- **Vibrotactile aids:** For a totally deaf and blind.

Education of Deaf

- For deaf child—residential and day school
- For child with moderate hearing loss—integrated in normal school with preferential seating ahead in class, use of radio hearing aid (microphone and transmitter worn by teacher, receiver and amplifier by child).

Chapter 17

Facial Nerve and its Disorders

■ INTRODUCTION

Q. Write a short note/essay on facial nerve and its branches.

The facial nerve is a mixed nerve, having both motor and sensory roots. There are two efferent and two afferent pathways.

Components of the Facial Nerve

Efferent pathway		Afferent pathway	
Special visceral	General visceral	Special visceral	General visceral
Forms the motor root	Supplies secretomotor fibers	Brings taste sensation from the anterior two-thirds of tongue and the plate	Brings general sensation from the concha, posterosuperior part of external canal, and the tympanic membrane
Supplies all muscles of the second branchial arch	Lacrimal, submandibular and sublingual glands	Chorda tympani and greater superficial petrosal nerves are afferent fibers	It also brings proprioceptive sensation from the facial muscles

Course of Facial Nerve (Fig. 1)

The motor nucleus is situated in the pons and receives fibers from the precentral gyrus. The upper part of the nucleus which innervates the muscles of forehead receives fibers from both the cerebral hemisphere whereas the lower part of the nucleus which supplies the lower face received crossed fibers from one hemisphere only.

The motor fibers originate from the nucleus of VIIth nerve, hook around the nucleus of VIth nerve, and received the sensory root of nerve of Wrisberg. Facial nerve leaves the brain at the pontomedullary junction, travels through posterior cranial fossa to enter the internal acoustic meatus, it enters the bony facial canal, and exits through the stylomastoid foramen where it crosses the styloid process and divides into terminal branches.

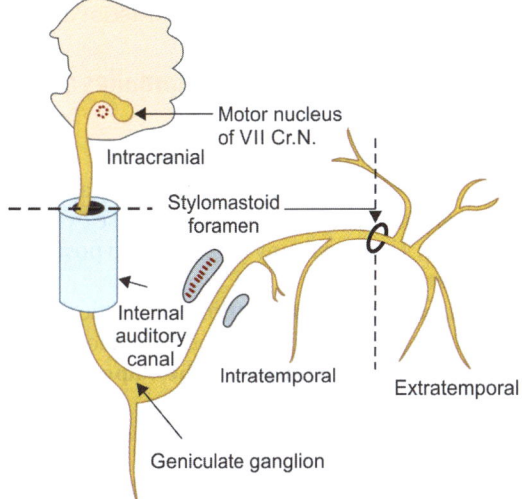

Fig. 1: Course of facial nerve.

The course can be divided into three parts:
1. **Intracranial part:** It is 15–17 mm in length and extends from the pons to internal acoustic meatus.
2. **Intratemporal part:** Extends from the internal acoustic meatus to the styloid foramen.
   It is further divided into:
   ➤ *Meatal segment:* It lies within the internal acoustic meatus. It is about 8–10 mm in length.
   ➤ *Labyrinthine segment:* It extends from the fundus of meatus to the geniculate ganglion and takes a posterior turn and forms a genu. The nerve is thinnest in this segment and the bony canal is also the narrowest. Thus edema or inflammation can easily compress the nerve and cause paralysis.

- *Tympanic or horizontal segment:* It is about 11 mm in length and extends from the geniculate ganglion to the pyramidal eminence and lies just above the oval window and below the lateral semicircular canal.
- *Mastoid or vertical segment:* It extends from the pyramid to stylomastoid foramen. It is about 13 mm in length.
3. **Extracranial part:** It extends from the stylomastoid foramen to the termination of its peripheral branches.

Branches of Facial Nerve (Fig. 2)

- **Greater superficial petrosal nerve:**
  - Arises from the geniculate ganglion.
  - It carries secretomotor fibers to the lacrimal and glands of nasal mucosa and palate.
- **Nerve to stapedius:**
  - Arises from the second genu to supply the stapedius muscle.
- **Chorda tympani:** Arises from the middle of the vertical segment. It passes between the incus and neck of malleus and leaves the tympanic cavity through a petrotympanic fissure.
  - It carries secretomotor fibers to submandibular and sublingual and brings taste from the anterior two-thirds of tongue.
- **Communicating branch:** It joins auricular branch of vagus to supply the concha, retroauricular groove, posterior meatus, and the outer surface of tympanic membrane.
- **Posterior auricular nerve:** This branch supplies muscles of the pinna, occipital belly of occipitofrontalis, and communicates with auricular branch of the vagus.
- Muscular branches supply the stylohyoid and posterior belly of digastric.
- **Peripheral branches:** The nerve trunk divides into upper temporofacial and lower cervicofacial branches.
- The cervicofacial further divides into—temporal, zygomatic, buccal, mandibular, and cervical branches to supply all the muscles of facial expression.

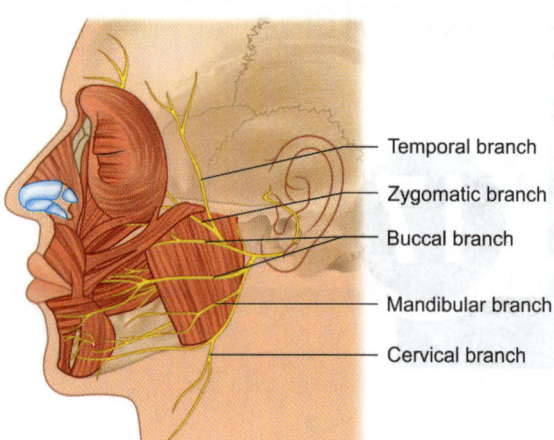

Fig. 2: Facial nerve course and branching.

Blood Supply of Facial Nerve

The facial nerve receives blood supply from four vessels. All the arteries form an external plexus that lies in the epineurium and feeds a deeper intraneural internal plexus:
- Anterior-inferior cerebellar artery supplies the intracranial segment.
- Labyrinthine artery supplies the nerve in internal auditory canal. It is a branch of the anterior-inferior cerebellar artery.
- Superfiacial petrosal artery branch of middle meningeal artery supplies geniculate gangion and its adjacent regions
- Stylomastoid artery branch of posterior auricular artery supplies mastoid and tympanic segment

Anatomical Variations and Anomalies of Facial Nerve

- **Bony dehiscence:**
  - It is the absence of bony cover and is the most common anomaly and occurs most commonly in the tympanic segment.
  - It is prone to injury during surgery and gets easily involved in the middle ear infections.
  - The dehiscent nerve may prolapse over the stapes making approach to stapes difficult.
- **Hump:** The nerve may make a hump posteriorly near the horizontal canal making it vulnerable to injury during mastoid surgery.
- **Bifurcation and trifurcation:** The vertical part of facial nerve divides into two or three branches, each occupying a separate canal and exiting through individual foramen.
- **Bifurcation and enclosing the stapes:** The nerve divides proximal to an oval window—one part passing above and the other below it and then reuniting.
- **Between oval and round windows:** Just before oval window the nerve crosses the middle ear passing between oval and round windows.

■ FACIAL NERVE INJURY

Q. Discuss facial nerve injury.

The nerve injury may be:
- **Neurapraxia:** It is characterized by a partial obstruction of flow of axoplasm through the axons.
- **Axonotmesis:** It is characterized by axonal injury.
- **Neurotmesis:** It is characterized by injury to the nerve

Sunderland Classification of Nerve Injury

It is based on anatomical structure of the nerve:
- **First degree**: Partial block of axoplasm flow. No morphological changes are seen. There is complete recovery.
- **Second degree**: There is loss of axons but the endoneurial tubes remain intact and recovery is good. The axons grow into their respective tubes.
- **Third degree**: There is an injury of endoneurium. Synkinesis occurs during recovery as axons of one tube grow into another.
- **Fourth degree**: There is injury of the perineurium causing partial resection of the nerve. Scarring will impair the regeneration of fibers.
- **Fifth degree**: There is injury of epineurium causing complete nerve transection.

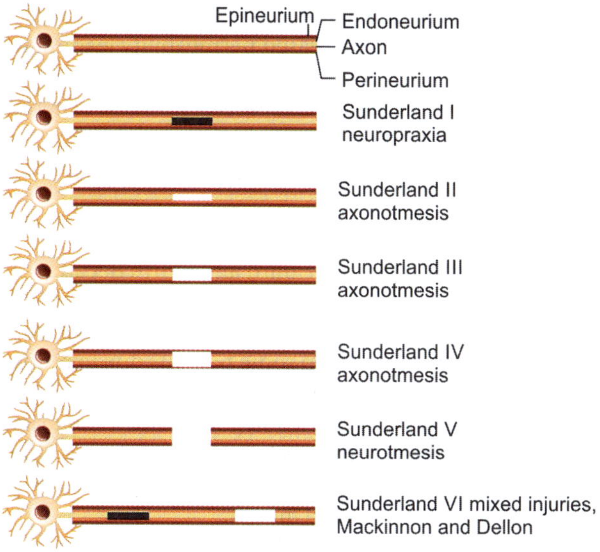

Fig. 3: Sunderland classification of nerve injury.

Diagnostic Tests

Q. Discuss electrodiagnostic and topodiagnostic tests for facial nerve.

Electrodiagnostic Tests

They help to differentiate between neurapraxia and degeneration of the nerve. They are also helpful to predict the prognosis and indicating the time for surgical decompression of the nerve.
- **Minimal nerve excitability test:** The nerve is stimulated with increasing intensity till facial twitch is just noticeable and is then compared with the normal side. The test is positive for degeneration when the difference between the two is >3.5 Amp. This test cannot detect degeneration of fibers in the initial 48–72 hours.
- **Maximal stimulation test:** This test determines the current level which gives the maximal facial movement instead of measuring the threshold of stimulus. The response is graded as equal, decreased, or absent.
- **Electroneuronography (ENoG):** It is a type of evoked electromyography. The bipolar stimulating electrical nodes are placed over the stylomastoid foramen, mastoid tip, and the nasolabial groove, and supramaximal electrical stimulation is given. The amplitude and latency of compound muscle action potential are measured and the percentage of degenerating fibers is calculated and compared to the normal side and if it is <10% of the normal side, it implies that there is >90% of axonal loss. This test is most useful between 4 and 21 days of the onset of complete paralysis.
- **Electromyography (EMG):** This test is done to elicit the motor activity of facial muscles. The needle electrodes are inserted in the orbicularis oculi and orbicularis oris muscles. The recordings are done at rest and during voluntary contraction of the muscle. This test is useful to plan for the reanimation procedure.

EN4.16: Describe the clinical features, investigations, and principles of management of facial nerve palsy.

■ FACIAL NERVE PARALYSIS

Q. Write a short note/essay on facial nerve palsy/Bell's palsy.

The cause of facial paralysis may be central or peripheral in origin. Peripheral lesions are more common and involved the nerve in the intracranial, intratemporal, or extratemporal parts.

Idiopathic

Bell's Palsy

It is defined as idiopathic, peripheral facial paralysis or paresis of acute onset. It is the most common cause of facial paralysis (60–75%). Risk of Bell's palsy is more in diabetics and during pregnancy. A positive family history is seen in 6–8%.

Etiology

- **Viral infection:** Most of the evidence supports the viral etiology due to herpes simplex, herpes zoster or the Epstein–Barr virus.

- ❖ **Vascular ischemia:** It may be primary or secondary. Cold or emotional stress-induced primary ischemia whereas secondary ischemia is due to increased permeability leading to exudation of fluid, edema, and compression of microcirculation of the nerve.
- ❖ **Hereditary:** The fallopian canal is narrow due to hereditary predisposition. This makes the nerve susceptible to compression with the slightest edema.
- ❖ **Autoimmune disorder:** T lymphocyte changes have been observed.

Clinical Features

- ❖ **Age:** It is common in the third and fourth decades of life.
- ❖ **Sex:** It is seen equally in both sexes.
- ❖ Patient presents with sudden onset of facial asymmetry and is unable to close his eye.
- ❖ Epiphora may be seen in some patients due to reflex increase in the secretions of the secretory glands due to exposure of sclera and eversion of the lower eyelid due to palsy.
- ❖ It may be associated with dull pain in the retroauricular region.
- ❖ Inability to wrinkle the forehead on the affected side.
- ❖ There may be intolerance to noise due to stapedial paralysis or loss of taste due to involvement of chorda tympani.
- ❖ Drooping of the angle of mouth.
- ❖ Drooling of saliva and liquids on attempts to drink.
- ❖ Inability to blow or whistle.
- ❖ Loss of taste due to the involvement of the chorda tympani nerve.
- ❖ **Bell's phenomenon**: The eyeball turns upwards in a forceful attempt to close the eye.
- ❖ **Diagnosis:** It is always by exclusion. All other causes of peripheral facial paralysis should be excluded.
- ❖ Nerve conduction study is done to monitor nerve degeneration.

Topodiagnosis (localizing the site of a lesion) helps to establish the etiology and the site of decompression of nerve, if required.

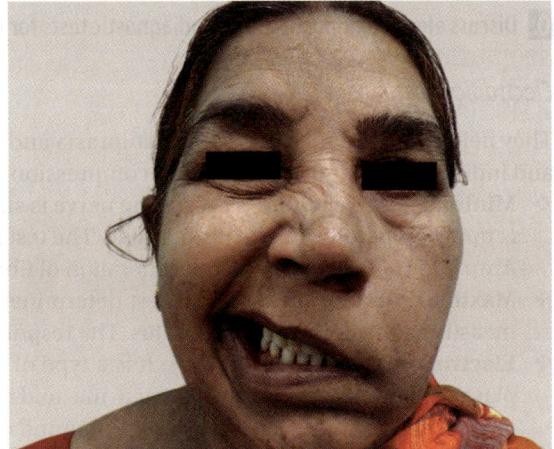

Fig. 3: Facial palsy with a deviation of angle of mouth.

General Treatment

- ❖ Reassurance
- ❖ Relief of pain by analgesics.
- ❖ Care of the eye to protect from exposure to keratitis.
- ❖ Physiotherapy or regular massage of the facial muscles.

Medical Management

- ❖ **Steroids:** Prednisolone is the drug of choice. The adult dose is 1 mg/kg/day in a divided dose given twice a day for 5 days. Patients are seen on the fifth day and the drug is tapered over the next five days. Contraindications to use of steroids include pregnancy, diabetes, hypertension, peptic ulcer, pulmonary tuberculosis, and glaucoma.
- ❖ Antivirals like acyclovir are given for 5 days.

Surgical Treatment

Nerve decompression relieves pressure on the nerve fibers and thus improves the microcirculation of the nerve.

Prognosis

About 85–99% of the patients recover fully. Incomplete recovery is seen in 10–15% of the patients.

Melkersson Syndrome

It is an idiopathic disorder consisting of a triad of facial paralysis, swelling of lips, and fissured tongue. Treatment is the same as for Bell's palsy.

Infections/Inflammatory

- ❖ Chronic otitis media—cholesteatoma and granulation tissues.
- ❖ Mastoiditis
- ❖ Herpes zoster oticus/Ramsay Hunt syndrome: It is characterized by facial paralysis along with vesicular rash in the external auditory canal and pinna.

- Acute suppurative otitis media.
- Mumps
- Tuberculosis
- Syphilis
- Leprosy
- Mucormycosis

Trauma

- **Fractures of the temporal bone:** The fracture may be longitudinal, transverse, or mixed. Paralysis may be due to hematoma, fracture fragment impinging on the facial nerve, transection of the nerve, or edema of the nerve due to trauma. Facial paralysis is seen as more common in transverse fracture. It can be immediate or delayed in onset. It is managed surgically in the form of decompression to remove the offending cause.
- **Iatrogenic cause:**
  - Facial nerve may be injured during ear surgeries such as tympanoplasty, stapedotomy, and mastoid surgeries. Sometimes, an ear pack may cause paralysis due to pressure on a dehiscent nerve. In such cases, the ear pack should be removed immediately.
  - Facial nerve may be injured during parotid surgeries. It may also as part of the surgery in cases of malignancy.

Neoplasms

- **Intratemporal neoplasms:**
  - Facial nerve palsy is seen in cases of tumors of the external ear, middle ear, glomus tumor, rhabdomyosarcoma, and metastatic tumors of the temporal bone. Facial nerve neuroma occurs along the course of nerve and causes paralysis.
- **Tumors of parotid:**
  - Facial paralysis is seen most commonly with malignant tumors of the parotid. Sometimes, benign tumors may cause facial paralysis as well.

Systemic Diseases

Facial paralysis may be seen in systemic diseases and hence diagnosis needs exclusion of diseases such as diabetes mellitus, hypothyroidism, leukemia, sarcoidosis, and Wegener's granulomatosis.

Investigations

- **Pure tone audiometry:** It is normal in Bell's palsy, conductive deafness is seen in middle ear infections or tumors. Sensorineural hearing loss is seen in mumps or acoustic neuroma.
- **Impedance and stapedial reflex:** Performed only in cases of Bell's palsy. Impedance is within normal limits. Stapedial reflex is absent due to the involvement of nerve in stapedius muscle.
- **CT scan of the brain and temporal bone:** To locate the site of lesion in tumors and trauma **(Fig. 4)**.
- **Facial nerve function tests:**
  - Electrodiagnostic
  - Topodiagnostic tests

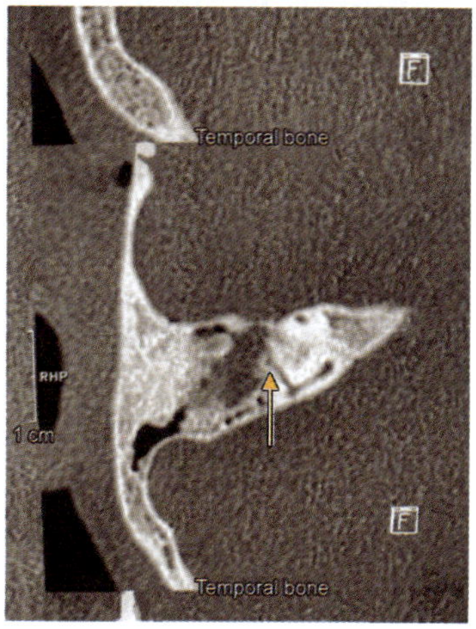

Fig. 4: High-resolution computed tomography (HRCT) temporal bone (arrow) showing fracture temporal bone with trauma to facial nerve.

Localization of Facial Lesion

- **Central facial paralysis:**
  - It causes paralysis of only the lower half of face on the contralateral side, forehead movements are preserved as the frontalis muscle receives bilateral innervation. It is seen in cerebrovascular accidents, tumors, or abscesses.
- **Peripheral facial paralysis:**
  - There is ipsilateral paralysis of all the facial muscles on the involved side. There is a loss of frontal wrinkling, weakness of upper eyelid, and inability to purse the lips or whistle.
  - Associated paralysis of VIth nerve suggested of a lesion at the level of nucleus.
  - A lesion at the cerebellopontine angle presents with vestibular and auditory impairments.
  - Lesions outside the temporal bone affects only the motor functions of the nerve.

Topodiagnostic Tests for Intratemporal Lesions

- **Schirmer test:** A strip of filter is hooked in the lower fornix of each eye and the amount of wetting of stripped is measured and compared. Lesions proximal to the geniculate ganglion showed decreased lacrimation as the secretomotor fibers to lacrimal gland leave at the geniculate ganglion via a greater superficial petrosal nerve **(Fig. 5)**.
- **Stapedial reflex**: It is a loss in lesions above the nerve to stapedius. It is tested by tympanometry.
- **Taste test**: Impaired taste sensation indicates that the lesion is above the chorda tympani.
- **Submandibular salivary flow test**: It also measures function of the chorda tympani. It is measured by passing into a polythene tube into both Wharton ducts and drops of saliva counted during one minute.

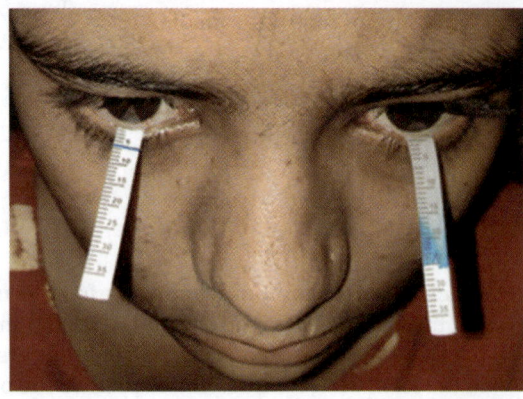

Fig. 5: Positive Schirmer's test with a difference in lacrimation.

Complications of Facial Paralysis

- Incomplete recovery
- **Exposure keratitis**: Eye remained open due to facial paralysis, there is evaporation of tear films causing dryness and keratitis, and corneal ulcer. This can be prevented by the use of artificial tears, eye ointment, and proper cover of the eye using tape tarsorrhaphy.
- **Synkinesis**: There is twitching of angle of mouth on closing the eye and vice versa. This is due to cross innervations of the nerve fibers.
- **Tics and spasms**: They are the result of faulty regeneration.
- **Contractures:** There is fibrosis of atrophied muscles or fixed contraction of a group of muscles.
- **Frey's syndrome:** There is sweating and flushing of skin over the parotid during mastication.
- **Gustatory lacrimation**: This is due to faulty regeneration of parasympathetic fibers which supply lacrimal glands instead of the salivary glands. There is unilateral lacrimation with mastication.

HYPERKINETIC DISORDERS OF FACIAL NERVE

Q. Write short note on hyperkinetic disorders of facial nerve.

- **Hemifacial pain**: It is characterized by repeated, uncontrollable twitching of facial muscles on one side. It is due to irritation of the nerve because of a vascular loop at the cerebellopontine angle.
  It is of two types:
  - Idiopathic where cause is not known. It is treated by a selective section of the branches of facial nerve in the parotid or by puncturing the facial nerve with a needle in its tympanic segment.
  - Secondary where the cause is known. Acoustic neuroma, congenital cholesteatoma, or glomus tumor are the common causes. Microvascular decompression through the posterior fossa craniotomy has given good results. Botulinum toxin injection to the affected muscle to block the neuromuscular junction by preventing release of acetylcholine.
- **Blepharospasm**: It is characterized by twitching and spasms of orbicularis oculi muscles on both sides and causes functional blindness. The cause is thought to lie in the basal ganglia. It is treated by Botulinum injection.

SURGERY OF FACIAL NERVE

- **Decompression:** The bony canal is exposed to relieve of the edema, and hematoma, or remove the fracture fragment impinging on the nerve.
- **End-to-end anastomosis:** This procedure is suitable for extratemporal part of the nerve where there is a minimal gap between the severed ends of the nerve.
- **Nerve graft**: This procedure is done when the severed ends cannot be opposed by end-to-end anastomosis. A nerve graft can be taken from the greater auricular, lateral cutaneous nerve of thigh, or the sural nerve.
- **Hypoglossal-facial anastomosis:** It is anastomosis of the hypoglossal nerve to the severed peripheral end of the facial nerve. It improves the muscle tone and permits some movements of facial nerve but causes atrophy of tongue on that side.
- **Plastic procedures:** They are used to improve cosmetic appearance when nerve grafting is not feasible or has failed. The procedure includes facial slings, face-lift operation or slings of the masseter, and temporalis muscle.

Chapter 18

Benign Conditions and Malignant Tumors of External Ear and Middle Ear

■ TUMORS OF EXTERNAL EAR

Classification

Q. Classify benign and malignant tumors of external ear.

	Benign	*Malignant*
Pinna	**Cysts** a. **True cysts:** Sebaceous cyst, preauricular cyst and fistula, dermoid cyst, epidermal implantation cyst b. **Pseudocysts:** Lesions of the cartilaginous external ear: ❖ Darwin's tubercle ❖ Rheumatoid arthritis ❖ Gout ❖ Chondroma ❖ Calcinosis ❖ Ossification of the auricle **Tumors:** ❖ Ceruminoma ❖ Keratosis obturans ❖ Keloid ❖ Papilloma or verrucous wart ❖ Keratoacanthoma ❖ Cutaneous horns ❖ Nevi ❖ Lipoma ❖ Xanthoma ❖ Myomas and fibromas ❖ Myxomas ❖ Mixed salivary gland type tumors ❖ Adenoma ❖ Vascular tumors—congenital strawberry mark, cavernous hemangioma, compact hemangioma ❖ Lymphangioma	❖ Squamous cell carcinoma ❖ Basal cell carcinoma ❖ Malignant melanoma
External auditory canal	**Hyperostosis:** Osteoma, exostoses, ceruminoma Papilloma	❖ Squamous cell carcinoma ❖ Basal cell carcinoma ❖ Malignant melanoma ❖ Adenocarcinoma ❖ Adenoid cystic carcinoma ❖ Basal cell carcinoma ❖ Sarcoma ❖ Malignant ceruminoma

Malignant Tumors

- Auricle (80–85%)
- External auditory canal (EAC) (10–15%)
- Middle ear mastoid (5–10%)

Benign Lesions of Pinna

Pseudocyst

Q. What is a pseudocyst and its treatment?

- Fluid collection into a tissue space without epithelial lining
- It can be a seroma or hematoma
- **Causes:** Trauma or cystic degeneration of a tumor
- Drainage is necessary for hematoma to prevent cartilage necrosis
- Drainage—incision on posterior aspect of auricle and compression dressings on anterior aspect of auricle to prevent reaccumulation of fluid, thus maintaining natural contour.

Preauricular Cyst

Q. Describe a preauricular sinus or cyst and its treatment.

- A congenital anomaly.
- Results from faulty union of hillocks of His during the development of pinna (first and second branchial arch derivatives).
- Unilateral/bilateral, a pit-like depression or small opening in front of the crus of a helix or above the tragus.
- This depression may lead to a cyst or has a branching tract lined by squamous epithelium which when blocked results in a retention cyst.
- It presents with a cyst that is infected with scanty foul discharge.
- It can be seen in syndromes associated with sensorineural deafness.
- **Treatment:** Surgery is indicated if symptomatic or for unsightly swelling. Cyst or sinus tract must be excised completely to avoid recurrence.

Note: Preauricular tags with or without cartilage are similar congenital anomalies that can be removed for cosmetic reasons.

Sebaceous Cyst

Q. What is a sebaceous cyst and its treatment?

- Retention cysts of sebaceous glands
- **Common site:** Postauricular sulcus or around the lobule region.
- Symptoms are present when the cyst becomes very large or gets infected, with occasional definable cyst apex.
- Removal is indicated—if a secondary infection, for cosmetic reasons, or if malignant degeneration is suspected.
- **Treatment:** Total surgical excision, with the capsule intact for preventing recurrence.

Dermoid Cyst

Q. Write a short note on dermoid cyst.

- **Congenital cysts**—a form of teratoma with a fibrous wall lined with stratified squamous epithelium and containing hair follicles, sweat glands, and sebaceous glands.
- **Presents as**—a round, spongy mass behind the pinna, over the upper part of the mastoid process
- Two theories—(a) An embryologic ontologic misplacement of cells, suggesting that teratoma represents the intrauterine displacement of normal cells that have escaped the influence of the primary organizer. (b) Second theory proposes the entrapment of normal tissue by improper fusion of tissues during development.
- **Treatment**—removed for cosmetic purposes.

Epidermal Implantation Cyst

Q. What is an incisional cyst or epidermal implantation cyst?

- Occurs following incision or trauma in the region of the ear—due to implantation of squamous epithelium into subcutaneous tissue

- The products of the secretory cells of implanted sweat or sebaceous glands produce secretions filling the cyst.
- Surgical removal—cosmetic or when doubt exists concerning the benign nature of the lesion.

Kerotosis Obturans

Q. What is keratosis obturans? Describe the etiology, presentation, and treatment of the condition.

- Desquamating epithelium of the bony part of external auditory canal forms a keratotic mass called keratosis obturans.
- **Etiology:** Accumulation of squamous epithelium and debris due to faulty migration of squamous epithelial cells from the surface of the tympanic membrane and the adjacent canal, which intermix with cerumen forming a mass.
- Appears pearly white and glistening (like middle ear cholesteatoma)—hence also called cholesteatoma of the external auditory canal.
- **Symptoms:** Pain is the common presenting symptom
  - Conductive hearing loss
  - Otorrhea
- **Treatment:** Periodic removal of accumulated debris, which can be difficult and painful for the patient, may require general anesthesia.
- Topical therapy for associated otitis externa
- For obstinate cases—in failure of prolonged conservative measures fail—**canaloplasty surgery.**

Keloid

Q. Write a short note on keloid.

- **Definition:** Keloid is a smooth, pink, rounded scar-like pedunculated benign tumor formed by connective tissue hypertrophy that invariably follows trauma like—piercing of pinna for ornaments or incision in the skin.
- **Etiology:** Secondary to a defect in collagenase causing overgrowth of collagen as opposed to a hypertrophic scar composed of immature collagen that has failed to convert from the tertiary to the quaternary form.
- **Risk factors:**
  - Females
  - Genetic susceptibility.
  - Following surgical or radiation therapy for carcinoma of the auricle
  - Black race
- **Treatment:** Surgical excision with an injection of triamcinolone into the surgical site or immediate postoperative low dose radiation of 300 rads. Complete eradication is difficult because of the tendency for recurrence. Recent reports indicate successful treatment using the CO_2 laser.

Hemangioma

Q. What is a hemangioma? Describe the types.

- Congenital tumors involving auricle in childhood. Other parts of face and neck may also be involved.
- **Two types:**
  1. **Capillary hemangioma:** A mass of capillary-sized blood vessels and may present as a **"port-wine stain."**
  2. **Cavernous hemangioma (also called strawberry tumor):** It consists of endothelial-lined spaces filled with blood. It increases rapidly during the first year but regresses thereafter, and may completely disappear by the fifth year. This lesion is usually an irregular, soft, bright-red or deep purple, a papular nodular mass that is easily compressible. It increases in size when the patient strains. For persistent lesions or those that tend to bleed or ulcerate, reconstructive or laser surgery may be indicated.

Papilloma

Q. Write a short note on papilloma affecting pinna/external auditory canal.

- Also called a wart
- **Presentation:** Cauliflower-like tufted outgrowth or flat grey plaque, with a rough surface.
  Papillomas are rare in the external auditory canal. It should be differentiated from a polyp and malignant growth
- **Etiology:** Viral—provokes local hypertrophy of the papillae
- **Treatment:** Surgical excision or curettage with cauterization of the base—cryosurgery

Cutaneous Horn/Keratoacanthoma

Q. Write a short note on cutaneous horn and keratoacanthoma.

- **Cutaneous horn:**
  - **Horn-shaped tumor:** Benign projection of unusually cohesive accumulation of keratin
  - **Site:** Helix of pinna
  - Elderly people
  - **Treatment of choice:** Surgical excision with histological examination (to rule out squamous cell carcinoma)
- **Keratoacanthoma:**
  - Benign tumor—resembling malignancy clinically
  - Presents as raised nodule—resembles squamous cell carcinoma
  - Rapid growth to the size of a 1 cm diameter or more within 4–6 weeks
  - Mostly occur as a solitary lesion, predilection for sun-exposed areas
  - **Treatment:**
    - Single lesion—excision
    - Multiple lesions—rule out the possibility of squamous cell carcinoma—treatment with retinoic acid.

Benign Tumors of the External Auditory Canal

Osteoma

Q. What is an osteoma? How do you treat it?

- **A single, bony hard, and smooth pedunculated tumor**—rare tumor
- Invariably occurs unilaterally—it may resemble a foreign body or a cyst
- **Site of origin**—cancellous bone of the posterior wall of the osseous meatus
- **Symptoms**—conductive hearing loss and discomfort:
  - If untreated—complete occlusion of the meatus and secondary infection
- **Palpation**—it can be done using a cotton-tipped wire applicator—hard, bony consistency
- **Treatment**—surgery in every case—drilling out the lesion or fracture at its base

Exostoses

Q. Describe the clinical features and treatment of exostoses of ear.

- Most commonly encountered tumors of the external auditory canal
- Presentation:
  - Usually bilateral
  - Multiple smooth sessile bony swellings in the deeper part of the meatus near tympanic membrane
  - In large lesions—retention of wax and debris, impaired hearing
- Arise from compact bone
- **Risk factors:**
  - Meatus exposed to repeated cold water, e.g., divers, swimmers in salt water
  - Males: Female—3:1
  - Other factors—chronic irritation from infection, eczema, or trauma
- **Mechanism:**
  - Bony ear canal—exposed to hypothermia → early thickening of the anterior and posterior bony canal walls → V-shaped meatus
  - Small rounded nodules on the superior bony wall adjacent to the annulus (asymptomatic) → enlarged blocking the meatus → obstruction/reduced hearing/accumulation of cerumen or debris à fullness of ear, secondary infected causing otorrhea and otalgia
- **Treatment:**
  - Small, asymptomatic—no treatment
  - Larger one—surgery:
    - Removal with a high speed drill to restore normal size of the meatus.
    - It may lie close to the facial nerve when present deep in the meatus—avoid gouge and hammer to prevent facial injury
- **Prevention:**
  - Surfer's and swimmers—vented ear plugs
  - Divers—should use a hood

CHAPTER 18: Benign Conditions and Malignant Tumors of External Ear and Middle Ear

Ceruminoma

Q. Write a short note on ceruminoma and its treatment.

- Tumor of modified sweat glands—secrets cerumen
- **Presentation:**
  - Smooth, firm, skin covered polypoidal swelling in outer meatus
  - Generally attached to posterior or inferior wall
  - Obstructs the meatus—causes retention of wax or debris
- Malignant type: Benign type—2:1
- **Treatment:**
  - Tendency to recur
  - *Surgery:* Wide local excision, with regular follow-up
  - Postoperative radiotherapy: If malignant suspicion on histology

Malignant Tumors Affecting External Ear

Q. Describe the malignant tumors of pinna and the external ear canal (EAC) in brief.

	Pinna	EAC
Squamous cell carcinoma	❖ **Risk factors:** Male, 50 years, prolonged exposure to direct sunlight, fair complexion ❖ **Site:** Helix commonly, 6 times more common on auricle than the canal ❖ **Presentation:** Painless nodule or an ulcer with everted edges and indurated base. Grows extremely slowly. ❖ **Metastasis** to lymph node—very late ❖ **Treatment:** ➤ Small lesions, no nodal metastasis—locally excised with 1 cm margin ➤ Large lesions, within 1 cm of EAC or with regional nodal metastasis—a chemosurgical technique by Moh's—use of zinc chloride followed by frozen sections for serial assessment of adequate margins ➤ For large fungating carcinomas—complete pinna amputation with en bloc removal of the parotid gland and cervical nodes ➤ Radiotherapy—combined with surgery or for recurrence	❖ **Risk factors**—long standing ear discharge ❖ **Presentation**—blood-stained mucopurulent or purulent discharge and severe earache ❖ **Examination**—an ulcerated area in the meatus or a bleeding polypoidal mass or granulations ❖ Facial nerve paralysis due to local extension of disease ❖ Regional lymph node involvement (preauricular, infra-auricular, postauricular, upper deep cervical) ❖ **Treatment:** Enbloc wide surgical excision with postoperative radiation
Basal cell carcinoma	❖ **Risk factors:** Male, 50 years ❖ **Site:** Helix and tragus ❖ **Presentation:** More common on the face than SCC than on the auricle. Nodule with a central crust bleeds on crust removal, ulcer—raised or beaded edges. Lesion extends circumferentially—may penetrate deeper into the skin—involving the underlying cartilage or the bone (locally aggressive) ❖ Lymph node metastases do not occur ❖ **Treatment:** ➤ Superficial lesions not involving cartilage—radiation (avoids cosmetic deformity) ➤ Lesions involving cartilage—surgical excision ➤ Extensive lesions—combination surgery and radiation	❖ Rarely arise from meatus ❖ Clinical features—similar to squamous cell variety ❖ Diagnosis only on biopsy ❖ **Treatment:** Wide surgical excision with postoperative radiation
Melanoma	❖ **Site:** Anywhere on the auricle ❖ **Risk factors:** Male, light complexion, exposure to sun ❖ **Presentation:** Small rounded darkly pigmented tumor of nevus. With a rapid increase in size and ulceration with increased pigmentation and bleed. Local discomfort or pain ❖ **Metastasis**—is seen in 16–50% of the cases ❖ **Treatment**—surgery is the choice: ➤ Superficial lesion <1 cm diameter, over the helix—wedge resection and primary closure ➤ Superficial lesion >1 cm, infiltrative melanoma, posterior auricular surface lesion, recurrence—resection of pinna, parotidectomy, and radical neck dissection	Rare

(EAC: external auditory canal; SCC: squamous cell carcinoma)

Sarcoma

Q. Write a short note on sarcoma of ear.

- **Origin:** Malignant tumor of mesoblastic derivation.
- Rapidly multiplying cells resemble those of connective tissue.
- **Various types:** Chondrosarcoma, fibrosarcoma, osteosarcoma, myxosarcoma, lymphosarcoma
- **Presentation:** As round and nodular swellings, rapid increase in size may be the first sign that arouses suspicion
- **Treatment:**
  - **Well-differentiated sarcoma**—excision may give a permanent cure
  - **Undifferentiated sarcoma in EAC**—rapid growth and destruction—can become fatal

■ TUMORS OF THE MIDDLE EAR AND MASTOID

Classification

	Benign	Malignant
Primary	Glomus tumor	Carcinoma, sarcoma
Secondary		❖ From adjacent areas, e.g., nasopharynx, external meatus, and the parotid. ❖ Metastatic, e.g., from carcinoma of bronchus, breast kidney, thyroid, prostate, and gastrointestinal tract.

Glomus Tumor

Q. What is a glomus tumor? and write about its cells of origin.

- Also called chemodectoma or non-chromaffin paraganglioma
- Most common benign neoplasm of middle ear.
- Slow growth
- Although benign histologically—can grow aggressively and cause multiple cranial nerve palsies.
- Cell of origin—**glomus bodies:**
  - They are distributed along with the parasympathetic nerves at skull base, neck, and thorax.
  - The glomus bodies resemble carotid body in structure, made of chemoreceptor tissue
  - Neural crest derivatives
  - In the temporal bone, they are found in the adventitia of jugular bulb and along any part of the glossopharyngeal (on the promontory) and vagus nerve.
- Consists of paraganglionic cells derived from the neural crest.
- Branchiomeric paraganglioma includes—jugulotympanic and intercarotid types
- Can be associated with other carotid body tumors
- The location of these tumors at the base of the skull—difficult exposure and removal

Pathology

Q. Write a short note on macroscopic and microscopic features og glomus tumor.

- **Macroscopically:**
  - Well defined, thin fibrous capsule
  - Jugulotympanic paragangliomas are—ovoid, lobulated structures
  - Hypervascular tumor—bleeds profusely with minimal trauma (vascular spaces are devoid of contractile elements)
  - Locally invasive:
    - Destruction of bone— becomes soft and hemorrhagic
    - Facial nerve involvement
- **Microscopically:**
  - Found in close relation with either **Jacobson's nerve or Arnold's nerve**
  - Blood supply—ascending pharyngeal artery
  - Sheets of epithelioid ovoid cells interspersed in highly vascular stroma with thin-walled vessels lacking contractile muscles.
  - Chief cells—contain cytoplasmic granules that store catecholamines

CHAPTER 18: Benign Conditions and Malignant Tumors of External Ear and Middle Ear

Clinical Features

Q. What is the site of origin of glomus tumors? Describe its pattern of growth and the related clinical features.

Clinical Features

- Middle age (40–50 years).
- Female: Male—5:1
- Benign, nonencapsulated, extremely vascular neoplasm.
- Growth—is very slow for several years

Site of Origin

- **Glomus jugulare**—arises from the dome of jugular bulb
- **Glomus tympanicum**—arises from the promontory of the middle ear (Fig. 1)

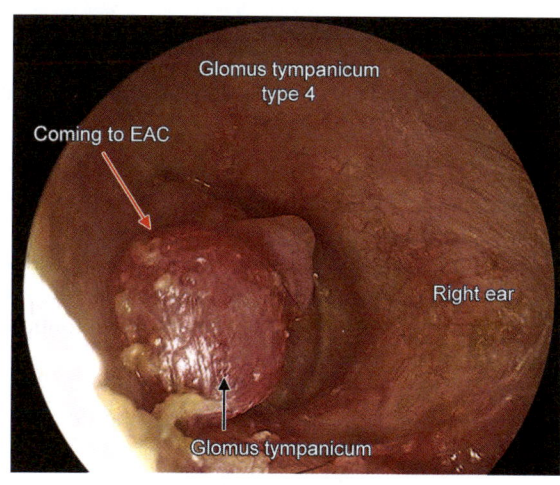

Fig. 1: Glomus tympanicum.

Pattern of growth of the above two tumors and the clinical features associated are as follows:

Filling the middle ear
- 90% cases—ear symptoms
- **Symptoms**—earliest—hearing loss and tinnitus
- Slowly progressive conductive hearing loss
- Swishing character, pulsatile tinnitus synchronus with the pulse
- Otoscopy: "Rising sun sign"—tumor arising from floor seen as red reflex through intact tympanic membrane
- "Brown sign" ear canal pressure raised by seigelisation—tumor pulsates and then blanches

EAC polyp mastoid
- Perforates the tympanic membrane to protrude as a polyp
- Symptom—profuse bleeding (spontaneous/even with slight trauma)
- Otorrhea—in secondary infections
- Otoscopy—red vascular polyp filling the EAC and bleeds profusely on manipulation or biopsy

Labyrinth, petrous pyramid
- Symptoms—dizziness, vertigo, and facial paralysis

Jugular foramen skull base
- Can extend to lumen of IJV and sigmoid sinus
- IX and XII cranial nerve palsies—at later stages
- **Symptoms:** Dysphagia, hoarseness of voice, unilateral soft palate paralysis, pharyngeal weakness and vocal cord palsy (CN IX and X). Weaknes of ipsilateral sternocleidomastoid and trapezius (CN XI), atrophy of ipsilateral tongue (CN XII)

Eustachian tube
- To nasopharynx as mass

Posterior and middle cranial fossa
- Symptoms of raised ICT
- Audible bruit: At all stages—auscultation with stethescope over the mastoid region—systolic bruit
- Features of catecholamine secreting tumors—headache, sweating, palpitation, hypertension, and anxiety

Metastasis
- Lungs and bone (4% of cases)
- Lymph nodes

*****Rule of 10s:** 10% of the tumors—are familial, 10%—multicentric, and 10%—functional, i.e., secrete catecholamines.

Investigations and Assessment

Q. Describe the available investigations for accurate diagnosis of glomus tumor.

Radiological Investigations

- **Plain X-ray mastoid:**
  - Clouding of middle ear and mastoid
    Phelp's sign: Absence of normal bony crest between carotid artery and the jugular fossa—seen in glomus jugulare.
- **Computed tomography (CT) scan**—gives the relation of a tumor with bony anatomy and erosion of the bone:
  - Bone window, 1 mm thin cuts—to differentiate between glomus jugulare and tympanicum (erosion of caroticojugular spine in glomus jugulare)
  - Rising Sun sign: Behind the eardrum
  - Other differential diagnoses of rising sun sign—(differentiated on CT scan):
    - Glomus tympanicum
    - High jugular bulb
    - Carotid artery aneurysm
    - Aberrant carotid artery
    - Cholesterol granuloma
    - Metastatic disease
- **Angiography:**
  - Digital subtraction angiography with contrast is used.
  - Shows blood supply of the tumor. Helps to identify coexisting glomus (can be multiple)
  - Helps in preoperative embolization
  - Retrograde venography—by catheterizing the IJV—differentiates between glomus tympanicum and glomus jugulare
- **Magnetic resonance imaging (MRI) scan:**
  - To know—soft tissue extent of tumor, skull base erosion, extension into the IJV and venous sinuses
  - Salt and pepper appearance due to mixed intensities inside of the tumor
- **Brain perfusion and flow studies:**
  - Done when carotid artery is under compression
  - To assess the opposite carotid flow and the circle of Willis
  - Thus assessing the risk of stroke during surgery, and the need for surgical replacement of the carotid

Endocrine Assessment

24 hours urine vanillylmandelic acid (VMA) and metanephrines assessment—raised.

Biopsy

- Avoided if suspicious of glomus tumor. It can also injure the aberrant carotid or high riding jugular bulb.
- Maybe done in doubtful cases to rule out squamous cell carcinoma in operative settings.

Management

Q. Discuss the treatment modalities for glomus tumor.

Treatment Options

- **Observation:** Patient is reassured and followed up if:
  - Elderly patient (60–70 years age)
  - CT scan showing smaller tumors with slow growth
- **Primary radiotherapy:**
  - Used in—inoperable, residual, or recurred tumor or in elderly to prevent extensive skull base surgery.
  - Effects—tumor shrinks and bleeding stops, tinnitus, and vertigo may improve
  - Radiation fibrosis—in 6–12 months
  - Endarteritis obliterans and thrombosis of some areas

- ➤ *Dose:* 2,000–3,000 rads
- ➤ *Complications:* Cerebral necrosis, osteoradionecrosis of temporal bone
- ❖ **Embolization:**
  - ➤ All glomus jugulare are embolized
  - ➤ Preoperatively—to reduce vascularity
  - ➤ Inoperable cases—postradiation
- ❖ **Surgical removal:** Various approaches depending on the extent of tumor.

Approach	Indication	Exposure
❖ Transcanal approach	❖ Glomus tympanicum—of limited extent ❖ Margins of the lesion are visible along the entire circumference	❖ Tympanotomy with tympanomeatal flap
❖ Hypotympanic approach	❖ Tumors limited to promontory extending to hypotympanum	❖ Hypotympanum is exposed by drilling the inferior bony tympanic ring to expose the lower limit of the tumor
❖ Post auricular → extended facial recess approach	❖ Tumor with indistinct margins	❖ Complete mastoidectomy ❖ Facial recess opened and extended through chorda tympani ❖ Exposure of hypotympanum between the facial nerve and the tympanic annulus ❖ Tumor removal from—ossicular chain, facial nerve, IJV, Eustachian tube
❖ Transtemporal approach	❖ Tumors confined to jugular foramen and Infra labyrinthine region	❖ Preserves EAC and ossicular anatomy
❖ Fisch's modified infratemporal fossa approach	❖ For large glomus jugulare tumors—extending to ICA, infratemporal fossa and intracranial extensions	❖ Mastoidectomy, extended facial recess approach with mastoid tip removal ❖ Removal of all middle ear structures lateral to the stapes ❖ Removal of TMJ
❖ Transcondylar approach	❖ Tumors extending towards foramen magnum ❖ Recurrence of glomus jugulare	❖ Approach to cervicocranial junction ❖ With exposure of the occipital condyle

(EAC: external auditory canal; ICA: internal carotid artery; TMJ: temporomandibular joint)

- ❖ Combination of the above modalities

Carcinoma of the Middle Ear and Mastoid

Q. Describe etiology, pathology, evaluation, and treatment of the carcinoma of middle ear and the mastoid.

Incidence: 1:20,000 (rare condition)

Most common primary malignancy of middle ear.

Etiology

- ❖ **Age:** 40–60 years
- ❖ Females
- ❖ Associated chronic irritation from long standing ear discharge (in 75% of cases)
- ❖ Radical mastoid cavities
- ❖ Primary carcinoma of mastoid air cells—in radium dial painters

Pathology

- ❖ Squamous cell carcinoma—most common variety.
- ❖ Glandular variety—occasional adenocarcinoma may be seen

Spread of Tumor

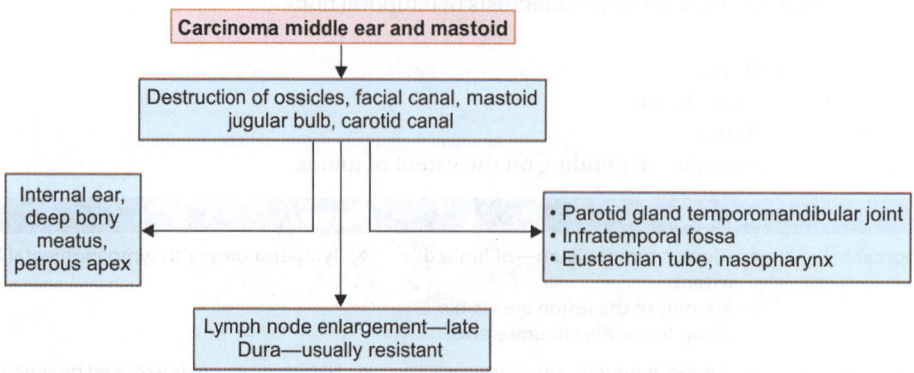

Clinical Features in Elderly Patient that Arouses Suspicion of Malignancy

- Chronic foul—smelling blood stained discharge with granulation or polyp
- Severe pain—more in the night
- Facial palsy
- Hearing loss
- Vertigo

Investigations

- **Biopsy**—definitive
- **Imaging**—CT scan of temporal bone, angiography

Treatment: Surgery + Radiotherapy

- **Surgery:** Radical mastoidectomy, subtotal or total petrosectomy
- **Radiotherapy alone:** For palliation when tumor involves cranial nerves, nasopharynx, or has gone intra cranially.

Rhabdomyosarcoma

Q. Write a short note on rhabdomyosarcoma.

- Rare tumor
- Mostly occur in children
- **Origin:** Pluripotent mesenchyme, embryonic muscle tissue
- **Presentation:** Early stage—chronic suppurative otitis media with discharge, polyp, or granulations. Facial palsy—early
- **Diagnosis:** Biopsy
- **Treatment:**
  - Combination of radiation and chemotherapy—treatment of choice
  - Small localized lesion—surgery.

Secondaries to Middle Ear

Q. What are the secondaries metastasizing to the middle ear?

- Tumors extending from the surrounding tissues to the middle ear cleft—external auditory canal, parotid gland, or nasopharynx
- Distant metastasis to temporal bone from carcinomas of—kidney, breast, prostate, bronchus, and gastrointestinal tract

Chapter 19

Vestibular Schwannoma

EN4.12: Describe the clinical features, investigations and principles of management of Acoustic neuroma.

■ DEFINITION

Q. What is vestibular schwannoma? State its site of origin.
- It is also called—acoustic neuroma or neurilemmoma
- It is a benign, extremely slow-growing, well-circumscribed, and encapsulated tumor of cranial nerve VIII, arising from the Schwann cells.
- It comprises 80% of cerebellopontine angle tumors and 10% of all brain tumors. Age: 40–60 years, occurs in both sexes.
- The nerve of origin—vestibular nerve > cochlear nerve
  - Inferior > superior vestibular nerve

■ PATHOLOGY

Q. Describe the pathology—gross and microscopy of vestibular schwannoma.

Macroscopically
- Well circumscribed, encapsulated
- **Color and consistency**—it depends on size and degree of degeneration—typically pinkish gray, rubbery consistency.
- **Large tumors**—they are often mottled due to hemorrhage and fibrosis. Cystic in case of necrosis and degeneration.

Microscopically
- Arises at the junction of Schwann cells and neuroglial supporting cells
- Tumor arising from nerve sheath—compresses the underlying nerve rather than invading it.
- Typical histological pattern:
  - **Antoni A:** Compact and cellular with the whirling appearance of cells called Verocay bodies.
  - **Antoni B:** Loose and less cellular, with a spongy appearance.
  - As the tumor grows—myxoid areas, necrosis, and fibrosis are seen.

PART 1: Diseases of ENT, Head and Neck

■ ACOUSTIC NEUROMA

Q. State the origin and growth pattern of acoustic neuroma. What are the clinical features according to involvement by the tumor?

❖ **Origin:** Internal auditory canal (IAC)—enlarging the porus and extending into the cerebellopontine angle (CPA)

Origin-IAC
- Fills the internal acoustic canal and widens the porus by resorption, compressing the vestibulocochlear nerves
- Earliest and most common presenting symptoms—progressive retrocochlear SNHL with tinnitus (unilateral)
- Poor speech discrimination—out of proportion to hearing loss (characteristic of aoustic neuroma)

Cerebellopontine angle
- Stretching and displacement of the CN VII and VIII, causing their thinning and anteroinferior cerebellar artery compression
- Symptoms CN VII—Hitzelberger sign— hypoesthesia of posterior meatal wall (sensory fibers affected early and motor are affected in later stages), loss of taste, and reduced lacrimation
- Vestibular symptoms (not in initial stage) —mainly as imbalance and unsteadiness, not vertigo

Superiorly- CN V Inferiorly- CN IX, X, XI
- Stretching and thinning of—CN V, VI and inferiorly lower cranial nerves
- Earliest nerve to be involved—CN V: Symptoms—loss of corneal sensation, paresthesia of face—indicates tumor is approximately 2.5 cm in size
- Lower CN paralysis—hoarseness of voice, dysphagia

Cerebellum
- Compression of cerebellum—positive cerebellar signs, dysdiadochokinesia, and ataxic gait

Brainstem and fourth ventricle
- Compression and displacement of brainstem and fourth ventricle→hydrocephalus
- Raised intracranial tension—late feature—headache, nausea, vomiting, diplopia (CN VI involvement), papilledema, and blurring of vision

Tentorium
- Obstructs cochlear aqueduct

(CN: cranial nerve; SNHL: sensorineural hearing loss)

■ CLASSIFICATION

❖ **Intracanalicular:** Confined to internal auditory canal (IAC)
❖ **Small:** <1.5 cm
❖ **Medium:** 1.5–4 cm
❖ **Large:** >4 cm

■ DIAGNOSIS AND MANAGEMENT

Q. How will you diagnose the tumor? Describe the examination and investigations required. Write a note on its treatment.

Examination

❖ **Otological examination:** Ear examination, tuning fork tests—sensorineural hearing loss (SNHL).
❖ **Eye examination:** Corneal sensitivity and nystagmus.
❖ **Postural tests:** Romberg's test, Unterberger's test, and tandem walking.

- **Cerebellar signs:** Finger nose test, heel knee test intention tremors, dysdiadochokinesia
- **Cranial nerve examination**

Investigations

Audiometric Studies

- **Pure tone audiometry**—SNHL—marked in higher frequencies
- **Speech discrimination**—poor (disproportionate to hearing loss)
- **Roll over phenomenon**—further reduction in speech discrimination when increasing loudness of the sound beyond a particular limit.
- **Short increment sensitivity index (SISI) score**—0–20%
- **Stapedial reflex decay**—shows retrocochlear type of lesion
- **Auditory brainstem response (ABR):** >90% sensitivity in the diagnosis of vestibular schwannoma—interaural wave V latency of >0.2 milliseconds

Vestibular Testing

- **Caloric test**—diminished response
- **Electronystagmography (ENG)**—is useful to identify the nerve of origin

Imaging Studies

- **Plain X-rays**—transorbital, Towne's, submentovertical view, Stenver's view—helpful in extracanalicular or larger tumors
- **CT scan**—tumor as small as 0.5 cm into the posterior fossa can be detected
- **Gadolinium-enhanced magnetic resonance imaging (MRI) (Figs. 1 to 3):**
  - Gold standard
  - **T2 weighted high resolution**—detect even intracanalicular tumor
  - Sensitive to detect as small as 1–2 mm size tumors
  - When MRI contraindicated—gaseous contrast computed tomography (CT) or posterior fossa myelography
- **Vertebral angiography**—to differentiate acoustic neuroma from other tumors when doubt exists.

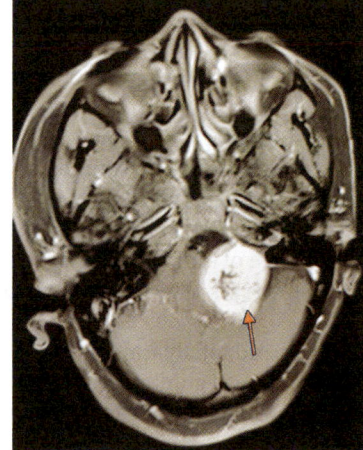

Fig. 2: MRI of brain and ear axial cut showing large CP angle tumor (acoustic neuroma).
(CP: cerebellopontine angle; MRI: magnetic resonance imaging)

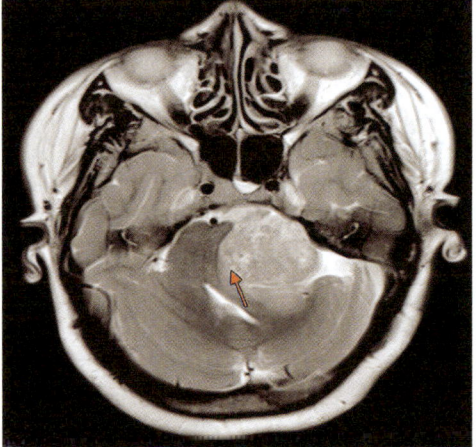

Fig. 1: MRI of brain and ear axial cut showing large CP angle tumor (acoustic neuroma).
(CP: cerebellopontine angle; MRI: magnetic resonance imaging)

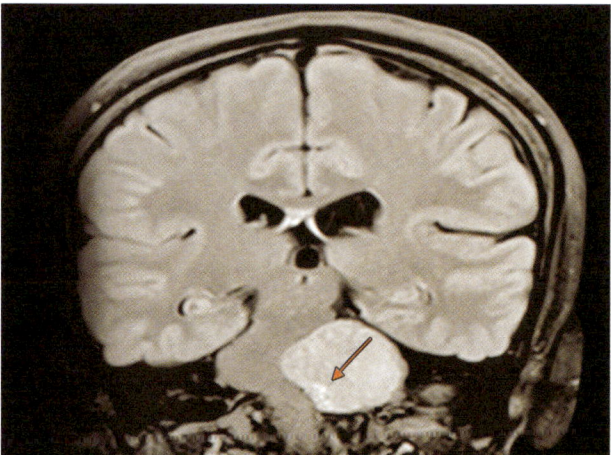

Fig. 3: MRI brain and ear coronal cut showing large CP angle tumor (acoustic neuroma).
(CP: cerebellopontine angle; MRI: magnetic resonance imaging)

◼ DIFFERENTIAL DIAGNOSIS

- ❖ Cochlear pathology, e.g., Meniere's disease should be ruled out
- ❖ Other posterior fossa/cerebellopontine angle tumors—meningioma, epidermoids, nonvestibular schwannoma, and primary cholesteatoma.

◼ TREATMENT

Observation

It is recommended in very small tumors, elderly >65 years, and medically unfit. Magnetic resonance imaging is obtained regularly to assess the growth rate (first at 6 months, followed by yearly).

Surgery

The treatment of choice. Various approaches are used for tumor removal, depending on its size:
- ❖ Middle cranial fossa approach—for tumors of 1–1.5 cm only
- ❖ Translabyrinthine approach—all sizes of tumors can be removed
- ❖ Retrosigmoid/suboccipital approach—all sizes, hearing preserved
- ❖ Combined translabyrinthine—suboccipital approach

Radiotherapy

- ❖ Conventional radiotherapy—no role
- ❖ Gamma knife surgery (cobalt 60 sources):
  - ▹ Stereotactic radiotherapy
  - ▹ Radiation is converged on the tumor, thus preventing surrounding tissue damage.
  - ▹ Causes shrinkage of tumor and restriction of its further growth.
  - ▹ Used when surgery is not possible due to contraindication or the patient refusing the surgery
- ❖ CyberKnife:
  - ▹ More accurate and totally frameless
  - ▹ Uses real-time image guidance
  - ▹ Computer-controlled robotic technology

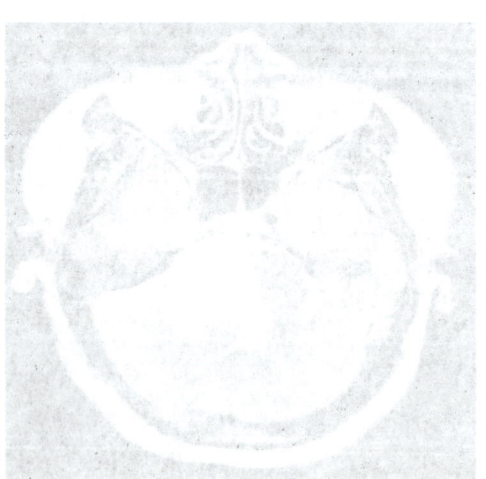

Section 3: Rhinology

Chapter 20

History Taking and Examination of Nose and Paranasal Sinuses

EN2.1: Elicit document and present an appropriate history in a patient presenting with an ENT complaint.

■ DEMOGRAPHICS

Importance of
- ❖ **Age—younger:**
  - Nasopharyngeal angiofibroma
  - Rhinosporidiosis
  - *Elderly:* Carcinoma maxilla
- ❖ **Sex—male:**
  - Nasopharyngeal angiofibroma
  - Rhinosporidiosis
  - *Female:* Atrophic rhinitis
- ❖ **Address—rhinosporidiosis:**
  - Along coastal areas in tropical countries like India, Bangladesh, Sri Lanka
  - *Rhinoscleroma:* Rural areas of India, South Africa, Europe
- ❖ **Occupation—farmers:**
  - Rhinosporidiosis
  - *Dusty environment:* Vasomotor rhinitis

■ HISTORY TAKING

It must include the details of all the complaints, mentioned in the **chief complaints**, that start with appearance of first symptom and extend up to time of consultation.

Common Complaints of Nose and PNS

Sl. No.	Main complaints	Sl. No.	Associated complaints
1.	Nasal discharge: Anterior/postnasal drip	1.	Fever
2.	Nasal obstruction/blockage	2.	Headache
3.	Nasal stuffiness and congestion	3.	Vomiting
4.	Recurrent sneezing/itching	4.	Change in voice (hypernasal and hyponasal)
5.	Nose bleed	5.	Facial pain/pressure
6.	Crusting	6.	Snoring
7.	Decrease or altered smell	7.	Epiphora
8.	Swelling over nose	8.	Exophthalmos
9.	Foul smell	9.	Deafness
10.	Nasal deformity/injury		

History of Present Illness

It consists of:
- Mode of onset (sudden/gradual)
- Preceding events causing onset
- Course of symptoms (progressive/constant/fluctuant and continuous or intermittent)
- Aggravating and relieving factors
- Accompanying complaints and treatment taken
- **Unilateral disorder:** Note site and side
- **Any associated systemic diseases:** Diabetes, hypertension, coronary artery diseases

> **EN4.21:** Elicit document and present a correct history, demonstrate and describe the clinical features, choose the correct investigations and describe the principles of management of nasal obstruction.

Nasal Obstruction

Q. Enumerate causes of unilateral nasal obstruction.

Nasal obstruction can be unilateral or bilateral common cause include:

Unilateral Nasal Obstruction

Causes of unilateral nasal obstruction

Vestibular	Nasal cavity	Sinuses	Nasopharynx
• Furuncle • Vestibulitis • Stenosis of nares • Atresia • Nasoalveolar cyst • Papilloma • Squamous cell carcinoma	• Foreign body • Deviated nasal septum (DNS) • Hypertrophic turbinates • Concha bullosa • Antrochoanal polyp • Synechiae • Rhinolith • Bleeding polypus of septum • Benign and malignant tumors of nose • Unilateral atrophic rhinitis	• Benign and malignant tumors of paranasal sinuses • Sinusitis unilateral	• Unilateral choanal atresia

Bilateral Nasal Obstruction

Q. Enumerate causes of bilateral nasal obstruction.

Causes of bilateral nasal obstruction.

Vestibular	Nasopharynx	Nasal cavity
• Bilateral vestibulitis • Collapsing nasal alae • Stenosis of nares • Congenital atresia	• Adenoid hypertrophy • Large choanal (polyp) • Thornwald's cyst • Soft palate and posterior pharyngeal wall adhesions • Large benign/malignant tumor • Nasopharyngeal angiofibroma	• Acute/chronic sinusitis • Acute/chronic rhinosinusitis • Rhinitis medicamentosa • Allergic rhinitis • Hypertrophic turbinates • DNS • Nasal polypi (ethmoidal polyp) • Atrophic rhinitis (rhinitis sicca) • Septal hematoma **(Fig. 1)**/abscess • Bilateral choanal atresia

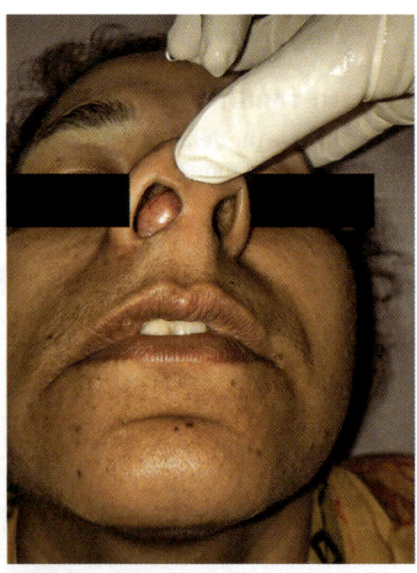

Fig. 1: Showing mass on the right septum occupying right nostril.

Differential Diagnosis of Nasal Obstruction

Q. Discuss differencial diagnosis between unilateral and bilateral nasal obstruction.

Age group	Causes of unilateral nasal obstruction	Causes of bilateral nasal obstruction
Children	❖ Malformations ❖ Foreign bodies ❖ Benign and malignant tumors ❖ Antrochoanal polyp ❖ Septal deviation	❖ Malformations ❖ Inflammatory ❖ Chronic rhinosinusitis with/without polyp ❖ Adenoid hypertrophy ❖ Turbinate hypertrophy
Teenagers	❖ Malformations ❖ Angiofibroma and benign or malignant tumors ❖ Unilateral chronic rhinosinusitis ❖ Antrochoanal polyp ❖ Septal deviation ❖ Concha bullosa	❖ Rhinitis of different causes (allergic, hormonal) ❖ Malformations ❖ Inflammatory ❖ Chronic rhinosinusitis with/without polyp ❖ Adenoid hypertrophy ❖ Turbinate hypertrophy
Adults	❖ Benign or malignant tumors ❖ Unilateral chronic rhinosinusitis ❖ Antrochoanal polyp ❖ Septal deviation ❖ Concha bullosa	❖ Rhinitis of different causes ❖ Chronic rhinosinusitis benign and malignant tumors ❖ Turbinate hypertrophy ❖ Systemic diseases ❖ Empty nose syndrome ❖ Valvular insufficiency

Nasal Discharge

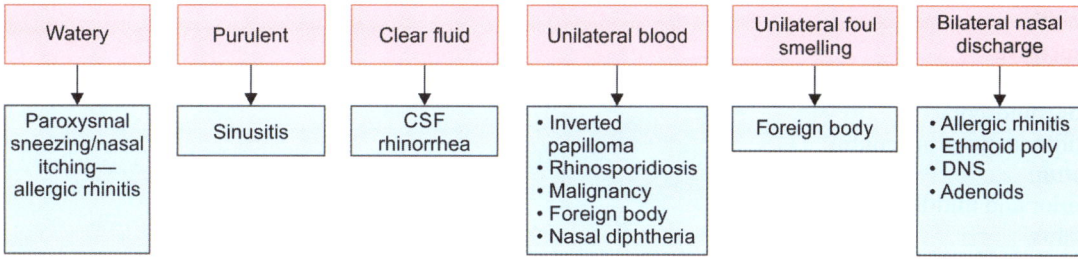

Epistaxis

- ❖ Most common site of nosebleed
  - ▷ *Children:* Little's area
  - ▷ *Adult:* Woodruff's area
- ❖ Intractable bleeding in case of young anemic adolescent male indicates juvenile nasopharyngeal angiofibroma
- ❖ Hypertension is the most common cause of bleeding in elderly people, although malignancy should also be ruled out.

Headache

- ❖ Sinusitis is one of the common causes of headache.
  - ▷ Frontal sinusitis
    - ♦ Brown pain/frontal headache
  - ▷ Maxillary sinusitis
    - ♦ Patient complaints of pain/pressure or fullness in maxillary/cheek region and upper dental area
  - ▷ Ethmoidal sinusitis
    - ♦ Pain over medial canthus and side of nose
  - ▷ Occipital sinusitis
    - ♦ Occipital headache is associated with sphenoid sinus infection
- ❖ **Sluder's neuralgia:** Anterior ethmoidal neuralgia patient with deviated nasal septum when the deviated septum touches middle turbinate, they develop pain in region of eyebrows and nasal bone.

Altered Sense of Smell

- ❖ Hyposmia
  - ▷ Partial loss of smell in cases of nasal disturbances

- ❖ Hyperemia
  - ➢ Increase in sense of smell
  - ➢ In case of pregnancy epilepsy
- ❖ Anosmia
  - ➢ Absence of smell
  - ➢ Neural pathology
- ❖ Presbyosmia
  - ➢ Hyposmia that occurs in old age
- ❖ Cacosmia
  - ➢ Perception of putrid odor empyema of maxillary sinus
- ❖ Parosmia
  - ➢ Perversion of sense of smell

EN2.2: Demonstrate the correct technique of examination of the nose and paranasal sinuses including the use of nasal speculum.

EXAMINATION OF NOSE AND PARANASAL SINUSES (PNS)

- ❖ Examining a nose does not require much instruments. Anterior rhinoscopy is enough for assessing nasal cavity septum and inferior turbinate. Nasal endoscopy allows through evaluation of intranasal anatomy and pathology which is little difficult with standard anterior rhinoscopy and head mirror/light examination.
- ❖ Examination of nasal cavity includes physical examination of external nose, vestibule, anterior rhinoscopy, functional examination of nose.

Examination:
- ❖ **External nose**
- ❖ **Vestibule**
- ❖ Anterior rhinoscopy
  - ➢ Thudicum nasal speculum
  - ➢ Septum
  - ➢ Inferior and middle turbinates
  - ➢ Meatus
  - ➢ Floor of nasal cavity
    - ♦ Topical nasal decongestant
    - ♦ Probe test
    - ♦ Posture test
- ❖ **Posterior rhinoscopy**
- ❖ **Patency of nasal cavity**
  - ➢ Spatula test
  - ➢ Cotton wool test
  - ➢ Alar nasi movements
- ❖ **Sense of smell**
- ❖ **Paranasal sinuses**
  - ➢ Tenderness
  - ➢ Transillumination
  - ➢ Endoscopic examination

External Nose

It needs proper palpation and inspection for the osseocartilaginous framework and deformity and skin lesions.

See for any:
- ❖ Injuries—with or without nasal/skull fracture
- ❖ Swelling—dermoid, furuncle, septal abscess cyst
- ❖ Scars—surgery or trauma
- ❖ Ulcers—rodent ulcer
- ❖ Neoplasm—rhinophyma, squamous cell carcinoma herpes zoster/simplex
- ❖ Deformity—hump, deviated nose
- ❖ Cartilaginous enlargement—chondroma or chondrosarcoma

Vestibule

It is the anterior lined part of nasal cavity having hairs (vibrissae) cavity examination by lifting the tip of the nose.

See for any: Furuncle, crusting, dislocated caudal end of the septal; cysts, tumors, fissure (chronic rhinitis).

Anterior Rhinoscopy (scan QR code)

Q. Write a short note on anterior rhinoscopy.

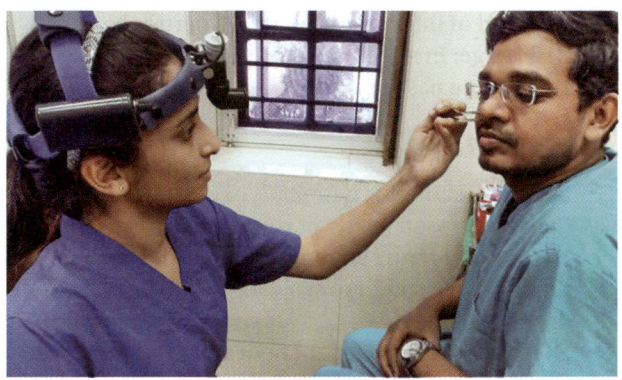

Fig. 2: Showing anterior rhinoscopy examination of nose using speculum.

- Examined using thudicum nasal speculum, held between left hand, helps in widening the vestibule, blades of septum are inserted in the vestibule, less sensitive area and should not touch the septal mucosa, which is very sensitive and vascular **(Fig. 2)**.
- The nasal septum is closed while introducing and opened during examination and remains partially open when removing from the nose.
- On examination, patients head needs to be turned in different directions to examine the different sites in the nose, septum, inferior turbinate and meatus middle turbinate and meatus and floor of the nose **(Fig. 3)**.
- **In nasal cavity look for:**
  - *Narrowing*: Septal deviation, hypertrophy of turbinate, any polyp
  - Wide nasal cavity (atrophic rhinitis)
  - Any discharges, crusting
  - Foreign body
- **Septum:** Deviation **(Fig. 4)** or spurs, perforation, ulcer growth (rhinosporidiosis, hemangioma), swelling (hematoma/abscess), bony destruction (syphilis)
- **Floor of nose:** Cleft palate or fistula, swelling, neoplasm, granulation
- **Inferior and middle turbinate:**
  - Enlarged and swollen (hypertrophic rhinitis, concha bullosa)
  - Congested in inflammation
  - Small and rudimentary—atrophic rhinitis
- **Inferior and middle meatuses:** Discharge/polyps in middle meatus
- **Probing:** Site of attachment, consistency, mobility, sensitiveness of mass, bleeding on touch

Posterior Rhinoscopy

Q. Write a short note on posterior rhinoscopy.

Indications

- **Posterior choana:** Atresia, polyp

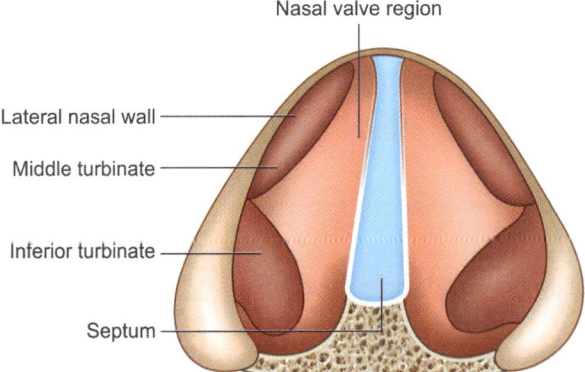

Fig. 3: Structures seen on anterior rhinoscopy.

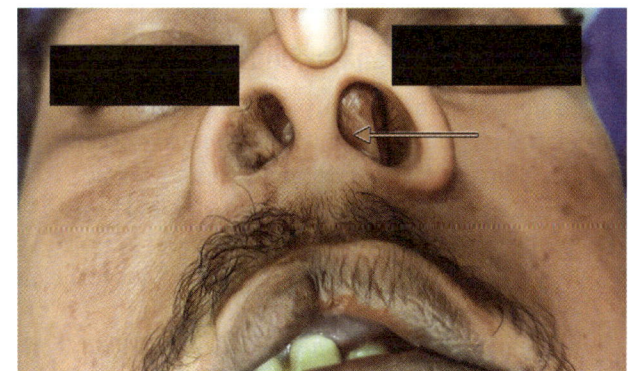

Fig. 4: Showing caudal deviation on examination of nose.

- **Post end of inferior turbinate:** Hypertrophy
- **Discharge:** In middle meatus
- To examine nasopharynx

Steps (scan QR code)

- Includes examining nasopharynx and posterior part of nasal cavity by posterior nasal mirror (St. Clair Thompson posterior rhinoscopy mirror) patient opens his mouth and breathes quietly.
- **Postnasal mirror:** Warmed but not to be hot, better check on back of hand before introducing. This is done in order to avoid fogging of mirror, alternative option is cleaning mirror with savlon or rub the mirror against the buccal mucosa.
- Examiner depresses the patient's tongue with depressor held in left hand and introduces **posterior rhinoscopy mirror**, should be held in right hand like a pen and carried behind the soft palate; without touching the posterior 1/3rd of tongue (to avoid gag reflex). Reflected light from head mirror illuminates the area of nasopharynx and examiner sees the reflected image of postnasal space in mirror **(Fig. 5)**.

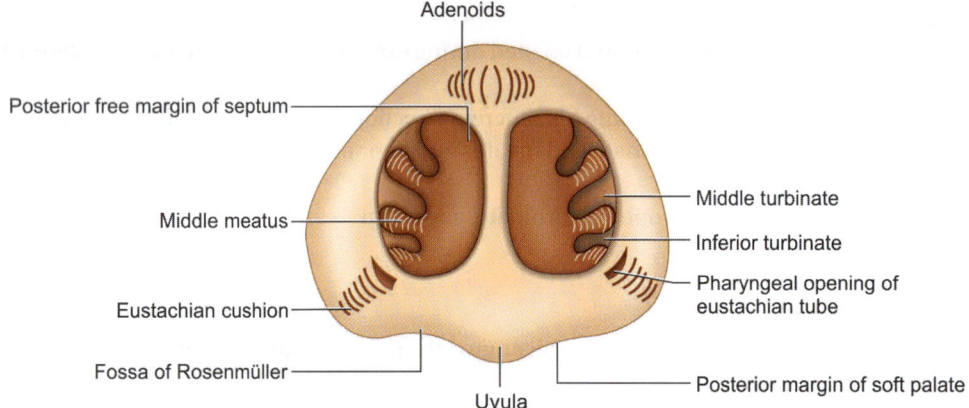

Fig. 5: Structures seen on posterior rhinoscopy.

Note: Superior turbinates are not seen on anterior as well as posterior rhinoscopy. Superior turbinates are seen on diagnostic nasal endoscopy (Refer to chapter on FESS for diagnostic endoscopy).

Functional Examination of Nose

To look for patency of nasal cavities:
- **Spatula test (scan QR code):** Clean cold stainless steel tongue depressor is held below the nose while the patient exhales area of mist formation on either side is compared **(Fig. 6)**.
- **Cotton wool test:** A fluffy of cotton is held between each nostril and each movements indicates the nasal blow of while the patient inhales and exhales.
- **Alae nasi movements:** Incase of inspiratory obstruction alae nasi collapse onto the septum.
- **Cottle's test (scan QR code):** It is done for abnormality of nasal value check of affected side is drawn laterally and upwards and the patient breathes quietly, any improvement in nasal airway the test is positive, indicates nasal value compromise **(Fig. 7)**.

Examination of Paranasal Sinuses

- Examined by inspection, palpation, transillumination
- Maxillary, frontal and anterior ethmoids—drains in middle meatus
- Posterior ethmoids drain into superior meatus
- Sphenoid sinus opens into sphenoethmoid recess
- **Tenderness:** Can be elicited by pressure
    - *Frontal sinus:* Anterior wall and floor above the medial parts of eyebrow and above the medial canthus **(Fig. 8)**
    - *Anterior ethmoids sinuses:* Medial wall of orbit just behind the root nose **(Fig. 9)**
    - *Maxillary sinus:* Anterior wall over the check lateral to nose **(Fig. 10)**

CHAPTER 20: History Taking and Examination of Nose and Paranasal Sinuses

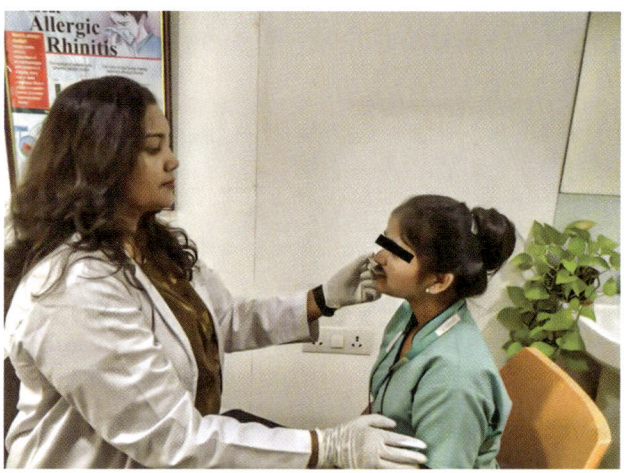

Fig. 6: Showing cold spatula test for nasal obstruction and nasal airflow.

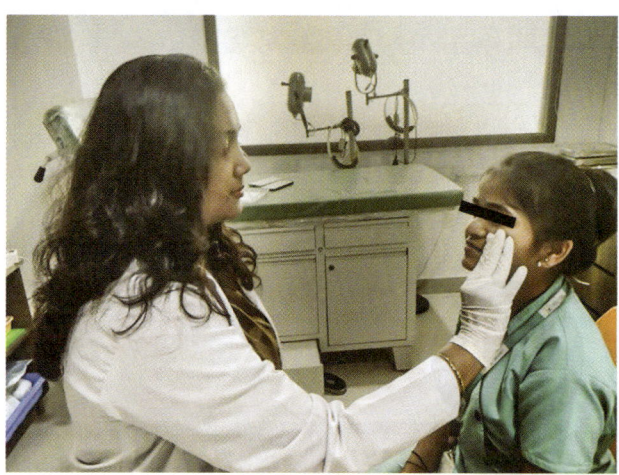

Fig. 7: Showing Cottle's test.

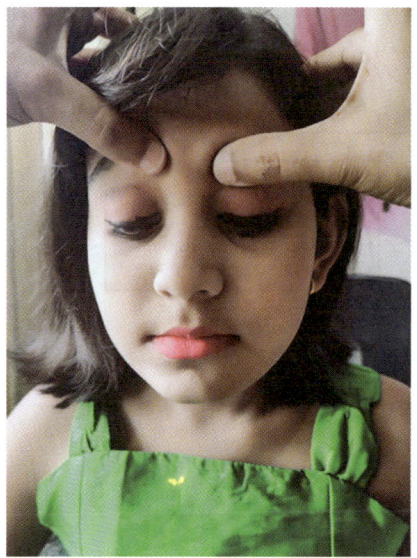

Fig. 8: Showing frontal sinus palpation.

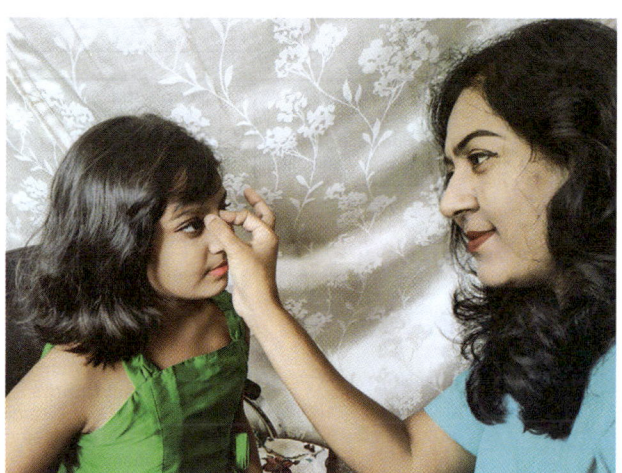

Fig. 9: Showing ethmoid sinus palpation.

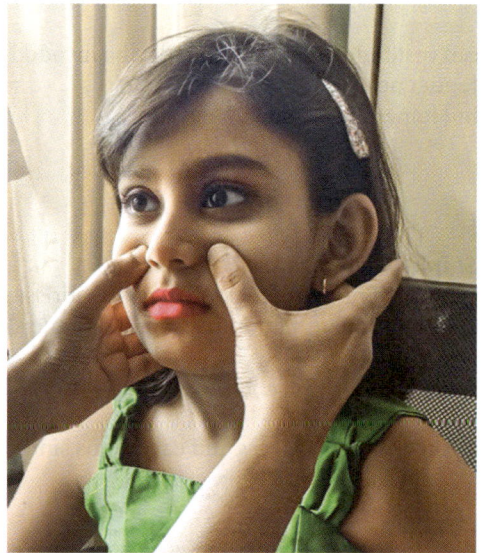

Fig. 10: Showing maxillary sinus palpation.

Chapter 21

Diseases of External Nose

Q. Enumerate the diseases of external nose.

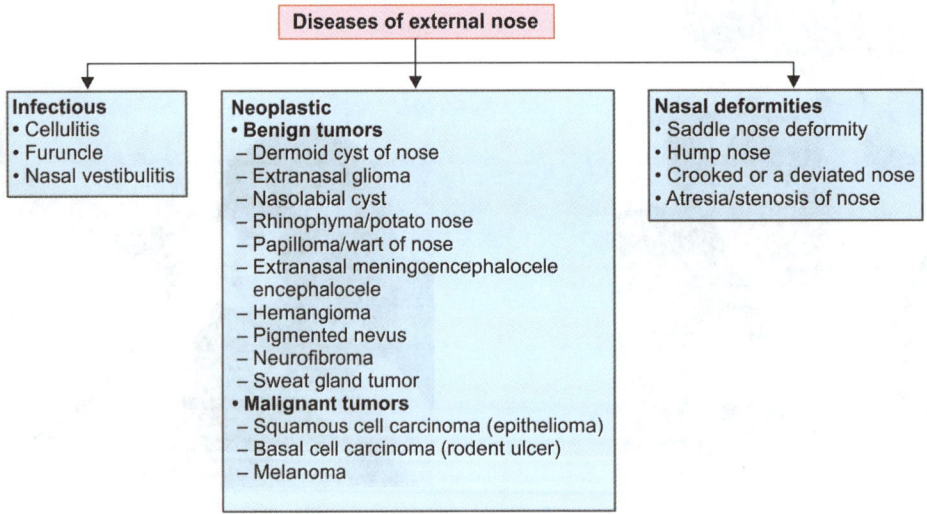

■ CELLULITIS

- It is an extension of infection from nasal vestibule, the nasal skin may be invaded by streptococci or staphylococci.
- **Clinical features:** Red, swollen, and tender nose
- **Treatment:** Systemic antibacterials, hot fomentation, and analgesics.

■ FURUNCLE OR BOIL

Q. Write short note on furuncle/boil on nose.

- Acute infection of the hair follicle by ***Staphylococcus aureus (S. aureus).***
- **Predisposing factors**—trauma from picking of nose or plucking of nasal vibrissae.
- **Clinical features**—tender and painful lesion. Inflammation may spread to the skin of nasal tip and dorsum which may become red and swollen.
- **Management**—warm compression, analgesics, topical, and systemic antibiotics. If a fluctuant area appears, incision and drainage can be done.
- **Complications**—cellulitis of the upper lip or septal abscess and cavernous sinus thrombosis.

■ NASAL VESTIBULITIS

Q. Write short note on nasal vestibulitis.

- It is diffuse dermatitis of nasal vestibule.

- **Predisposing factors**—nasal discharge due to any cause such as rhinitis, sinusitis, or nasal allergy, coupled with trauma of handkerchief.
- **Causative organism**—*S. aureus*
- **Acute form**—vestibular skin is red, swollen, and tender, crusts and scales cover an area of skin erosion or excoriation.
- **Chronic form**—induration of vestibular skin with painful fissures and crusting.
- **Management**—cleaning of nasal vestibule of all crusts and scales with cotton applicator soaked in hydrogen peroxide and application of antibiotic and steroid ointment.

SADDLE NOSE DEFORMITY (FIG. 1)

Q. Write short note on saddle nose.

- **Etiology:** Nasal trauma, excessive removal of septum in submucous resection, destruction of septum by: hematoma, abscess, leprosy, tuberculosis, syphilis.
- **Management:** The deformity can be corrected by augmentation rhinoplasty by filling the dorsum with cartilage, bone, or synthetic implant. If deformity involves both cartilage and bone, a cancellous bone from iliac crest is the best **(Fig. 2)**.

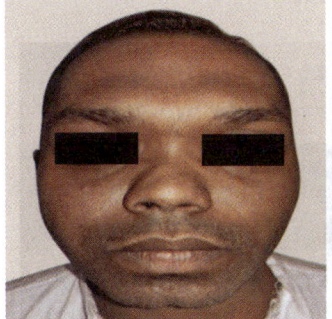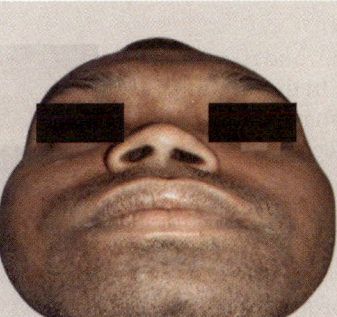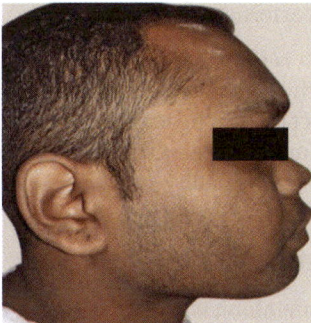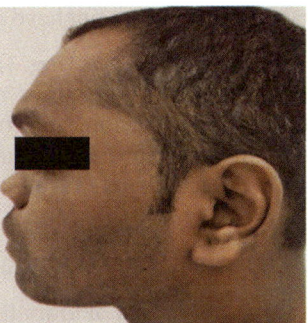

Fig. 1: Preoperative images of saddle nose deformity.

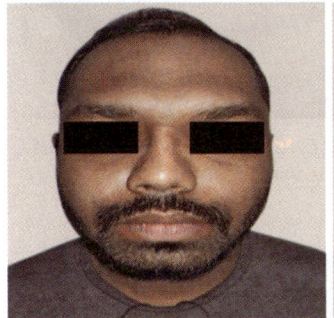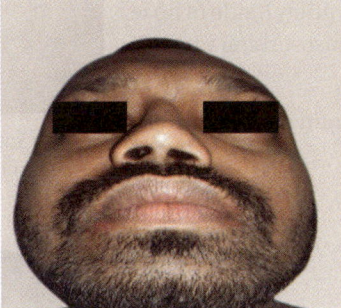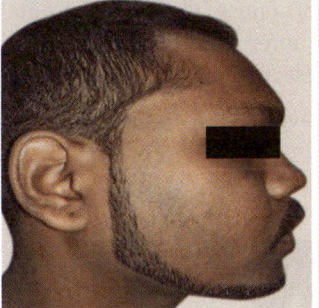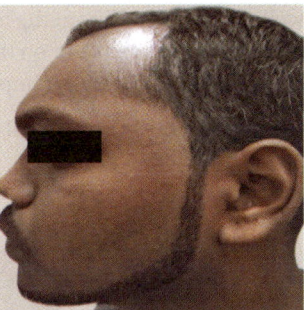

Fig. 2: Postoperative images of saddle nose deformity.

HUMP NOSE DEFORMITY (FIG. 3)

Q. Write short note on hump nose.

- It can involve the bone or cartilage or both bone and cartilage.
- **Management:** Reduction rhinoplasty—it consists of exposure of nasal framework by careful raising of the nasal skin by a vestibular incision, removal of a hump, and narrowing of the lateral walls by osteotomies to reduce the widening left by hump removal.

CROOKED OR A DEVIATED NOSE (FIG. 4)

Q. Write short note on crooked nose/deviated nose.

- In a crooked nose, the midline of dorsum from frontonasal angle to tip is curved in a C or S-shaped manner. In a deviated nose the midline is straight but deviated to one side.

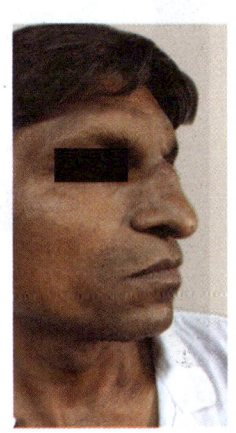

Fig. 3: Hump nose.

- **Etiology:** Traumatic, an injury sustained during birth, and neonatal period or childhood.
- **Management:** Rhinoplasty or septorhinoplasty

CONGENITAL TUMORS

Q. Enumerate congenital tumors of external nose.

Q. Write short note on:
a. Dermoid cyst of nose.
b. Encephalocele/Meningoencephalocele.
c. Glioma.

Dermoid Cyst

Simple dermoid: Midline swelling under the skin but in front of nasal bones. It does not have an external opening.

Dermoid with a sinus (Fig. 5): It is seen in infants and children, and is represented by a pit or sinus in the midline of dorsum of nose. In those with intracranial extension, sinus tract passes through the cribriform plate or foramen caecum and is attached to dura or has other intracranial connections. Meningitis can occur if infection travels along this path.

Encephalocele or Meningoencephalocele

It is the herniation of brain tissue along with its meninges through a congenital bony defect **(Fig. 6)**.

An extranasal meningoencephalocele presents as a subcutaneous pulsatile swelling in the midline at the root of nose **(Fig. 7)** (nasofrontal variety), side of nose (nasoethmoid variety), or on the anteromedial aspect of orbit (naso-orbital variety).

Swelling shows cough impulse and is reducible.

Management: Neurosurgical, severing the tumor stalk from brain and repairing the bony defect.

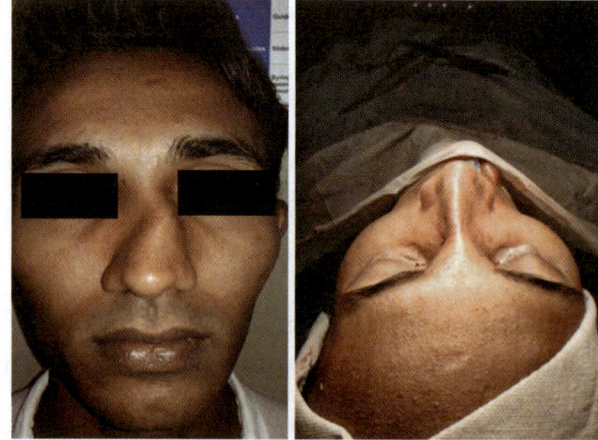

Fig. 4: Preoperative and intraoperative image of a crooked nose.

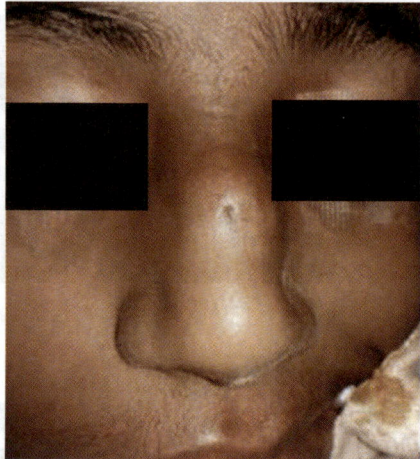

Fig. 5: Soft cystic swelling over dorsum of nose with fistula opening.

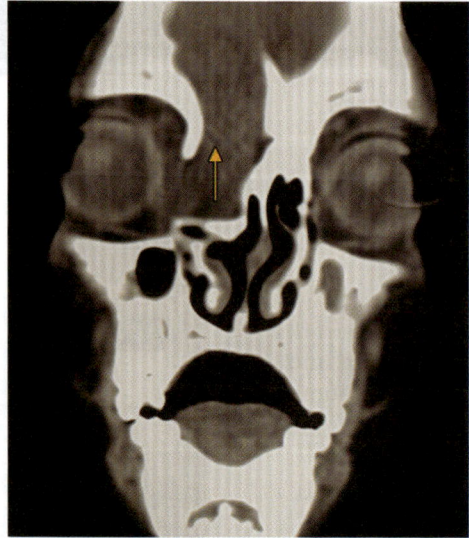

Fig. 6: Computed tomography (CT) scan of nose showing herniation of brain tissue along with its meninges through a congenital bony defect.

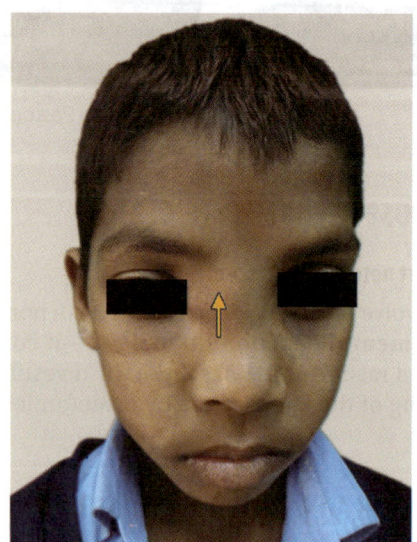

Fig. 7: Meningoencephalocele.

Glioma (Figs. 8 and 9)

It is a nipped-off portion of encephalocele during embryonic development. Most of them are extranasal and present as firm subcutaneous swelling on the bridge, side of the nose, or near the inner canthus. Some of them are purely intranasal (30%).

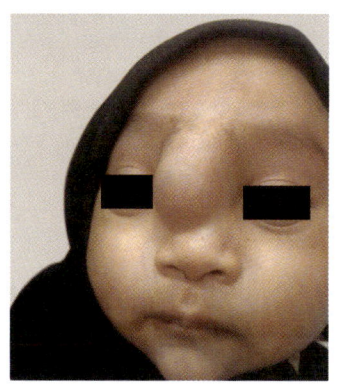

Fig. 8: Nasal glioma.

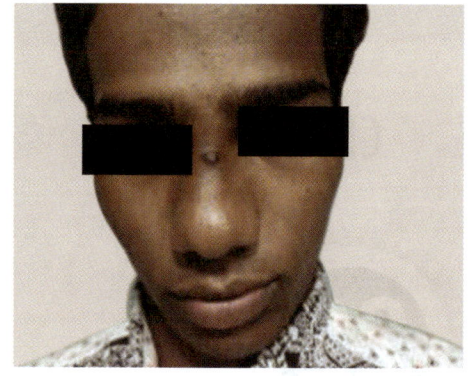

Fig. 9: Fistula opening with sebaceous discharge and hair seen in the opening.

■ BENIGN TUMORS

Q. Enumerate benign tumors affecting external nose. Write short note on rhinophyma.

- Rhinophyma
- Hemangioma
- Pigmented nevus
- Neurofibroma
- Sweat gland tumor

Rhinophyma (Fig. 10)

- Also called potato tumor.
- It is a slow growing benign tumor due to hypertrophy of Sebaceous gland of tip of nose.
- Seen in long standing case of acne rosacea.
- It presents as a pink, lobulated mass over nose with superficial vascular dilation, and mostly affects men past middle age.

Management: Paring down the bulk of tumor with sharp knife or carbon dioxide laser. Complete excision of tumor and raw area skin grafting is also done.

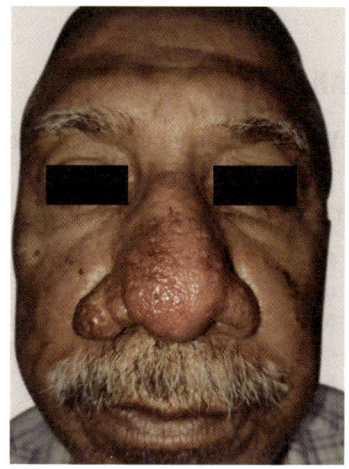

Fig. 10: Rhinophyma of nose.

■ MALIGNANT TUMORS

Q. Enumerate malignant tumors affecting external nose. Write a short note on (a) basal cell carcinoma, (b) squamous cell carcinoma.

- Basal cell carcinoma
- Squamous cell carcinoma
- Melanoma

Basal Cell Carcinoma (Rodent Ulcer) (Fig. 11)

- Most common malignant tumor involving skin of nose
- **Age group involved:** 40–60 years, affects male and female equally.
- **Common site:** Tip and ala of nose
- **Presentation:** Cyst or papulo-pearly nodule or an ulcer with rolled edges. Slow growing, underlying cartilage, or bone may get invaded.
- **Management:** Early lesion can be cured by cryosurgery, irradiation, or surgical excision with 3–5 mm of healthy skin around palpable borders of tumor.
- Extensive lesions are excised and surgical defect closed by local or distant flaps.

Squamous Cell Carcinoma

- Second most common malignant tumor
- **Age group:** 40–60 years
- **Presentation:** Infiltrating nodule or an ulcer with rolled out edges affecting side of nose or columella.
- **Management:** Early lesion respond to radiotherapy. Advanced lesion require surgical excision and plastic repair of defect.

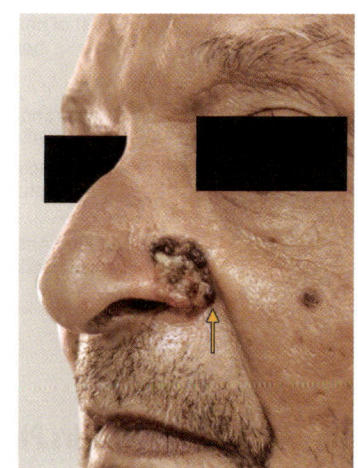

Fig. 11: Basal cell carcinoma (rodent ulcer) of external nose.

Chapter 22

Nasal Septum and its Diseases

ANATOMY

Q. Write a short note on (a) anatomy of nasal septum, (b) Little's area/Kiesselbach's plexus.

Parts of Nasal Septum (Fig. 1)

1. **Columellar septum:** It is formed of columella containing the medial crura of alar cartilages united together by fibrous tissue and covered on either side by the skin.
2. **Membranous septum:** It consists of a double layer of skin with no bony or cartilaginous support. It lies between the columella and caudal border of septal cartilage.
3. **Septum proper:**
    - **Bony and cartilaginous parts**
    - Its principal constituents are:
        - Perpendicular plate of ethmoid
        - Vomer
    - Large septal cartilage wedged between two bones anteriorly.

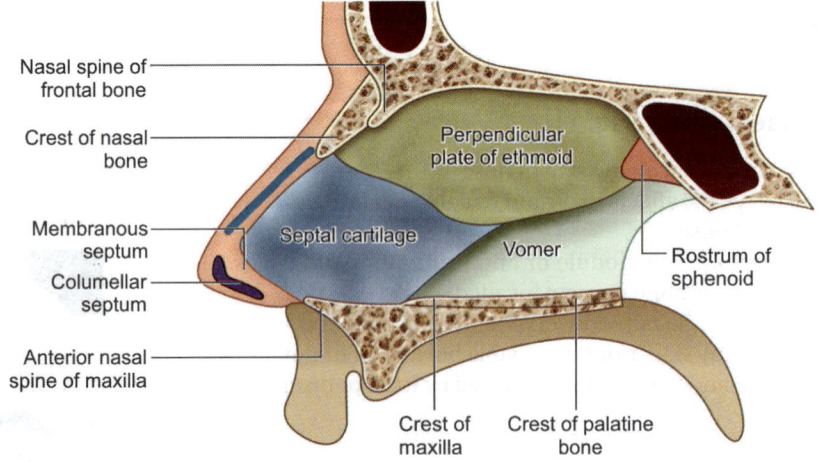

Fig. 1: Parts of the nasal septum.

Little's Area or Kiesselbach's Plexus (Fig. 2)

- It is the most common site for epistaxis.
- It is the vascular area in the anteroinferior part of nasal septum.
- It is also the site for origin of hemangioma of nasal septum.

CHAPTER 22: Nasal Septum and its Diseases

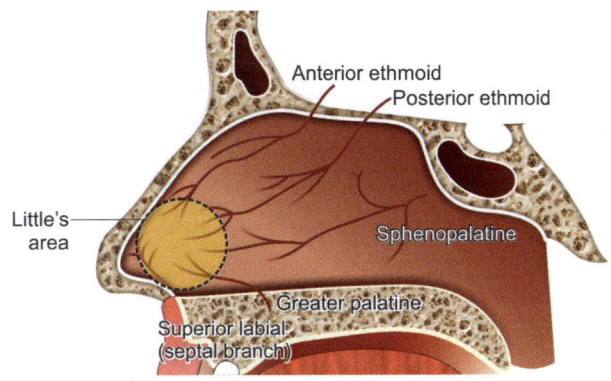

Fig. 2: Little's area.

EN4.22: Describe the clinical features, investigations, and principles of management of DNS.

DEVIATED NASAL SEPTUM (DNS)

Q. Write a short note/essay on deviated nasal septum and discuss its types, clinical features and management.

Etiology

- Trauma
- **Developmental error:** Unequal growth between the palate and the base of the skull may cause buckling of nasal septum.
- **Racial factors:** Caucasians are more affected than black Americans
- **Hereditary factors:** Several members of the same family may have deviated nasal septum (DNS)

Types of DNS

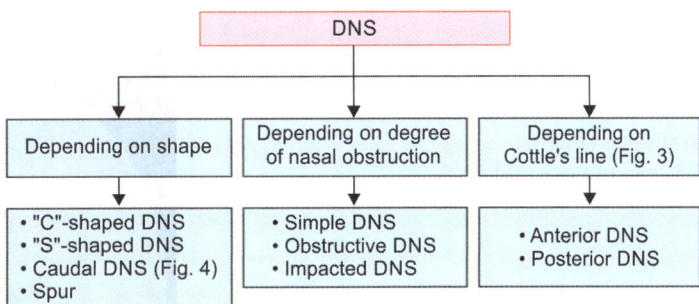

- **Anterior dislocation:** Septal cartilage may be dislocated into one of the nasal chambers.
- **C-shaped deformity:** Septum is deviated in a single curve to one side.
- **S-shaped deformity:** Such a deformity will cause bilateral nasal obstruction.
- **Spurs.** A spur is a shelf-like projection often found at the bony cartilaginous junction. A spur may press on the lateral wall and give rise to a headache **(Fig. 5)**.
- **Simple:** Mild DNS
- **Obstructive:** Nasal obstruction relieved by putting nasal decongestant drops.
- **Impacted:** Nasal obstruction does not get relieved on putting nasal decongestants.

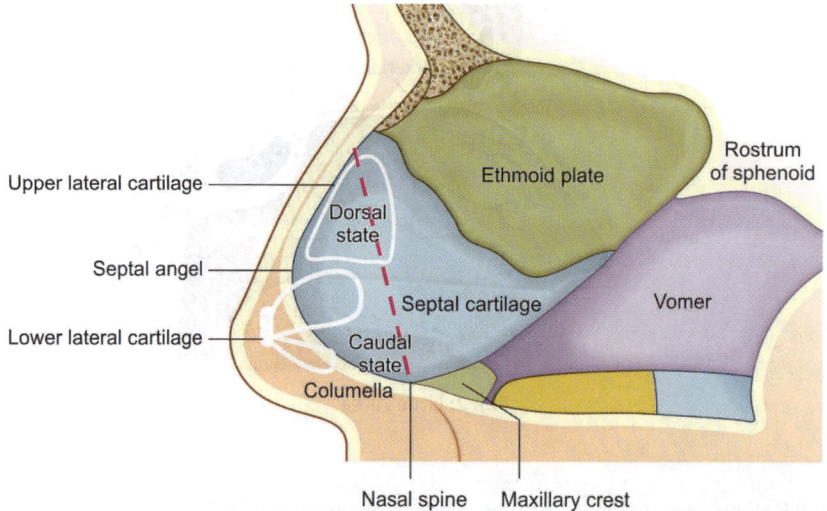

Fig. 3: Cottle's line.

Clinical Features

- **Nasal obstruction:** Depending on the type of septal deformity the obstruction may be unilateral or bilateral. **Cottle test** is used in the nasal obstruction due to abnormality of the nasal valve. In this test, the cheek is drawn laterally while the patient breathes, if the nasal airway improves on the test side the test is positive and indicates an abnormality of the vestibular component of the nasal valve.
- **Headache:** Deviated septum, especially a spur may press on the lateral wall and give rise to pressure headache.
- **Sinusitis:** Deviated septum may obstruct the sinus ostia resulting in poor ventilation of the sinuses.
- Epistaxis
- **Anosmia:** Failure of the inspired air to reach the olfactory region may result in total or partial loss of smell.
- **Middle ear infections:** DNS also predisposes to middle ear infections.

Investigations

- Routine blood investigations, bleeding profile, bleeding time, and clotting time.
- X-ray of nose and paranasal sinuses (PNS).
- Computed tomography (CT) scan of nose and PNS.

Treatment

Medical

Antihistaminics, nasal decongestant drops, and antibiotics are given to reduce nasal symptoms.

Surgical

- Minor degree of septal deviation with no symptom are commonly seen in people and requires no treatment. Surgery is indicated only when the deviated septum causes mechanical obstruction.

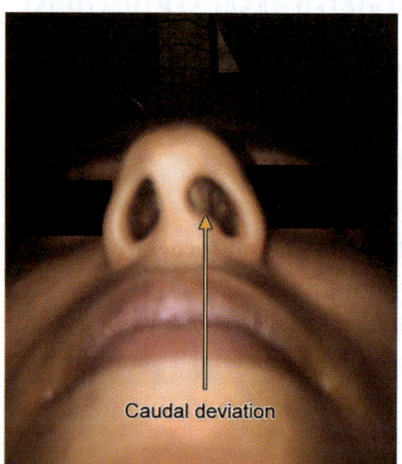

Fig. 4: Caudal deviation.

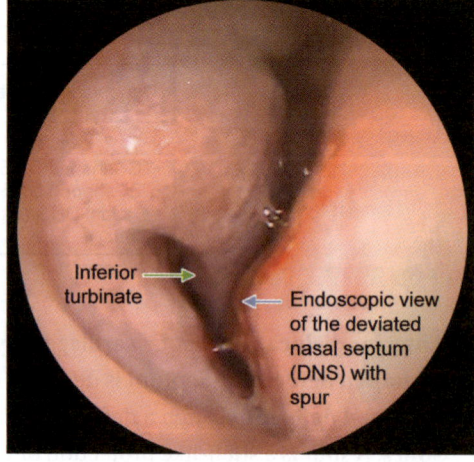

Fig. 5: Endoscopic view of the deviated nasal septum (DNS) with spur.

- ❖ **Submucous resection surgery**: It consists of elevation of mucoperichondrial and mucoperiosteal flaps on either side of the septal framework by a single incision made on one side of the septum, removing the deflected parts of bony and cartilaginous septum and then repositioning of the flaps.
- ❖ **Septoplasty**: It is a conservational surgery, much of the septal framework is preserved. Only the most deviated part is removed. Mucoperiosteal and mucoperichondrial flaps are raised only on one side of the septum retaining the mucosa and blood supply of the other side.

■ SEPTAL HEMATOMA

Q. Write a short note on septal hematoma.

Etiology

It is a collection of blood under the perichondrium or periosteum of nasal septum. It often results from nasal trauma or septal surgery.

Clinical Features

- ❖ Bilateral nasal obstruction is the most common presenting symptom.
- ❖ This may be associated with frontal headache and a sense of pressure over the nasal bridge.

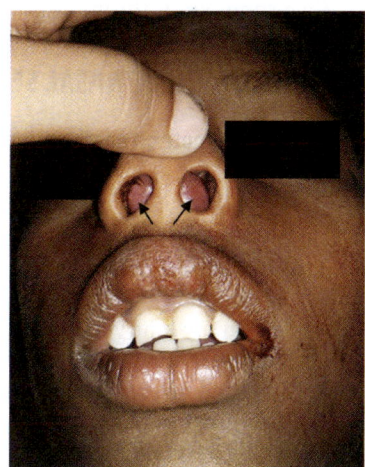

Fig. 6: Nasal septal hematoma.

Examination

Reveals smooth rounded swelling of septum in both the nasal fossae **(Fig. 6)**.

Treatment

Small hematomas can be aspirated with a wide bore needle. Larger hematomas are incised and drained by a small anteroposterior incision parallel to nasal floor. Following drainage, nose is packed on both sides to prevent reaccumulation. Systemic antibiotics should be given to prevent septal abscess.

■ SEPTAL ABSCESS

Q. Write a short note on septal abscess.

Etiology

- ❖ It results from secondary infection of septal hematoma.
- ❖ Occasionally, it follows furuncle of nose or upper lip.

Clinical Features

- ❖ Bilateral nasal obstruction with pain and tenderness over the bridge of nose.
- ❖ Fever with chills and frontal headache.
- ❖ Skin over nose may be red and swollen.
- ❖ **Examination:** Smooth bilateral swelling of the nasal septum. Septal mucosa is congested.
- ❖ Submandibular lymph nodes be enlarged and tender.

Treatment

Abscess should be drained as soon as possible. Incision is made in the most dependent part of abscess and a piece of septal mucosa excised. Pus and necrosed pieces of cartilage are removed by suction. Systemic antibiotics are started as soon as diagnosis has been made and continued at least for a period or 10 days.

Complications

- ❖ Necrosis of septal cartilage often results in depression of the cartilaginous dorsum in the supratip area and may require augmentation rhinoplasty 2–3 months later.
- ❖ Necrosis of septal flaps may lead to septal perforation.
- ❖ Meningitis
- ❖ Cavernous sinus thrombosis

■ PERFORATION OF NASAL SEPTUM

Q. Write a short note on nasal septum perforation.

Etiology

- ❖ **Traumatic perforation**:
  - ▹ Accidental or direct trauma to nose and face is the most common cause.
  - ▹ Iatrogenic injury to mucosal flaps during SMR, septoplasty, and following nasal surgeries.
  - ▹ Cauterization of septum with chemicals or galvanocautery for epistaxis
  - ▹ Habitual nose picking.
- ❖ **Pathological perforation**: Septal abscess, nasal myiasis, rhinolith, chronic granulomatous conditions such as lupus, tuberculosis, and leprosy.
- ❖ **Drugs and chemical**: Prolonged use of steroidal nasal spray and cocaine addicts
- ❖ **Idiopathic**

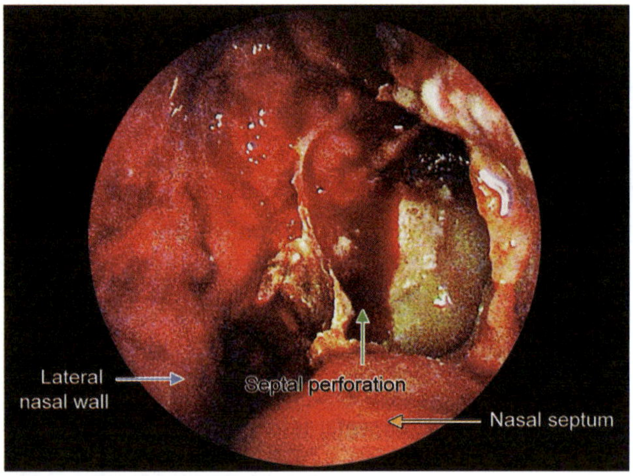

Clinical Features

- ❖ Small anterior perforations cause whistling sound during inspiration or expiration.
- ❖ Larger perforations develop crusts which obstruct the nose or cause severe epistaxis when removed **(Fig. 7)**.
- ❖ Atrophic rhinitis changes can be seen.
- ❖ External nasal deformity like saddle nose and supratip depression can be seen.
- ❖ Maggots can be seen on anterior rhinoscopy.

Fig. 7: Septal perforation.

Treatment

- ❖ Inactive small perforations can be surgically closed by plastic flaps.
- ❖ Large perforations are difficult to close. Their treatment is aimed to keep nose crust free by alkaline nasal douches and application of a bland ointment.
- ❖ Sometimes a thin silastic button can be worn to get relief from the symptoms.

Chapter 23

Acute and Chronic Rhinitis and Sinusitis and its Complications

EN4.26: Elicit document and present a correct history demonstrate and describe the clinical features, choose the correct investigations and describe the principles of management of acute and chronic rhinitis.
EN4.32: Elicit document and present a correct history demonstrate and describe the clinical features, choose the correct investigations and describe the principles of management of acute and chronic sinusitis and its complications.

■ RHINOSINUSITIS

Q. Write a short note/essay on rhinosinusitis and discuss its various types.

Definition

Inflammation of mucosa of sinuses and nasal mucosa. In acute rhinosinusitis symptoms last for <4 weeks.

Classification

- Acute rhinosinusitis
- **Subacute rhinosinusitis**: Duration 4–12 weeks
- **Chronic rhinosinusitis**: Duration for <12 weeks.
- **Recurrent rhinosinusitis**: Four or more episodes/year, each lasting for 7–10 days or more with complete resolution in between the episodes.

Clinical Features

- Symptoms associated with rhinosinusitis include:
  - Nasal obstruction
  - Nasal discharge/congestion
  - Facial pain or pressure
  - Hyposmia or anosmia
  - Other symptoms include cough, fever, halitosis, fatigue, dental pain, and pharyngitis

Acute Viral Rhinosinusitis (Common Cold, Coryza)

Q. Write a short note on acute viral rhinosinusitis.

It is **caused by respiratory viruses**, usually the common cold viruses such as rhinovirus, influenza, and parainfluenza. They spread by aerosolized droplets through coughing and sneezing.

Clinical Features

- Nasal congestion
- Rhinorrhea
- Sneezing
- Low-grade fever

Treatment

Symptomatic treatment like the use of nasal decongestants and antihistamines. Analgesics to relieve headache, myalgia, and fever.

Complications

The disease is self-limiting, if the bacterial infection supervenes or if the patient is immunocompromised, it can convert to bacterial rhinosinusitis and also cause pharyngitis, bronchitis, and pneumonia.

Acute Bacterial Rhinusinusitis

Q. Write a short note on acute viral rhinosinusitis.

Most common bacteria responsible are **Streptococcus pneumoniae, Hemophilus influenzae, Staphylococcus aureus (S. aureus).**

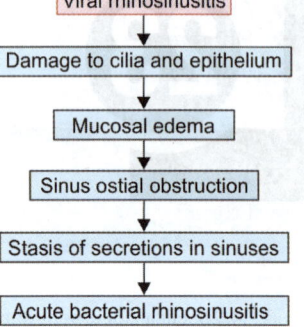

Clinical Features

- Nasal obstruction
- Purulent rhinorrhea
- Facial pain and pressure
- Hyposmia and anosmia
- Cough
- Fever
- Headache
- Dental pain and halitosis

Diagnosis

- Made when symptoms of acute viral rhinosinusitis persist or worsen beyond 10 days.
- **Nasal endoscopy** may reveal purulent discharge in the osteomeatal complex.
- **A swab** can be taken from the middle meatus to establish culture and sensitivity of bacteria.
- **Antral puncture** washes can be taken for culture and antibiotic sensitivity.

Treatment

- **Analgesics**
- **Antibiotics**: A short course of antibiotics can cut down the course of disease.
- **Saline irrigation**: They help to thin the mucus, wash out bacteria, and give symptomatic relief, antihistaminics
- **Decongestants**: Give relief from acute bacterial rhinosinusitis.
- **Intranasal steroids**: They are anti-inflammatory in nature and are used to relieve edema and associated allergy and cut down the course of disease.

Acute Maxillary Sinusitis

Q. Write a short note on acute maxillary sinusitis.

Etiology

- Viral rhinitis followed by bacterial invasion
- Diving and swimming in contaminated water
- Dental infections
- Trauma to the sinus such as compound fractures, penetrating injuries, or gunshot wounds.

Clinical Features

- **Constitutional symptoms:** Fever, general malaise, and body ache
- Headache
- Pain over the upper jaw may be referred to as gums or teeth pain, is also referred to as supraorbital region.
- Tenderness
- Redness and edema of the cheek
- Postnasal discharge

Diagnosis

- **Transillumination test**: Affected sinus will be found opaque.
- **X-rays:** X-ray paranasal sinuses (PNS) Water's view will show either opacity or a fluid level in the involved sinus.

Treatment

- **Antimicrobial drugs**: Ampicillin and amoxicillin are quite effective and cover a wide range of organisms.
- **Nasal decongestant drops**: Xylometazoline or oxymetazoline to decongest sinus ostium and encourage drainage.
- Steam inhalation
- Analgesics
- Hot fomentation
- **Antral lavage**: Lavage is done only when medical treatment has failed and that too is only under the cover of antibiotics.

Complications

- Acute maxillary sinusitis
- Frontal sinusitis
- Osteomyelitis of maxilla
- Orbital cellulitis

Acute Frontal Sinusitis

Q. Write a short note on acute frontal sinusitis.

Etiology

- Viral infections followed by bacterial invasion
- Entry of water into the sinus during diving/swimming
- External trauma to the sinuses

Clinical Features

- **Frontal headache**: It shows characteristic periodicity, comes up on waking, gradually increases, and reaches its peak by about mid-day and then starts subsiding. It is also called office headache.
- Tenderness
- Edema of the upper eyelid
- Nasal discharge (purulent)

Treatment

- Antimicrobials
- Decongestion of the sinus ostium
- Analgesics

Complications

- Orbital cellulitis
- Osteomyelitis of frontal bone
- Meningitis
- Chronic frontal sinusitis

Acute Ethmoid Sinusitis

Q. Write a short note on acute ethmoid sinusitis.

Acute ethmoiditis is often associated with infection of other sinuses.

Clinical Features

- Pain is localized over the bridge of the nose, medial, and deep to the eye
- Edema of the lids
- Nasal discharge
- Swelling of the middle turbinate

Treatment

Medical treatment is the same as for acute maxillary sinusitis.

Complications

- Orbital cellulitis and abscess
- Visual deterioration and blindness
- Cavernous sinus thrombosis
- Extradural abscess

Chronic Rhinosinusitis

It is a chronic inflammatory disease of nasal and paranasal sinus mucosa where symptomatology has continued beyond 12 weeks.

Chronic Rhinosinusitis (CRS) without Polyps

Q. Write a short note on chronic rhinosinusitis without polyps.

It is bacterial in origin. Organisms involved are *S. aureus, Pseudomonas aeruginosa,* and *Klebsiella pneumoniae.*

Predisposing Factors

- **Structural deformities**: Deviated nasal septum, concha bullosa, prominent agger nasi which comprise the osteomeatal complex leading to sinusitis.
- Impairment of mucociliary clearance
- Cystic fibrosis and young syndrome
- Osteomyelitis
- Dental infection
- Asthma
- Allergy

Pathophysiology

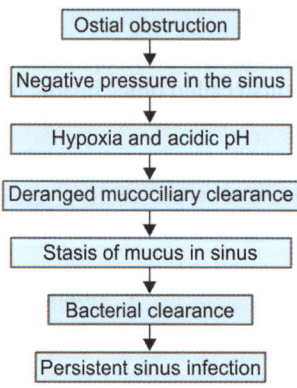

Clinical Features

- Nasal obstruction
- Nasal or postnasal discharge
- Facial pain and pressure
- Disturbance of smell
- Edema of nasal mucosa in the anterior or the posterior osteomeatal complex
- Purulent discharge

Treatment

Medical

- Antibiotics
- **Saline irrigation:** They help to wash out bacteria and also disrupt biofilms
- Topical decongestants
- Steroid sprays
- Antihistaminics

Surgical

Functional endoscopic sinus surgery (FESS) is used for those who fail medical treatment.

Chronic Rhinosinusitis (CRS) with Polyposis

Q. Write a short note on chronic rhinosinusitis with polyposis/nasal polyps.

- Polyp formation in the nose and sinuses can be due to the infection processes or systemic disorders such as primary ciliary dyskinesia, cystic fibrosis, asthma, and Churg–Strauss syndrome.
- Symptomatology is similar to that seen in CRS.
- Examination of the nose shows multiple nasal polyps **(Fig. 1)**.

Diagnosis

- It can be made on history, physical examination, and imaging studies.
- Computed tomography (CT) scan of PNS reveals the extent of the disease.

Treatment

Medical

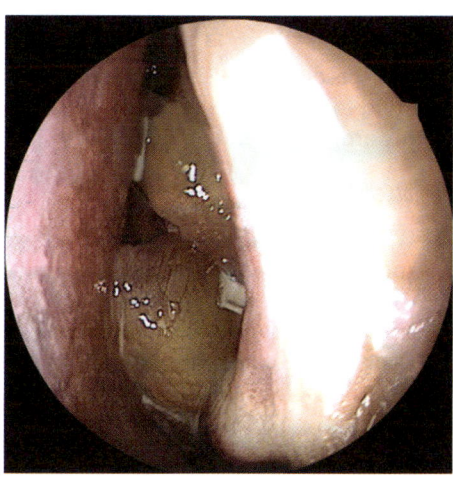

Fig. 1: Nasal endoscopic view of rhinosinusitis with polyps.

- Systemic steroids
- Steroidal nasal sprays
- Management of allergies
- Nasal irrigations
- Antibiotics

Functional Endoscopic Sinus Surgery

- It is the latest development of endoscopic surgeries.
- Rigid endoscopes provide better illumination and magnification and permit the visualization of structures situated at different angles.

Microsurgical Instruments

Which permit precise and limited surgery, directed at specific sites, to remove the obstruction to the sinus.

Complications of Sinusitis

Q. Describe the complications following sinusitis.

Local Complications

- Mucocele
- Osteomyelitis
- Mucous retention cyst
- Osteomyelitis

Mucocele

- The sinuses are commonly affected by mucocele in the order of frequency are the frontal, ethmoid, maxillary, and sphenoid.
- **Etiology:** Chronic obstruction to sinus ostium resulting in accumulation of secretions which slowly expand and destroy its bony walls.
- **Mucocele of frontal sinus**: Usually present in the superomedial quadrant of orbit and displaces the eyeball forward, downward, and laterally.
- Swelling is cystic and nontender, egg shell crackling may be elicited. Patient presents with headache, diplopia, and proptosis.
- Treatment is frontoethmoidectomy with free drainage of frontal sinus into the middle meatus.

Orbital Complications

Q. Write a short note on orbital complications with sinusitis.

- Preseptal inflammatory edema of lids
- Subperiosteal abscess
- Orbital cellulitis
- Orbital abscess **(Fig. 2)**
- Orbital apex syndrome

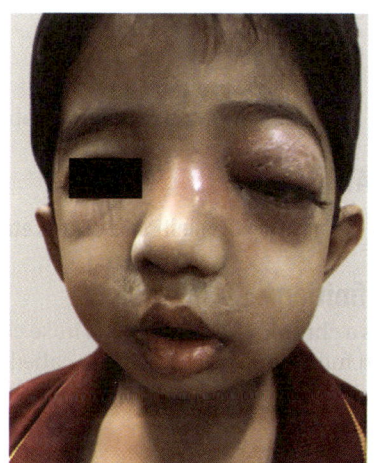

Fig. 2: Orbital abscess due to rhinosinusitis.

PART 1: Diseases of ENT, Head and Neck

Subperiosteal Abscess

Pus collects outside the bone under the periosteum. A subperiosteal abscess from ethmoid forms on the medial wall of orbit and displaces the eyeball forward, downward, and laterally.

Orbital Cellulitis (Fig. 3)

- When pus breaks through the periosteum and finds its way into the orbit, it spreads between the orbital fat, extraocular muscles, vessels, and nerves.
- Clinical features include edema of lids, exophthalmos, chemosis of conjunctiva, and restricted movements of eyeball.
- Orbital cellulitis is potentially dangerous because of the risk of meningitis and cavernous sinus thrombosis.

Orbital Apex Syndrome

It is superior orbital fissure syndrome with additional involvement of the optic nerve and maxillary division of trigeminal.

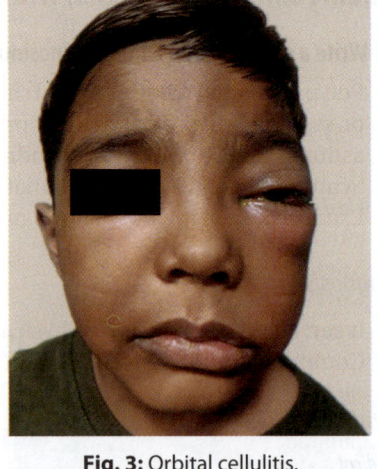

Fig. 3: Orbital cellulitis.

Intracranial Complications

Q. Write a short note on intracranial complications of sinusitis.

- Cavernous sinus thrombosis
- Meningitis
- Extradural abscess
- Subdural abscess
- Brain abscess **(Fig. 4)**

Cavernous Sinus Thrombosis

- Infections of PNS, particularly those of ethmoid and sphenoid, and orbital complications from these sinus infections cause thrombophlebitis of the cavernous sinus.
- Clinical features:
  - Swollen eyelids with chemosis and proptosis of eyeball
  - Total ophthalmoplegia
  - Pupil becomes dilated and fixed, the optic disk shows congestion and edema with diminution of vision.
- **Investigations**: CT scan of nose + PNS + orbital cuts + brain
- **Treatment**: It consists of intravenous (IV) antibiotics and attention to the focus of infections, drainage of infection ethmoid or sphenoid sinus.

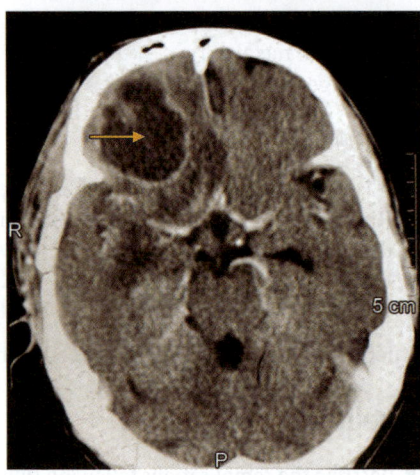

Fig. 4: Computed tomography (CT) scan of brain showing frontal lobe abscess due to rhinosinusitis.

Descending Infections

- Otitis media
- Pharyngitis and tonsillitis
- Persistent laryngitis and tracheobronchitis

ATROPHIC RHINITIS

Q. Define atrophic rhinitis and discuss etiopathology and management of atrophic rhinitis.

Definition

It is a chronic inflammation of nose characterized by atrophy of nasal mucosa and turbinate bones. The nasal cavity is roomy and full of foul-smelling crusts called Ozaenae.

Types

```
                    Atrophic rhinitis
                   /                \
         Primary atrophic rhinitis   Secondary atrophic rhinitis
```

Primary Atrophic Rhinitis

Q. Write a short note on primary atrophic rhinitis.

Etiology

- Hereditary factors
- **Endocrine disturbances:** Disease starts at puberty, and involves females more than males. The crusting tends to reduce after menopause.
- **Racial factors:** White and yellow races are more susceptible than natives of equatorial Africa.
- **Nutritional deficiency:** Deficiency of vitamin A and D, iron, or some other dietary factors.
- **Infective:** *Klebsiella ozaenae*, diphtheroids, and *Proteus vulgaris*

Pathology

- Ciliated columnar epithelium is lost and is replaced by stratified squamous epithelium. There is atrophy of seromucinous glands. There is obliterative endarteritis and periarteritis of terminal arterioles in Type I.
- There are dilated capillaries worsened by estrogen in Type II
- The bone of turbinates undergoes resorption causing widening of nasal chambers.

Clinical Features

- Symptoms:
  - Foul smell from nose
  - Anosmia (merciful)
  - Nasal obstruction due to large crusts filling the nose
  - Epistaxis
- Signs:
  - Greyish black, green, and yellow dry crusts in the nasal cavity.
  - Roomy nasal cavity and nasopharynx can be visualized through anterior nares
  - Pale nasal mucosa, shriveled, and shrunken turbinates
  - Septal perforation
  - Dermatitis of the nasal vestibule

Treatment

Medical

- Nasal irrigation and removal of crusts: Warm normal saline or an alkaline nasal douche solution made by dissolving a teaspoonful of powder containing sodium bicarbonate 1 part, sodium biborate 1 part, sodium chloride 2 parts in 280 mL of water used to irrigate the nasal cavities. The solution is run through one nostril and comes out from the other irrigations are done two or three times a day but later once in every 2 or 3 days.
- **25% glucose in glycerine:** It inhibits the growth of proteolytic organisms which are responsible for the foul smell.
- **Local antibiotics:** Streptomycin/rifampicin
- **Kemicetine antiozaenae solution:** Chloramphenicol, estradiol, vitamin D_2
- **Estradiol sprays:** It helps to increase the vascularity of nasal mucosa and regeneration of seromucinous glands.
- Placental extract injected submucosally may provide some relief.
- **Systemic use of streptomycin:** Effective against *Klebsiella* organisms.
- Potassium iodide tablets and nasal solution

Surgical

- **Young's operation:** Both nostrils are closed completely just within the nasal vestibule by raising flaps. They are opened after 6 months or later. In these cases, the mucosa may revert to normal, and crusting reduced.
- **Modified Young's operation:** To avoid the discomfort of bilateral nasal obstruction, modified procedure aims to partially close both the nostrils. 2 mm opening is kept in one nostril for breathing.
- **Gadre's double breasting:** Double nasal flap mucosal and skin at mucocutaneous junction and closed.
- **Raghav Sharan's operation:** Antral mucosal transplantation into nasal cavity. Parotid ducted transplanted in maxillary sinus mucosa.
- Cervical sympathectomy

- Stellate ganglion block
- Sphenopalatine ganglion block
- **Lautenslager operation:** Fracture and medial displacement of lateral nasal wall
- **Ghosh vestibuloplasty:** Raising a lateral shelf from nasal vestibular flap to cover turbinates
- **Narrowing the nasal cavities:** Wison's operation—submucosal injection of Teflon paste.

Nasal closure	Volume reduction	Denervation	Salivary irrigation
Young	Lautenslager	Cervical sympathectomy	Parotid duct implantation
Modified Young	Ghosh vestibuloplasty	Stellate ganglion block	
	Sublabial implants	Sphenopalatine ganglion block	

Secondary Atrophic Rhinitis

Q. Write a short note on secondary atrophic rhinitis.

- Specific infections such as syphilis, lupus, and leprosy may cause destruction of nasal structures leading to atrophic changes.
- Atrophic rhinitis can also result from long standing purulent sinusitis
- Radiotherapy to nose
- Iatrogenic:
  - Excessive surgical removal of turbinates
  - Septoplasty
  - Submucosal resection (SMR)
- Maggots in the nose **(Fig. 5)**
- Severe deviated nasal septum (DNS) on one side

■ FUNGAL INFECTION OF SINUSES

Q. Describe various fungal infections affecting sinuses.

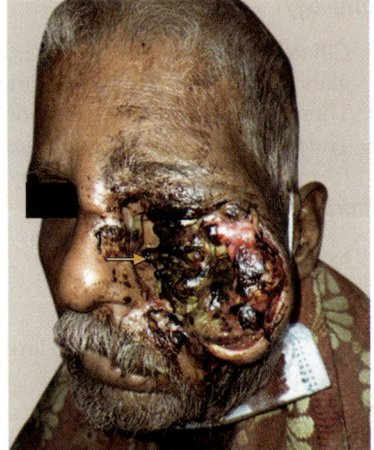

Fig. 5: Excessive maggots involving nose, paranasal sinuses, and orbit.

Fungal Ball

- It is due to implantation of fungus into an otherwise healthy sinus which on CT shows a hyperdense area with no evidence of bone erosion or expansion.
- Maxillary sinus is the most common involved followed by sphenoid, ethmoid, and frontal.
- Treatment is surgical, removal of fungal ball and adequate drainage of sinus. No antifungal therapy is required.

Allergic Fungal Sinusitis

Q. Write a short note on allergic fungal sinusitis.

- It is an allergic reaction to the causative fungus.
- It presents with sinonasal polyposis and mucin.
- It contains eosinophils, Charcot–Leyden cells, and fungal hyphae.
- No invasion of sinus mucosa by fungus.
- CT is suggestive of hyperdense areas and mucosal thickening.
- There may be expansion of sinuses or bone erosion due to pressure, but no fungal invasion.
- **Treatment:** Endoscopic surgical clearance of the sinuses with provision of drainage and ventilation. Systemic steroids can be used.

Chronic Invasive Sinusitis

Q. Write a short note on chronic invasive sinusitis.

- Fungus invades the nasal mucosa.
- There is bone erosion by the fungus
- Patient presents with chronic rhinosinusitis.
- CT scan of nose and paranasal sinuses shows thickened mucosa with opacification of sinus and bone erosion.
- Patient may have an intracranial or intraorbital invasion.
- Histopathology shows fungal invasion of submucosa and granulomatous reaction with multinucleated giant cells.

Fulminant Fungal Sinusitis

Q. Write a short note on fulmitant fungal sinusitis.

- Acute presentation and seen mostly in immunocompromised or diabetic individuals.
- Common species are **Mucor** and **Aspergillus.**
- Mucor causes rhinocerebral disease. Invasion of blood vessels, *Mucor* fungus causes ischemic necrosis presenting as black eschar.
- It involves turbinates, palate, sinuses, and intraorbital invasion may be present **(Fig. 6)**.
- It spreads to the face, eyes, skull base, and the brain. The treatment is surgical debridement and IV amphotericin B.
- *Aspergillus* infection can also cause acute fulminant sinusitis with tissue invasion. Such patients present with acute sinusitis and develop sepsis and other sinus complications sinuses and intraorbital invasion may be present on MRI **(Figs. 7A and B)** and diagnostic nasal endoscopy **(Fig. 8)**.
- Treatment is antifungal therapy and surgery.

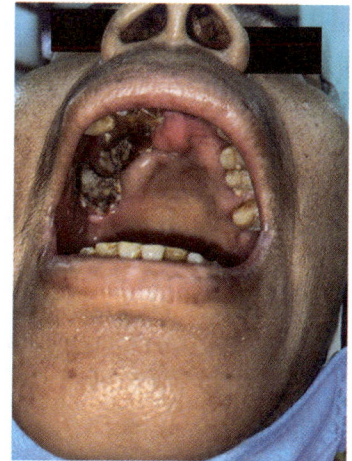

Fig. 6: Palatal mucormycosis following nasal mucormycosis.

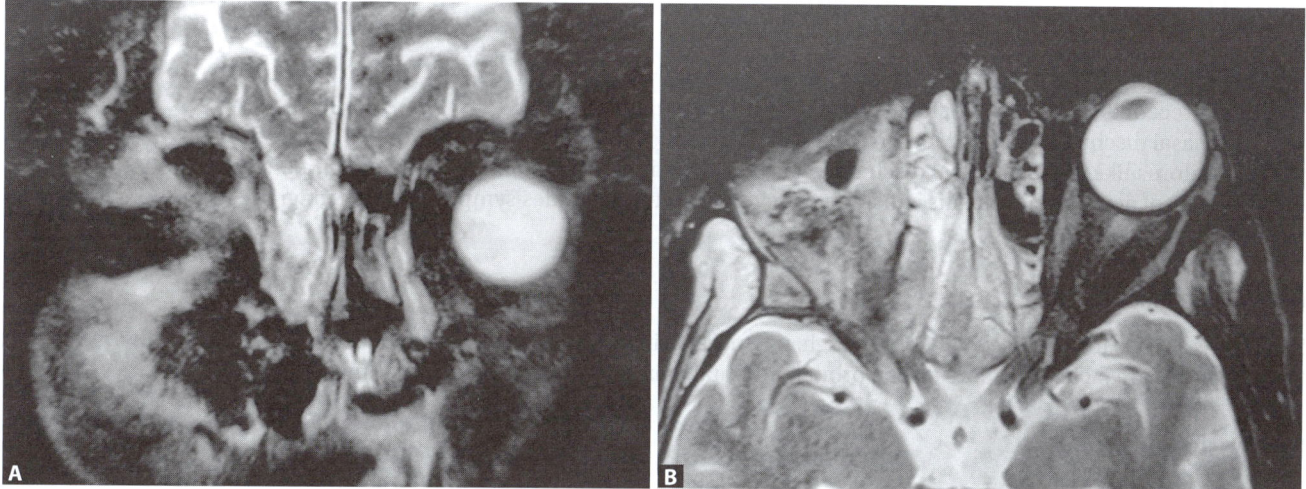

Figs. 7A and B: Magnetic resonance imaging (MRI) showing extensive mucormycosis of paranasal sinuses and orbit.

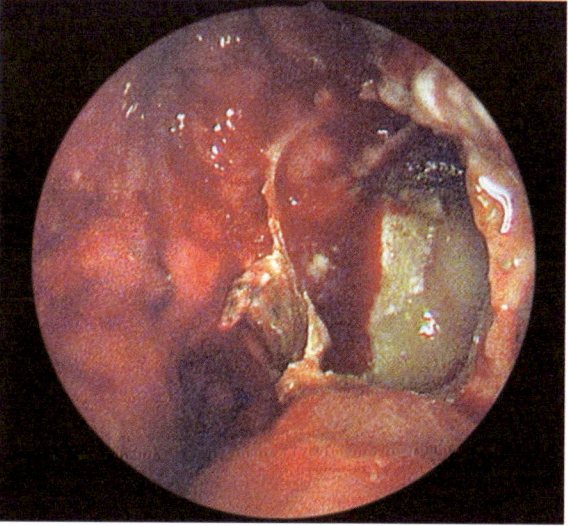

Fig. 8: Nasal endoscopic view of septal perforation with black crust of mucormycosis.

PEDIATRIC RHINOSINUSITIS

It is multifactorial disease.
There are predisposing factors and increasing age factor, c ourse of disease which classifies it in different types:
- **Acute**: 10 days to less than 3 weeks
- **Subacute**: 3 weeks to less than 12 weeks
- **Chronic**: More than 12 weeks
- **Recurrent**: Complete resolution occurs in between episodes which are 3 or more in 6 months or more than 4 in 1 year.

Pathophysiology
- Obstruction in drainage pathway of sinuses.
  - Stasis of secretions leading to sinus disease
- Anatomic obstruction can be due to turbinate hypertrophy, concha bullosa. Septal deviations, polyps, spur, enlarges adenoids, infection
- Other conditions may increase incidence of sinus disease includes allergy, air pollution, smoke, gastroesophageal reflux disease (GERD)

Clinical Features

Acute Rinosinusitis
- Often preceded by viral upper airway respiratory infection.
- Clear nasal discharge often recedes in 5 days.
- If symptoms like purulent nasal discharge, nasal obstruction, facial pain, day time cough persist for more than 10days diagnosis of acute rhinosinusitis considered. Severe infection includes symptoms like high grade fever more than 40° C and periorbital edema.

Chronic Rhinosinusitis

Symptoms are nasal discharge, night time cough, postnasal drip, nasal obstruction, headache persist for more than 12 weeks. Other features are facial pain, sore throat, orbital or dental pain, low grade fever and asthma.

Diagnosis
- Clinical
- Diagnostic nasal endoscopic examination
- Culture of nasal , sinus secretions
- Allergic assessment
- CT scan of paranasal sinuses (limited coronal cuts)

Treatment

Medical Therapy
- **Acute rhinosinusitis:** Antibiotics (amoxycillin, azithromycin, cefuroxime, clarithromycin)
- **Chronic rhinosinusitis**: Antibiotics for 3 weeks.
- **Topical nasal spray:** Mometazone, fluticasone propionate

Surgical Treatment
- Adenoidectomy
- Functional endoscopic sinus surgery (FESS)

Chapter 24

Allergic, Vasomotor Rhinitis and Nonallergic Rhinitis

> **EN4.25**: Elicit document and present a correct history, demonstrate, and describe the clinical features, choose the correct investigations and describe the principles of management of vasomotor rhinitis.

■ VASOMOTOR RHINITIS

Q. Write short note/essay on vasomotor rhinitis.

It is nonallergic rhinitis but clinically resembles nasal allergy with symptoms of nasal obstruction, rhinorrhea, and sneezing.

Pathogenesis of Vasomotor Rhinitis

- Parasympathetic stimulation causes vasodilation, engorgement, and excessive secretions from nasal glands, sympathetic stimulation causes vasoconstriction and shrinkage of the mucosa.
- The autonomic nervous system is under the control of the hypothalamus and therefore emotions play a great role in vasomotor rhinitis. Autonomic system (ANS) is unstable in cases of vasomotor rhinitis.

Symptomatology and Signs

- Paroxysmal sneezing
- Excessive rhinorrhea
- Nasal obstruction
- Postnasal drips
- Nasal mucosa over the turbinates is hypertrophic and congested or in some cases normal.

Complications

Long-standing cases may develop:
- Nasal polyps
- Hypertrophic rhinitis and sinusitis.

Treatment

Medical

- Avoidance of physical factors that stimulate symptoms, e.g., humidity and blast of air or dust
- Antihistamines and oral nasal decongestion provide relief from symptoms
- Topical steroids
- Systemic steroids in severe cases.

Surgical

- Causes of nasal obstruction are corrected, e.g., polyp, deviated nasal septum, and reduce size of nasal turbinates.
- **Vidian neurectomy** is done in cases of excessive rhinorrhea not corrected by medical therapy.

PART 1: Diseases of ENT, Head and Neck

EN4.24: Elicit document and present a correct history, demonstrate, and describe the clinical features, choose the correct investigations and describe the principles of management of allergic rhinitis.

ALLERGIC RHINITIS

Q. Write short note/essay on allergic rhinitis.

Types

- **Seasonal:** Symptoms in and around a particular season.
- **Perennial:** Symptoms are present throughout the year.

Etiology

- **Inhalant allergen:** Pollen, dust mites, cockroaches, and dust mites from animals **(Fig. 1)**.
- **Genetic predisposition:** There is a risk of 20% if one parent suffers from allergic rhinitis and 47% if both parents suffer from allergic rhinitis.
- **Common allergen:** Pollen and dust, dust mites, food substances such as mushrooms and fungus growing over damp walls, nuts such as almonds and peanuts, industrial smoke, pollution, and certain medications like penicillin.

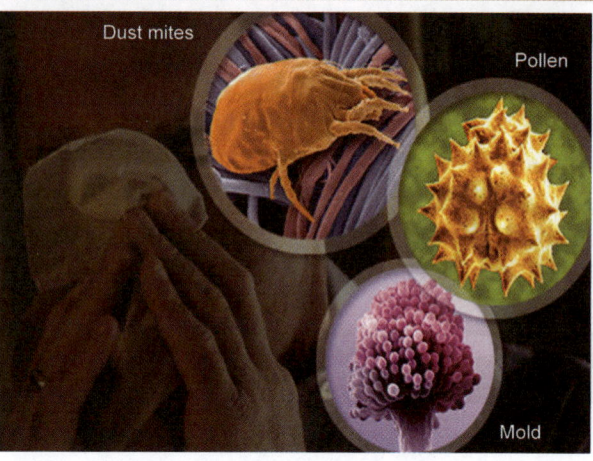

Fig. 1: Sources of nasal allergy.

Pathogenesis

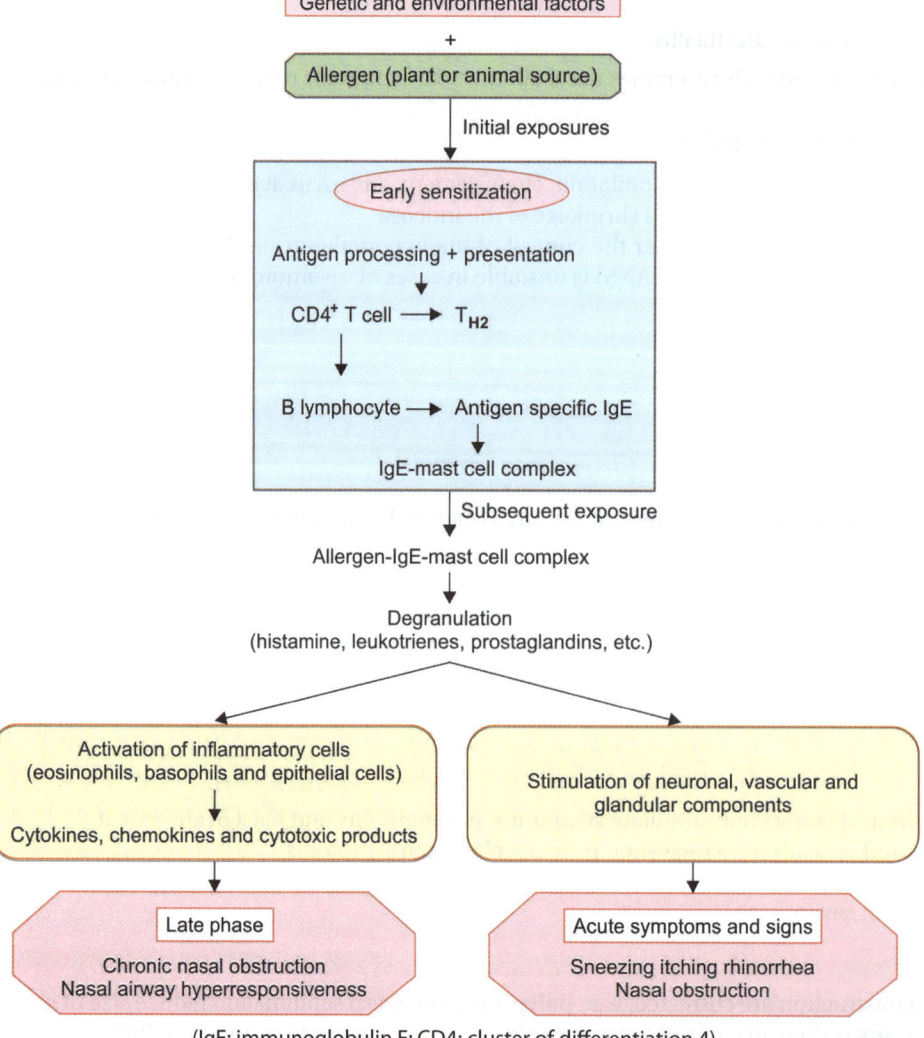

(IgE: immunoglobulin E; CD4: cluster of differentiation 4)

Clinical Features

Symptoms

- **Seasonal nasal allergy:** Paroxysmal sneezing, nasal obstruction, watery nasal discharge, and itching in the nose, eyes, and pharynx.
- **Perennial allergy:** Persistent stuffy nose, loss of smell, postnasal drip, chronic cough, frequent cold.

Signs

- **Nasal signs—allergic salute:** A black line across the middle of dorsum of nose due to constant upward rubbing of the nose. Pale and edematous nasal mucosa, watery or mucoid nasal discharge.
- **Ocular signs:** Eyelid edema, congestion, cobblestone appearance of the conjunctiva, and allergic shiners.
- **Otologic signs:** Retracted tympanic membrane and serous otitis media.
- **Pharyngeal signs:** Granular pharyngitis
- **Laryngeal signs:** Hoarseness and edema

Classification

Allergic rhinitis and its impact on asthma (ARIA) Guidelines 2019.

Intermittent
- <4 days/week
- <4 consecutive weeks

Persistent
- >4 days/week
- >4 consecutive weeks

Mild
- Normal sleep
- No impairment of daily activities, sport, and leisure
- Normal work and school
- No troublesome symptoms

Moderate-severe
- One or more items
- Abnormal sleep
- Impairment of daily activities, sport, and leisure
- Abnormal work and school
- Troublesome symptoms

Investigations

- **Total and differential count:** Peripheral eosinophilia
- **Nasal smear:** Large number of eosinophils are seen.
- Specific immunoglobulin E (IgE) measurements
- **Radioallergosorbent test:** It is an in vitro test and measures specific IgE antibody concentrations in patient's serum.
- **Skin prick test:** A drop of concentrated allergen solution is placed on the volar surface of the forearm and a sharp needle is pricked into the dermis through the drop. A positive reaction is manifested by the formation of a central wheal and a surrounding zone of erythema within 10–15 minutes.

Complications

- Recurrent sinusitis
- Formation of nasal polyps
- Serous otitis media
- Orthodontic problems
- Bronchial asthma

Treatment

- Avoidance of allergen
- Treatment with drugs
- Pharmacotherapy:
  - **Antihistaminics:** For control of rhinorrhea, sneezing, and nasal itch.
  - **Sympathomimetic drugs:** Alpha-adrenergic drugs constrict blood vessels and reduce nasal congestion and edema. They are used in combination with antihistaminics such as chlorpheniramine, cetirizine, levocetirizine, loratadine, desloratadine, and bilastine to counteract drowsiness.
  - **Corticosteroids:** For control of symptoms and used in acute episodes that have not been controlled by other measures.
  - Systemic steroids in oral tablet form and/or local steroidal nasal sprays are given. Oral steroids contain methylprednisolone and deflazacort. Nasal steroidal sprays contains—fluticasone, mometasone, azelastine.
  - **Sodium cromoglycate:** It is used as a 2% solution for nasal drips or sprays, it stabilizes mast cells and prevents them from degranulation despite the formation of IgE—antigen complex.
  - **Leukotriene receptor antagonist:** Montelukast, zafirlukast, and palookas. They block cysteinyl leukotriene-type receptors.
  - **Anti IgE:** Omalizumab, reduces the IgE level and has an anti-inflammatory effect.

Immunotherapy

- Use of allergy shots in the body to make the body familiar to the allergen.
- Not very cost-effective and immediate local and systemic allergic reactions.

NONALLERGIC RHINITIS

Types

Nonallergic rhinitis with eosinophilia syndrome (NARES)
- Drug-induced rhinitis
- Rhinitis medicamentosa
- Honeymoon rhinitis
- Emotional rhinitis
- Hormone-related rhinitis (hypothyroidism, menstruation, puberty, pregnancy)
- Gustatory rhinitis
- Occupational rhinitis
- Nonairflow rhinitis
- Idiopathic or vasomotor rhinitis

Etiological Classification of Nonallergic Rhinitis

Medicines: Local and systemic	Topical decongestants (medicamentosa), antihypertensive beta blockers, aspirin, nonsteroidal anti-inflammatory (NSAID), oral contraceptives, psychotropic
Hormonal	Hypothyroidism, acromegaly, puberty, menstruation, postmenopausal
Irritant and corrosives	Dust, fumes, smoke, gases, chemical, pollution. Acids, organophosphates
Smell	Cosmetics, perfumes, fragrances, cleaning agents, deodorizers
Taste	Gustatory rhinitis due to hot and spicy food
Occupational	Body spray, latex, paint, insecticides, grains
Environmental	Humidity, aviation, altitude, weather, barometric
Local: Trauma, infection, tumors, structural	DNS, septal perforation. Nasal valve collapse, turbinate and adenoid hypertrophy, choanal atresia, rhinosinusitis, polyps, inverted papilloma, rhinoscleroma, malignancy
Emotional	Anxiety, tension, hostility, humiliation, grief
Substance abuse	Alcohol, nicotine, cocaine
Exercise	Sedentary lifestyle
Decreased nasal flow	Tracheostomy, laryngectomy
Atrophic changes	Atrophic rhinitis, infection, aging, surgery
Systemic diseases	Sjogren's syndrome, Kartagener's syndrome, Wegner's granulomatosis, Young's syndrome, systemic lupus erythematosus, cystic fibrosis, Horner's syndrome
Idiopathic	Vasomotor rhinitis, rhinitis with eosinophilia

Investigations
- Absolute eosinophilic count
- Nasal smear cytology
- Skin and in vitro allergy test
- Acoustic rhinometry to measure nasal patency

Treatment

Medical
- Avoidance of inciting factors
- Antihistaminics and oral decongestants
- Steroidal nasal spray
- Systemic steroids
- Exercise
- Tranquilizers
- Psychological counseling

Surgery
- Reduction of turbinate hypertrophy
- Vidian neurectomy
- Removal of polyps
- Correction of DNS

Chapter 25

Nasal Polyp

EN4.27: Elicit document and present a correct history, demonstrate and describe the clinical features, choose the correct investigations and describe the principles of management of nasal polyps.

■ DEFINITION

Q. Define nasal polyps. Discuss etiopathogenesis, clinical features, investigations and management of nasal polyps.

Nasal polyps are non-neoplastic masses of edematous sinonasal mucosa. There are two types of nasal polyps—(1) antrochoanal and (2) ethmoidal.

■ ETIOLOGY

Exact etiology is not known. It is a manifestation of the following:
- Rhinosinusitis
- Allergic fungal sinusitis
- Cystic fibrosis—a disorder of ciliary motility
- Kartagener's syndrome—bronchiectasis, sinusitis, situs invertus, and ciliary dyskinesia
- Woakes' syndrome—bronchiectasis and nasal polyp
- Young's syndrome—sinupulmonary disease and azoospermia
- Bernoulli's phenomenon—suction effect near the sinus osteum, pulls the sinus mucosa into the nose due to pressure drop or negative pressure near the constriction

■ PATHOLOGY

Columnar ciliated epithelium turns into transitional or squamous type with submucosal edema and eosinophils.

■ CLINICAL FEATURES

History

Nasal polyps present with unilateral or bilateral nasal obstruction.

Symptoms

- Unilateral/bilateral nasal obstruction
- Nasal discharge—watery/mucoid/purulent
- Increased sneezing
- Itching of nose
- Partial or complete anosmia
- Headache/pain over sinus areas
- Change in voice, nasal twang (rhinolalia clausa)

Signs

Smooth, globular, painless, pale pedunculated, or sessile nasal mass is seen on anterior rhinoscopy.

Antrochoanal vs Ethmoidal Polyp

Q. What are the differences between antrochoanal and ethmoidal polyp?

	Antrochoanal polyp (Figs. 1 and 2)	Ethmoidal polyp (Fig. 3)
Age	Common in children	Common in adults
Side	Unilateral	Unilateral
Etiology	Infective	Allergy
Origin	Maxillary sinus	Ethmoidal sinus
Shape	Dumbbell (nasal, antral part)/trifoliate (nasal, antral, and nasopharyngeal part)	Grape like masses
Growth	Towards anterior nares	Towards posterior choana

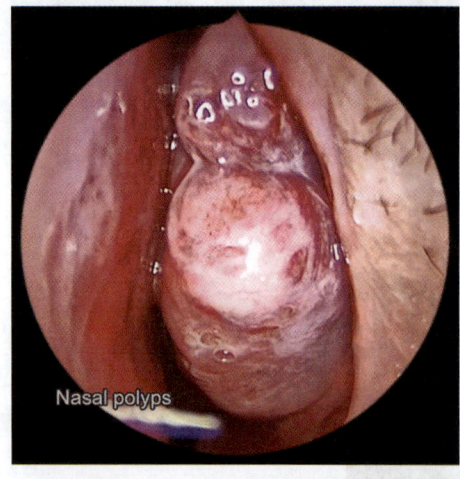

Fig. 1: Endoscopic view of the antrochoanal nasal polyp.

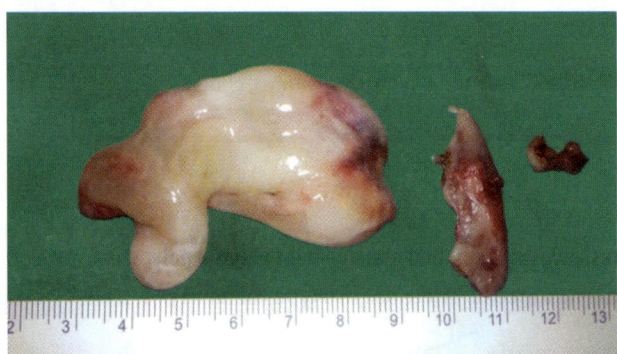

Fig. 2: Antrochoanal nasal polyp (dumbbell shape).

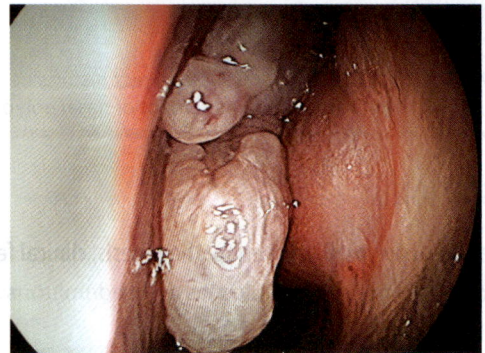

Fig. 3: Nasal endoscopic view of ethmoidal polyp.

■ MANAGEMENT

Investigations

- ❖ X-ray of the nose and paranasal sinuses:
  - ➢ Water's view: Suggestive of opacity in maxillary sinus and nasal cavity
  - ➢ Caldwell's view: Suggestive of—opacity in the maxillary and or ethmoidal sinuses
- ❖ Computed tomography (CT) scan of nose and paranasal sinuses—soft tissue opacity in ethmoidal/maxillary sinus, nasopharynx, and nose.

Treatment

	Antrochoanal polyp	Ethmoidal polyp
Medical	❖ Antibiotics and antihistaminic drugs ❖ Nasal decongestant drops (oxymetazoline/xylometazoline)	❖ Antihistaminic tablets, systemic steroids ❖ Nasal steroidal spray (fluticasone, azelastine, mometasone)
Surgical	Recent functional sinus surgery (FESS)	Recent FESS
	Outdated: Caldwell Luc surgery and nasal polypectomy	Outdated: Intranasal polypectomy and external ethmoidectomy

■ DIFFERENTIAL DIAGNOSIS OF NASAL OBSTRUCTION

- ❖ Nasal polyp
- ❖ Hypertrophied middle turbinate
- ❖ Angiofibroma
- ❖ Pediatric nasal masses such as encephalocele, Thornwald cyst, and nasal glioma

Tip to differentiate nasal polyp from other nasal swelling: Probe test is helpful. Probe can be passes all along the swelling and polyp is painless and does not bleed on touch. On putting nose drops turbinate it shrink in size whereas polyp does not shrink.

Chapter 26

Epistaxis

EN4.28: Elicit document and present a correct history, demonstrate and describe the clinical features, choose the correct investigations and describe the principles of management of epistaxis.

■ INTRODUCTION

Q. What is epistaxis? Write a note on its etiology and classification.

Epistaxis means bleeding from the nose.

Reasons of Bleeding

- ❖ Vascular organ secondary to incredible heating/humidification requirements
  - ➢ Vasculature runs just under mucosa (not squamous)
  - ➢ Arterial to venous anastomoses
  - ➢ Internal carotid artery (ICA) and external carotid artery (ECA) blood flow
- ❖ Blood supply of nasal septum **(Fig. 1)**

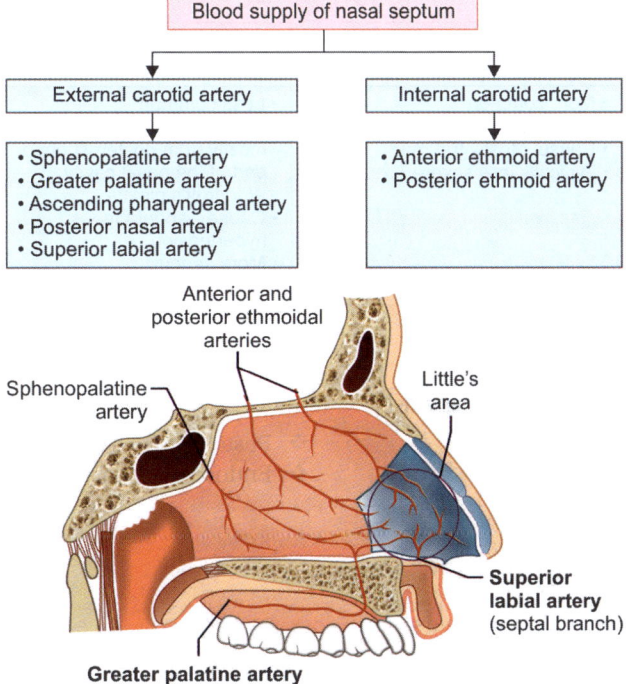

Fig. 1: Blood supply of nasal septum.

PART 1: Diseases of ENT, Head and Neck

ETIOLOGY OF EPISTAXIS

Local	General	Idiopathic
Adults: Trauma, nasal fractures - Iatrogenic nasal injury functional endoscopic sinus surgery - Rhinoplasty - Nasal reconstruction In children—nose picking, foreign body, and nasal diphtheria (one-third with chronic bleeds have coagulation disorder)	Disorder of blood and blood products: Leukemia, thrombocytopenia, vitamin K deficiency	Adults
Deviated nasal septum	**Old age:** Cardiovascular system: Hypertension, mitral stenosis, and arteriosclerosis	
Infections: Acute sinusitis, viral rhinitis, granulomatous lesions, crust forming lesions, (atrophic rhinitis), adenoiditis, TB	Liver disease: Hepatic cirrhosis	
Foreign bodies	Kidney disease: Chronic nephritis	

- Middle age: Neoplasm of nose and PNS
- Benign lesions:
  ➢ Hemangioma
  ➢ Inverted papilloma
  ➢ Juvenile nasopharyngeal
  ➢ Angiofibroma
- Malignant lesions (carcinoma and sarcoma)
  ➢ SCCA
  ➢ Adenocarcinoma
  ➢ Melanoma
  ➢ Esthesioneuroblastoma
  ➢ Lymphoma
	Drugs: Anticoagulant therapy, excessive use of analgesics and salicylates, vicarious epistaxis	

(PNS: peripheral nervous system; SCCA: squamous cell carcinoma; TB: tuberculosis)

CLASSIFICATION OF EPISTAXIS

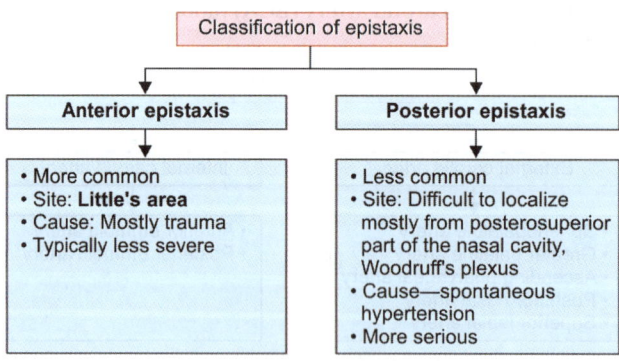

MANAGEMENT OF EPISTAXIS

Q. How will you manage the case of bleeding nose/epistaxis?

- First aid
- Cauterization
- Anterior nasal packing
- Posterior nasal packing
- Endoscopic cauterization

General Measures and First Aid in Epistaxis

- Local compression with thumb and index fingers.
- Cold compression

- Reassure the patient
- Blood pressure and pulse rate monitoring
- Maintenance of hemodynamics

Cauterization

Useful in anterior epistaxis when the bleeding point has been localized. Bleeding point can be cauterized with silver nitrate or electrocautery.

Anterior Nasal Packing (Figs. 2A to C)

Q. Write a short note on anterior nasal packing.

Traditional—Vaseline Gauze Packing

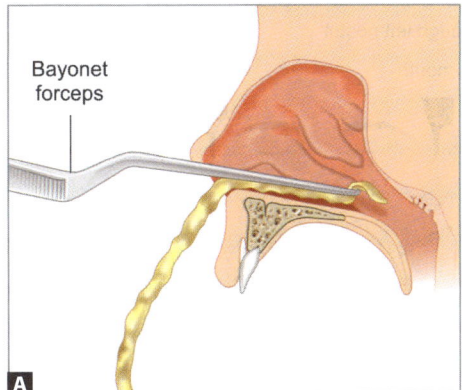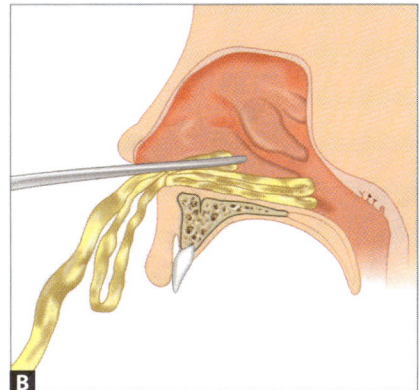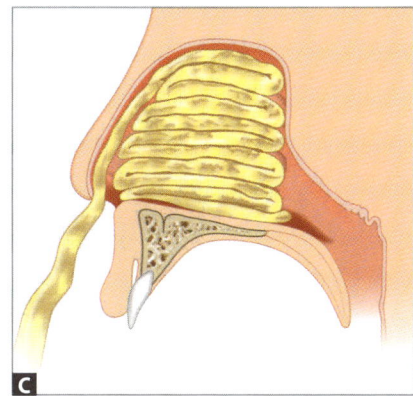

Figs. 2A to C: Anterior nasal packing.

- 1 m gauze (2.5 cm wide in adults and 1.2 cm wide in children) soaked in liquid paraffin is used for both nasal cavity.
- First, few centimeters of gauze are folded upon itself and inserted along the floor, and then the whole nasal cavity is packed tightly by layering the gauze from floor to roof and from before backward. A pack can usually be removed after 48 hours. Systemic antibiotic coverage is given to prevent sinus infection and toxic shock syndrome.

Recent Modifications: Netcell and Gelfoam (Figs. 3 and 4)

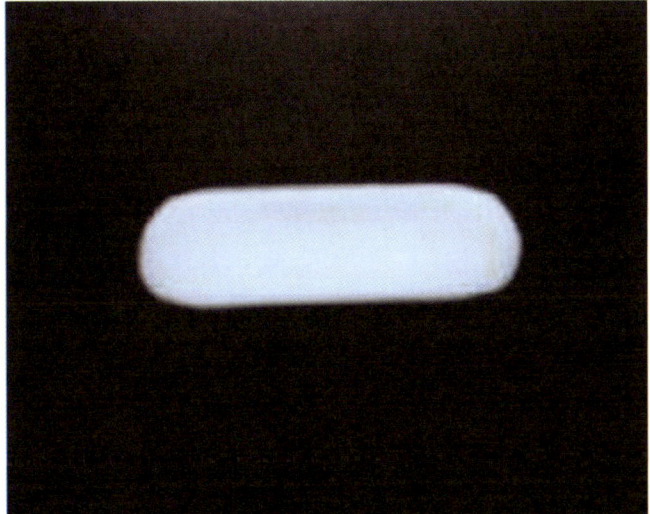

Fig. 3: Netcell.

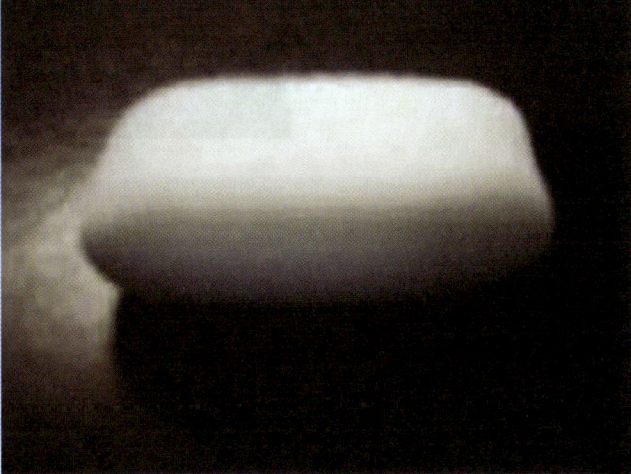

Fig. 4: Gelfoam.

Posterior Nasal Packing (Fig. 5)

Q. Write a short note on posterior nasal packing.

Traditional—Vaseline Gauze Packing

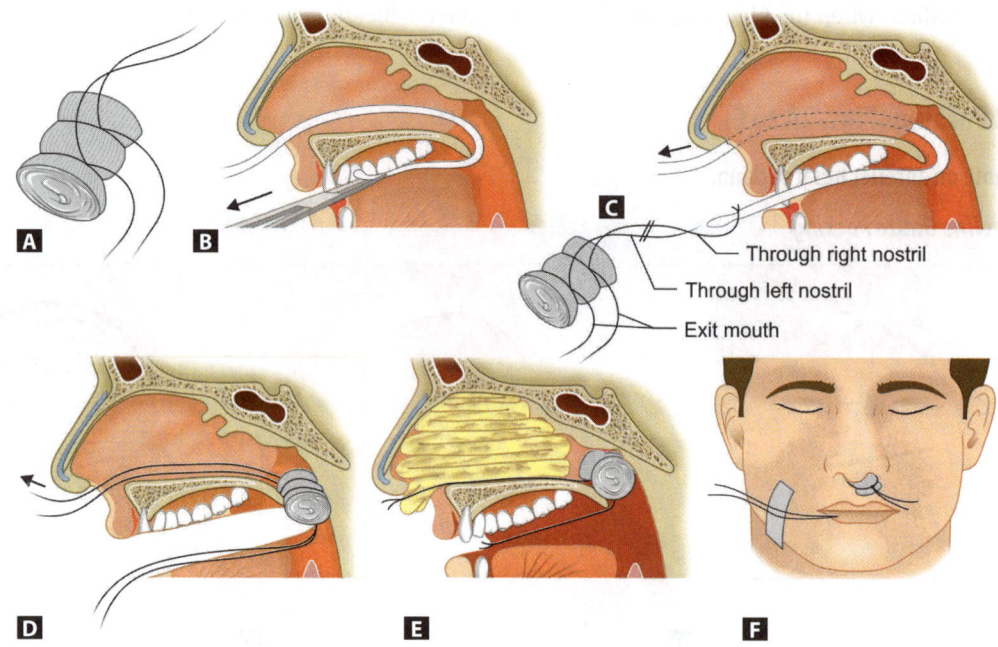

Figs. 5A to F: Posterior nasal packing.

Recent Modifications: Tampons (Fig. 6)

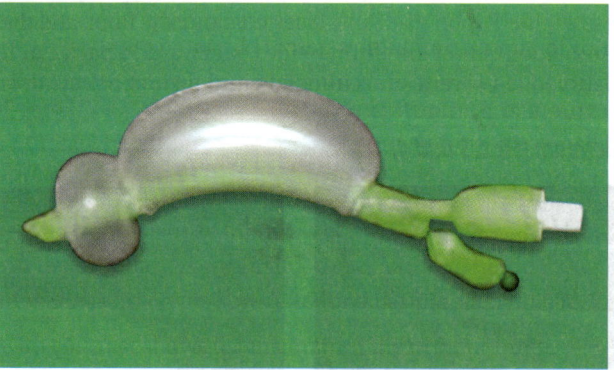

Fig. 6: Tampons.

Ligation of Vessels

- External carotid
- Maxillary artery
- Ethmoidal arteries

Embolization

Done by an interventional radiologist through femoral artery catheterization. Internal maxillary artery is localized and the embolization is performed with absorbable gelfoam or polyvinyl alcohol or coils.

Chapter 27

Facial Trauma

EN4.30: Describe the clinical features, investigations and principles of management of trauma to the face and neck.

■ INTRODUCTION

Injuries of face may involve soft tissues, bones, or both.
Causes:
- Automobile accidents
- Sports
- Personal accidents
- Assaults
- Fights

■ MANAGEMENT

Q. How do you manage a case of facial trauma?

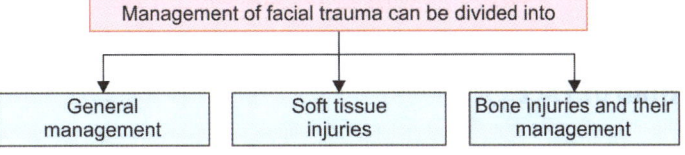

Management of facial trauma can be divided into: General management, Soft tissue injuries, Bone injuries and their management.

General Management
- **Airway:** Maintenance of airway → Highest priority.
  Can be obstructed by:
  - Loss of skeletal support
  - Aspiration of foreign bodies, blood, or gastric contents
  - Swelling of tissues
    Airway is secured by intubation or tracheostomy.
- **Hemorrhage:** Injuries of face may bleed profusely.
  Bleeding should be stopped by pressure or ligation of vessels.
- **Associated injuries:** Injuries of head, chest, abdomen, neck, larynx, cervical spine, or limbs should be attended too.

Soft Tissue Injuries and their Management

Facial Lacerations
- Wound thoroughly cleaned of any dirt, grease, or foreign matter.
- Lacerations closed by accurate approximation of each layer.

Parotid Gland and Duct

Q. How do you manage parotid gland injury?

Damaged structure	Plan
Parotid tissue (if exposed)	Suturing
Duct	❖ Both ends of duct identified and sutured over polyethylene tube with fine suture ❖ The tube is left for 3 days to 2 weeks
Facial nerve	If severed, facial nerve is exposed by superficial parotidectomy and cut ends are approximated with 8–0 or 10–0 silk under magnification

Bone Injuries and their Management

Q. How do you divide face into various regions?

Face can be divided into three regions:
1. **Upper third:** Above level of supraorbital ridge.
2. **Middle third:** Between supraorbital ridge and upper teeth.
3. **Lower third:** Mandible and lower teeth.

Facial Fractures

Q. What are the various fractures of face and what all bony structures are involved?

Upper third	Middle third	Lower third
❖ Frontal sinuses ❖ Supraorbital ridge ❖ Frontal bone	❖ Nasal bones and septum ❖ Naso-orbital area ❖ Zygoma ❖ Zygomatic arch ❖ Orbital floor ❖ Maxilla ❖ Le Fort I (transverse) ❖ Le Fort II (pyramidal) ❖ Le Fort III (craniofacial disjunction)	❖ Mandible: ➤ Alveolar process ➤ Symphysis ➤ Body ➤ Ascending ramus ➤ Condyle ❖ Temporomandibular joint

■ FRACTURES OF UPPER THIRD OF FACE

Frontal Sinus

Q. Write a short note/essay on frontal sinus fractures and its management.

Frontal sinus fractures may involve anterior wall, posterior wall, or nasofrontal duct.

Anterior Wall Fractures

❖ Depressed or comminuted
❖ Defect is mainly cosmetic

Posterior Wall Fractures

It may be accompanied by:
❖ Dural tears
❖ Brain injury   ⎤ Neurosurgical consultation
❖ Cerebrospinal fluid (CSF) rhinorrhea ⎦ is required

 Treatment: Dural tears are repaired with temporalis fascia—small sinus defects—obliterated with fat

> Sinus is approached through a wound in the skin if that is present, or through a brow incision
> ↓
> Bone fragments are elevated, taking care not to strip them from periosteum
> ↓
> Interior of sinus is always inspected to rule out fracture of posterior wall

Injury to Nasofrontal Duct

Complication
- Leads to → obstruction to sinus drainage → mucocele.
- *Treatment:* Make a large communication between sinus and nose.
  Small sinuses → obliterated with fat after removing sinus mucosa completely.

Supraorbital Ridge

Q. Write a short note on clinical features and management of supraorbital ridge fracture.

Clinical Presentation
- Periorbital ecchymosis
- Flattening of eyebrow
- Proptosis or downward displacement of the eye
- Impacted bone fragment in orbit

Treatment
Open reduction through an incision in brow or transverse skin line of forehead.

Fractures of Frontal Bone

Q. What are other associated injuries with frontal bone fracture?
- May be depressed or linear
- With or without separation
- Associated with orbital fracture
- Brain injury and cerebral edema → neurosurgical consultation

FRACTURES OF MIDDLE THIRD OF FACE

Nasal Bones and Septum

Q. Write a short note on most common bony fracture in face.
Q. Write a short note/essay of fractures of nasal bones/nasal septum.
- Most common due to projection of nose on face.
- Traumatic forces may act from front or side.
- Magnitude of force will determine depth of injury.

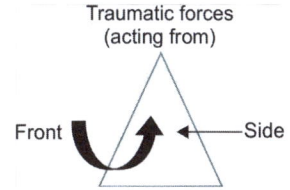

Types of Nasal Fractures

Depressed	Angulated
❖ Due to frontal blow ❖ Lower part of nasal bones which is thinner, easily gives way	Unilateral depression of nasal bone on same side or both nasal bones and septum with deviation of nasal bridge

❖ "Open-book fracture"
Collapsed nasal septum and splayed out nasal bones
	❖ Injuries of nasal septum:
	  ➤ Buckled
	  ➤ Dislocated
	  ➤ Fractured into several pieces

❖ Comminution of nasal bones ❖ Fracture of frontal processes of maxilla with flattening and widening of nasal dorsum	Septal hematoma may form

Clinical Features
- Swelling over nose
- Periorbital ecchymosis
- Tenderness

PART 1: Diseases of ENT, Head and Neck

- Nasal deformity
- **Depressed nasal bone:** Front/side/whole pyramid deviated to one side **(Fig. 1)**
- Crepitus
- Epistaxis
- Nasal obstruction → due to septal hematoma or fractured bony fragments.

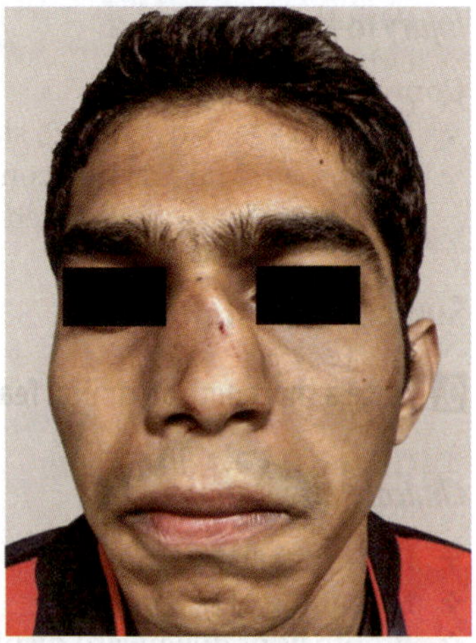

Diagnosis

- Physical examination
- X-rays:
  - Water's view
  - Right and left lateral views

Note: Patient should not be dismissed as having no fracture because X-rays did not reveal it.

Treatment

Best time to reduce a fracture:
- Before appearance of edema
  Or
- After it has subsided

Difficult to reduce a nasal fracture after 2 weeks because it heals by that time.

1. **Simple fractures** (undisplaced) without displacement → **No treatment**
2. **Closed reduction:**

Depressed fractures of nasal bones by frontal or lateral blow	Reduction by straight blunt elevator guided by digital manipulation from outside
Laterally, displaced nasal bridge	Reduced by firm digital pressure in opposite direction
Impacted fragments	Disimpaction with Walsham or Asch's forceps before realignment
Unstable fractures	Intranasal packing and external splintage

Note: Septal hematoma, if present, must be drained.

3. **Open reduction:** Early open reduction rarely required.
   - *Indication:* When closed methods fail
4. **Healed nasal deformities:** Healed nasal deformities can be corrected by rhinoplasty or septorhinoplasty.

Fig. 1: Depressed fracture of nasal bone.

Naso-orbital Fractures

Q. What is the mode of naso-orbital fracture? Write a note on its clinical features and management.

Mode of Fracture

- Direct force over nasion fractures nasal bones and displaces them posteriorly.
- Perpendicular plate of ethmoid, ethmoidal air cells, and medial orbital wall are fractured and driven posteriorly.
- **May involve:**
  - Cribriform plate
  - Frontal sinus
  - Frontonasal duct
  - Extraocular muscles
  - Eyeball
  - Lacrimal apparatus
  - Medial canthal ligament may be avulsed.

Clinical Features

- Telecanthus
- Bridge of nose is depressed and tip turned up (pug nose)

- Periorbital ecchymosis
- Orbital hematoma
- Cerebrospinal fluid (CSF) leak
- Displaced eyeball

Investigation

Three-dimensional (3-D) computed tomography (CT) face

Treatment

- **Closed reduction:** Fracture reduced with Asch's forceps, stabilized by a wire passed through fractured bony fragments and septum and tied over lead plates.
- **Open reduction:**
  - Indications
    - Extensive comminution of nasal and orbital bones.
    - Complicated by other injuries to lacrimal apparatus, medial canthal ligaments, and frontal sinus
  - Procedure:

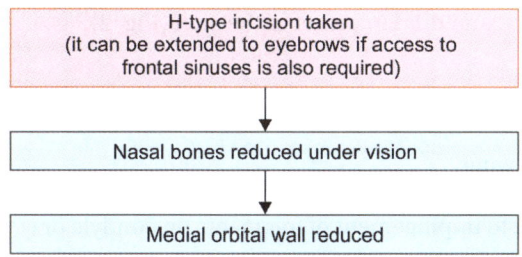

Fractures of Zygoma (Tripod Fracture)

Q. Write a short note on second most commonly fractured bone of face/fracture of zygoma/tripod fracture.

Zygoma is second most frequently fractured bone.
Mode: Direct trauma

Clinical Features

- Flattened malar prominence.
- Step deformity of infraorbital margin.
- Anesthesia in the distribution of infraorbital nerve.
- Trismus
- Oblique palpebral fissure, due to the displacement of lateral palpebral ligament.
- Restricted ocular movements, due to entrapment of inferior rectus muscle
- Periorbital emphysema

Diagnosis

- X-ray Water's view
- CT PNS + orbit

Treatment

Open reduction and internal wire fixation

PART 1: Diseases of ENT, Head and Neck

Procedure:

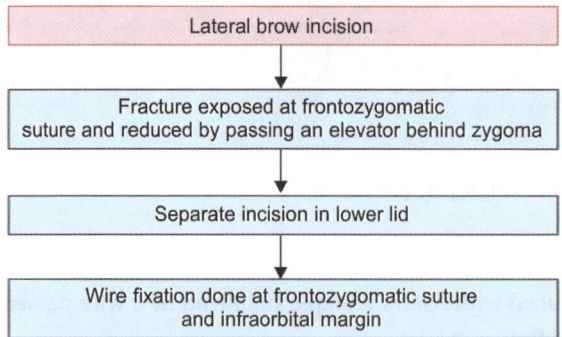

Fractures of Zygomatic Arch

Q. Write a short note on fracture of zygomatic arch.

- Zygomatic arch breaks into two fragments which get depressed.
- Three fracture lines, one at each end and third in center of the arch **(Fig. 2)**.

Clinical Features

- Depression in zygomatic arch area
- Pain aggravated by talking and chewing
- Trismus
- Limited mandible movements due to impingement of fragments on condyle or coronoid process.

Diagnosis

X-ray of skull:
- Submentovertical
- Waters' view
- CT face

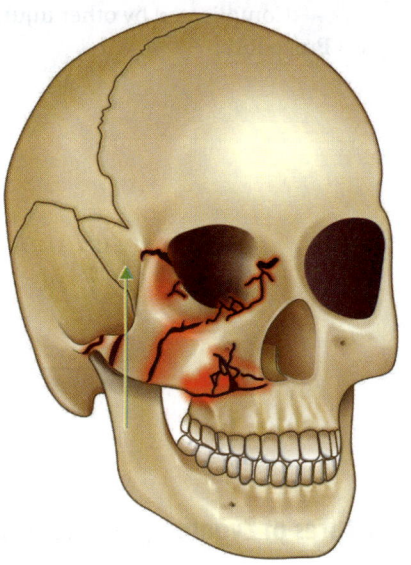

Fig. 2: Zygomatic fracture.

Treatment

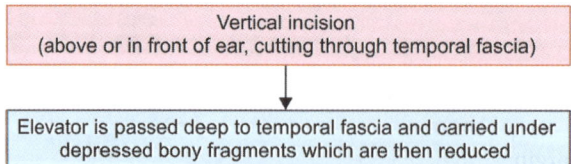

Fractures of Orbital Floor

Q. Write a short note on blow out fractures/orbital floor fractures.

"*Blow out fractures*": Isolated fractures of orbital floor when a large blunt object strikes globe.
Note: Zygomatic and Le Fort II maxillary fractures are always accompanied by fractures of orbital floor.

Clinical Features

- Diplopia
- Enophthalmos
- Ecchymosis of lid, conjunctiva, and sclera
- Hypoesthesia or anesthesia of cheek and upper lip, if infraorbital nerve is involved.

Diagnosis

- X-ray Water's view: **Tear drop sign (Fig. 3)** (convex opacity bulging into the antrum from above)
- CT orbit
- **Traction test:** Grasp globe and passively rotate it to check for restriction of its movements.
- Check for extraocular muscles: Ask patient to look up and down (entrapment of inferior rectus and inferior oblique muscles is diagnosed).

Treatment

Indications for surgery:
- Enophthalmos
- Persistent diplopia due to muscle entrapment

Two approaches:
- **Transantral:**
  - Orbital floor fractures reduced by a finger passed into antrum
  - Pack kept in antrum to support fragments.
- **Infraorbital:** Used alone or in combination with transantral approach
- If badly comminuted fracture of orbital floor:
  - Repair from:
    - Bone graft from the iliac crest
    - Nasal septum
    - Anterior wall of antrum
    - Silicon or Teflon sheets

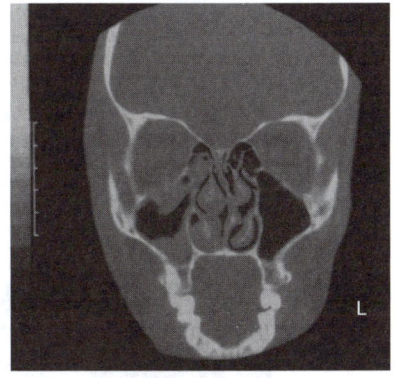

Fig. 3: Fracture orbital floor with hanging tear drop sign, air fluid level.

Fractures of Maxilla

Q. How do you classify fractures of maxilla? Write a note on its clinical features and management.

Classification

Classified into three types **(Fig. 4)**:

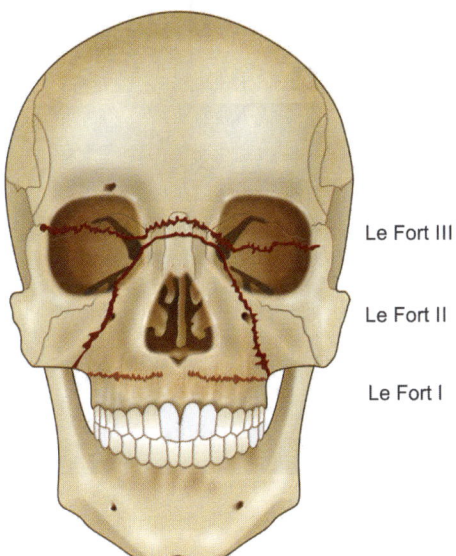

Fig. 4: LeFort I, II, and III fracture.

Le Fort I (transverse) (Fig. 5A)	Le Fort II (pyramidal) (Fig. 5B)	Le Fort III (craniofacial disjunction)
Fracture runs above and parallel to palate	Fracture passes through root of nose, lacrimal bone, floor of orbit, upper part of maxillary sinus and pterygoid plates	• Fracture line passes through root of nose, ethmofrontal junction, superior orbital fissure, lateral wall of orbit, frontozygomatic and temporozygomatic sutures and upper part of pterygoid plates
Crosses lower part of nasal septum, maxillary antrum, and the pterygoid plates	Cribriform plate is injured	• Complete separation of facial bones from cranial bones • Cribriform plate is injured

Clinical Features

- Malocclusion of teeth with anterior open bite
- Midface elongation
- Mobile maxillary fragments
- CSF rhinorrhea

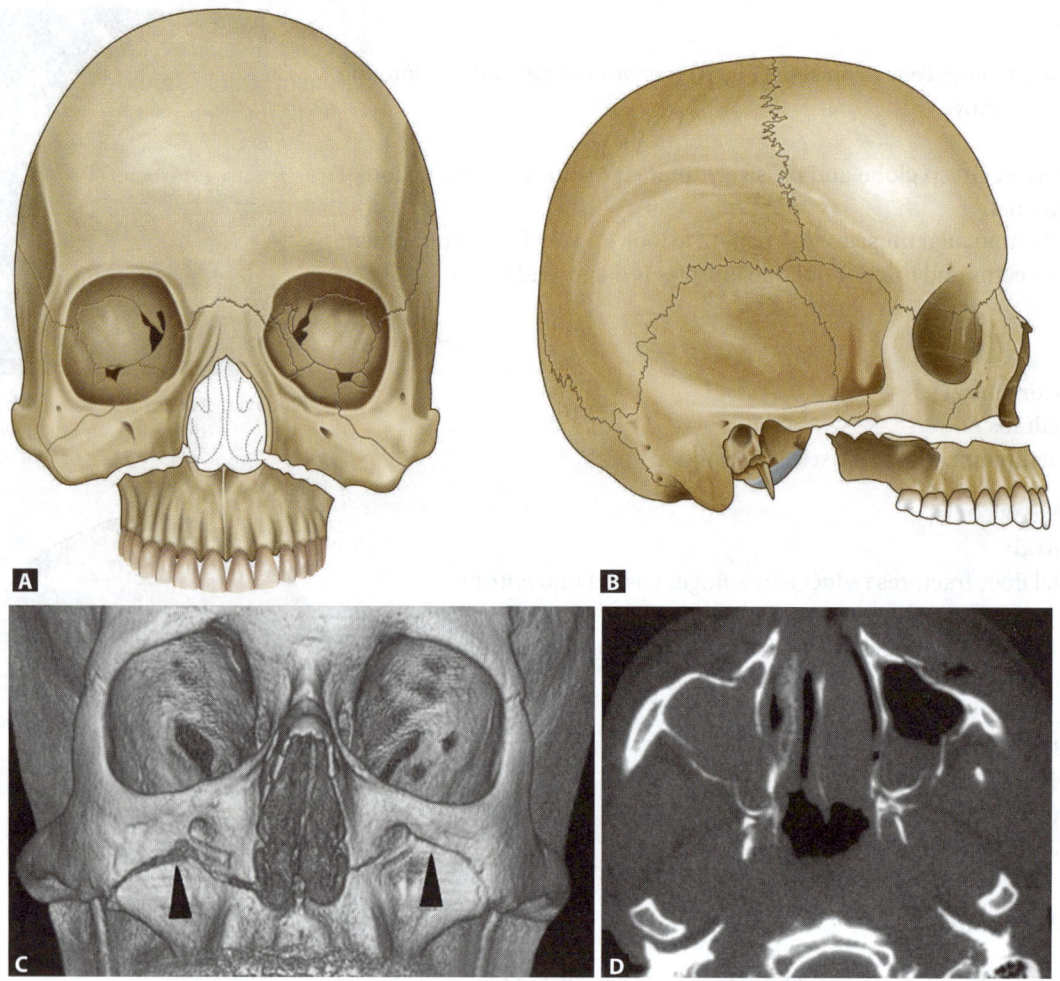

Figs. 5A to D: Le Fort I and II fractures.

Diagnosis

- X-ray
  - Water's view
  - Posteroanterior view
  - Lateral view
- 3-D CT face **(Figs. 5C and D)**

Treatment

- **General management:** Restore airway
  - Stop severe hemorrhage from maxillary artery
  - Associated intracranial and cervical spine injuries are treated.
- **Specific management:** Fixation of maxillary fractures can be achieved by:
  - Interdental wiring
  - Intermaxillary wiring using arch bars.
  - Open reduction and interosseous wiring as in zygomatic fractures.
  - Wire slings from frontal bone, zygoma, or infraorbital rim to the teeth or arch bars.

FRACTURES OF LOWER THIRD

Fractures of Mandible

Q. Classify mandibular fractures. Write a note on its presentation and management.

Classification

Dingmans's classification: Fractures of mandible are classified according to their location.

Mode: Direct trauma

Note: Condylar fractures caused by indirect trauma to chin or opposite side of body of mandible.

Displacement of mandibular fractures determined by:
- Pull of muscles attached to fragments
- Direction of fracture line
- Bevel of the fracture

- Condylar fractures→Most common
- Angle of mandible fracture
- Body
- Symphysis
- Ramus, coronoid and alveolar processes (uncommon)

(In decreasing order of frequency)

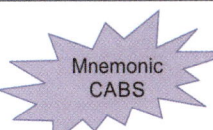

Mnemonic CABS

Clinical Features

In fractures of condyle		In fractures of angle, body, and symphysis
If fragments are not displaced	<ul><li>Pain</li><li>Trismus</li><li>Tenderness at site of fracture</li></ul>	<ul><li>Step deformity</li><li>Malocclusion of teeth</li><li>Ecchymosis of oral mucosa</li><li>Tenderness at site of fracture</li><li>Crepitus</li></ul>
If fragments are displaced	<ul><li>Malocclusion of teeth</li><li>Deviation of jaw to opposite side on opening mouth</li></ul>	Diagnosed by intraoral and extraoral palpation

Diagnosis

- X-ray skull posteroanterior (PA) view
  - Right and left oblique views of mandible
- Orthopantomogram (OPG) **(Fig. 6)**
- 3-D CT face

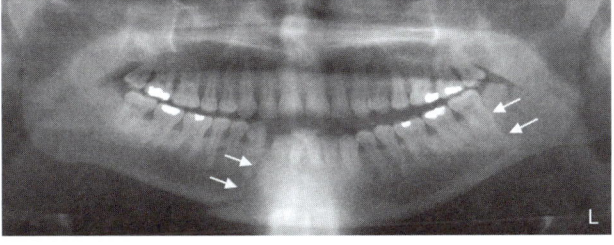

Fig. 6: Fracture mandible.

Treatment

For reduction and fixation of mandibular fractures.
- **Closed methods:**
  - Interdental wiring and intermaxillary fixation.
  - External pin fixation
- **Open methods:**

Fracture site is exposed and fragments fixed by direct interosseous wiring

Further strengthened by wire tied in a figure-of-eight manner

Intermaxillary fixation with arch bars and rubber bands is also done. Immobilization of mandible beyond 3 weeks, in condylar fractures, can cause ankylosis of temporomandibular joints. Therefore, intermaxillary wires are removed and jaw exercises started

If occlusion is still disturbed

Intermaxillary wires reapplied for another week and process repeated till bite and jaw movements are normal

Note: Sometimes, open reduction and interosseous wiring may be required in adult edentulous patients with bilateral condylar fractures or in fractures of children

Chapter 28

Granulomatous Diseases of Nose

EN4.34: Describe the clinical features, investigation and management of granulomatous diseases of nose.

CLASSIFICATION

Q. Classify granulomatous diseases of nose.

Specific			Nonspecific	
Bacterial	**Fungal**	**Parasitic**	**Neoplastic**	**Inflammatory**
Tuberculosis	Rhinosporidiosis	Leishmaniasis	Sinonasal lymphoma	Sarcoidosis
Leprosy	Candidiasis			Wegener's granulomatosis
Syphilis	Aspergillosis			Eosinophilic granuloma
Yaws	Mucormycosis			Giant cell reparative granuloma
Rhinoscleroma				Cholesterol granuloma
				Allergic granulomatosis
				Plasma cell granuloma

RHINOSCLEROMA

Q. Describe etiopathogenesis, clinical features, and treatment of rhinoscleroma.

Hebra: He first reported the condition.
Mikulicz: He described histology.
Von Frisch: He discovered *Klebsiella rhinoscleromatis (K. rhinoscleromatis)*.

Etiology

It is a chronic granulomatous disease **caused by gram negative bacillus called *K. rhinoscleromatis* or Frisch bacillus**.

Pathology

The disease starts in the nose and extends to nasopharynx, oropharynx, larynx, trachea, and bronchi. The mode of infection is unknown.

Clinical Features

- **Atrophic stage:** It resembles atrophic rhinitis and is characterized by a foul-smelling purulent nasal discharge and crusting.
- **Granulomatous stage:** Granulomatous nodules form in the nasal mucosa. Disease may extend into sinuses, nasopharynx, larynx, trachea, nasolacrimal system, and even intraorbitally and intracranially.
- **Cicatricial stage:** This causes stenosis of nares, distortion of upper lip, adhesions in nose, nasopharynx, and oropharynx. There is also subdermal infiltration of lower part of external nose and upper lip giving a **woody feel**.

Hebra nose: Nasal enlargement, cartilage destruction, hyperplastic alae, and the tip of nose.

Diagnosis

- Biopsy shows infiltration of submucosa with plasma cells, lymphocytes, eosinophils, Mikulicz cells, and Russell bodies **(Fig. 1)**.
- Mikulicz cells are large foam cells with a central nucleus and vacuolated cytoplasm containing bacilli.
- Russell bodies are homogeneous eosinophilic inclusion bodies found in the plasma cells.
- **Microbiological:** Demonstration of *K. rhinoscleromatis*.
- **Immunohistochemical:** *Klebsiella* capsular antigen III.

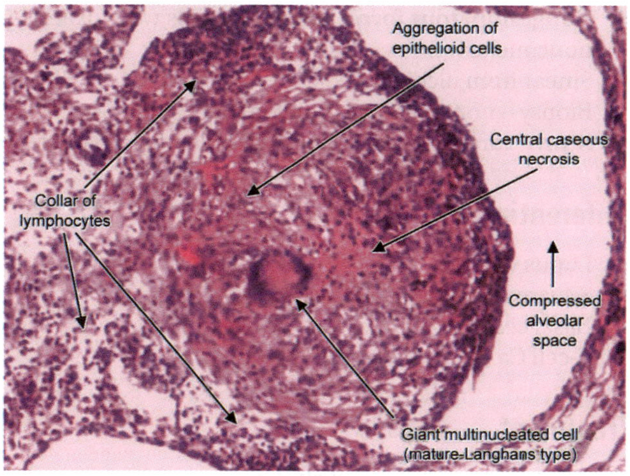

Fig. 1: Granulomatous diseases of the nose.

Treatment

- **Streptomycin** (1 g/day) and tetracycline (2 g/day) are given together for a minimum period of 4–6 weeks and repeated if necessary after 1 month.
- **Steroids** can be combined to reduce fibrosis.
- Surgical treatment may be required to establish the airway and correct nasal deformity.
- **Radiation:** Destroys the organisms—3,000–3,500 Gy for 3 weeks.

SYPHILIS

Q. Write a short note on syphilis and its effects on nasal structures.

Etiology

May be venereal or congenital caused by *Treponema pallidum (T. pallidum)*.

Clinical Features

- **Acquired**: It occurs as:
  - **Primary**: It manifests as the primary chancre of the vestibule of nose.
  - **Secondary**: It manifests as simple rhinitis with crusting and fissuring in the nasal vestibule. Diagnosis is suggested by the presence of mucous patches in the pharynx, skin rash, fever, and generalized lymphadenitis.
  - **Tertiary**: Typical manifestation is the formation of gumma on nasal septum. Septum is destroyed in both its bony and cartilaginous parts. Perforation may also appear in the hard palate. There is an offensive nasal discharge with crusts.
- **Congenital:**
  - **Early form:** It is seen in the first 3 months of life and manifests as snuffles. Soon the nasal discharge becomes purulent.
  - **Late form**: Usually manifests around puberty. Clinical picture is similar to that seen in the tertiary stage of acquired syphilis. **Gummatous lesions destroy the nasal structures.**
  - **Hutchinson's triad**: Notched central incisors **(Fig. 2)**, interstitial keratitis, and sensorineural hearing loss.

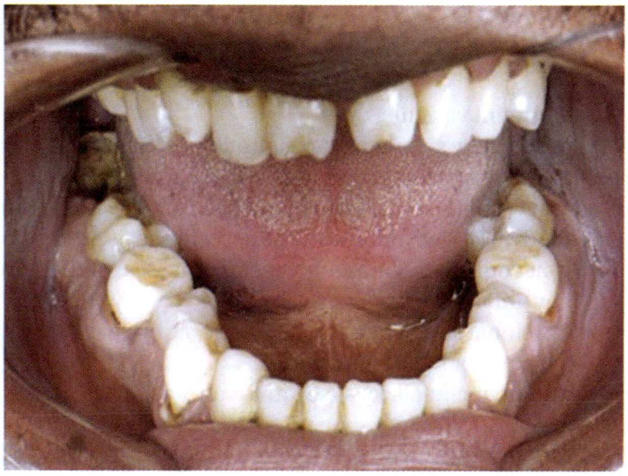

Fig. 2: Hutchinson's teeth in syphilis.

Diagnosis

- Serological test—venereal disease research laboratory (VDRL) and biopsy of tissue with stains to demonstrate *T. pallidum*.
- Serological tests for syphilis (positive in 90%) and tests for mycobacteria

- ❖ **Nongummatous form:** Staining of cells with alkaline phosphatase and periodic acid-Schiff (PAS) if serological tests are nonconclusive.
- ❖ Smear from ulcer/node
- ❖ Biopsy—noncaseating granulomas
- ❖ X-ray—rarefaction of bones with a blurring of cortical outline.

Differential Diagnosis

- ❖ Lupus vulgaris
- ❖ Squamous cell carcinoma (Ca)
- ❖ Basal cell Ca
- ❖ T-cell Ca

Treatment

- ❖ **Penicillin is the drug of choice:** Benzathine penicillin 2.4 million units intramuscular (IM) every week for 3 weeks with a total dose of 7.2 million units.
- ❖ Alternatively, tetracycline or doxycycline for 2 weeks.
- ❖ Nasal crusts are removed by irrigation with an alkaline solution.
- ❖ The cosmetic deformity is corrected after the disease becomes inactive.

Complications

Syphilis can lead to vestibular stenosis, perforations of nasal septum and hard palate, secondary atrophic rhinitis, and saddle nose deformity.

■ TUBERCULOSIS

Q. Write a short note on tuberculosis manifestations in ENT.

- ❖ Primary tuberculosis of the nose is rare. Most times it is secondary to lung tuberculosis.
- ❖ Most common sites involved are anterior part of the nasal septum and anterior end of inferior turbinate.
- ❖ First, there is nodular infiltration followed later by ulceration and perforation of nasal septum in the cartilaginous part.

Clinical Forms

Vulgaris

Most frequent variant
- ❖ Produced by scratching or aspiration of tubercular bacilli
  Characteristic lesion: Lupus nodule (apple-jelly nodules). It is a low-grade tuberculosis infection commonly affecting the nasal vestibule or the skin of the nose and face. The skin lesion manifests characteristically as brown, gelatinous nodules called apple-jelly nodules. In the vestibule, it presents as chronic vestibulitis.
- ❖ Rosaceous granulations or vegetant masses on the skin of the nose
- ❖ Itchy and bleeding nasal scabs
- ❖ Occasional septal perforations perforation may occur in the cartilaginous part of nasal septum.
- ❖ Mistaken for squamous cell Ca
- ❖ Lesion paucibacillary—negative cultures in 50%.

Pseudotumor Form

- ❖ Slow development
- ❖ Scarce virulence
- ❖ Produced by inoculation by scratching
- ❖ Generally not associated with pulmonary lesions
- ❖ **Clinical presentation:**
  ➢ Nasal obstruction
  ➢ Mucopurulent rhinorrhea
  ➢ Edematous, granulomatous lesions nasal septum, and inferior turbinates
- ❖ **Differential diagnosis:** Malignancies—biopsy is mandatory.

Ulcerated Forms

- Rarer and more serious
- **Etiology:** Hematogenic dysfunction in severe pulmonary tuberculosis (TB)
- Rapidly progressive
- Superficial ulcers and crusts are seen on the surface
- Cartilaginous septal perforation, scarring of external nose
- Rich in bacilli—cultures-positive.

Diagnosis

- Blanching of tissue
- Histopathology—caseating granuloma, acid-alcohol fast bacilli
- Mantoux test
- Chest X-ray
- Sputum for acid-fast bacillus (AFB)
- Bacterial culture
- Polymerase chain reaction (PCR).

Treatment

- Antitubercular drugs
- Extrapulmonary TB regimen
- 2 HRZE + 4 HR
- Multidrug-resistant tuberculosis (MDR-TB) regimen for treatment failures
- Plastic repair of deformities.

LEPROSY

Q. Write short note on leprosy and its effects on nasal structures.

Causative Agent

Mycobacterium leprae

Clinical Presentation

- **Early form:** Mucosal infiltration and abnormal drying
- **Intermediate form:**
  - Mucosal thickening and increased nasal secretions
  - Nasal crusts
- **Late form:**
  - Ulcer
  - Secondary infection
  - Cartilaginous septal perforation and saddle nose deformity
  - Decreased sensitivity and hyposmia

Infection starts in anterior part of nasal septum and anterior end of inferior turbinate. Initially, there is excessive nasal discharge with red and swollen mucosa. Later, crusting and bleeding supervene. A nodular lesion on the septum may ulcerate and cause perforation. Later, there may be depression of the bridge of nose and destruction of anterior nasal spine with retrusion of the columella.

Treatment

Treated with dapsone, rifampin, and isoniazid. Reconstruction procedures are required when the disease is inactive.

RHINOSPORIDIOSIS

Q. Describe etiopathogenesis, clinical features, and treatment of rhinosporidiosis.

Causative Agent

Rhinosporidium seeberi

Epidemiology

- In India, the disease is more common in the southern states. It is prevalent in the states of Tamil Nadu, Kerala, Madhya Pradesh, Chhattisgarh, and Andhra Pradesh.
- **Life cycle:** Three stages have been recognized in the life cycle of the organism—(1) trophic stage, (2) development of sporangium, and (3) production of endospores.

Clinical Features

- The disease mostly affects the nose and nasopharynx **(Fig. 3)**, other sites such as the lip, palate, conjunctiva, epiglottis, larynx, trachea, bronchi, skin, vulva, and vagina may also be affected.
- The disease is acquired through contaminated water of ponds, and also frequently by animals. In the nose, the disease presents as a leafy, polypoidal mass, pink to purple in color, and attached to the nasal septum or lateral wall. Sometimes, it extends into the nasopharynx and may hang behind the soft palate **(Fig. 4)**. The mass is very vascular and bleeds easily on touch. Its surface is studded with white dots representing the sporangia.
- In the early stage, patient may complain of nasal discharge which is often blood-tinged, and nasal stuffiness.

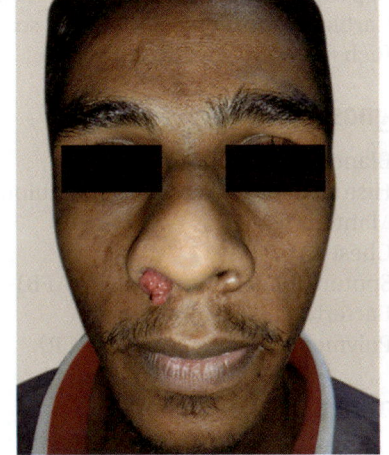

Fig. 3: Rhinosporidiosis of nose.

Diagnosis

This is made on **biopsy**. It shows several sporangia, oval or round in shape and filled with spores which may be seen bursting through its chitinous wall.

Treatment

- Complete excision of the mass with a diathermy knife and cauterization of its base.
- Recurrence may occur after surgical excision.
- Dapsone can be used.

ASPERGILLOSIS

Q. Write a short note on aspergillosis.

Causative Agent

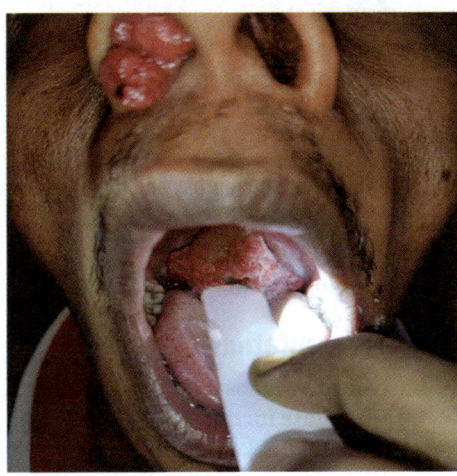

Fig. 4: Rhinosporidiosis of the nose extending to nasopharynx and oropharynx.

Aspergillus niger, *Aspergillus flavus*, *Aspergillus fumigatus*.
They invade nasal tissues when the hosts defense mechanisms are compromised due to immunosuppressant drugs.

Clinical Features

- Acute/subacute rhinitis or sinusitis
- Black or grayish membrane is seen in the nasal mucosa. Exploration of maxillary sinus reveals a fungus ball containing semisolid cheesy white or blackish material.

Treatment

Surgical debridement of the involved tissues and antifungal drugs, e.g, amphotericin B.

MUCORMYCOSIS

Q. Write a short note on mucormycosis.

- **Predisposing factors:** Uncontrolled diabetes mellitus and immunocompromised status.
- The infection spreads from nose and paranasal sinuses to orbit, cribriform plate, and brain.

- The rapid destruction associated with the disease is due to the affinity of the fungus to invade the arteries and cause endothelial damage and thrombosis.
- Typical finding is the presence of black necrotic mass filling the nasal cavity and eroding the septum **(Fig. 5)** and hard palate **(Fig. 6)**.
- Treatment is by amphotericin B and surgical debridement.
- Mucormycosis is confirmed by diagnostic nasal endoscopy, nasal swab sent for culture and histopathology reporting. MRI is also one of the diagnostic Tool for extensive mucormycosis involving orbit and intracranial cavity, brain **(Fig. 7)** apart from nose and paranasal sinuses.

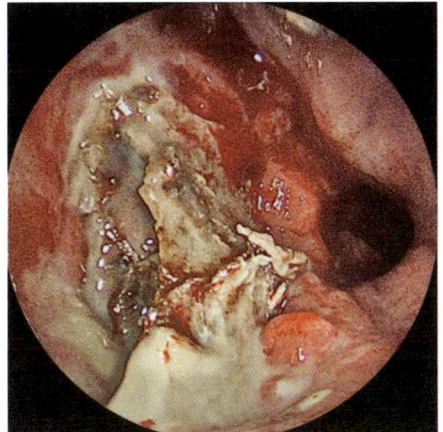
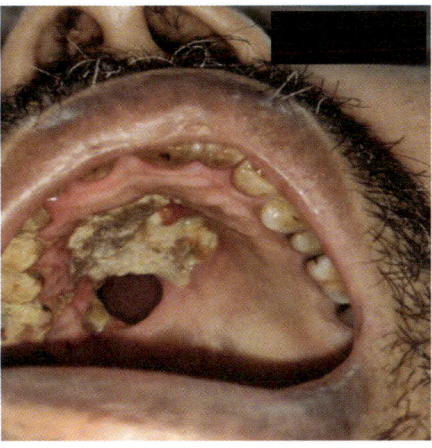
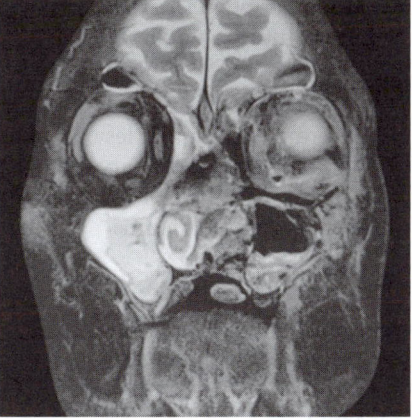

Fig. 5: Endoscopic view of nasal mucormycosis with crusting and bony erosion.

Fig. 6: Palatal perforation in mucormycosis.

Fig. 7: Magnetic resonance imaging (MRI) of nose showing mucormycosis involving maxillary, ethmoidal, and frontal sinus involvement with intracranial extension.

YAWS

Q. Write a short note on Yaws.

- Extragenital and treponemal infection
- **Caused by *Treponema pertenue***
- Occurs in tropical countries
- Usually begins in childhood
- Clinical features:
  - Papillomatous and ulcerated skin nodules
  - Subsequent involvement of lymph nodes and bone
  - Gummatous destruction within the nose and paranasal sinuses (PNS)
- **Treatment:** Penicillin.

ACTINOMYCOSIS

Q. Write a short note on actinomycosis.

- **Caused by *Actinomyces israelii***
- >50% occur in the head and neck region, usually cervicofacial tissue
- Nose and PNS are rarely involved—most common—maxillary antrum

Clinical Features

- Granular lesions in nose
- Erosion of bone at the early stage
- Brawny swelling of the cheek with fistulae
- Irrigation may reveal foul pus-containing causative organisms
- Sulfur granules surrounded by purulent exudate
- Diagnosis confirmed if gram-positive filaments identified in sulfur granules

Treatment

Penicillin is a drug of choice, erythromycin/clindamycin.

LEISHMANIASIS

Q. Write short note on Leishmaniasis.

- Also called American leishmaniasis/espundia
- Widespread in tropical and subtropical countries
- **Mucocutaneous form affects the nose:** Caused by *Leishmania braziliensis*
- Nasal implantation by fingers; lesion develops at the site of inoculation

Clinical Features

- Ulcerative or nodular lesions involving anterior nares, spread to nasal fossa and upper lip
- It may involve nasopharynx and cause destruction
- **Chronic condition:** Midfacial destruction and death from bronchopneumonia
- Regional lymphadenitis

Diagnosis

- **Biopsy:** *Leishmania donovani (L. donovani)* bodies in reticuloendothelial cells and ulcer discharge
- **Differential diagnosis:** Tuberculosis—numerous inflammatory cells and few organisms

Treatment

- Acute condition: antimony compounds
- Amphotericin
- Local cleaning and curettage

SARCOIDOSIS

Q. Write short note on Sarcoidosis.

Etiology: Unknown

Clinical Features

- Nose-affected frequently
- Nasal skin involvement (Lupus pernio):
  - Granulomatous plaques occupying full thickness of dermis—bulbous red/violet lesions **(Fig. 8)**
- Nasal bones involvement:
  - Nasal bridge swollen
  - X-ray shows translucent deposits
- Nasal mucosa involvement:
  - Septum and inferior turbinates
  - Obstruction, mucopurulent/blood-stained discharge
  - Yellow or grayish slightly raised nodules with crusting
  - Anterior septal perforation, saddling of nose, synechiae, and stenosis
  - May spread to the sinus and orbit

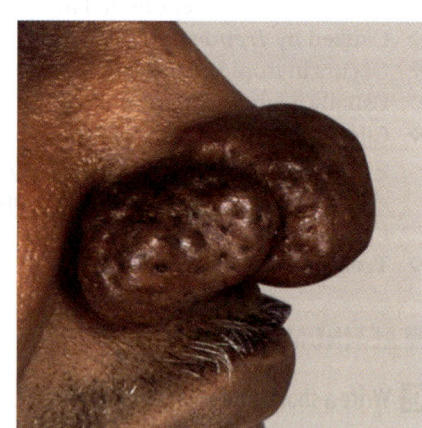

Fig. 8: Cutaneous sarcoidosis.

Investigations

- Erythrocyte sedimentation rate (ESR) and serum calcium
- Serum angiotensin-converting enzyme (increased by 83%)
- Chest X-ray—hilar lymphadenopathy
- X-ray PNS—rarefaction with cystic and punctate osteolysis
- **Kveim test**—role controversial
  Diagnosis by exclusion of other causes of granulomatous changes

- ❖ **Histopathology**:
  - ➢ Granulomas smaller than Wegener's granulomatosis
  - ➢ Epithelioid tubercles without caseation converted into hyaline fibrous tissue
  - ➢ Central necrosis without caseation
  - ➢ **Schaumann bodies**

Treatment

- ❖ Spontaneous remission
- ❖ Alkaline douches and betamethasone drops
- ❖ Systemic therapy:
  - ➢ Oral steroid
  - ➢ Methotrexate 5 mg once a week for 3 months
  - ➢ Hydroxy chloroquine 250 mg on alternate days for 9 months
- ❖ Surgery exacerbates the condition.

WEGENER'S GRANULOMATOSIS

Q. Write short note on Wegener's granulomatosis.

Clinical Features

- ❖ Adolescence to the eighth decade; mostly under 25 years
- ❖ Most common in the respiratory tract and kidneys
- ❖ Nonspecific general symptoms—malaise, pyrexia, and weight loss with minimal physical findings initially
- ❖ Nose and sinuses involved in 80% of patients
- ❖ Granuloma of the upper respiratory tract are most common presenting feature
- ❖ Epistaxis, nasal obstruction, and bloody crusts
- ❖ Destruction of nasal bones—nasal collapse **(Fig. 9)**
- ❖ No gross destructive changes in midfacial skin as seen in T-cell lymphomas and basal cell carcinomas.

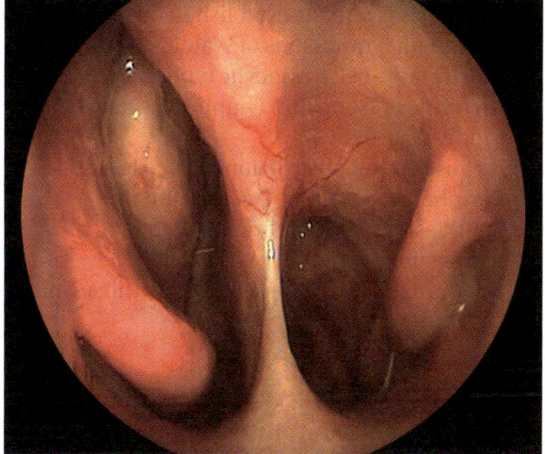

Fig. 9: Septal perforation with atrophy of left middle turbinate in Wegener's granulomatosis.

Investigations

- ❖ Mandatory
  - ➢ ESR, antineutrophil cytoplasmic autoantibody, cytoplasmic (c-ANCA), chest X-ray, urine examination, and pulmonary function tests (PFT)
- ❖ Case-specific
  - ➢ Sinus X-rays
  - ➢ Renal biopsy
- ❖ ESR >80, positive nasal findings/chest X-ray changes—**steroid and cytotoxics**

Nasal biopsy:
- ❖ Mandatory in nasal involvement with clinical suspicion
- ❖ Wegener's triad:
  - ➢ Necrotizing granulomatous inflammation of the respiratory tract
  - ➢ Systemic or focal necrotizing vasculitis
  - ➢ Necrotizing glomerulonephritis
- ❖ Epithelial cell granulomas
- ❖ Multinucleated giant cells with numerous eosinophils

Treatment

- ❖ Steroids and cytotoxics—prolonged remission
  - ➢ *Initial dose:* Prednisolone 60–80 mg/day + cyclophosphamide 2 mg/kg or azathioprine 200 mg/day, then tapered off
- ❖ Treatment to start on suspicion—do not wait for a biopsy report
- ❖ ESR the most useful to monitor response to treatment, c-ANCA also used

PART 1: Diseases of ENT, Head and Neck

- Renal function tests to monitor the renal status
- Plasma exchange and immunoglobulin (Ig) infusion

SINONASAL LYMPHOMA

Q. Write short note on sinonasal lymphoma.

- Also called nonhealing midline granuloma/midfacial destructive lesion
- Three types in nose:
  - Generalized lymphoma of the sinonasal tract
  - Lymphomas of Waldeyer's ring
  - Peripheral and extranodal sinonasal lymphoma
- Generalized lymphoma involving nasal tract
- Rare in nose and PNS
- Destruction of facial structures rare
- Diagnosis is already established on lymph node biopsy
- Malignant lymphomas of Waldeyer's ring
- Mostly large cell histiocytic type
- All forms of Hodgkin's lymphomas may occur
- Mildly destructive
- It causes nasal obstruction, epistaxis, and swelling of the maxillary area
- Peripheral, sinonasal T-cell lymphoma
- First described by McBride (1896)
- Uncertain etiology
- Slow progressive destruction of the nose and midfacial region by a chronic inflammatory response

Clinical Features

- **Prodromal phase:**
  - Persistent nasal obstruction and rhinorrhea—many years
- **Activity phase:**
  - Necrosis of nasal cavity
  - Purulent discharge, crusting, and tissue loss
  - Progressive destruction of midfacial region, extending into pharynx, orbit, and skull base
- **Terminal phase:**
  - Severe hemorrhage
  - Gross mutilation of the face
  - Death due to systemic metastasis
- **Histopathology:**
  - Atypical cell infiltrates dispersed in necrotic areas—good biopsy essential
  - Fresh tissue biopsy essential
  - Infiltrates of polymorphic and neoplastic atypical lymphocytes arranged in necrotizing angioinfiltrative growth pattern
  - Positive immunohistochemical reactivity to T-cell markers
- Granulomas and giant cells are not present
- Thrombosis and necrosis common

Treatment

- **Radical dose radiotherapy:** >5,500 cGy with wide-field coverage
- Chemotherapy is controversial, may be used to prevent disseminated lymphoma
- Surgical debridement with reconstruction

EOSINOPHILIC GRANULOMA

Q. Write short note on eosinophilic granuloma.

- A localized form of "Histiocytosis X"
- Hyperplasia of Langerhans cell-type histiocytes
- Predominantly occur in bone most commonly in the skull
- Mainly affects the young children

Presentation
- Painful swelling of involved bone
- Cervical lymphadenopathy
- Toothache, gum ulceration, and loose teeth

Radiological Evaluation
Punched out bony lesions—produce a dramatic appearance in jaw.

Histopathology
- Numerous histiocytic cells and eosinophils with associated fibrosis
- More eosinophils and a better prognosis
- Numerous histiocytic cells and eosinophils with associated fibrosis
- More eosinophils and a better prognosis

Treatment
- Unifocal disease—curettage/excision + radiotherapy
- Generalized disease— surgery + radiotherapy + chemotherapy
- Alpha interferon and bone marrow transplantation have also been tried successfully

GIANT CELL REPARATIVE GRANULOMA
- Common in children and young adults
- Benign osseous lesions
- Histology—giant cells without multiple nuclei
- Complete excision to prevent a recurrence

CHOLESTEROL GRANULOMA
- Most common in mastoid air cells and paranasal sinuses (frontal sinus most common)
- Granulomatous reaction to cholesterol crystals precipitated in tissue following hemorrhage
- **Histopathology:** Granulation tissue containing foreign body type giant cells surrounding clefts created by cholesterol crystals

Treatment: Surgical excision.

ALLERGIC GRANULOMATOSIS
- As described by Churg and Strauss
- Asthma associated with pulmonary infiltrates
- Nasal lesions—rhinitis, polyp formation, and septal perforation
- **Nasal biopsy:** Necrotizing granulomas surrounded by an abundance of eosinophils, giant cells, and plasma cells without vasculitis
- **Treatment:** Systemic and local corticosteroids, polyp removal

Disease	Presentation	Part of the nose involved	Histopathology
Tuberculosis	Ulcers/polyps	Anterior part	Caseating granulomas
Leprosy	Crusting, ulcers, and nasal deformity	Anterior part and anterior nasal spine	Noncaseating granulomas
Syphilis	Nasal deformity, chancre, gumma	Bony involvement	Granulomas with necrosis
Rhinoscleroma	Nodular mass and Hebra nose	Soft tissue	Mikulicz cells, Russell bodies
Rhinosporidiosis	Leafy polypoidal mass	Mucosa	Sporangia
Leishmaniasis	Ulcerative lesions	Anterior portions	Leishmania donovani (LD) bodies
Sarcoidosis	Nodules and lupus pernio	Bone, skin, and mucosa	Noncaseating granulomas, Schaumann bodies
Wegener's granulomatosis	Nasal destruction	Bone	Noncaseating granulomas
T-cell lymphoma	Midface destruction	Bone	Necrotizing angioinvasive lesions

Chapter 29

Neoplasms of the Nasal Cavity and Paranasal Sinuses

EN4.33: Describe the clinical features, investigations and principles of management of tumors of nose, nasopharynx and paranasal sinus.

■ CLASSIFICATION

Q. Classify tumors of maxillary region/neoplasms affecting nasal cavity.

Tissue of origin	Benign tumors	Malignant tumors
Epithelial	❖ Inverted papilloma ❖ Squamous cell papilloma ❖ Salivary gland adenomas	❖ Squamous cell carcinoma ❖ Sinonasal undifferentiated carcinoma ❖ Lymphoepithelial carcinoma ❖ Adenocarcinoma ❖ Salivary gland carcinomas ❖ Malignant melanoma
Neuroendocrine	None	Carcinoid tumors
Soft tissue	❖ Myxoma ❖ Leiomyoma ❖ Hemangioma ❖ Schwannoma ❖ Neurofibroma ❖ Juvenile angiofibroma ❖ Hemangiopericytoma ❖ Telangiectasias ❖ Angiomas	❖ Fibrosarcoma ❖ Rhabdomyosarcoma ❖ Angiosarcoma ❖ Peripheral nerve sheath tumor
Bone and cartilage	❖ Fibrous dysplasia ❖ Osteoma ❖ Osteoblastoma ❖ Chondroma ❖ Ameloblastoma	❖ Chondrosarcoma ❖ Osteosarcoma ❖ Chordoma
Hematological	None	❖ Lymphoma (non-Hodgkin's) ❖ Langerhans cell histiocytosis
Germ cell tumors	Dermoid cyst	❖ Teratoma ❖ Sinonasal yolk sac tumor
Neuroectodermal	None	Olfactory neuroblastoma (esthesioneuroblastoma)

Cysts of Nose and Paranasal Sinus (PNS)

❖ Congenital cysts, i.e., Thornwaldt's cyst **(Figs. 1 and 2)**
❖ Mucoceles and pyoceles
❖ Cystic odontomas
❖ Dermoids
❖ Bone cysts

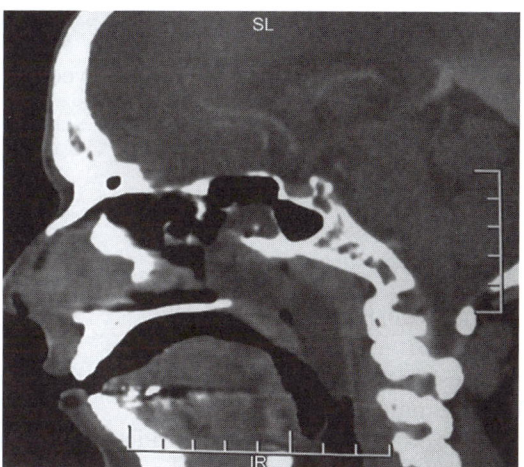

Fig. 1: Computed tomography (CT) scan showing Thornwaldt's cyst.

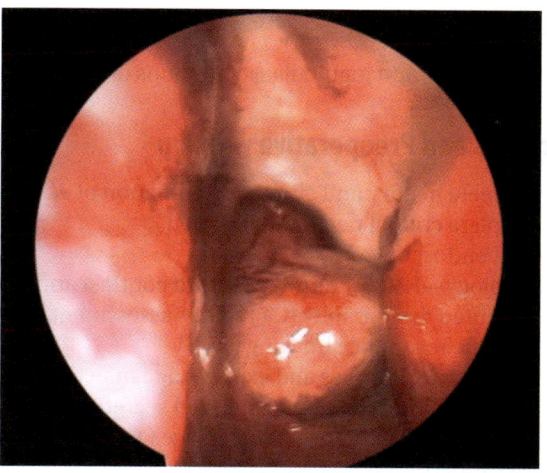

Fig. 2: Nasal endoscopic view of Thornwaldt's cyst.

Congenital soft tissue swellings of the nasal cavity:
- Encephaloceles
- Meningoencephaloceles
- Gliomas

SINONASAL MALIGNANCY

Q. Write a short note on sinonasal malignancy.

Incidence

0.5–1/1 lakh population. Account for 1% of all malignancies and 3–5% of all head and neck cancers. Male: Female = 2:1.

Types

Primary epithelial tumors are the most common type with squamous cells.
  Carcinoma as being the most common subtype.

Maxillary sinus tumors are the most common (55%) followed by the nasal cavity (35%), ethmoid sinuses, and rarely frontal and sphenoid sinuses (1%).

Etiology

- Inhalation of carcinogens—responsible for 40% of sinonasal malignancies.
  - Hardwood (wood dust) exposure—risk of adenocarcinoma
  - Softwood (wood dust) exposure—risk of squamous cell carcinoma (SCC).

African mahogany is the most carcinogenic among all the types of woods.
- Nickel—increases the risk of developing sinonasal SCC 250-folds.
- Smoking also increases the risk of these cancers in synergism with wood dust.
- Chromium, polycyclic hydrocarbons, aflatoxin, mustard gas, thorotrast.
- Radiation, viral, and genetic causes.

Ohngren's Line and its Significance

Ohngren's line is a line running from the medial canthus of the orbit to the angle of the mandible.
  It is used to separate the sinonasal tumors into two groups.
  Tumors above the line were more aggressive, poorly differentiated, and hence had a bad prognosis while tumors below the line were less aggressive, better differentiated, and hence had a good prognosis.

Lymph Nodes

Submandibular and jugulodigastric groups of lymph nodes are the most common group of lymph nodes involved.

Diagnosis and Preoperative work up

- Complete history and clinical examination of ear, nose, and throat doctor (ENT)
- Complete cranial nerve examination
- Nasal endoscopy
- Radiology—HRCT (1 mm) cuts with contrast and MRI
  Computed tomography (CT) scan—assessment of osseous margins of the skull base and sinus walls
  Magnetic resonance imaging (MRI):
  - Soft-tissue masses and extension of infectious or malignant processes outside the confines of the paranasal sinuses.
  - Better differentiation of retained secretions and hemorrhage from the tumor.
  - MRI (T1 and T2)-weighted image (1 mm cuts) of the sinonasal cavity, orbit, skull base, and the adjacent intracranial compartment.
  - Positron emission tomography (PET) scan—to see for metastases if any.
- Biopsy—performed once the radiological investigation is done.

Concerning Clinical Feature

- Conductive hearing loss/middle ear effusion
- Visual loss, diplopia/ophthalmoplegia, pain in eye movement, chemosis
- Clear rhinorrhea
- Facial paresthesia
- Loose teeth—dental paresthesia
- Facial asymmetry
- Oronasal/oroantral fistula
- Palpable cervical nodes
- Reduced neck range of motion

■ INVERTED PAPILLOMA OF NOSE

Q. What are the other names of inverted papilloma of nose? Mention its etiopathogenesis, clinical features, and management.

- Transitional cell papilloma
- Ringertz tumor
- Schneiderian papilloma
- Soft papilloma
- Fungiform papilloma
- Cylindrical cell papilloma
- Papillary sinusitis
- Sinonasal type papilloma

Etiology

Human papillomavirus (HPV).

Pathogenesis

Thickening of the epithelial layer with infolding and formation of solid hyperplastic papillomatous mass which grows into the stroma rather than in an exophytic manner. The basement membrane is intact.

Clinical Features

- Males > Females
- Age group: 40–70 years
- Unilateral almost always

- Benign tumor but has a malignant potential
- Prone to recurrence and potential for local destruction of tissues.
- Site of origin—lateral wall of the nose—middle meatus area.
- Arises from the Schneiderian membrane of the nose, i.e., nonolfactory mucosa of the nose.
- Other sites of origin—frontal sinus, sphenoid sinus, or lateral wall of the maxillary sinus.

Clinical Presentation

- Unilateral nasal obstruction, nasal discharge, and epistaxis.
- Orbital invasion—proptosis, diplopia, and lacrimation.

On nasal endoscopy—seen as soft pale polypoidal mass resembling nasal polyp.

Management

Investigations

CT scan and MRI scan to see the extent of the mass and its origin.

Surgery

Complete excision of the mass **(Fig. 3)** with cauterization/drilling of the underlying tissue/bone from which it arises to avoid recurrence.

Approach for Surgery

- Endoscopic approach—medial maxillectomy by modified Denker's approach.
- Open/external approach—lateral rhinotomy or sublabial degloving approach if the mass is extensive and complete excision by endoscopic approach is not possible.

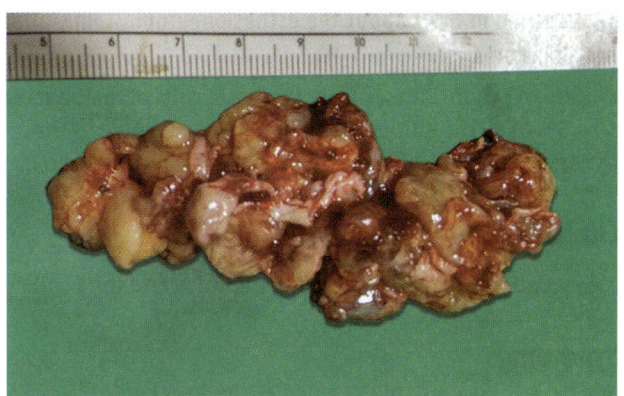

Fig. 3: Postoperative image of inverted nasal papilloma specimen.

■ HEMANIGIOMA

Q. What are the types of hemangioma which present as nasal mass?

Two types are described:
1. Capillary hemangioma
2. Cavernous hemangioma.

Capillary Hemangioma

- Soft, smooth, and dark reddish in color, and pedunculated or sessile tumor
- Origin—nasal septum (anterior part)
- Clinical features—nasal obstruction and epistaxis
- Diagnosis—diagnostic nasal endoscopy (DNE)
- Treatment—local excision with the cuff of surrounding mucoperichondrium

Cavernous Hemangioma

- Arises from the turbinates on the lateral wall of the nose.
- Treatment—surgical excision with cryotherapy. Radiation in case of large tumors.

■ INTRANASAL MENINGOENCEPHALOCELE

Q. Describe in brief about intranasal meningoencephalocele.

Herniation of the brain tissues and meninges through the foramen cecum (primitive tract between the anterior cranial fossa and the nasal space) or cribriform plate.

Clinical Features

- Seen in infants and young children
- Smooth polyp between the septum and middle turbinate **(Fig. 4)**
- Increases in size on crying/straining
- Managed by craniotomy—stalk is severed from the brain with repair of bony and dural defect.
- Intranasal mass removed by endoscopic approach in the second sitting.

■ ESTHESIONEUROBLASTOMA

Q. Describe in brief about the esthesioneuroblastoma/olfactory neuroblastoma.

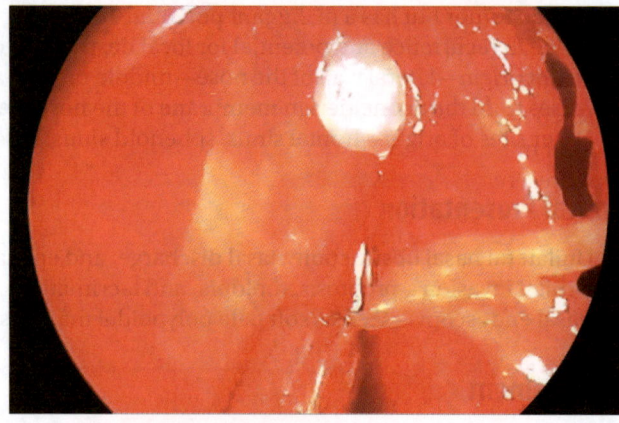

Fig. 4: Endoscopic view of meningoencephalocele.

- Site of origin—arises from the basal cells of the olfactory epithelium in the upper third of nose.
- <5% of all the sinonasal malignancies. Females > males
- Age group—bimodal—2 peaks at 20 years and then 50 years

Clinical Features

Neuroendocrine tumor secreting peptides and thus causing paraneoplastic.

Syndromes

Cushing's syndrome, inappropriate antidiuretic hormone secretion, or hypertension produced by vasoactive peptides are reported.
- Is one of a group of small round blue cell tumors.
- Unilateral nasal obstruction and epistaxis.
- Orbit invasion—proptosis, headache, epiphora, diplopia, and blurred vision.
  Lymph node metastasis in 10–15% of cases.

Diagnosis

Diagnostic nasal endoscopy (DNE)—friable cherry red mass in the upper third of nasal cavity.

Investigation

- High-resolution computed tomography (HRCT) scan may show destruction or erosion of the cribriform plate or orbital wall.
- Magnetic resonance imaging with contrast shows extension into the orbit or brain.

Pathology

- Low grade with the formation of pseudorosettes or high grade with nuclear pleomorphism but no rosette formation.
- ***Hyams, et al.*** developed a four-point histological grading system for olfactory neuroblastoma (OAN) based on features:
- The degree of differentiation, the tumor architecture, mitotic index, nuclear polymorphism, fibrillary nature of the matrix, and tumor necrosis.

Treatment

- Craniofacial resection with radiation and/or chemotherapy.
  Craniofacial resection approaches:
  - Osteoplastic flap
  - Facial approach through lateral rhinotomy/midfacial degloving approach.

NASAL DERMOID

Q. How does a nasal dermoid present?

❖ Nasal dermoid presents as widening of the upper part of nasal septum with splaying of nasal bones and hypertelorism.
❖ A pit or sinus is seen in the midline of the nasal dorsum with hair protruding **(Figs. 5A and B)** from the opening which represents its ectodermal origin.

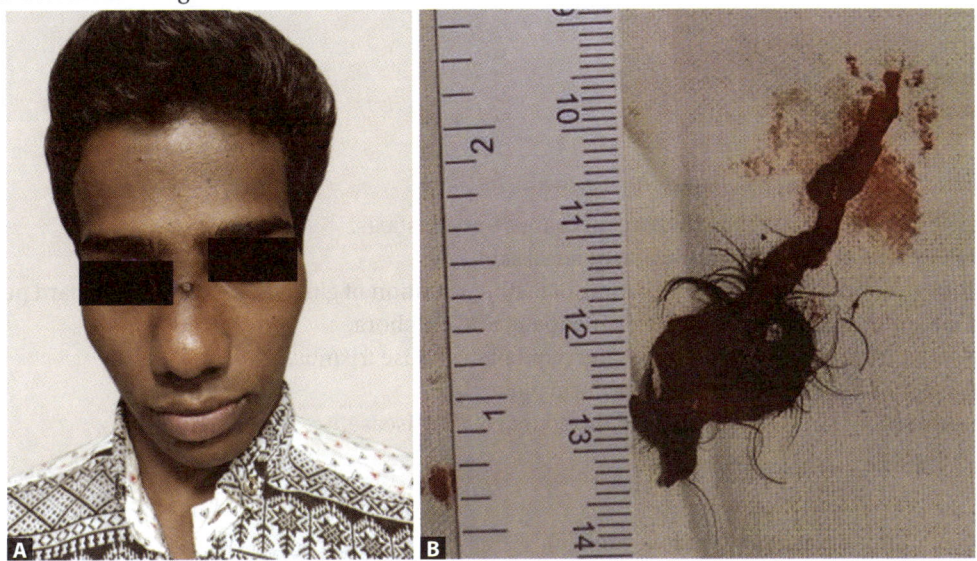

Figs. 5A and B: Clinical picture of nasal dermoid and excised nasal dermoid with hair.

CARCINOMA NASAL CAVITY

Q. Describe in brief about the carcinoma of the nasal cavity/nose-pickers cancer.

Squamous cell carcinoma is the most common variety followed by adenoid cystic carcinoma or adenocarcinoma.

Incidence and Etiology

❖ Age group—50-70 years of age. Males > females
❖ Site of origin—an extension of maxillary/ethmoid carcinoma.
❖ Risk factors:
  ▸ Transformation of Schneiderian papillomas into SCC. Incidence—14.6%
  ▸ Smoking
  ▸ Inhalational carcinogens
  ▸ Radiation

Sites

It arises from the following common sites:
❖ **Lateral wall:** Most commonly involved site. Presents as a polypoid mass in the lateral wall of nose. 50% gets developed on the turbinates **(Fig. 6)**.
❖ **Vestibular:** It arises from the lateral wall of the vestibule and extends into columella, nasal floor, and upper lip with secondaries to parotid nodes **(Fig. 7)**.
❖ **Septal:** It arises from the mucocutaneous junction. It causes burning and soreness.

Management

Surgery plus radiotherapy.

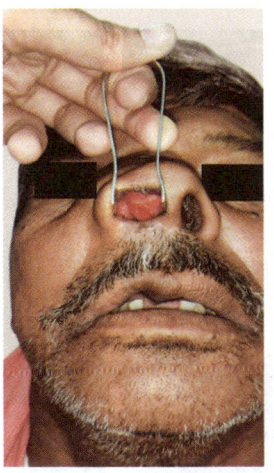

Fig. 6: Nasal mass (carcinoma).

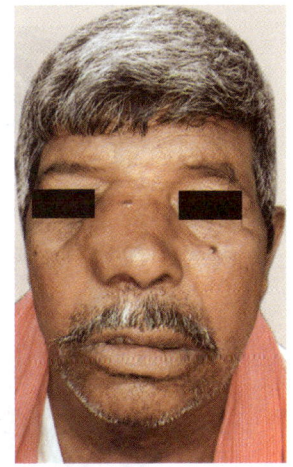

Fig. 7: Nasal carcinoma with bony destruction and hypertelorism.

CARCINOMA MAXILLARY SINUS

Q. What are the clinical features and management for maxillary sinus carcinoma?

Clinical Features

- Nasal stuffiness
- Blood stained nasal discharge
- Facial paresthesia/pain
- Epiphora
- Loose teeth

Late features depend upon the spread and extent of growth:

Medial spread to nasal cavity—nasal obstruction, discharge, and epistaxis.
Anterior spread—swelling of cheeks and invasion of facial skin.
Inferior spread into alveolus—dental pain, loosening of teeth, ulceration of gingiva, and swelling in hard palate.
Superior spread into orbit—proptosis, diplopia, ocular pain, and epiphora.
Posterior spread into pterygomaxillary fossa and pterygoid plates cause trismus.
Intracranial spread—through ethmoids and cribriform plate.
Lymph node metastases are rare and occur late in the course of the disease.

Investigations

- Nasal mass biopsy (antral wash samples for cytology).
- X-ray nose suggestive of positive Hondusa's sign with widening in the space between maxillary tuberosity and temporomandibular (TM) joint of the affected side.
- CT scan of nose and paranasal sinuses (shows soft tissue mass in maxillary sinus with bony destruction).

Treatment

Surgery for T1 and T2 maxillary carcinoma; while T3 and T4 lesions require surgery plus radiotherapy. Chemoradiation (chemotherapy + radiation) is used for large and inoperable tumors.

Surgical Techniques

- Partial maxillectomy—medial maxillectomy which involves clearance of lateral wall of nose with ethmoid sinuses. Palatal resection with alveolus for tumors of oral cavity involving hard palate.
- Total maxillectomy—total removal of the upper jaw along with the tumor (**Figs. 8A and B**)
- Extended maxillectomy—required when tumor is beyond the upper jaw—craniofacial resection is done
- Open approach-Weber-Ferguson-Longmire incision is used (**Figs. 9A and B**).

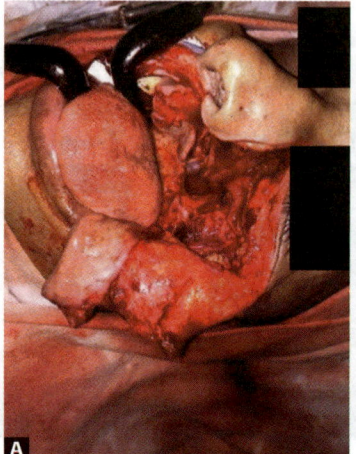
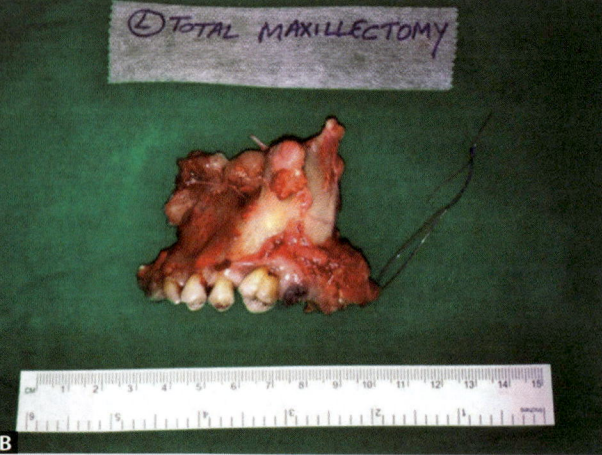

Figs. 8A and B: Total maxillectomy specimen after excision of maxilla.

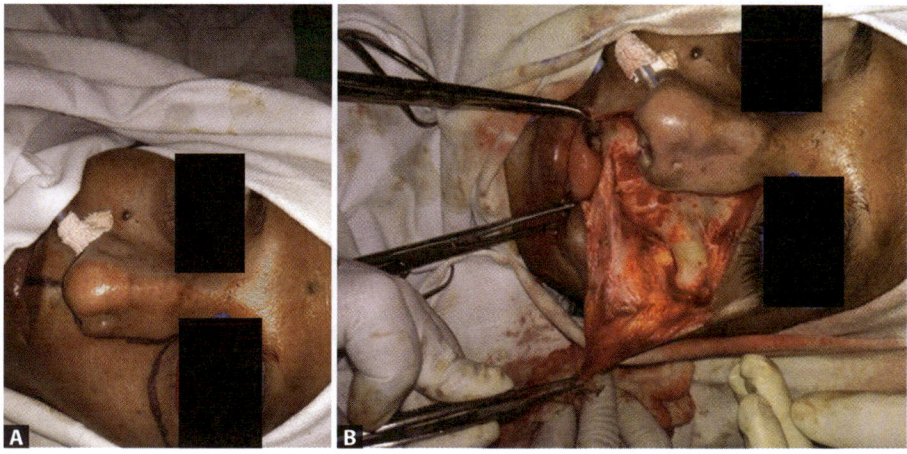

Figs. 9A and B: Weber–Ferguson incision and elevation of flap over maxilla.

ETHMOID SINUS MALIGNANCY

Q. Write the clinical features and management of ethmoid sinus malignancy.

- Extension of maxillary sinus carcinoma.
- Primary ethmoid sinus malignancy is very rare.
- Early features—nasal obstruction, blood-stained nasal discharge, and retro-orbital pain.
- Late features—broadening of nose root, lateral displacement of eyeball, and diplopia.
- Very late feature—extension through cribriform plate cause meningitis.
- CT scan—to know the extent of the disease. Preoperative radiation is followed by total ethmoidectomy by lateral rhinotomy approach (external approach).
- If a cribriform plate is involved then—is combined approach by neurosurgeon and ENT surgeon by craniofacial resection.

BENIGN NEOPLASMS OF PARANASAL SINUSES

Q. Enumerate the commonly seen benign neoplasms of paranasal sinuses.

- Osteomas
- Fibrous dysplasia
- Ossifying fibromas
- Ameloblastoma

Note: Frontal sinus is the most common site amongst all the sinuses.

Section 4: Laryngology, Head and Neck

Chapter 30

History and Examination of Oral Cavity, Throat, Head and Neck

EN2.1: Elicit document and present an appropriate history in a patient presenting with an ENT complaint.
EN2.2: Demonstrate the correct technique of examining the throat including the use of a tongue depressor.
EN2.2: Demonstrate the correct technique of examination of neck including elicitation of laryngeal crepitus.

ORAL CAVITY

Oral cavity extends from the lips to the level of anterior tonsillar pillars. Structures included are:

- Lips
- Buccal mucosa
- Gums and teeth
- Hard palate
- Anterior two-third of tongue
- Floor of mouth
- Retromolar trigone

History Taking

- Pain
- Disturbance of salivation
- Disturbance of taste
- Trismus—Restricted mouth opening
- **Lesion over oral cavity:** Ulcers, swelling, ankyloglossia
- **Xerostomia:** Dryness of mouth due to oral breathing, radiotherapy, or generalized oral lesions
- **Halitosis:** Bad breath
- Bleeding from oral cavity
- Drooling of saliva
- **Change in voice:** Hoarse voice, breathy voice, hot potato speech, husky voice
- **Difficulty in breathing:** Breathing through oral cavity, noisy breathing
- **Swallowing:** Painful (odynophagia), difficulty in swallowing (dysphagia), dysphagia to solid/liquid
- **Aspiration:** Coughing while drinking liquids

Examination

Lips

To examine both lips—upper and lower, by inspection and palpation. Each lip has an outer (cutaneous), an inner (mucosal) surface, and a vermillion border. Look for any swellings **(Fig. 1)**, vesicles, ulcers, crusts, scars, unilateral, or bilateral clefts.

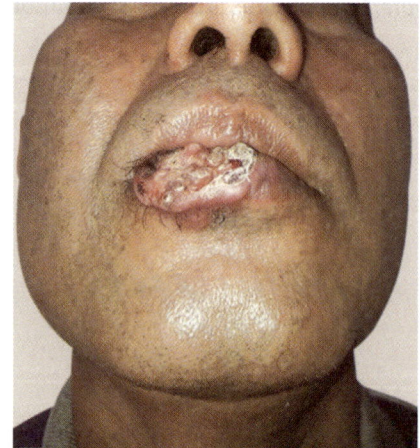

Fig. 1: Ulceroproliferative growth over lower lip suggestive of carcinoma of lip.

Buccal Mucosa

Examine it by explaining the procedure to the patient, asking him to open the mouth and by retracting the cheek with a **tongue** depressor. Examine the mucosa of cheek and vestibule of mouth for:
- Change in color
- Change in surface appearance, e.g., ulceration, vesicles or bullae, white striae, blanched appearance with pigmentation, atrophic changes in mucosa, and swelling or growth
- Opening of parotid duct is seen opposite the upper second molar tooth. Look for any redness, swelling around that area.

Lesions which can be seen: Ulcers, tumors, white patches (leukoplakia), black patches (melanoplakia), red patches (erythroplakia), fibrosis, proliferative, and ulcerative growth (malignancy)

Gums and Teeth

Are examined in both the upper and lower jaws. Outer surface of gums is examined by retracting the cheeks and lips and the inner surface by pushing the tongue away with a tongue depressor.
Look for:
- Red and swollen gums
- Ulcerated gums covered with a membrane
- Hyperplasia
- **Growths:** Benign or malignant neoplasms
- Loose teeth (carcinoma of maxilla)
- Carious infected tooth or teeth
- Malocclusion
- Fractures of mandible or maxilla, abnormalities of temporomandibular joint

Hard Palate

Look for:
- Cleft palate
- Oronasal fistula
- High-arched palate/bulge
- Bony growth in midline
- Mass or ulcer (minor salivary gland tumors (**Fig. 2**)/malignancy)
- Palatal perforation/defect (mucormycosis, carcinoma of maxilla, or palate)

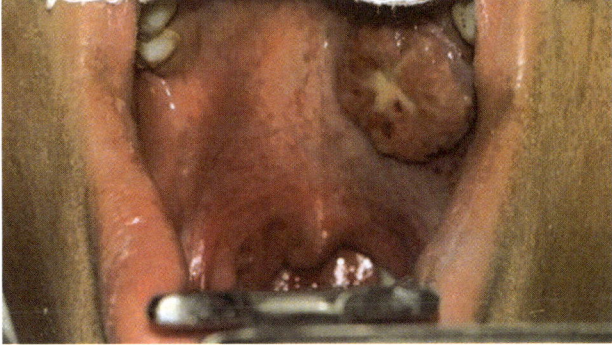

Fig. 2: Tumor over hard palate.

Tongue

Only oral tongue (anterior two-third) is included in the oral cavity. First, examine the tongue in its natural position and then ask the patient to protrude it, move it to the right and left and then up.
- Examine the tip, dorsum, lateral borders, and under surface.
- **Look for:**
  - Large size
  - Inability to protrude
  - Deviation on protrusion (**Fig. 3**) suggestive of carcinoma tongue
  - Bald tongue
  - Fissures
  - Ulcers (**Fig. 4**)
  - White thick patch (**Fig. 5**)
  - Proliferative growth
  - Hemangioma (**Fig. 6**)

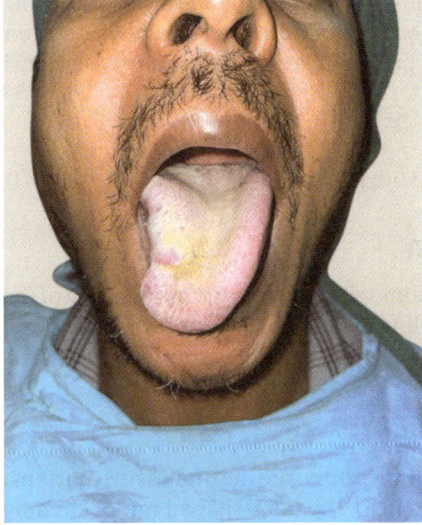

Fig. 3: Deviation of tongue on one side in carcinoma of tongue.

Floor of Mouth

Examine anterior part which lies under the tongue and two lateral gutters. Lateral gutters are better examined by two tongue depressors; one retracting the tongue and the other, the cheek.

PART 1: Diseases of ENT, Head and Neck

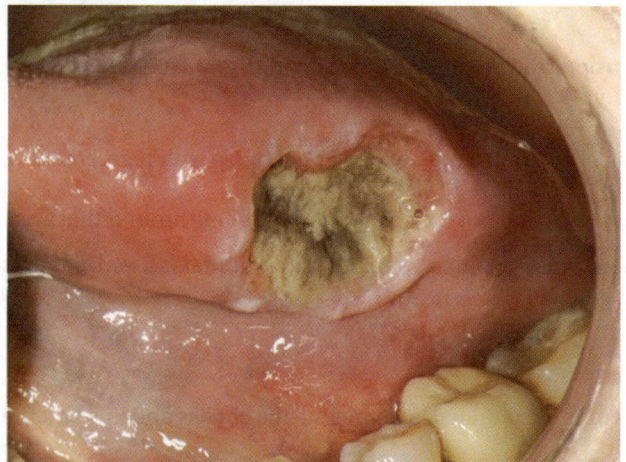

Fig. 4: Ulcer over lateral border of tongue.

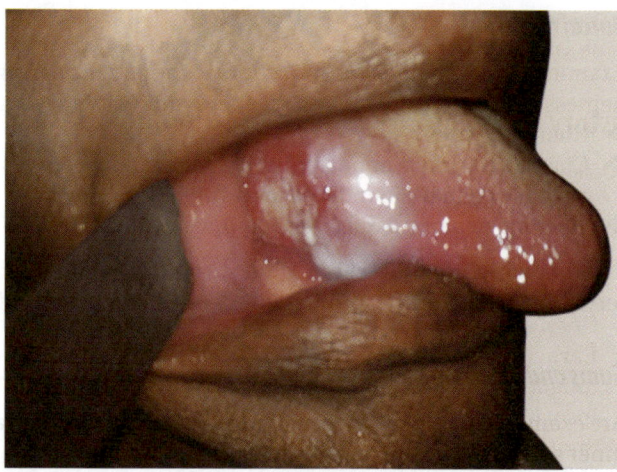

Fig. 5: Whitish patch and thickening over lateral border of tongue.

- Opening of the submandibular duct is seen as a raised papilla on either side of the frenulum.
- Look for:
  - Short frenulum
  - Scar
  - Ulcer
  - Swelling

Retromolar Trigone

Look for the inflammation due to impaction of last molar tooth or a malignant lesion of this area.

Anterior and Posterior Pillar

Look for any congestion, ulcers, (tonsillitis, quinsy)

Tonsils

Hypertrophy (unilateral/bilateral), congestion (tonsillitis), ulcers, cysts, tonsillolith, grayish/white membrane over tonsillitis, peritonsillar swelling (quinsy/peritonsillar abscess)

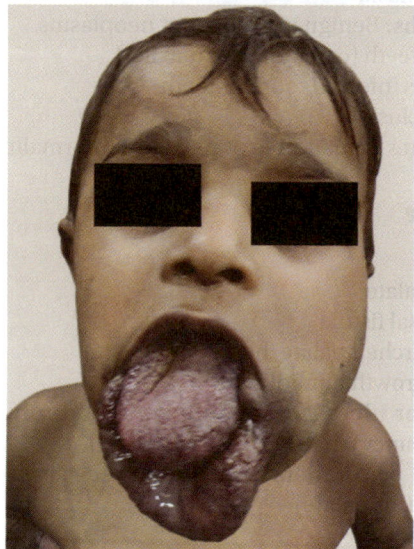

Fig. 6: Hemangioma of lower lip and tongue.

Uvula

Enlarged, congested, shifted to one side, ulcers/tumors over uvula

Palpation

- All lesions of the oral cavity, particularly of the tongue, floor of mouth, cheek, lip, and palate must be palpated.
- A swelling in the floor of mouth should be examined by bimanual palpation, to differentiate a swelling of submandibular salivary gland from that of submandibular lymph nodes (salivary gland tumors are bimanually palpable/ballotable).

■ OROPHARYNX

Oropharynx lies opposite the oral cavity. Starts at the level of anterior pillars, bounded above by the junction of hard and soft palate, and below by the V-shaped row of circumvallate papillae.

Structures included in it are:

- Tonsils and pillars
- Soft palate

- Base of tongue
- Posterior pharyngeal wall

History

A disease of the oropharynx can disturb swallowing, phonation, respiration, and hearing.

A patient with disease of oropharynx presents with one or more of the following complaints:
- Sore throat
- Odynophagia (painful swallowing)
- Dysphagia (difficulty in swallowing)
- **Change in voice:** Hyper or hyponasality, hot potato voice
- **Earache:** Benign ulcers or malignant lesions of the base of tongue, tonsil, pillars and palate cause referred pain in the ipsilateral ear
- Snoring
- Halitosis (bad smell from the mouth)
- **Hearing loss:** A conductive hearing loss due to Eustachian tube dysfunction
- Congestion, granulations
- Mass in oropharynx (carcinoma oropharynx, antrochoanal polyp)
- Postnasal discharge
- **Abnormal appearance:** Patient may notice an abnormal finding while looking at his throat in the mirror and then consult an ENT surgeon.

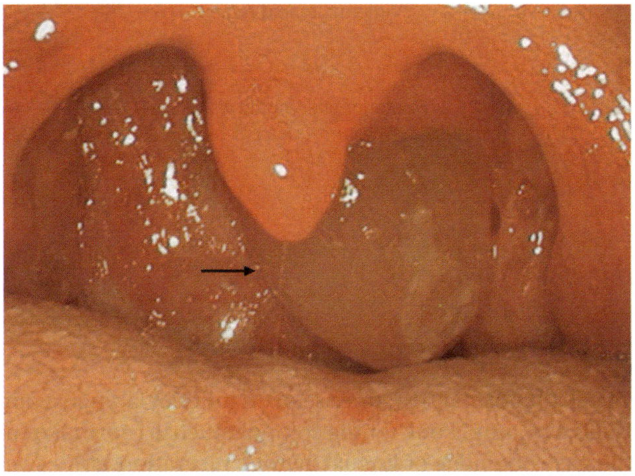

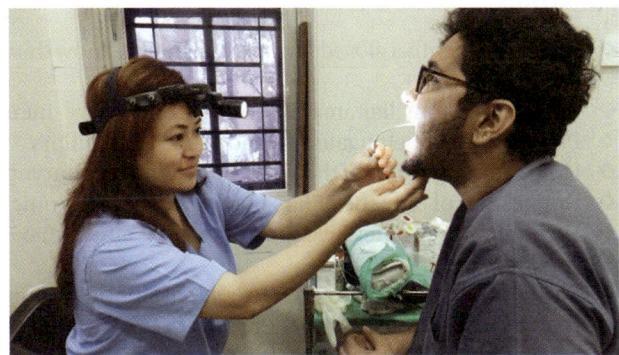

Fig. 7: Antrochoanal polyp coming in oropharynx.

Examination

- First, examine the oropharynx by asking the patient to open the mouth widely. Look for mass: Polyp **(Fig. 7)** and postnasal drip
- Tongue depressor along with Headmirror with Bull's Eyelamp/Headlight **(Fig. 8)** is used when it is required to displace the tongue to one side to examine tonsillolingual sulcus, or to press on the tonsils to look for the contents of tonsillar crypts.
- The base of tongue is examined by laryngeal mirror.

Soft Palate

Look for redness (peritonsillitis), bulge or swelling.

Fig. 8: Examination of oral cavity using tongue depressor and headlight.

Uvula

Normally, uvula is in the midline. It becomes edematous and **displaced to the opposite side in peritonsillar abscess.** Note movements of soft palate when the patient says "Aa." Deviation of the uvula and soft palate to the healthy side is a sign of vagal paralysis. A bifid uvula may be a sign of submucous cleft palate. In such cases, a notch can be palpated in the hard palate at its junction with soft palate in the midline.

Posterior Pharyngeal Wall

Posterior pharyngeal wall can be seen directly. Look for lymphoid nodules (granular pharyngitis), purulent discharge trickling down the posterior pharyngeal wall (sinusitis), hypertrophy of lateral pharyngeal bands just behind the posterior pillars (chronic sinusitis), thin glazed mucosa, and crusting (atrophic pharyngitis).

Base of Tongue and Valleculae

Posterior one-third of tongue forms the base of tongue and lies between the V-shaped row of circumvallate papillae and the valleculae. Valleculae are two shallow depressions, which lie between the base of tongue and the epiglottis. Base of tongue and valleculae are best examined by indirect laryngoscopy.

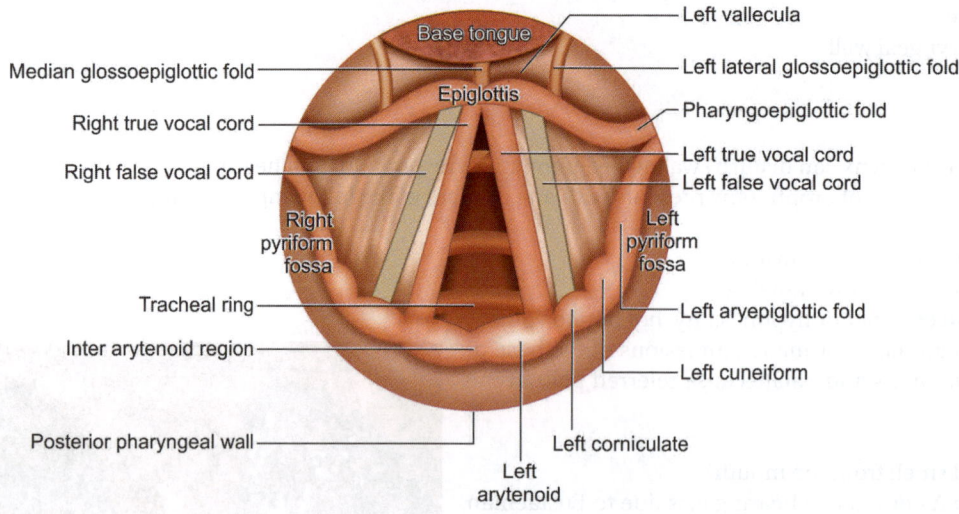

Fig. 9: Indirect laryngoscopy (IDL).

Indirect Laryngoscopy (scan QR code)

Check for normal structures seen on indirect laryngoscopy (Fig. 9) using head light/head mirror and Bull's eye lamp. Look for the color of mucosa (normal or congested); prominent veins, varicosities at the base of tongue or lingual thyroid, ulceration, solid swelling, and cystic swelling.

Palpation

- Of the tonsil with a gloved finger is essential to know the consistency of the mass (hard in malignancy or tonsillolith)
- Pulsation in tonsillar area (internal carotid artery aneurysm)
- Palpation for an elongated styloid process (b) pillars.
- Uniform congestion of the pillars, tonsils, and pharyngeal mucosa is seen in acute tonsillitis.
- Congestion of only the pillars may be a sign of chronic tonsillitis.
- Ulceration or proliferative growth may be an extension of malignancy from the tonsil base of tongue or the retromolar trigone.
- **Palpation of base of tongue:** Extent of tumor which infiltrates deeper into the tongue is better appreciated by palpation than by inspection. If the patient fails to relax sufficiently, palpation should be done under general anesthesia.
- When palpating any structure in the oropharynx in a child, the examiner should invaginate the patient's cheek between his teeth with finger of the opposite hand to prevent biting on the examiner's finger.

■ LARYNX AND LARYNGOPHARYNX

History

A patient with disease of the larynx presents with one or more of the following complaints:
- **Disorders of voice,** e.g., hoarseness aphonia, puberphonia, or easy fatiguability of voice
- Respiratory obstruction
- Cough and expectoration
- Repeated clearing of throat, pain in throat
- Dysphagia (difficulty in swallowing)
- Mass in the neck

Examination

- External examination of larynx
- Indirect laryngoscopy

- Flexible or rigid fiberoptic endoscopy
- Assessment of voice
- Assessment of cervical lymph nodes

External Examination of Larynx

Both inspection and palpation are employed. Look for:
- Redness of skin
- Bulge or swelling
- Widening of larynx
- Surgical emphysema
- Change in contour or displacement of laryngeal structures

Palpate the hyoid bone, thyroid cartilage, thyroid notch, cricoid cartilage, and the tracheal rings.

Movements of larynx: Normally, larynx moves with deglutition. It can also be moved from side-to-side producing a characteristic grating sound **(laryngeal crepitus) (scan QR code)**. Fixity of larynx indicates inflammation or infiltration of growth into the surrounding structures. Loss of laryngeal crepitus is due to postcricoid carcinoma.

Indirect Laryngoscopy

Q. Write short note on indirect laryngoscopy.

- **Technique:** The procedure is explained to the patient and consent is taken. Patient is seated opposite the examiner. He should sit erect with the head and chest leaning slightly toward the examiner. He is asked to protrude his tongue which is wrapped in gauze and held by the examiner between the thumb and middle finger. Gauze piece is used to get a firm grip of the tongue and to protect it against injury by the lower incisors.
- **Laryngeal mirror (size 4–6)** which has been warmed and tested on the back of hand is introduced into the mouth and held firmly against the uvula and soft palate. Light is focused on the laryngeal mirror and patient is asked to breathe quietly. To see movements of the cords, patient is asked to take deep inspiration (abduction of cords), say "Aa" (adduction of cords) and "Eee" (for adduction and tension). Movements of both the cords are compared.

Indirect laryngoscopy permits examination of structures of the oropharynx, larynx, and laryngopharynx (Fig. 10)

- **Larynx:** Epiglottis, aryepiglottic folds, arytenoids, cuneiform and corniculate cartilages, ventricular bands, ventricles, true cords, anterior commissure, posterior commissure, subglottis, and rings of trachea
- **Laryngopharynx:** Both pyriform fossae, postcricoid region, posterior wall of laryngopharynx
- **Oropharynx:** Base of tongue, lingual tonsils, valleculae, medial and lateral glossoepiglottic folds

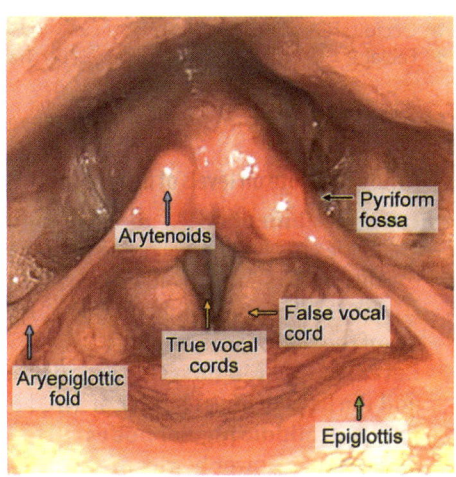

Fig. 10: Laryngeal inlet.

Methods of defogging of laryngeal mirror:
- Heating mirror surface of laryngeal mirror with spirit lamp and check the temperature with back of palm
- Never heat metallic surface of mirror with spirit lamp
- Deep the mirror in Savlon solution
- Rub against the mucosa of cheek

Flexible or Rigid Fiberoptic Endoscopy

Q. Write short note on flexible/rigid fiberoptic endoscopy.

- **Flexible endoscopy:** In difficult cases, where laryngeal examination cannot be performed with a mirror due to anatomical abnormalities or intolerance of mirror by the patient, a flexible rhinolaryngoscope can be used. It is passed through the nose under local anesthesia and gives a good view of the larynx, laryngopharynx, subglottis, and even upper trachea. It is an OPD procedure.
- **Rigid endoscopy:** For this purpose, a rigid fiberoptic telescope is used. It gives a clear, wide-angle view of the larynx and laryngopharynx. It is also an outdoor procedure. Local anesthesia may be required for patients with an active gag reflex.
- **Stroboscope:** A stroboscope is a device which emits light in pulses and the frequency of pulses can be set by the examiner. If frequency of pulses is same at which vocal cords are moving, the latter appear stationary giving more time to study the cord. If frequency of pulses is more or less than that of vocal cord movements, the cords are seen in slow motion. Stroboscopes are synchronized with rigid or **fiberoptic endoscopes** and the vocal cord movements can be recorded on video (**video stroboscopy**).
- **Stroboscopy** has been found very useful in diagnosis of laryngeal paralysis, completeness of glottic closure during phonation, very small early laryngeal cancer, vocal cord scarring, laryngeal cyst versus polyp, and sulcus vocalis.

Assessment of Voice

The examiner should make note of the quality of voice of the patient when he is speaking, whether it is hoarse, rough, breathy, bitonal, dysphonic, whispered, or feeble.

EXAMINATION OF NECK

Lymph Nodes of the Head and Neck

Neck nodes are inspected and then palpated with fingers.

Classification of Lymph Nodes of the Head and Neck

Q. Write a short note on lymph nodes of head and neck.

Lymph nodes of the head and neck		
1. **Upper horizontal chain of nodes**	2. **Lateral cervical nodes**—nodes, superficial and deep to sternocleidomastoid muscle and in the posterior triangle	3. **Anterior cervical nodes**
❖ Submental ❖ Submandibular ❖ Parotid ❖ Postauricular (mastoid) ❖ Occipital ❖ Facial	❖ Superficial external jugular group ➢ Deep group ➢ Internal jugular chain (upper, middle and lower groups) ➢ Spinal accessory chain ➢ Transverse cervical chain	❖ Anterior jugular chain ❖ Juxtavisceral chain ➢ Prelaryngeal ➢ Pretracheal ➢ Paratracheal

Classification of Neck Nodes According to Level (Fig 11)

Q. Write short note on levels of neck nodes.

❖ **Level I: Submental (IA) and submandibular (IB)**
  ➢ Nodes IA, submental nodes, which lie in the submental triangle, i.e., between right and left anterior bellies of digastric muscles and the hyoid bone
  ➢ Nodes IB, submandibular nodes, lying between anterior and posterior bellies of digastric muscle and the lower border of the body of mandible
❖ **Level II: Upper jugular nodes**—they are located along the upper third of jugular vein, i.e., between the skull base above and the level of lower border of hyoid bone (or bifurcation of carotid artery) below.
❖ **Level III: Middle jugular nodes**—they are located along the middle third jugular vein, from the level of hyoid bone above, to the level of lower border of cricoid cartilage (or where omohyoid muscle crosses the jugular vein) below.
❖ **Level IV: Lower jugular nodes**—they are located along the lower third of jugular vein; from lower border of cricoid cartilage to the clavicle. Virchow's node is included into this level.

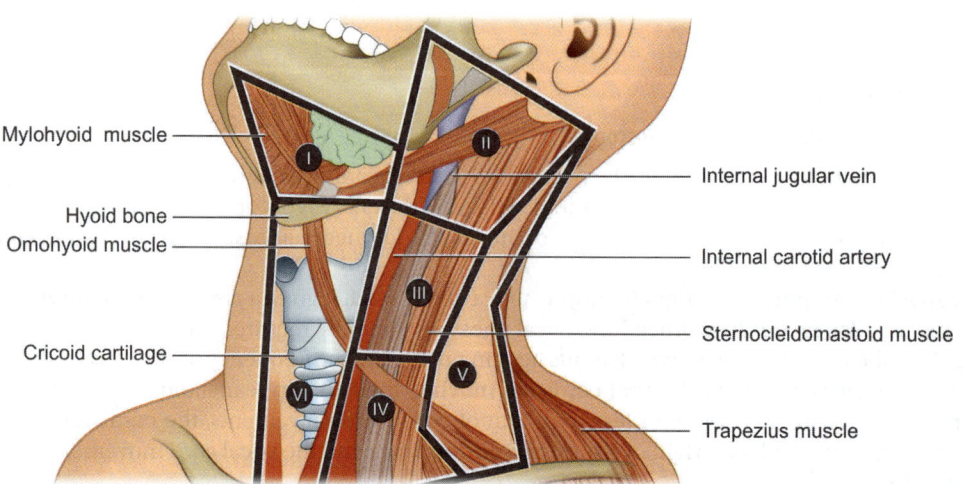

Fig. 11: Neck triangles and neck nodes.

- **Level V: Posterior cervical group**—they are located in the posterior triangle, i.e., between posterior border of sternocleidomastoid (anteriorly), anterior border of trapezius (posteriorly), and the clavicle below. They include lymph nodes of spinal accessory chain, transverse cervical nodes, and supraclavicular nodes. Level V nodes are further subdivided into upper, middle, and lower, corresponding to planes that define levels II, III, and IV.
- **Level VI: Anterior compartment nodes**—they are located between the medial borders of sternocleidomastoid muscles (or carotid sheaths) on each side, hyoid bone above, and suprasternal notch below. They include prelaryngeal, pretracheal, and paratracheal nodes.
- **Level VII:** They are located below the suprasternal notch and include nodes of the upper mediastinum.

Examination of Neck Nodes

Examination of neck nodes is important, particularly in head and neck malignancies and a systematic approach should be followed.

Neck nodes are better palpated while standing at the back of the patient (Fig. 12). Neck is slightly flexed to achieve relaxation of muscles. The nodes are examined in the following manner so that none is missed.

- **Upper horizontal chain:** Examine submental, submandibular, parotid, facial, postauricular, and occipital nodes
- **External jugular chain:** It lies superficial to sternomastoid.
- **Internal jugular chain:** Examine the upper, middle, and lower groups. Many of them lie deep to sternomastoid muscle which may need to be displaced posteriorly.
- Spinal accessory chain
- Transverse cervical chain
- Anterior jugular chain
- **Juxtavisceral chain:** Prelaryngeal, pretracheal, and paratracheal nodes.

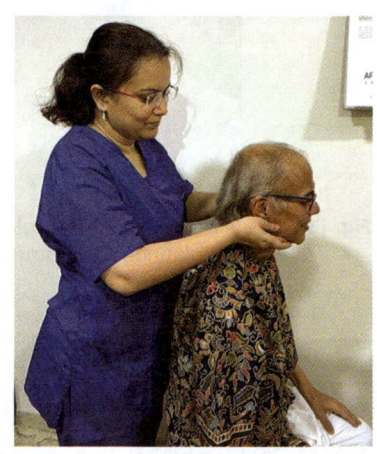

Fig. 12: Examination of neck nodes.

Medial and lateral groups of retropharyngeal lymph nodes are seen from behind. Node of Rouviere is the uppermost node of the lateral group.

When a node or nodes are palpable, look for the following points:
- Location of nodes
- Number of nodes
- Size
- **Consistency:** Metastatic nodes are hard; lymphoma nodes are firm and rubbery; hyperplastic nodes are soft. Nodes of metastatic melanoma are also soft.
- Discrete or matted nodes
- **Tenderness:** Inflammatory nodes are tender.
- Fixity to overlying skin or deeper structures. Mobility should be checked both in the vertical and horizontal planes.

Differential Diagnosis of Neck Swelling

Anterior neck swellings	Lateral neck swellings

Digastric triangle, carotid triangle, muscular triangle
- Thyroglossal cyst **(Fig. 13)**
- Thyroid swelling **(Fig. 17)**
	- Occipital triangle
	- Lymph nodes:
	  - Inflammatory: Neck sinus **(Fig. 14)**
	  - Neoplastic: Benign or malignant swellings **(Fig. 15)**
	  - Cystic hygroma **(Fig. 16)**

- Submandibular sialadenitis or tumors
- Submandibular lymph nodes
  - Inflammatory
  - Neoplastic
  - Metastatic
- Jugular lymph nodes
- Plunging ranula
- Branchial cyst
- Thyroid swelling
- Carotid body tumor
- Parotid tail swelling
- Parapharyngeal tumor
- Laryngocele
- Pharyngeal pouch
	Supraclavicular triangle
	- **Metastatic nodes from infraclavicular primaries**
	  - Breast
	  - Lung
	  - Gastrointestinal (GI) tract
	  - Kidney
	  - Ovary, testis
	- Subclavian aneurysm
	- Cystic hygroma
	- Cervical rib

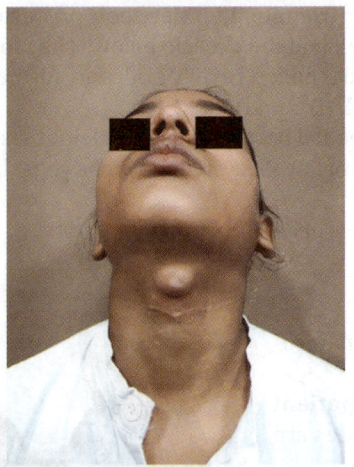

Fig. 13: Midline neck swelling, thyroglossal cyst (swelling moves with deglutition and protrusion of tongue).

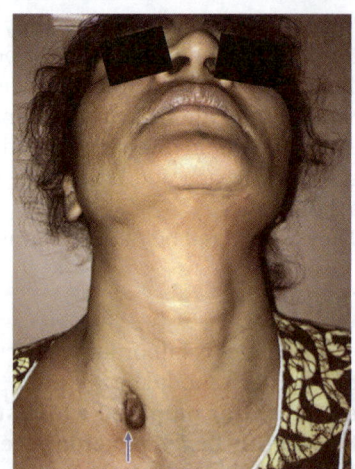

Fig. 14: Sinus in the neck.

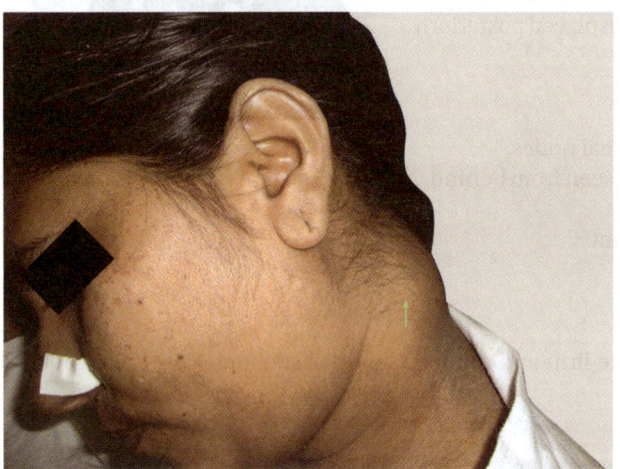

Fig. 15: Swelling in the posterior triangle of neck.

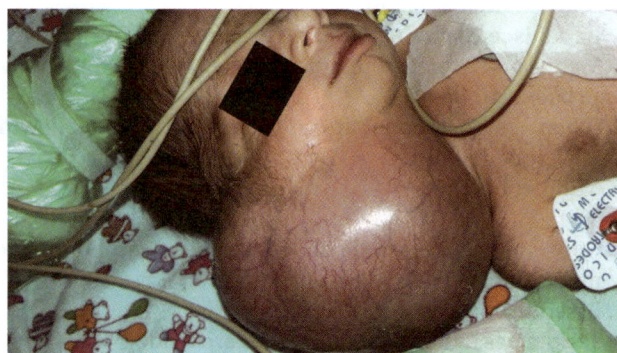

Fig. 16: Cystic hygroma of neck.

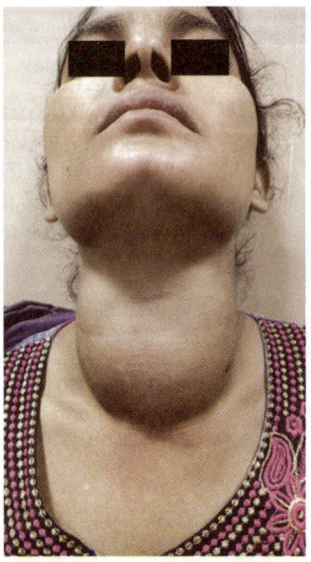

Fig. 17: Anterior neck midline swelling (goiter).

Chapter 31

Disorders and Tumors of Oral Cavity

COMMON DISORDERS OF ORAL CAVITY

Q. Enumerate the common disorders/benign conditions of the oral cavity.

- Oral ulcers/mucositis
- Angular cheilitis
- Stomatitis
- Oral submucous fibrosis (OSMF)
- Geographical tongue
- Fissured tongue
- Ankyloglossia (tongue-tie)
- Median rhomboid glossitis
- Fordyce spots
- Nicotine stomatitis
- Hairy tongue

ORAL ULCERS

Etiology

Q. Discuss various etiological causes of oral ulcers in brief.

- Infections
- Immune disorders
- Trauma
- Neoplasms
- Skin disorders
- Blood disorders
- Drug allergy
- Vitamin deficiencies
- Systemic disorders
- Following cancer therapy

Infections

- **Viral:**
  - Coxsackievirus infection (herpangina)
  - Herpes simplex virus infection (HSV)
  - Hand-foot-mouth disease
- **Bacterial:**
  - Acute necrotizing ulcerative gingivitis (Vincent's angina)
  - Tuberculosis
  - Syphilis
  - Actinomycosis
- **Fungal:**
  - Candidiasis

Candidiasis

The two forms of candidiasis which are present as ulcers in the oral cavity as:
- **Thrush:** White gray patches on the oral mucosa and tongue tend to bleed on the removal. It is seen in immunocompromised conditions

❖ **Chronic hypertrophic candidiasis (CHC):** It is a white patch that cannot be wiped off. It involves mainly the buccal mucosa behind the angle of the mouth.

Treatment

❖ For thrush—local application of antifungal mouth paint such as nystatin/clotrimazole.
❖ In case of extensive involvement/systemic involvement along with the oral cavity—tablet fluconazole/ketoconazole.
❖ For chronic hyperplastic candidiasis (CHC)—excision

Traumatic Ulcers

❖ **Physical causes:** Cheek bite
  ➢ Jagged tooth
  ➢ Ill-fitting dentures
  ➢ Pencil/toothbrush injury
❖ **Chemical causes:** Aspirin burns
  ➢ Silver nitrate
  ➢ Phenols
  ➢ Poisoning (caustic/acids)
❖ **Thermal causes:** Hot fluids/food
  ➢ Reverse smoking

Skin Disorders

❖ Lichen planus
❖ Mucous membrane pemphigoid
❖ Erythema multiforme
❖ Bullous pemphigoid
❖ Systemic lupus erythematosus (SLE)
❖ Chronic discoid lupus erythematosus (DLE)

Blood Disorders

❖ Leukemia
  ➢ Agranulocytosis
  ➢ Pancytopenia
  ➢ Cyclical neutropenia
  ➢ Sickle cell anemia

Common Malignancies

❖ Squamous cell carcinoma (SCC)
❖ Carcinoma of minor salivary glands
❖ Non-Hodgkin's lymphoma (NHL)

Immune Disorders

❖ Aphthous ulcers
❖ Behcet's syndrome

APHTHOUS ULCERS

Q. Write short note/essay on aphthous ulcers.

Common Sites Affected by Aphthous Ulcers

❖ Inner surfaces of the lips
❖ Buccal mucosa
❖ Tongue
❖ Floor of the mouth
❖ Soft palate

Characteristics

- They are usually multiple and recurrent in nature
- Involvement of movable mucosa and sparing of hard palate and gingiva
- No fever, malaise, and enlargement of cervical nodes

Different Forms

- **Minor form**—more common and are multiple
  - 2–10 mm in size
  - Central necrotic area with a peripheral halo. Heals without a scar
- **Major form**—very big ulcers, and mostly solitary
  - 2–4 cm in size
  - It heals with a scar

Proposed Etiologies

- Idiopathic
- Autoimmune disorder
- Nutritional deficiency
- Viral/bacterial infection
- Food allergies
- Hormonal changes
- Stress

Treatment Options

- Topical application of steroids
- Cauterization with 10% silver nitrate
- Tetracycline dissolved in water—mouth rinse
- Lignocaine jelly for local application

ERYTHEMA MULTIFORME

The distinctive clinical presentation of the erythema multiforme is hemorrhagic crust formation on the lips.

LICHEN PLANUS

Q. What are the clinical forms of the lichen planus (LP)?

- **Reticular form:** A white striae forming lace-like pattern seen on the bilateral buccal mucosa.
  - Usually asymptomatic—requires no treatment
- **Erosive form:** Painful ulceration on the buccal mucosa, gingiva, or lateral aspect of the tongue. The periphery is keratotic.
  - Treatment—local steroids

MUCOSITIS

Clinical presentation of radiation mucositis:
- Erythema → spotty mucositis → large ulcers with slough
- Clinical presentation of chemotherapy induced mucositis.
- Erythema → edema → ulceration

PREMALIGNANT LESIONS AND CONDITIONS

Q. Enumerate premalignant lesions and conditions of the oral cavity.

- **Premalignant lesions:**
  - Leukoplakia

- Erythroplakia
- Melanosis and mucosal hyperpigmentation
- Nicotine stomatitis
- Candidiasis
- Carcinoma in situ
❖ **Premalignant conditions:**
- OSMF
- Oral lichen planus
- Actinic keratosis
- Syphilis
- DLE
- Sideropenic dysphagia [Plummer-Vinson syndrome (PV) syndrome]

LEUKOPLAKIA

Q. Define leukoplakia. Write note on etiological factors, clinical presentation and treatment.

Leukoplakia is defined as a clinical white patch that cannot be characterized clinically or pathologically as any other disease.

Etiological Factors

- ❖ Smoking
- ❖ Tobacco chewing
- ❖ Betel nut chewing
- ❖ Alcohol abuse with smoking
- ❖ Ill-fitting dentures
- ❖ Cheek bite
- ❖ In association with hyperplastic candidiasis, OSMF or PV syndrome

Common Oral Subsites

- ❖ Buccal mucosa with alveolus (it is most common in India)
- ❖ Oral commissures
- ❖ Floor of mouth
- ❖ Gingivobuccal sulcus (GBS)
- ❖ Tongue
- ❖ Mucosal surfaces of the lips

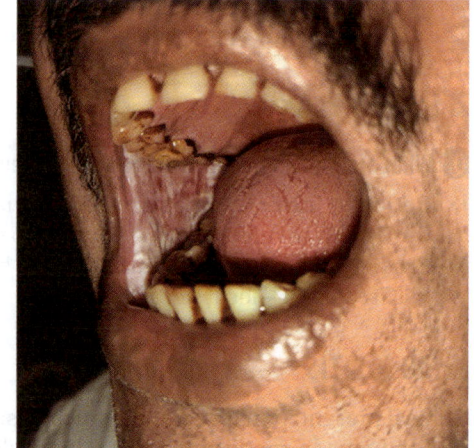

Fig. 1: Leukoplakia patch on the right buccal mucosa.

Clinical Features

Age group involved—is 40–50 years most commonly. Males:females—3:1

Clinical types of the leukoplakia are as follows:
- ❖ Homogenous—smooth/wrinkled white patch **(Fig 1)**.
  - The association with malignancy is rare.
- ❖ Nodular (speckled)—white patches/nodules resting on an erythematous base.
  - The association with malignancy is high.
- ❖ Erosive—mixed with erythroplakia, it has erosions and fissures.
  - The association with malignancy is highest.

About 25% of leukoplakia show some form of dysplasia.
- ❖ Chances of leukoplakia turning into malignancy is 1–17.5%. On average 5% become malignant.

Treatment

- ❖ Removal of causative agent/stimulus—lesion disappears spontaneously
- ❖ Suspicious small lesions—surgical excision with laser/cryotherapy
- ❖ Lesions with higher malignant potential—biopsy is taken

ERYTHROPLAKIA

Causes of red patch: It is due to the decreased keratinization and as a results the red vascular tissue shines through.

Common sites

- Lower alveolar mucosa, GBS, and floor of the mouth.
- Incidence of erythroplakia is 17 times higher than leukoplakia.

ORAL SUBMUCOUS FIBROSIS

Q. Define OSMF. Write note on its etiology, grading, clinical features and treatment.

Oral submucous fibrosis is a chronic insidious onset disorder characterized by juxtaepithelial deposition of fibrous tissue in the oral cavity and oropharynx **(Fig 2)**.

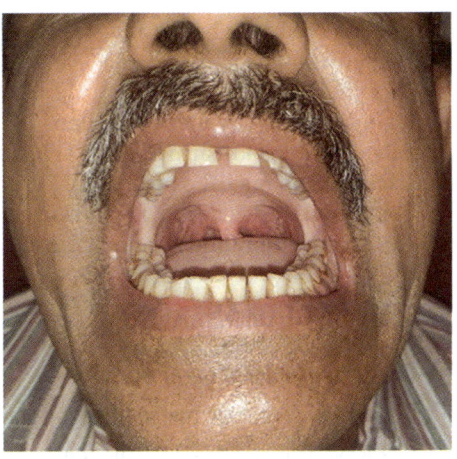

Fig. 2: Oral submucous fibrosis.

Etiology

Low socioeconomic status—related to the lifestyle, education, and access to medical care and diet.

- Tobacco chewing—a major risk factor
- Betel nut quid—an independent risk factor
- Alcohol—synergistic effect with tobacco
- Nutritional deficiency—vitamins and micronutrient deficiency
- Immune-mediated disorder—cell-mediated response to the betel nut
- Multifactorial—a combination of the above factors.

Pathogenesis

Increased production of collagen and its decreased degradation in subepithelial layers of oral mucosa brought about by the activated T-lymphocytes which cause reduced production of antifibrotic cytokines; and the macrophages which cause increased production of fibrogenic cytokines. Hence both processes result in increased collagen production.

Common Subsites

- Soft palate
- Faucial pillars
- Buccal mucosa

Clinical Features

The most commonly involved age group—is 20–50 years.

Symptoms:

- Constant burning sensation in the mouth
- Intolerance to spicy food especially chilies
- Soreness of the mouth
- Frequent vesicular eruptions on the pillars and palate
- Trismus
- Difficulty to protrude the tongue

Treatment

Medical

- Local injections of steroids mixed with injections of hyaluronidase for 8–10 weeks—weekly/biweekly injections
- Avoid irritants such as betel nut, tobacco, and pan
- Treat underlying anemia/vitamin deficiency
- Encourage jaw-opening exercises.

Surgical Treatment

It is required in advanced cases of trismus.

Options:
- Release of fibrotic bands and skin grafting
- Bilateral tongue flaps
- Nasolabial flaps
- Island palatal mucoperiosteal flap
- Bilateral radial forearm free flap (FRAFF)
- Excision and buccal pad fat graft
- Temporalis fascia flap and split skin graft
- Coronoidectomy and temporal muscle myotomy

TUMORS OF ORAL CAVITY

Q. Classify the tumor of the oral cavity.

Q. Discuss various benign tumors affecting oral cavity.

Q. Discuss various malignant lesions/tumors affecting oral cavity.

Benign tumor	Premalignant lesions	Malignant lesions
Soft tissue lesions: - Papilloma - Fibroma - Hemangioma - Lymphangioma - Torus - Pyogenic granuloma - Pregnancy granuloma - Granular cell tumor - Minor salivary gland neoplasms - Solitary fibrous tumor *Cystic lesions*: - Ranula - Mucocele - Dermoid	- Leukoplakia - Erythroplakia - Melanosis and hyperpigmentation of mucosa	Carcinoma oral cavity Squamous cell carcinoma (SCC) mostly *Cancers as per subsite*—(squamous lesions): - Carcinoma of lip - Carcinoma of the oral tongue - Carcinoma buccal mucosa - Carcinoma hard palate - Carcinoma alveolar ridge - Carcinoma floor of the mouth - Carcinoma retromolar trigone (RMT) *Nonsquamous lesions*: - Minor salivary gland tumor - Melanoma - Lymphoma - Kaposi sarcoma

Benign Tumors

Q. Discuss in brief various benign tumors affecting oral cavity.

Oral Papilloma

The most common sites of oral papillomas are soft and hard palate, uvula, tongue, and lips.

Oral Lymphangioma

The most common site of oral lymphangiomas is anterior two-thirds of the tongue.

Torus

- It is a submucosal bony outgrowth involving the hard palate or the mandible.
- Palatine torus is more common which presents as a narrow ridge, solitary nodule, or a lobulated mass.

Pyogenic Granuloma

The common oral sites involved in the pyogenic granuloma are gingivae, tongue, buccal mucosa, or lips.

Granular Cell Tumor

The site of predilection for the granular cell tumor is the tongue and tumor arises from the Schwann cells.

Congenital Epulis

It is a granular cell tumor involving the gums of future incisors in female infants.

Mucocele

Mucocele is a retention cyst of the minor salivary glands that appears as a soft cystic swelling, bluish in color most commonly seen on the lower lip. It is treated by excision.

Ranula

- Ranula is a cystic translucent swelling in the floor of the mouth **(Fig. 3)** which arises from the sublingual salivary gland due to obstruction of its duct. Small ranulas are excised while large ones require marsupialization.
- **Plunging ranula:** It is called so when the ranula extends into the neck.

Malignant Tumors

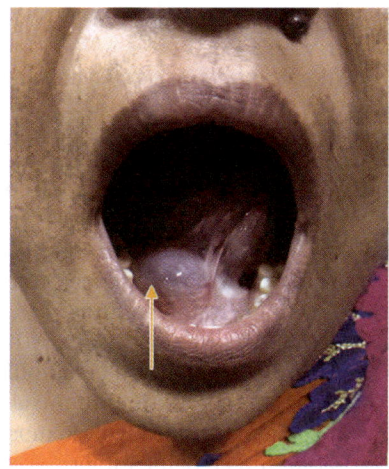

Fig. 3: Ranula.

Q. Write short note on non-squamous malignant tumors affecting oral cavity.

Melanoma

The most common subsites for oral cavity melanomas are palate and gingiva.

Lymphoma

- The most common subsite for oral cavity lymphoma is palatine tonsils.
- The most common variety of lymphoma seen in the oral cavity is non-Hodgkin's lymphoma.

Kaposi's Sarcoma

- It is a vascular tumor, multifocal in origin affecting the oral cavity and skin.
- Incidences high in acquired immunodeficiency syndrome (AIDS) patients
- Lesion appears as a reddish-purple nodule or plaque
- The most common site affected is a palate
- Microscopy—spindle cells with hemorrhagic cleft-like spaces
- Treatment—chemotherapy

Carcinoma of Oral Cavity

Q. Write short note on oral cavity carcinoma/squamous cell carcinoma.

Etiology

- Smoking
- Tobacco chewing
- Alcohol
- Dietary deficiencies—riboflavin deficiency
- Dental sepsis, jagged-sharp teeth
- Ill-fitting dentures

Clinical Presentation

- Mostly it is squamous cell carcinoma
- Males > females. Age group—40–60 years
- The most common site—lower lip **(Fig. 4)**
- Exophytic/ulcerative lesion
- Submental and submandibular lymph nodes (LN) groups involved—very late presentation
- Treatment—surgical excision with plastic repair of the defect
- Radiation therapy (RT) in early cases

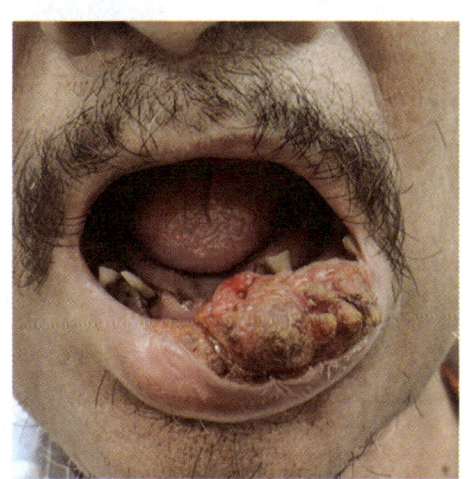

Fig. 4: Carcinoma of lip.

Carcinoma of the Buccal Mucosa

Q. Write short note on buccal mucosa carcinoma/squamous cell carcinoma affecting buccal mucosa.

Clinical Features

Squamous cell carcinoma is most common
- Sex predilection—M:F = 1:1
- The most common site—angle of mouth or the line of occlusion of upper and lower teeth **(Fig. 5)**
- Carcinoma is multicentric
- Gross appearance—exophytic (associated with erythroleukoplakia)/ulceroproliferative (deep-infiltration)
- Local spread—skin and muscle involvement. Masseter/buccinator muscle involved mostly
- Radial spread of the tumor:
    - Superior spread—maxilla and upper GBS (gingivobuccal sulcus)
    - Inferior spread—lower GBS, alveolar ridge, and gums
    - Anterior spread—the angle of mouth and lip
    - Posterior spread—retromolar trigon (RMT) and medial pterygoid **(Fig. 6)**
- LN spread—submandibular and upper jugular group of nodes involved
- Early lesions—asymptomatic and late lesions (deep infiltration)—pain and bleeding
- Trismus
- Fungating mass over a cheek, foul-smelling bleeding mass in the oral cavity—late feature

Treatment

- **Stage I:** Surgical excision
- **Stage II:** RT to lesion and nodes if a bone is spared
    - If bone is involved—surgery—involves excision of growth with segmental/marginal mandibulectomy with a reconstruction of the defect
- **Stage III and IV:** Surgery **(Fig. 7)** + reconstruction with skin/myocutaneous **(Fig. 8)**. Flaps + postoperative radiation.

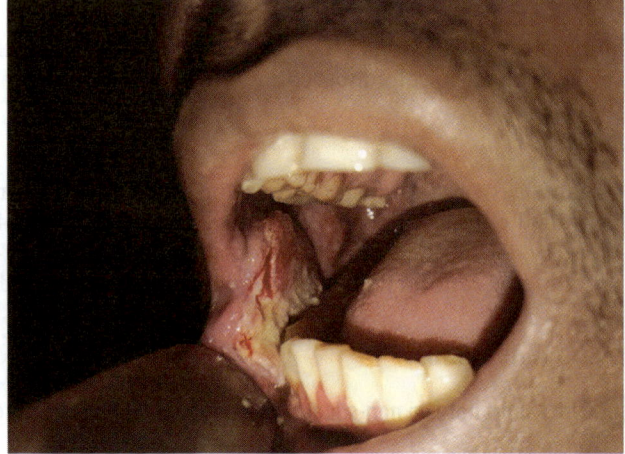

Fig. 5: Buccal carcinoma.

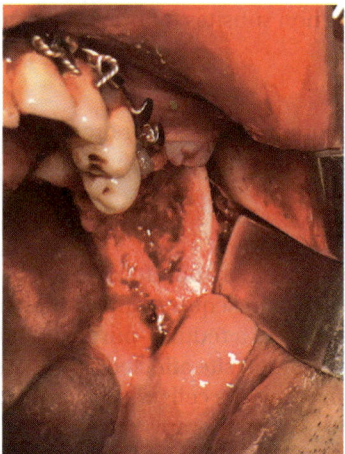

Fig. 6: The involvement of retromolar trigone (RMT).

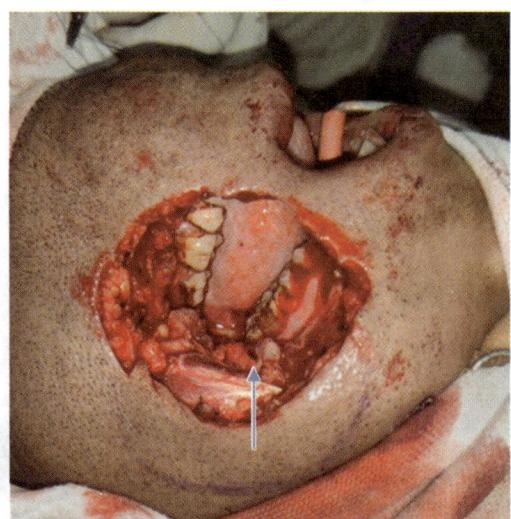

Fig. 7: Carcinoma cheek after wide local excision.

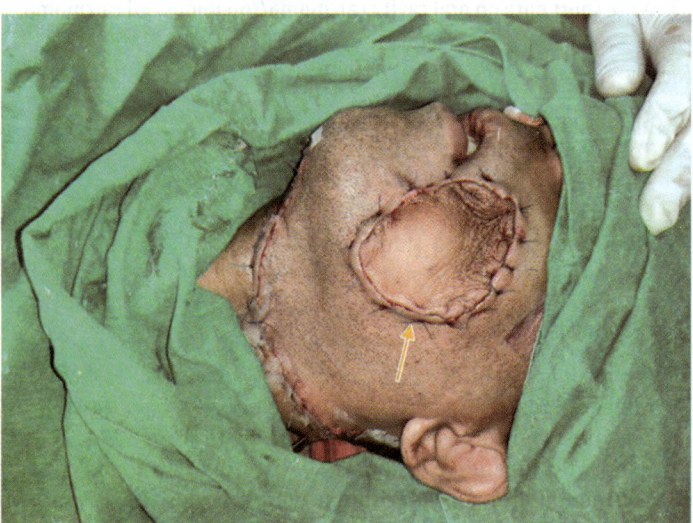

Fig. 8: Myocutaneous flap reconstruction in carcinoma cheek after excision of cheek tumor.

Carcinoma of Tongue

Q. Write in short note about the carcinoma of the tongue.

- Squamous cell carcinoma is most common
- The most common site—anterior two-thirds of the tongue—middle of the lateral border/ventral aspect of the tongue
- Sex predilection—males > females
- The most common age group involved is 50-70 years
- Local spread—intrinsic muscle involvement—causes ankyloglossia
  - It may spread to the floor of the mouth, alveolus, and mandible
- LN spread—from the lateral border of the tongue—spread to submandibular
  - LN and upper jugular group.
  - From the tip—spread to submental and jugulo-omohyoid group of LNs

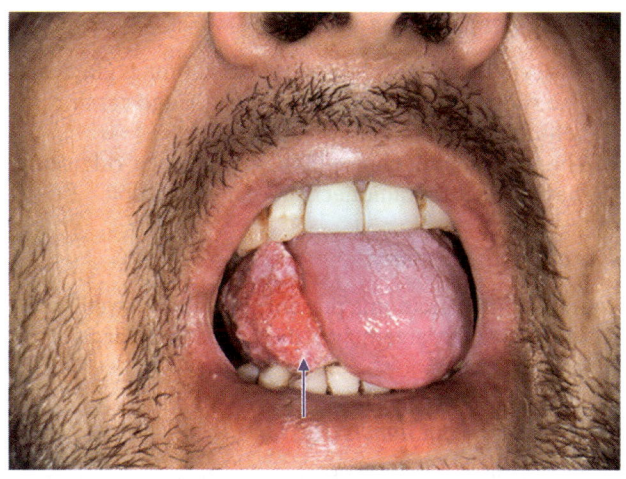

Fig. 9: Carcinoma of tongue with proliferative lesion.

Clinical Presentation

Three types:
1. Exophytic lesion **(Fig. 9)**
2. A nonhealing ulcer with rolled edges, grayish-white shaggy base with induration **(Fig. 10)**
3. A submucous nodule with induration of the surrounding tissues

Symptoms and Signs

- Early lesions—painless and asymptomatic
- Pain at the site of the tongue ulcer
- Otalgia
- A lump in the mouth
- Enlarged LNs in the neck—mass
- Dysphagia, difficulty in protruding the tongue
- Slurred speech and bleeding per oral

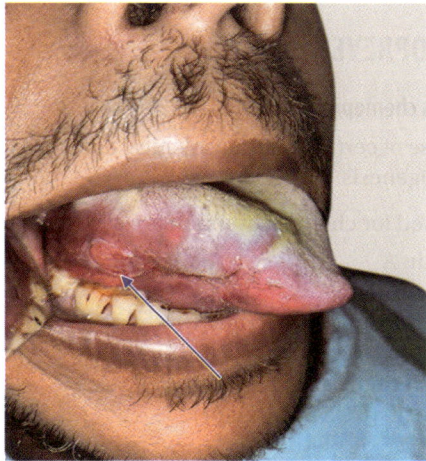

Fig. 10: Carcinoma of the tongue with an ulcerative lesion.

Treatment

- **Stage I (T1 N0):** Radiotherapy/surgery (hemiglossectomy/wide local excision) **(Fig. 11)**.
- **Stage II tumor:** Radiotherapy to lesion and nodes/surgery with neck dissection.
- **Stage III and IV:** There is combined surgery + RT with block dissection of the neck.

COMMANDO Operation

COMbined **MAND**ibulectomy and **N**eck **D**issection **O**peration is known as the COMMANDO Operation.

Carcinoma of Hard Palate

- The most common variety of carcinoma of hard palate is glandular followed by the squamous variety.
- The different clinical types of hard palate carcinoma:
  - Adenoid cystic carcinoma
  - Adenocarcinoma
  - Mucoepidermoid carcinoma

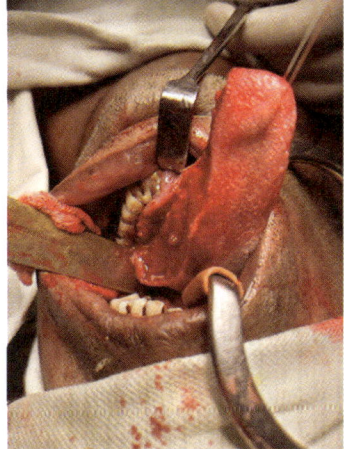

Fig. 11: Hemiglossectomy surgery intraoperative picture.

Alveolar Ridge Carcinoma

- The synonym for alveolar ridge carcinoma is gingival carcinoma
- The most common site for alveolar ridge carcinoma is lower jaw **(Fig. 12)** behind the first molar
- The treatment of choice (TOC) for alveolar ridge carcinoma is surgery as RT may cause osteoradionecrosis of the mandible.

Floor of Mouth Carcinoma

Floor of mouth carcinoma present clinically as swelling in the lateral aspect of the neck because of enlargement of the submandibular gland due to its duct obstruction by the lesion.

Minor Salivary Glant Tumors (Fig. 13)

- The most common site for minor salivary gland tumor is palate.
- The most common variety of minor salivary gland tumor is **adenoid cystic carcinoma.**

CHEMOPREVENTION

Q. What is chemoprevention?

It is the use of certain pharmacological agents to halt, delay or reverse the process of carcinogenesis.

Agents used for chemoprevention are as follows:

- Vitamin A
- Beta-carotene
- Alpha-tocopherol (vitamin E)
- Selenium
- 13-cis retinoic acid
- Celecoxib (COX-2 inhibitor)

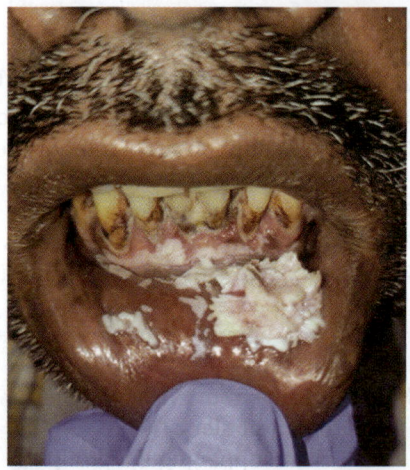

Fig. 12: Alveolar ridge carcinoma extending over the lower lip.

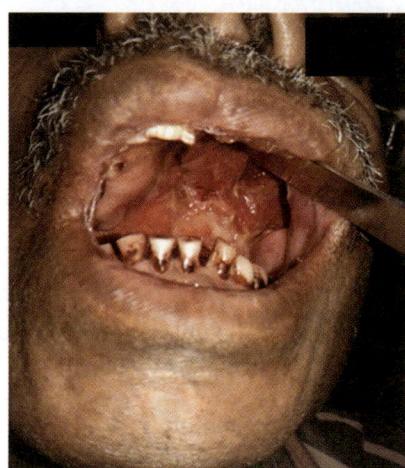

Fig. 13: Carcinoma of the hard palate with palatal perforation.

Chapter 32

Disorders and Tumors of the Salivary Glands

EN4.35: Describe the clinical features, investigations and principles of management of diseases of the salivary glands.

■ DISORDERS OF SALIVARY GLAND

Viral Parotitis/Mumps

Q. Write a short note on viral parotitis/mumps.

- Caused by paramyxovirus
- The incubation period for mumps is 2-3 weeks

Clinical Features

- Fever (up to 103°F)
- Malaise
- Anorexia
- Muscular pain
- Parotid swelling

Complications

- Orchitis—painful, tender testis on one or both sides
- Oophoritis—presents with abdominal pain but no sterility
- Pancreatitis—abdominal pain
- Aseptic meningitis/meningoencephalitis—headache, neck stiffness, and drowsiness
- Unilateral sensorineural hearing loss (SNHL)—sudden deafness common
- Myocarditis, nephritis, arthritis, and thyroiditis—late stages

Diagnosis

- Mainly diagnosis is clinical
- Supporting investigations are—serum and urinary amylase
- Serum immunoglobulin G (IgG)—indicative of past infection
- Serum immunoglobulin M (IgM)—indicative of recent infection

Treatment and Prevention

Treatment

- Proper hydration

❖ Rest
❖ Analgesics
❖ Cold compresses over the parotid to relieve pain
❖ Cold compresses and supports for the scrotum

Prevention

Measles, mumps, and rubella (MMR) vaccine to infants at 15 months of age

Acute Suppurative Parotitis (ASP) (Fig. 1)

Q. Write short note on acute suppurative parotitis/acute parotitis.

The usual causative organism for *Staphylococcus aureus*.

Clinical Features

❖ It is seen in elderly, debilitated, immunocompromised, and dehydrated patients.
❖ Sudden onset with excruciating pain and enlargement of the gland.
❖ Pain in movements of the jaw
❖ Fever
❖ Stensen's duct is swollen, red, and may express pus on gentle pressure

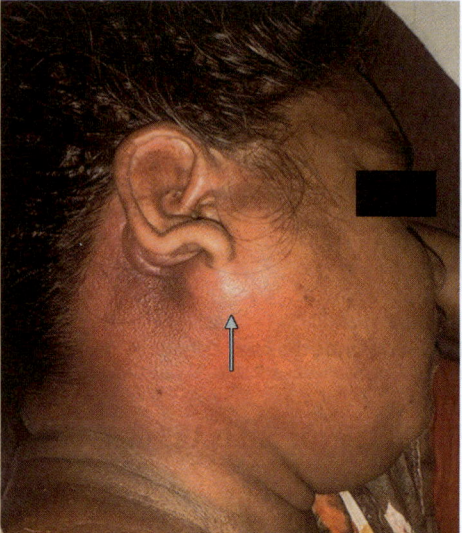

Fig. 1: Acute suppurative parotitis (ASP).

Investigations and Treatment

Investigations

❖ Whit cell count—shows leukocytosis
❖ Culture of blood and pus collected from the Stensen's duct

Treatment

❖ Intravenous (IV) antibiotics
❖ Adequate hydration—IV fluids
❖ Analgesics and anti-inflammatory agents to reduce pain and swelling
❖ Salivary flow promoting agents **(sialagogues)**—vitamin C chewable tablets
❖ Attention to oral hygiene—oral rinse with benzydamine rinses
❖ If fever not reducing and swelling increases despite antibiotics—incision and drainage should be done.

Sialectasis

Dilatation of the ductal system of the salivary gland leads to stasis of secretions which predisposes to infection.

Granulomatous Infections of the Salivary Glands

❖ Tuberculosis
❖ Sarcoidosis
❖ Actinomycosis
❖ Toxoplasmosis

Sialolithiasis

Q. Write a short note on sialolithiasis.

Calculi/stone formation in the ducts of submandibular or parotid glands; formed by the deposition of the calcium phosphate on the matrix of mucin or cellular debris. About 90% of stones are seen in the submandibular gland. About 10% are seen in the parotid gland.

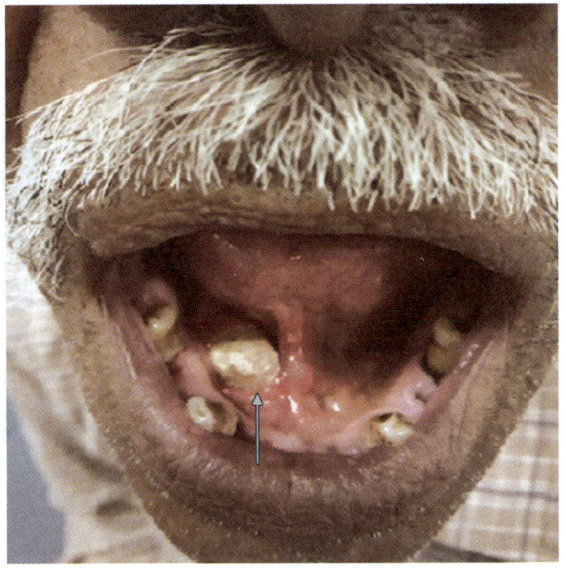

Fig. 2: Sialolith in submandibular gland duct.

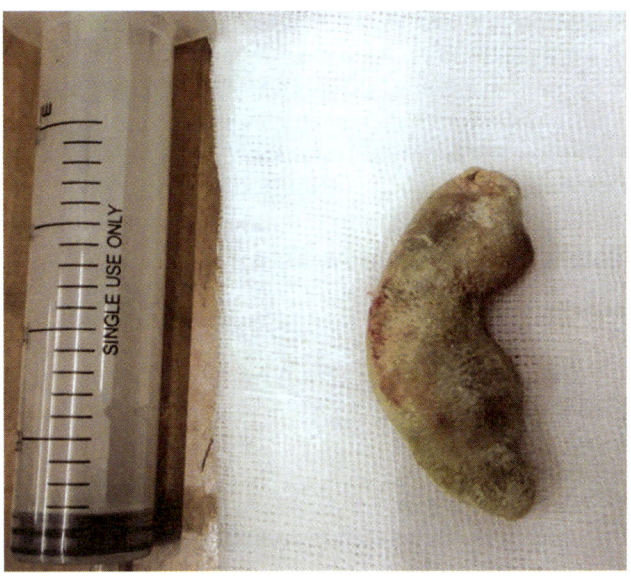

Fig. 3: Huge salivary stone (sialolith)/megalith.

Clinical Features

- Intermittent swelling of the gland and pain due to obstruction of salivary outflow obstruction
- Stone visible at the duct opening **(Figs. 2 and 3)** or can be palpated intraorally
- About 80% of stones are radiopaque—seen on X-rays
- Radiolucent stones are seen on sialography

Investigations and Diagnosis

- Contrast sialography
- Ultrasonography
- Magnetic resonance imaging (MRI)
- Digital subtraction sialography
- Sialoendoscopy
- X-rays

Sjogren's Syndrome

Q. What is Sjogren's syndrome? Write about its types and describe them in brief.

It is an autoimmune disorder affecting salivary glands and other exocrine glands of the body characterized by lymphoepithelial sialadenitis. Also known as sicca syndrome as **it presents with dry mouth and dry eyes.**

Types of Sjogren's Syndrome

- **Primary Sjogren's syndrome**—Male:Female = 1:1: Presents with xerostomia and xerophthalmia. Parotid gland is most commonly affected.
- **Secondary Sjogren's syndrome**—consists of three major components:
  1. Keratoconjunctivitis sicca—lacrimal gland is involved.
  2. Xerostomia—salivary glands and minor salivary glands are involved.
  3. Autoimmune connective tissue disorder—rheumatoid arthritis or systemic lupus erythematosus (SLE)
     Females—90% of the cases are found

Diagnosis

- History and clinical examination of dry eye and dry mouth

- Schirmer's test to show decreased tear production.
- Biopsy of the lower lip to prove minor salivary gland involvement.
- Sjogren's syndrome (SS)-A and SS-B antibodies titer
- ESR—usually raised
- Rheumatoid factor (RF) estimation
- Antinuclear antibodies (ANAs) estimation

Bilateral Parotid Gland Swelling (Fig. 4)

Causes are:
- Sarcoidosis
- Tuberculosis
- Diabetes
- Sjogren's syndrome
- Lymphomas
- Sialadenitis
- Human immunodeficiency virus (HIV)

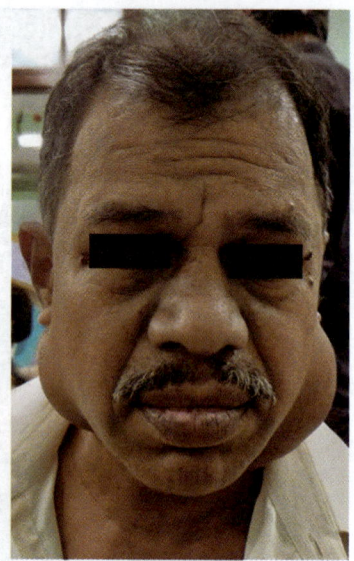

Fig. 4: Bilateral parotid gland swelling.

TUMORS OF THE SALIVARY GLANDS

Q. Classify tumors of the salivary glands.

Benign tumors	Malignant tumors
❖ Epithelial: 　➤ Pleomorphic adenoma 　➤ Adenolymphoma 　➤ Oncocytoma 　➤ Other adenomas	❖ Epithelial: 　➤ Mucoepidermoid carcinoma 　　– Low-grade 　　– High-grade 　➤ Adenoid cystic carcinoma 　➤ Acinic cell carcinoma 　➤ Adenocarcinoma 　➤ Malignant mixed tumor 　➤ Squamous cell carcinoma 　➤ Undifferentiated carcinoma
❖ Mesenchymal 　➤ Hemangioma 　➤ Lymphangioma 　➤ Lipoma 　➤ Neurofibroma	❖ Mesenchymal 　➤ Lymphoma 　➤ Sarcoma

Pleomorphic Adenoma

Q. Write a short note on pleomorphic adenoma.

- The most common benign salivary gland tumor.
- Tail of parotid gland and deep lobe of parotid gland are the two most common sites of origin.

Characteristic Features

- Benign tumor
- Slow growing, and encapsulated tumor
- Capsule is extremely thin in one area and incomplete in 50% of cases.
- More prone to spillage during surgery due to the thin capsules.
- It can affect parotid, submandibular, and minor salivary glands
- Age group—all age groups were affected with a peak in the sixth decade
- Females > males
- Mixed tumors—as tumors show both epithelial and mesenchymal elements on histology
- Stroma of the tumor may be mucoid, myxoid, fibroid, vascular, chondroid. or chondromyxoid
- Tumor sends pseudopods into the surrounding glands which may be left behind if it is only scooped.

Clinical Features

Pleomorphic Adenoma of Parotid Glands (Fig. 5)

- Steadily growing mass behind the angle of jaw, in front of the ear, or in the cheek
- On palpation—smooth, mobile, and painless.
- May cause discomfort by obstructing the salivary flow
- Deep lobe PAs can displace tonsil and palate medially and are often impalpable from outside
- **Very large parapharyngeal PAs can cause the following symptoms:**
  - Stertor
  - Sleep-disordered breathing
  - Affect quality of voice
  - Eustachian tube dysfunction

Pleomorphic Adenoma of Submandibular Gland

Present in the submandibular triangle and can be palpated bimanually at the floor of the mouth. They may increase in size at the time of the meals and go back to their original size once meals are over.

Pleomorphic Adenoma of Minor Salivary Glands

Of oral and pharyngeal mucosa present as submucosal swellings.

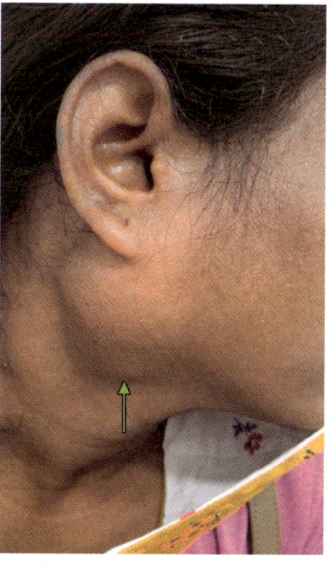

Fig. 5: Pleomorphic adenoma of the parotid gland.

Investigations and Diagnosis

- Ultrasound-guided fine needle aspiration cytology (FNAC)
- Core biopsy when FNAC shows malignancy
- **MRI/CT performed under the following circumstances (Fig. 6):**
  - Tumor >3 cm in size
  - Deep lobe/parapharyngeal space involvement
  - Suspicion of malignancy
- **The features on imaging suggestive of malignancy in salivary gland tumors:**
  - Irregular tumor capsule
  - Extracapsular invasion
  - Hypervascularity
  - Tumor necrosis

Symptoms and Signs Suggestive of Salivary Gland Malignancy

- Pain
- Paresthesia
- Rapid increase in the size of the swelling
- Facial nerve palsy
- Skin involvement and fixity
- Irregularity

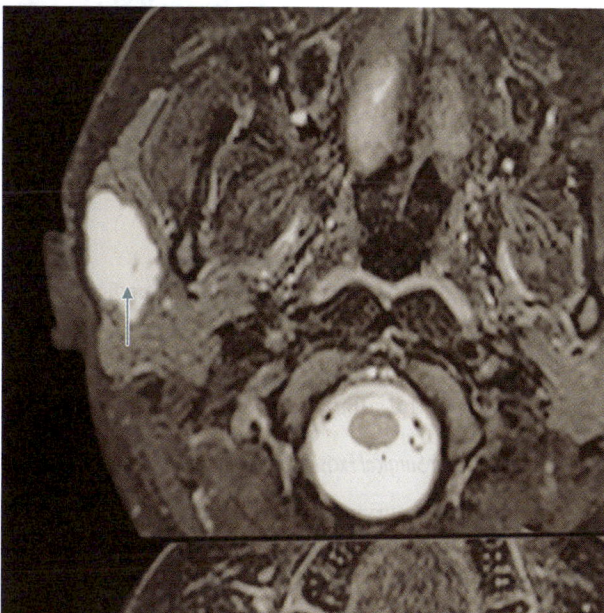

Fig. 6: Magnetic resonance imaging (MRI) of face and neck showing pleomorphic adenoma of the parotid gland.

Treatment

Surgical

- Extracapsular dissection
- Partial/superficial parotidectomy
- Total conservative parotidectomy
- Total parotidectomy
- Radical parotidectomy

Treatment of Choice for Pleomorphic Adenoma of Parotid Gland

Superficial parotidectomy (Figs. 7 to 9) wherein the tumor along with the adjacent cuff of normal tissue superficial to the facial nerve is removed. Also known as partial parotidectomy.

PART 1: Diseases of ENT, Head and Neck

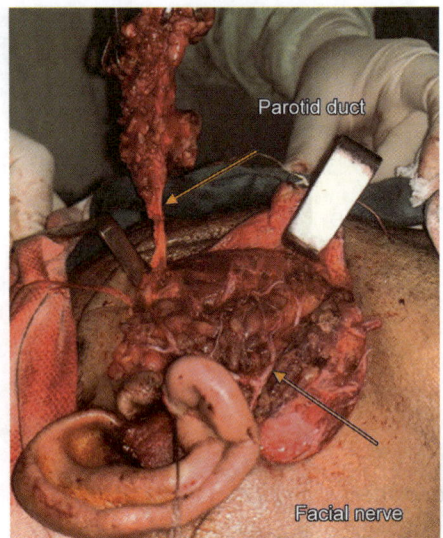

Fig. 7: Superficial parotidectomy surgery and dissected parotid gland.

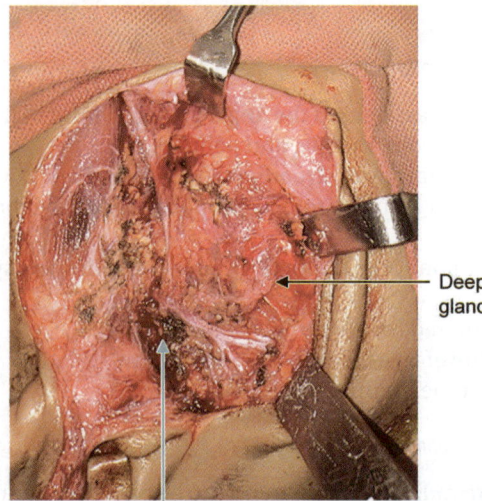

Fig. 8: Intraoperative picture of superficial parotidectomy.

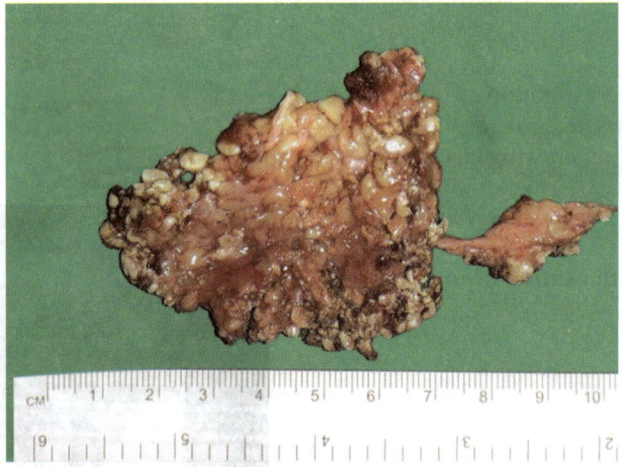

Fig. 9: Superficial parotidectomy specimen (postoperative).

Treatment of Choice for the Pleomorphic Adenoma of Submandibular Gland

Total resection of the submandibular gland is the treatment of choice.

Various Techniques for Surgical Excision of Pleomorphic Adenomas of Parapharyngeal Space

- ❖ Small tumors—cervical-parotid approach
- ❖ Larger tumors—transmandibulotomy/transpharyngeal approach
- ❖ Transoral robotic surgery (TORS) is an alternative

Skin Incision Used for Superficial Parotidectomy

Lazy "S" incision or modified Blair incision **(Fig. 10)**.

Surgical Landmarks to Locate Facial Nerves During Superficial Parotidectomy

- ❖ **Tragal pointer** (an inferior portion of the cartilaginous external auditory canal):
  - ▷ The facial nerve lies 1 cm inferior and deep to it.
  - ▷ **Tympanomastoid suture**: Facial nerve lies 10–12 mm deep and inferior to this at its point of exit from the skull.

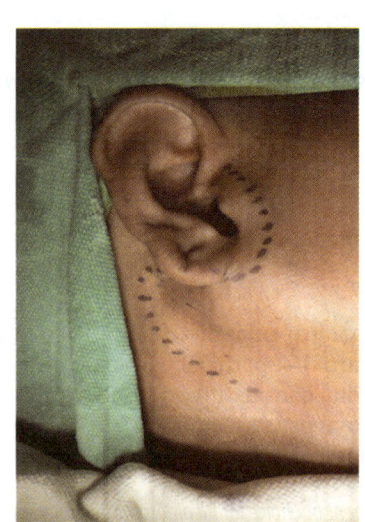

Fig. 10: Modified Blair incision.

➢ *The anterior border of the posterior belly of digastric muscle*: Facial nerve leaves the skull immediately anterior to the attachment of this muscle.

Surgery Rationale

- Definitive histology
- Continued growth if left untreated
- Small chance of malignant transformation

Warthin's Tumor

Q. Write a short note on Warthin's tumor/adenolymphoma/papillary cystadenoma lymphomatosum.

Also known as:

- Adenolymphoma
- Papillary cystadenoma lymphomatosum

Characteristic Features

- Benign tumor
- Rounded, encapsulated tumor, at times cystic with mucoid or brownish fluid **(Figs. 11 and 12)**.
- Form soft, painless swellings usually on the lower pole of the gland.
- Bilateral in only 10% of patients
- Age group affected: 50–70 years most commonly
- Male: female—1.6:1
- They involve the tail of the parotid.
- Histologically consists of lymphoid stroma and oncocytic epithelium. Hence, may arise from salivary duct inclusions of intraparotid or periparotid nodes.

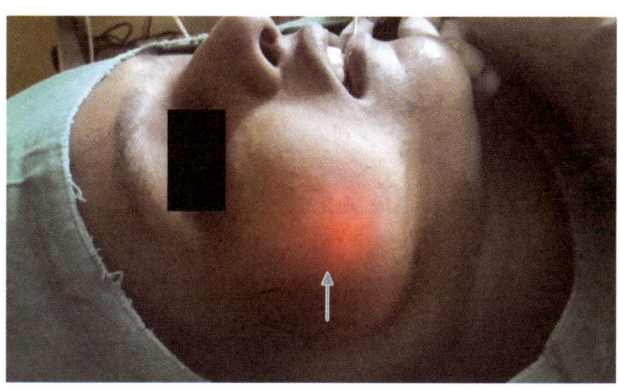

Fig. 11: Cystic parotid swelling with transillumination.

Treatment of Choice

Surgical excision via a partial/superficial parotidectomy.

Mucoepidermoid carcinoma

Q. Write a short note on mucoepidermoid carcinoma.

Characteristics Features

- Malignant tumor
- Slow-growing but can spread rapidly involving facial nerve and lead to death.
- Histology—areas of mucin-producing cells and epidermoid (squamous) cells.
- More the epidermoid element, the more is the malignant behavior of the tumor.
- **Low-grade tumors—less aggressive hence good prognosis—seen in children**
- **High-grade tumors—more aggressive hence poor prognosis—are seen in adults**.
- Behavior of mucoepidermoid carcinoma in minor salivary gland is more aggressive.

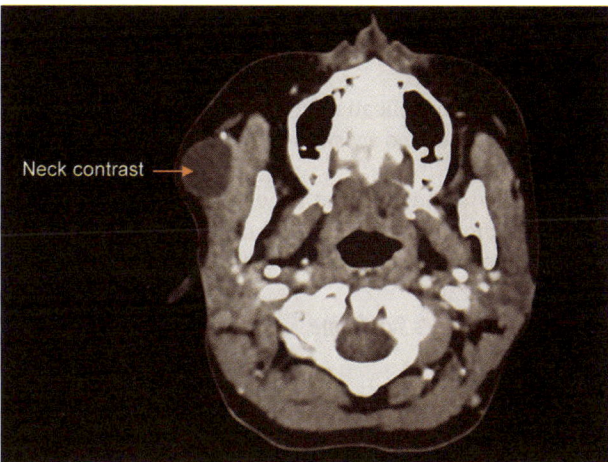

Fig. 12: Computed tomography (CT) scan of the face showing cystic parotid swelling (Warthin's tumor).

Treatment

- Low-grade tumors—treated by total parotidectomy by the preservation of facial nerve.
- High-grade tumors—treated by radical parotidectomy by sacrificing facial nerve. It may need neck dissection if neck nodes are involved.

Adenoid Cystic Carcinoma (Figs. 13 and 14)

Q. Write a short note on adenoid cystic carcinoma.

Characteristic Features

- Malignant tumor
- Slow growing but infiltrates widely into the tissue planes and muscles.
- Invades perineural space and lymphatics and thus causes pain and VIIth nerve paralysis.
- Local recurrences after surgery are common.
- Treatment—radical parotidectomy SOS neck dissection. Postoperative radiation if margins are positive.
- Superficial and deep lobe of parotid gland in carcinoma

Complications of the Superficial Parotidectomy Surgery

- Facial weakness
- Sensory loss due to damage to greater auricular nerve
- Cosmetic defect
- Frey's syndrome
- Salivary fistula/sialocele
- Stump neuroma of the greater auricular nerve
- Wound dehiscence/infection

Frey's Syndrome

Q. Write a short note on most common complication flowing parotid surgery/Frey's syndrome.

- Arises as a complication of parotid surgery
- It is characterized by sweating and flushing of the preauricular skin during mastication.
- It is due to the aberrant innervation of sweat glands by parasympathetic secretomotor fibers which are destined for parotid gland.
- Starch iodine test is the test to diagnose Frey's syndrome.

Treatment for Frey's Syndrome

- Reassurance
- Tympanic neurectomy of parasympathetic fibers at the level of the middle ear.
- Placement of fascia between the skin and underlying fat to prevent parasympathetic fibers from reaching the skin.
- Botulinum toxin (BOTOX).

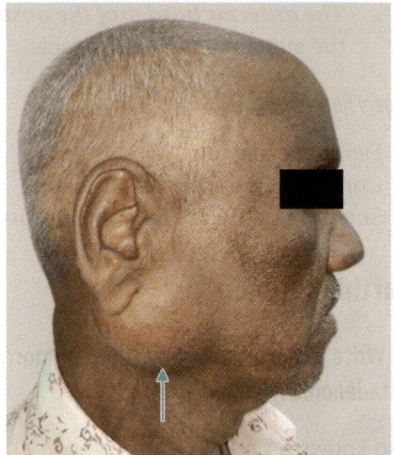

Fig. 13: Carcinoma of parotid.

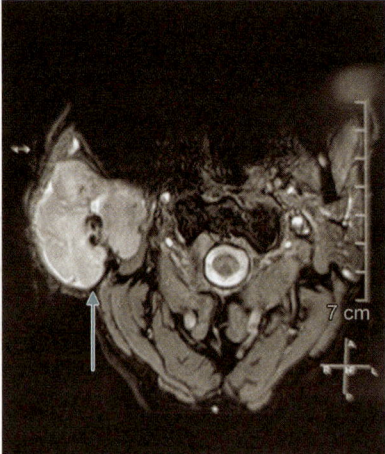

Fig. 14: Magnetic resonance imaging (MRI) showing tumor involvement.

Chapter 33

Acute and Chronic Tonsillitis

EN1.1: Describe the anatomy and physiology of ear, nose, throat, head and neck.

ANATOMY OF PALATINE TONSILS AND PHYSIOLOGY OF TONSIL

Q. Describe anatomy and physiology of tonsils.

- Tonsils are mass of lymphoid tissue located at tonsillar fossa.
- **Anterior relation:** Palatoglossal arch
- **Posterior relation:** Palatopharyngeal arch
- Palatine tonsils are two in number, each present medial and lateral surface and upper and lower pole.
- Epithelial lining of medial surface—stratified nonkeratinized squamous epithelium.
- Epithelium dips into tonsillar parenchyma to form tonsillar crypts opens on medial surface (15-20 number).
- Largest crypt (present near upper pole called crypta magna from second pharyngeal pouch)
- Lateral surface rest on tonsillar bed
- Tonsillar bed—(from medial to lateral) **(Fig. 1)**
    - Loose areolar tissue with paratonsillar vein
    - Pharyngobasilar fascia
    - Superior constrictor muscle
    - Buccopharyngeal fascia
    - Styloglossus
    - Glossopharyngeal nerve
    - Facial artery
    - Medial pterygoid muscle
    - Angle of mandible
    - Submandibular gland

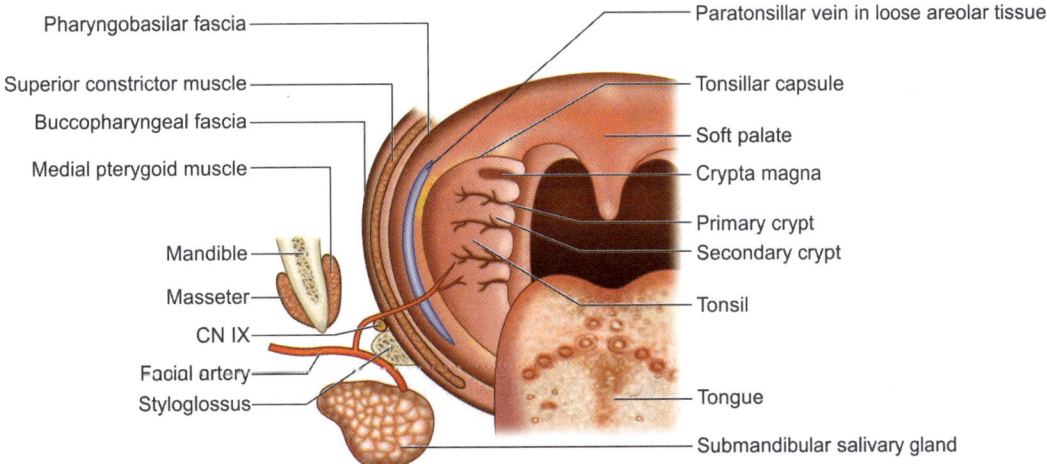

Fig. 1: Tonsillar bed structures.

PART 1: Diseases of ENT, Head and Neck

- ❖ **Nerve supply:** Tonsillar branch of glossopharyngeal nerve (result in referred pain to the middle ear)
  Arterial blood supply
  - ➢ Dorsal lingual branch—lingual artery
  - ➢ Tonsillar branch—facial artery
  - ➢ Ascending palatine artery—branch of the facial artery
  - ➢ Ascending pharyngeal artery—branch of the external carotid artery
  - ➢ Descending palatine branch—maxillary artery
- ❖ **Venous drainage:** Paratonsillar vein
  ↓
  Common facial vein and pharyngeal venous plexus
- ❖ **Lymphatic drainage:** Upper deep cervical and jugulodigastric (JD) lymph node (LN)
- ❖ **Function of tonsils (physiology)**—immunity provided by both humoral and cellular mechanism.
  - ➢ *Local immunity*—epithelial lining of tonsils and adenoid contain M cell, antigen presenting cells, on foreign organism intrusion antigen presented to lymphoid follicles.
    Lymphoid follicles have germinal centers rich in B cell on antigenic stimulation it forms plasma cells which produces antibodies.
  Macrophages in lymphoid follicle kills bacteria and viruses by phagocytic action
  - ➢ *Systemic immunity*—alerts body for wider response to infection.
    On high antigenic stimulation B cell of germinal center undergo hyperplasia enter circulation, antibodies increases phagocytic efficiency of neutrophils and macrophages.

> **EN4.38**: Elicit document and present a correct history, demonstrate and describe the clinical features, choose the correct investigations and describe the principles of management of acute and chronic tonsillitis.

■ ACUTE TONSILLITIS

Q. Write a short note/essay on acute tonsillitis.

Classification

Depending upon infection of any components of tonsil (Lining epithelium, crypts of tonsils and parenchyma), tonsillitis classified as:
- ❖ **Acute superficial/catarrhal tonsillitis**—infection of lining epithelium is a part of generalize pharyngitis (viral pharyngitis)
- ❖ **Acute follicular tonsillitis**—spread of infection from epithelium to tonsillar crypts, purulent material fills crypts, and present as yellowish spots on medial surface of tonsils at opening of crypts.
- ❖ **Acute membranous stage**—following follicular stage, purulent material from crypts coals to form membrane over tonsils.
- ❖ **Acute parenchymal stage**—infection from crypts spread to tonsillar parenchyma, result in tonsillar enlargement.

Etiology

- ❖ Age—affects frequently school going children
- ❖ Sex—affects equally
- ❖ **Causative organism:** Hemolytic streptococci most common organism
  - ➢ Staphylococci, pneumococci, and viral infection

Symptoms

- ❖ Sore throat
- ❖ **Pain in throat**—aggravated by swallowing, difficulty in swallowing due to **odynophagia** child refuses to eat and drink.
- ❖ **Fever with chills**
- ❖ **Earache**—referred pain to ear or due to acute otitis media (complication of tonsillitis)
- ❖ Constitutional symptoms—headache, malaise, and fever
- ❖ Acute abdominal pain—due to mesenteric lymphadenitis mimic acute appendicitis

Sign

- **Halitosis**—foul breath and coasted tongue
- **Oral cavity:**
  - Hyperemia of anterior tonsillar pillar, uvula, and soft palate
  - **Enlarged congested and swollen tonsils**—in sever enlargement tonsils meet midline (kissing tonsils) **(Fig. 2)**
  - **Yellowish spots** of purulent material on tonsillar surface—**acute follicular tonsillitis**
  - **Whitish membrane** over tonsils easily wiped out—acute membranous tonsillitis
  - Enlarged tender JD LN

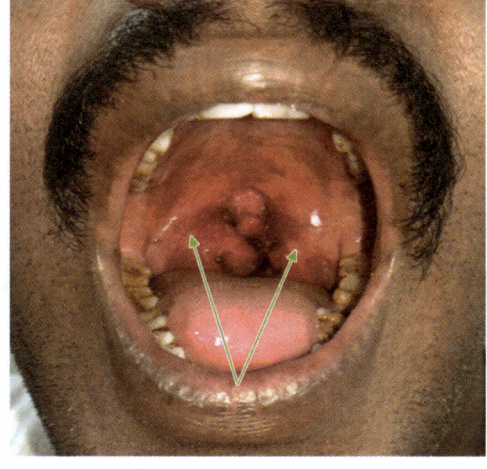

Fig. 2: Acute tonsillitis with congestion of anterior pillars and palatine tonsils.

Differential Diagnosis

- **Diphtheria**

Q. Write differences between acute membranous tonsillitis and diphtheria.

Acute membranous tonsillitis	Diphtheria
History of recurrent tonsillitis	History of exposure to diphtheria case
High-grade fever with chills	Normal/mild fever
Tachycardia proportion to fever	Tachycardia out of proportion to fever
Throat pain present	Absent
Membrane limited to tonsil Can be easily removed	Membrane (dirty gray) extend beyond tonsils It cannot be easily separated, leaves raw bleeding surface
Jugulodigastric (JD) lymph node (LN) enlarged and tender	Marked lymphadenopathy and bulls neck
Albuminuria absent	Present
Corynebacterium diphtheriae (C. diphtheriae) negative on swab	Positive

- **Vincent angina**—it is caused by spirochaete and *Bacillus fusiformis* ulcer present over one or both tonsils, leave irregular ulcer on tonsil on removal, RX—responds to penicillin
- **Infectious mononucleosis**—affect young adults
  - Highly suspicious on failure to antibiotic treatment.
  - **Lymphadenopathy of posterior triangle of neck** with splenomegaly
  - **Paul–Bunnell test (mono test)** show high titer of heterophile antibody
- **Agranulocytosis**—ulcer present over oropharynx along with tonsils with total leukocyte counts <2,000 mm^3, neutrophil <5%.
- **Leukemia**—in children, acute lymphoblastic is more common over myelogenous or chronic.
  In adult, nonlymphocytic is more common than lymphocytic.
- **Aphthous ulcer**—it involves any part of oral cavity, and is very painful.
- **Malignancy of tonsil**—unilateral tonsillar enlargement
- **Tonsillar trauma**—fingering, toothbrush, and pencil
- **Thrush** (candidiasis and moniliasis)—affect diabetic and immunocompromised patients curdy white patchy lesion, leaves ulcer on removal

Complications

- Peritonsillar abscess (quinsy)
- Parapharyngeal abscess
- Chronic tonsillitis
- Cervical abscess
- Acute otitis media (AOM)
- Rheumatic fever
- Acute glomerulonephritis
- Subacute bacterial endocarditis

Treatment

- Bed rest, plenty of fluid intake, and soft diet
- **Antibiotics—penicillin.** Penicillin allergic patient treated with erythromycin
- Analgesics antipyretic
- Warm saline gargles (soothing effect) and lozenges

CHRONIC TONSILLITIS

Q. Discuss etiopathology, clinical features and management of chronic tonsillitis.

Etiology

- Complication of acute tonsillitis
- Subclinical infection of tonsils following sinusitis, upper respiratory tract infection (URTI), and teeth.

Types

- **Chronic follicular**—yellow spots of cheesy material over tonsils
- **Chronic parenchymatous**—tonsils are enlarged which interfere with speech, deglutition, and respiration.
- Long-standing obstruction shows features of cor pulmonale
- **Chronic fibroid tonsillitis**—small fibrosed tonsils

Clinical Features

Symptoms

- Recurrent attacks of acute tonsillitis with variable interval in between attacks
- Halitosis and bad taste
- Difficulty in swallowing, breathing, and thick speech
- Chronic cough and throaty irritation

Signs

- Chronic parenchymatous tonsillitis—varying degree of tonsillar enlargement **(Fig. 3)**
- Chronic follicular tonsillitis—white cheesy follicular spots seen on tonsils
- Chronic fibroid tonsillitis—tonsils are small but Ervin-Moore sign positive—compression of anterior tonsillar pillar cheesy material oozes out from tonsillar crypts
- Flushing of anterior pillar and rest of oropharyngeal mucosa appears normal
- Enlargement of JD LN which becomes tender on acute attach of tonsillitis.

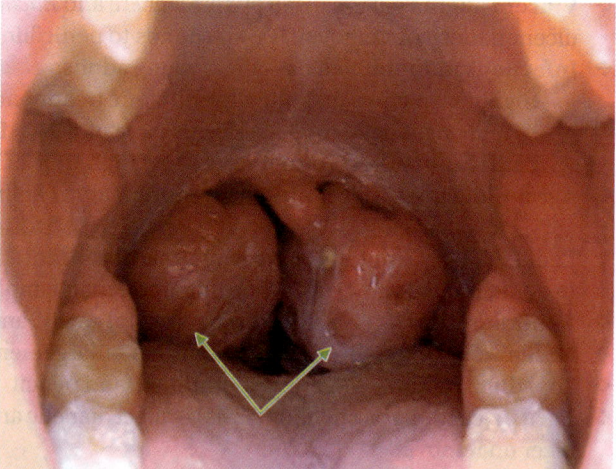

Fig. 3: Palatine tonsillar hypertrophy and congestion in chronics tonsillitis (arrows).

Brodsky Grading of Tonsillar Hypertrophy (Fig. 4)

It is based on projection of tonsil medially from anterior tonsillar pillar

Grade 0	Tonsil in fossa or removed
Grade 1+	Up to 25% projection in oropharynx
Grade 2+	Up to 25–50% projection in oropharynx
Grade 3+	Up to 50–75% projection in oropharynx
Grade 4+	Up to 75–100% projection in oropharynx

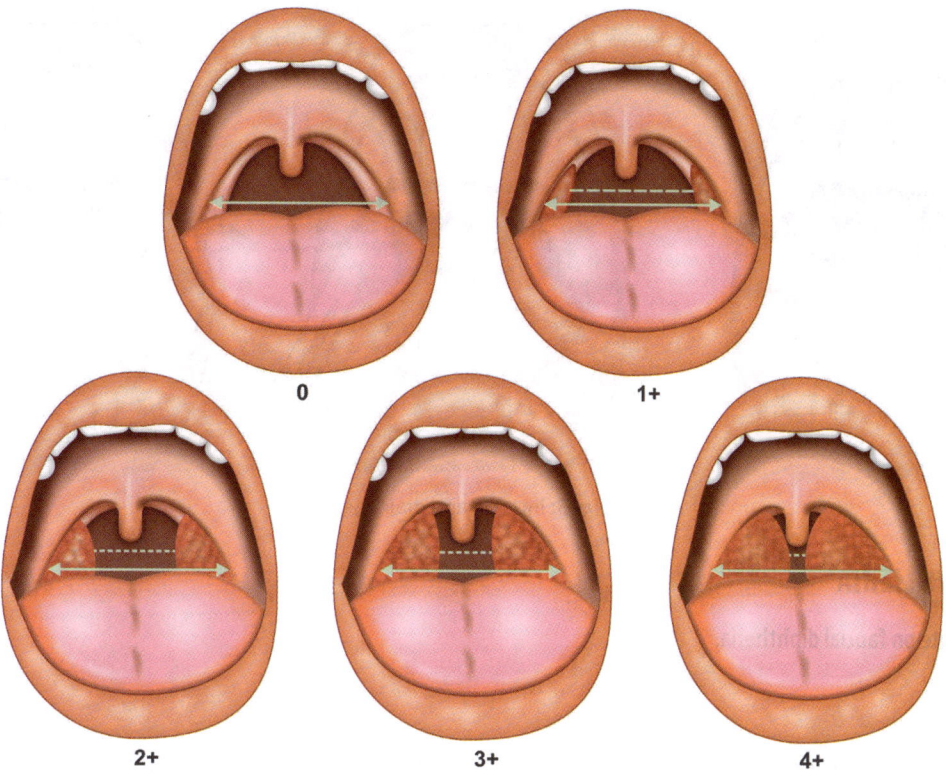

Fig. 4: Tonsillar grading.

Treatment

❖ The treatment of acute attack is mentioned above.
❖ To consider **for tonsillectomy surgery** when it affects swallowing, speech, breathing, and recurrent attack (*refer* Chapter 59)

■ TONSILLAR CYST

❖ Appears as a yellowish swelling over tonsil due to blockage of tonsillar crypts
❖ Usually seen in adults incidentally and it is symptomless

■ TONSILLOLITHS (CALCULI)

❖ Blockage of tonsillar crypts with chronic accumulation of debris
❖ **Later inorganic calcium and magnesium salts get deposited which forms stone, gradually increases in size.**
  ▹ It is seen more commonly in adults presented with foreign body sensation in throat, diagnosed with palpation and probing (gritty sensation)
  ▹ Treated—simple removal of stone or tonsillectomy

■ INTRATONSILLAR ABSCESS (QUINSY)

Following follicular tonsillitis crypts get obstructed, pus get accumulated in substance of tonsil, tonsil appears swollen inflamed with intense pain dysphagia.

Management

❖ Hospitalization, rehydration, intravenous (IV) antibiotic, incision and drainage of abscess **(Fig. 5)**, once acute attack subsided plan for tonsillectomy surgery
❖ After acute attack tonsillectomy is done after interval of 4 weeks—it is called **interval tonsillectomy.**

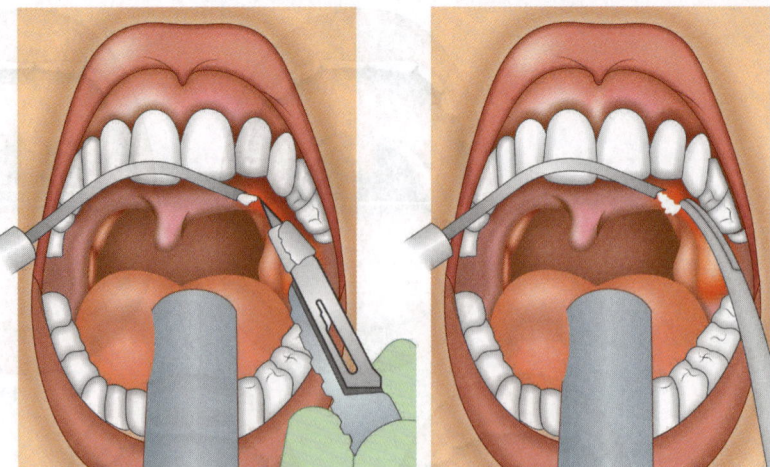

Fig. 5: Incision and drainage.

FAUCIAL DIPHTHERIA

Q. Write a short note on faucial diphtheria.

Etiology

It is caused by *Corynebacterium diphtheriae (C. diphtheriae)* (gram-positive bacilli), spread by droplet infection.

Clinical Features

- No age group is immune
- Affect oropharynx nasopharynx even larynx
- Dirty grayish membrane appear on oropharynx involving tonsils, soft palate, postpharyngeal wall, lymphadenopathy giving bull neck appearance, and fever with toxemia.
- Membrane may extend to larynx causes laryngeal obstruction (stridor).

Complication

- Exotoxin produced by *C. diphtheriae* have **cardiotoxic and neurotoxic action**
- **Cardiotoxic action:** Arrhythmia, myocarditis, and cardiac failure
- **Neurotoxic action:** Soft palate palsy and ocular palsy

Treatment

- To be started on the clinical assessment
- Aim to neutralize exotoxin by antitoxin by giving it intravenously
- Sensitivity to horse serum antitoxin checked by intracutaneous test before giving neutralizing dose
    - For membrane confined to tonsil (<48 hours) = 20,000–40,000 U IV infusion with saline for 60 minutes
    - For extensive membrane >48 hours = 80,000–120,000 U IV infusion with saline for 60 minutes

Antibiotics

- Benzyl penicillin 600 mg 6 hourly for 7 days
- Penicillin sensitive cases erythromycin 500 mg 6 hourly

Chapter 34

Adenoiditis (Nasopharyngeal Tonsil)

> **EN4.23**: Elicit document and present a correct history, demonstrate and describe the clinical features, choose the correct investigations and describe the principles of management of adenoids.

ANATOMY OF ADENOIDS

Q. Describe the anatomy of adenoids.

- **Location:** At junction of roof of the nasopharynx and posterior pharyngeal wall.
- **Epithelial lining:** A pseudostratified ciliated columnar epithelium
    - Transitional epithelium
    - Stratified squamous epithelium
- **Blood supply:**
    - Facial artery—ascending palatine branch
    - External carotid artery—ascending pharyngeal branch
    - Thyrocervical trunk—ascending cervical artery branch of inferior thyroid artery branch
- **Lymphatic:** Jugular lymph node via retropharyngeal, parapharyngeal nodes
- **Nerve supply:** It is through IX and X nerves
  (It is present at the birth and then increases in size till 5–6 years after puberty and tend to atrophy).

ADENOID HYPERTROPHY

Q. Write a short note/essay on adenoid hypertrophy.

Etiology

- **Physiological enlargement**—considers unhealthy if it produces symptoms
- **Infection**—recurrent rhinitis, sinusitis, and chronic tonsillitis may cause adenoid hypertrophy
- **Noninfective**—allergic rhinitis, allergy of the upper respiratory tract (URT) causing adenoid hypertrophy.

Clinical Features

- **Associated with nasal obstruction**
    - Mouth breathing, snoring, and drooling of saliva from the mouth
    - Infant—breathing and feeding cannot take place simultaneously resulting in difficulty in feeding and failure to thrive
    - Voice becomes flat and with loss of nasal quality, toneless (rhinolalia clausa)
    - Adenoid facies—narrow, pinched nose, high-arch palate, undershoot lower jaw, crowded irregular protruded teeth, drooling of saliva, expression-less face, and flattened chest.

PART 1: Diseases of ENT, Head and Neck

- ❖ **Associated with eustachian tube obstruction**
  - ➢ Retracted tympanic membrane
  - ➢ Serous otitis media
  - ➢ Recurrent acute otitis media (AOM)
  - ➢ Chronic suppurative otitis media (CSOM)
- ❖ **Associate with infection**
  - ➢ Nose-purulent nasal discharge due to recurrent rhinitis, and sinusitis. Wet bubbly nose due to obstruction to drainage of nasal secretion.
  - ➢ Recurrent pharyngitis, tonsillitis, postnasal drip
  - ➢ Aggravation of bronchial asthma, and bronchitis if present
- ❖ **General features**
  - ➢ Pulmonary hypertension on long-standing nasal obstruction
  - ➢ Nocturnal enuresis
  - ➢ Aprosexia—lack of concentration

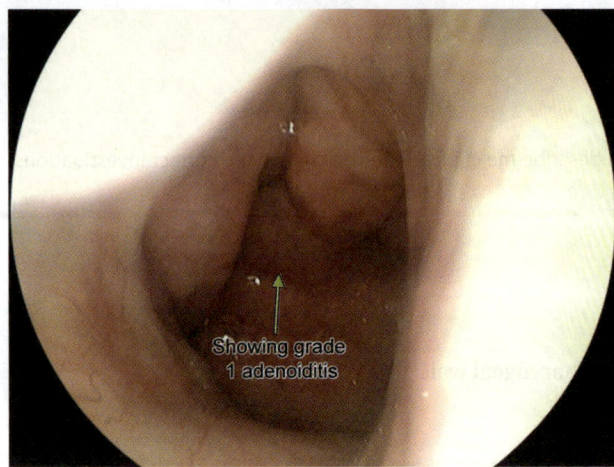

Fig. 1: Grade 1: Adenoiditis.

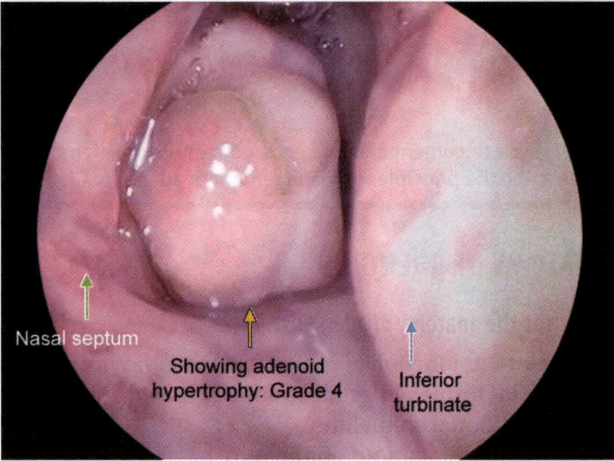

Fig. 2: Grade 4: Adenoid hypertrophy.

Grading of Adenoid Hypertrophy

Grade	Description
Grade I **(Fig. 1)**	Adenoid tissue filling one-third of the vertical portion of the choanae
Grade II	Adenoid tissue filling one-third to two-thirds of the vertical portion of the choanae
Grade III	From two-third to nearly complete obstruction of the choanae
Grade IV **(Fig. 2)**	Complete choanal obstruction

Adenoid Facies

Q. Write short note on adenoid facies/long face syndrome.

It is characterized by the following:
- ❖ An elongated face
- ❖ Retrognathic mandible
- ❖ Open mouth
- ❖ Pinched nose due to alar atrophy
- ❖ Open bite, crossbite, and protrusion of the maxilla
- ❖ Prominent and overcrowding of upper teeth
- ❖ High-arched palate due to the absence of molding action of the tongue
- ❖ Dull expression
- ❖ Dark circles under the eyes

Management

Diagnosis

- On the history of obstructive symptoms and clinical examination
- Posterior nasal rhinoscopy (structures seen on posterior rhinoscopy)
- Radiological—X-ray nasopharynx lateral view shows soft tissue shadow in the nasopharynx
- Examination under general anesthesia by digital palpation while performing tonsillectomy, adenoidectomy surgery to be done if necessary

Treatment

- Mild cases without significant symptoms conservatively
- Antibiotics in the acute phase
- Decongestant to establish breathing
- Steroidal nasal spray to control allergic etiological factor
- Breathing exercise
- Surgical treatment
- Adenoidectomy surgery is to be considered for severe and recurrent complaints, and obstructive symptoms. Coblation adenoidectomy using coblator and nasal endoscope **(Fig. 3)**.
- Grommet—to be considered for secretory otitis media with conductive hearing loss.

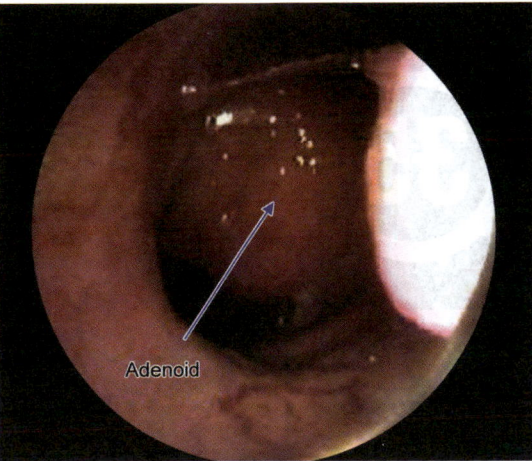

Fig. 3: Endoscopic view of enlarged adenoids through choana.

Chapter 35

Acute and Chronic Pharyngitis

ACUTE PHARYNGITIS

Q. Describe etiology, clinical features, and management of acute pharyngitis.

Etiology

Viral pharyngitis are more common cause for acute pharyngitis.

Acute streptococcal pharyngitis (group A beta-hemolytic streptococci) is important due to its etiology in rheumatic fever and poststreptococcal glomerulonephritis.

Causes of acute pharyngitis			
Viral	*Bacterial*	*Fungal*	*Miscellaneous*
Influenza Parainfluenza Adenovirus Measles Chickenpox Cytomegalovirus Epstein–Barr virus	Streptococci Gonococci Diphtheria	Candida albicans Chlamydia trachomatis	Parasitic

Clinical Features

- **Mild infection:** It is present with:
  - Discomfort in throat
  - Malaise
  - Mild fever
  - Congestion of the pharynx (without lymphadenopathy)
- **Moderate to severe infection:**
  - Throat pain (odynophagia)
  - Dysphagia
  - Fever and congestion
  - Erythematous mucosa
  - Tonsillar hypertrophy
  - Lymphadenopathy
- **Very severe infection (Fig. 1):**
  - Edema of uvula
  - Soft palate
  - Enlarged cervical lymph nodes
  - High-grade fever
  - Dysphagia
  - Odynophagia

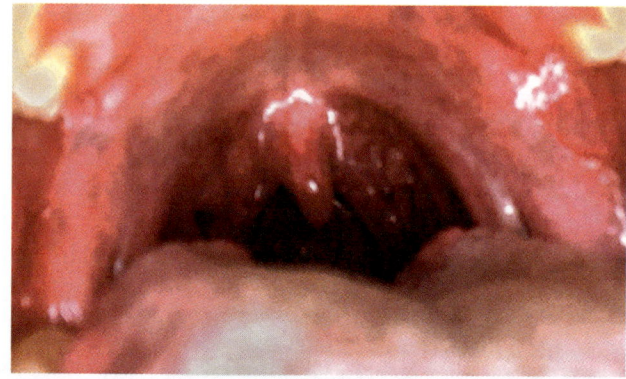

Fig. 1: Acute pharyngitis.

Management

Investigation

Throat swab—for diagnosis of bacterial pharyngitis

The most common organism found is group A streptococci (gram-positive cocci in a chain)

- *Corynebacterium diphtheriae (C. diphtheriae)* (gram-positive clubbed-shaped bacillus) cultured on Loeffler serum slope
- Failure of bacterial growth on culture suggests viral infection.

Treatment

- Bed rest
- Plenty of fluid intakes
- Warm saline gargles
- Lozenges
- Antibiotic
- Penicillin V oral 500 mg two times a day for 10 days.
- Amoxicillin oral 500 mg two times a day/250 mg three times a day.
- For penicillin-allergic patients
- Macrolid (erythromycin/azithromycin), cephalosporin class of antibiotics are used.
- *C. diphtheriae* (For treatment of tonsillitis due to *C. Diphtheria* refer to Chapters 33 and 39).
- Gonococcal infection treated with penicillin and tetracycline class of antibiotics.
- For pharyngeal candidiasis (oral thrush) nystatin is the drug of choice.

■ CHRONIC PHARYNGITIS

Q. Describe etiology, clinical features, and management of chronic pharyngitis.

Chronic inflammation of the pharynx is characterized by hypertrophy of mucosa, and subepithelial lymphoid follicles.

Etiology

- **Persistent infection of surrounding structures:** Chronic rhinosinusitis, chronic tonsillitis, and dental sepsis.
- Mouth breathing due to adenoid hypertrophy, nasal polyposis, and deviated nasal septum.
- Chronic irritation caused by smoking, tobacco chewing, chronic alcohol intake, environmental pollution

Clinical Features

Symptoms

- Foreign body sensation in the throat
- Chronic throat irritation
- Chronic cough
- Thick mucosal secretions

Signs

- **Chronic catarrhal pharyngitis:** Congested mucosa of the posterior pharyngeal wall, tonsilla pillars, and increased mucous secretions.
- **Chronic granular pharyngitis:** Edematous, thick pharyngeal mucosa hypertrophy of subepithelial lymphoid follicles appearing red nodules of pharyngeal mucosa edematous elongated uvula.

Treatment

- Eradicate infections of surrounding structures (management of chronic rhinosinusitis, correction of deviated nasal septum)
- Abstinence of chronic irritants (smoking, tobacco, and alcohol)
- Antacid in patients with reflux disease and diet modification.
- Mandl's paint is to be applied on pharyngeal mucosa for granular pharyngitis.
- Chemical cautery (10–25% sliver nitrate) of granules or electrocautery of nodules under general anesthesia.

Chapter 36

Head and Neck Space Infections

EN4.36: Describe the clinical features, investigations and principles of management of deep neck space Infection.

■ PAROTID ABSCESS

Suppuration of parotid space.

Q. What are the contents of parotid space and where does it lie? Write a short note on parotid abscess.

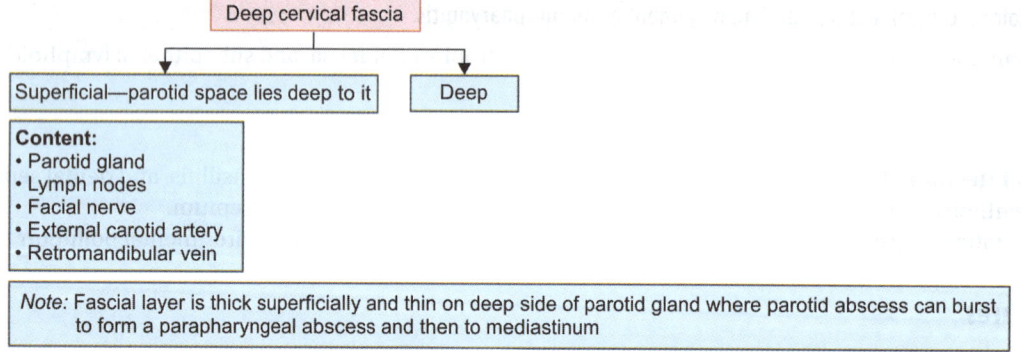

Note: Fascial layer is thick superficially and thin on deep side of parotid gland where parotid abscess can burst to form a parapharyngeal abscess and then to mediastinum

Etiology

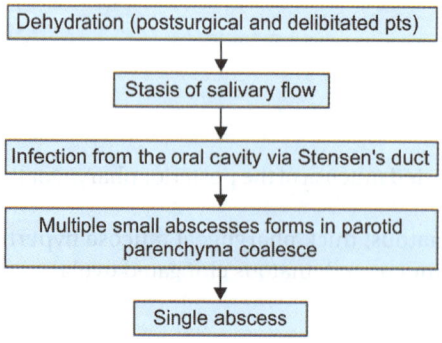

Bacteriology

- *Staphylococcus aureus*
- Streptococci
- Rarely gram-negative

Clinical Features

Usually follows 5–7 days after the operation.

General condition: Toxic, high fever, and dehydrated.

Local examination:
- Swelling, redness, induration, and tenderness in parotid area, at an angle of mandible.
- Usually unilateral, but bilateral may occur.
- Fluctuation is difficult to elicit due to the thick capsules.
- Stensen's duct opening congested and may exude pus on pressure over the parotid.

Diagnosis
- Ultrasound
- Computed tomography (CT) scan
- Aspiration of abscess can be done for culture and sensitivity of the causative organism.

Treatment
- Correct dehydration
- Improve oral hygiene and promote salivary flow
- Intravenous antibiotics are instituted.
- **Surgical drainage:**

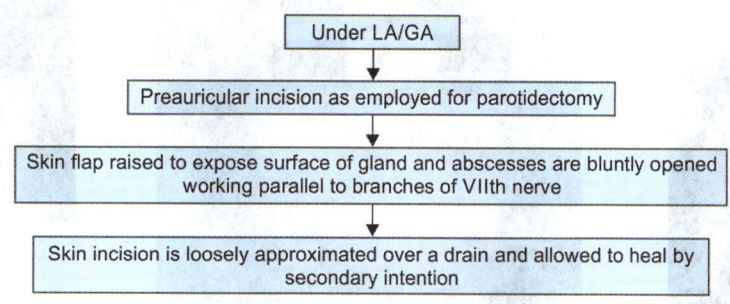

LUDWIG'S ANGINA

Q. What is Ludwig's angina? Write a short note/essay on its clinical features and treatment.

Applied Anatomy: Infection of Submandibular Space

Submandibular space:
- Mucous membrane of floor of mouth and tongue on one side
- A superficial layer of deep cervical fascia between hyoid bone and mandible on other

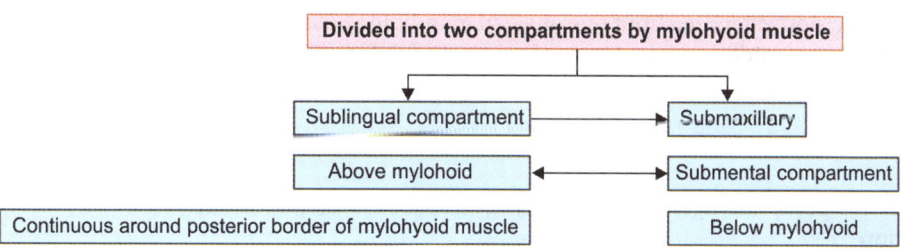

Etiology

- Dental infection—roots of premolar
- Roots of molar
- Submandibular sialadenitis
- Injuries of oral mucosa
- Fractures of mandible

Bacteriology

- Alpha-hemolytic streptococci
- Staphylococci
- Bacteroides groups
- *Haemophilus influenza* (rarely)
- *Escherichia coli*
- *Pseudomonas*

Clinical Features (Figs. 1 to 3)

- Odynophagia with varying degrees of trismus.
- If infection is localized to sublingual space: Swollen structures on the floor of the mouth

Submaxillary space:

- Swollen and tender
- Woody-hard feel
- Cellulitis
- Abscess
- Threatening of airway
- Laryngeal edema

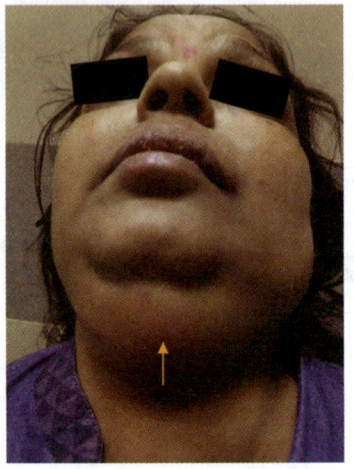

Fig. 1: Ludwig's angina.

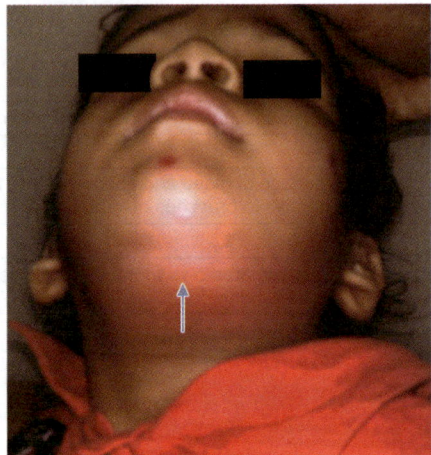

Fig. 2: Ludwig's angina in a child.

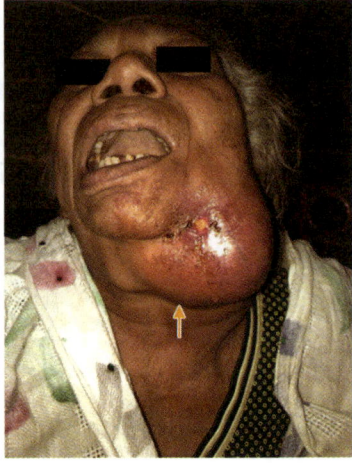

Fig. 3: Submandibular abscess.

Treatment

- Systemic antibiotics.
- **Incision and drainage of the abscess**.
    - **Intraoral**—if infection localized to sublingual space.
    - **External**—if infection involves submaxillary space.
        - Transverse incision extending from one angle of mandible to other
        - Vertical opening of midline musculature of tongue with a blunt hemostat.
- **Tracheostomy:** If airway is endangered.

Complications

- Spread of infection → parapharyngeal → retropharyngeal spaces → mediastinum
- Airway obstruction

- Septicemia
- Aspiration pneumonia

PERITONSILLAR ABSCESS (QUINSY)

Q. Write a short note/essay on peritonsillar abscess/quinsy.

Infection of peritonsillar space: Tonsil capsule → peritonsillar space ← superior constrictor muscle

Etiology

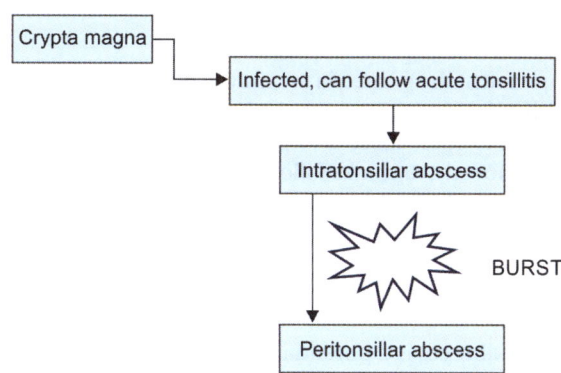

Bacteriology

- *Streptococcus pyogenes*
- *S. aureus*
- Anaerobes

Clinical Features

- **Adults;** rarely children though acute tonsillitis is more common in children.
- Unilateral, occasionally bilateral

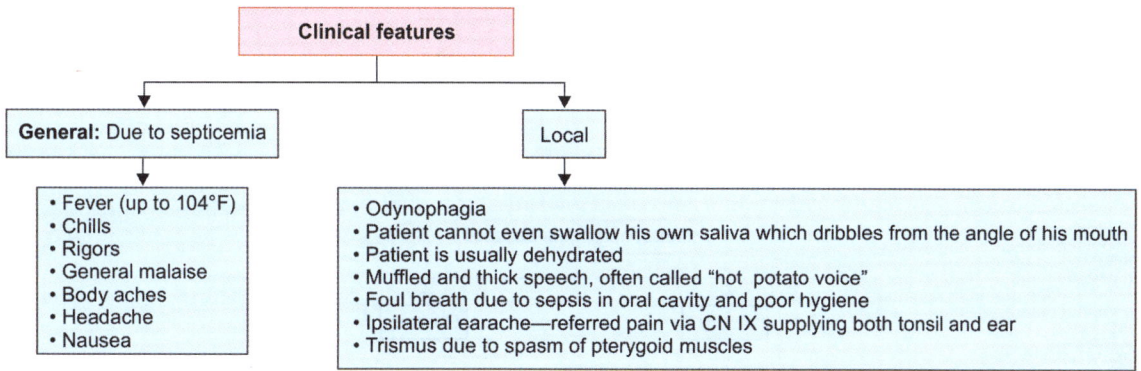

Examination

- Congested and swollen tonsil, pillars, and soft palate
  Note: Tonsil itself may not appear enlarged as it gets buried in edematous pillars
- Swollen and edematous uvula pushed to the opposite side.
- Bulging of the soft palate and anterior pillar above tonsil.
- Mucopus may be seen covering the tonsillar region.
- Cervical lymphadenopathy (jugulodigastric).
- Torticollis

Treatment

Medical
- *Hospitalization*
- *Intravenous fluids* to combat dehydration.
- *IV antibiotics*
- *Analgesics* like paracetamol is given for relief of pain and to lower the temperature.
- *Oral hygiene* should be maintained by saline/chlorhexidine mouthwashes or betadine gargles.

Surgical
If a frank abscess has formed, incision and drainage are required.
- **Incision and drainage:** Abscess opened at the point of a maximum bulge above upper pole of tonsil or just lateral to point of junction of an anterior pillar with a line drawn through the base of the uvula.
  Stab incision → sinus forceps inserted to open abscess → pus-drained
- Interval tonsillectomy. Tonsils are removed 4–6 weeks following an attack of quinsy.
- Abscess or hot tonsillectomy. It has the risk of rupture of abscess during anesthesia and excessive bleeding

Complications
Rare nowadays
- Parapharyngeal abscess (peritonsillar abscess is a potential parapharyngeal abscess).
- Laryngeal edema—tracheostomy
- Septicemia—other complications such as endocarditis, nephritis, and brain abscess may occur

■ RETROPHARYNGEAL ABSCESS

Q. Briefly describe the anatomy of retropharyngeal space. Write a note on retropharyngeal abscess.

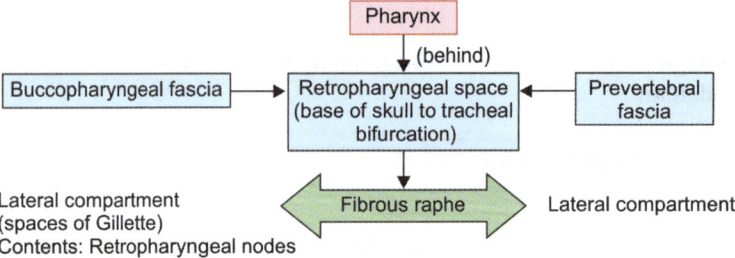

Types

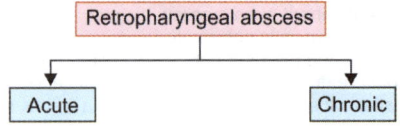

Acute Retropharyngeal Abscess

Q. What are the causes of acute retropharyngeal abscess? Write a note on its clinical features and treatment.

Etiology
- Children below 3 years
- Due to suppuration of retropharyngeal lymph nodes secondary to infection in:
  - Adenoids
  - Nasopharynx
  - Posterior nasal sinuses
  - Nasal cavity

- In adults, may result from:
  - Penetrating injury of the posterior pharyngeal wall
  - Or cervical esophagus
  - Pus from acute mastoiditis tracks along the undersurface of the petrous bone

Clinical Features

- *Dysphagia and dyspnea*
- *Stridor and* croupy *cough*
- *Torticollis*
- *Bulge in the posterior pharyngeal wall*—usually unilateral

Investigation

X-ray soft tissue, lateral view of the neck → widening of prevertebral shadow **(Fig. 4)**

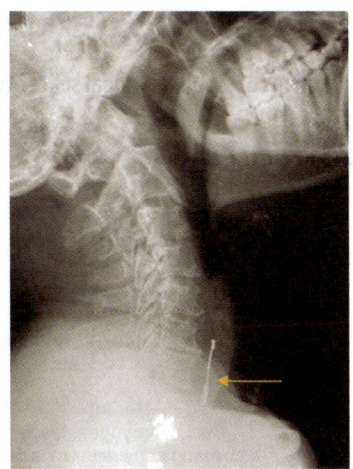

Fig. 4: X-ray of the neck showing (arrow) acute retropharyngeal abscess due to a metallic foreign body.

Treatment

- **Incision and drainage of abscess:** Usually done without anesthesia as there is a risk of rupture of abscess during:
  - Intubation
  - A child is kept supine with his/her head low
  - Mouth is opened with a gag
  - A vertical incision is given in the most fluctuant area of abscess.
  - Suctioning to prevent aspiration of pus.
- **Systemic antibiotics**

Chronic Retropharyngeal Abscess (Prevertebral Abscess)

Q. Write a short note on prevertebral abscess.

Prevertebral space: It lies between vertebral bodies posteriorly and prevertebral fascia anteriorly from the base to skull of the coccyx.

Etiology

Tubercular, central/midline in nature
- **Result of:**
  - Caries of cervical spine
  - Tuberculous infection of retropharyngeal lymph nodes secondary to tuberculosis of deep cervical nodes

Clinical Features

- Throat discomfort
- **Dysphagia:** It is present but not marked

On Examination

- Fluctuant swelling in posterior pharyngeal wall centrally or on one side of midline.
- Cervical tuberculous lymphadenopathy

Investigation

- X-ray cervical spine **(Fig. 5)**
- Magnetic resonance imaging (MRI) cervical spine

Treatment

- **Incision and drainage of abscess:** Vertical incision along anterior border of:
  - Sternomastoid (for low abscess)
  - Or along its posterior border (for high abscess).
- Full course of *antitubercular therapy*

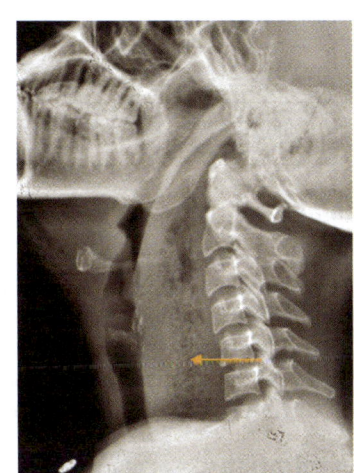

Fig. 5: X-ray of neck lateral view (arrow) showing retropharyngeal abscess.

PARAPHARYNGEAL ABSCESS (ABSCESS OF PHARYNGOMAXILLARY OR LATERAL PHARYNGEAL SPACE)

Q. What are synonyms of parapharyngeal space? Write short note on parapharyngeal abscess.

Parapharyngeal Space

Relations

Pyramidal in shape with its base at base of skull and apex at the hyoid bone.

Posterior
Prevertebral fascia covering prevertebral muscle and transverse processes of cervical vertebrae

Medial
Buccopharyngeal fascia covering constrictor muscles

Base
Apex

Lateral
Medial pterygoid muscle, mandible and deep surface of parotid gland

Q. Why infection of this space is dangerous?

Papharyngeal space ⇅ Communicates with

Spaces:
- Retropharynx
- Submandibular
- Parotid
- Carotid
- Visceral

Q. How is this space divided and infections are presented clinically?

Styloid process and the muscles attached to it divide parapharyngeal space into anterior and posterior compartments.

Parapharyngeal space

Anterior compartment
Medially: Tonsillar fossa
Laterally: Medial pterygoid muscle
Triad of symptoms:
- Prolapse of tonsil and tonsillar fossa
- Trismus (due to spasm of medial pterygoid muscle)
- External swelling behind angle of jaw marked odynophagia

Posterior compartment
Medially: Posterior part of lateral pharyngeal wall
Laterally: Parotid gland
Contents: Carotid artery jugular vein IXth, Xth, XIth, and XIIth cranial nerves sympathetic trunk upper deep cervical nodes
- Bulge of pharynx behind posterior pillar
- Paralysis of CN IX, X, XI, and XII and sympathetic chain
- Swelling of the parotid region minimal trismus or tonsillar prolapse

Note: Fever, odynophagia, sore throat, torticollis (due to spasm of prevertebral muscles) and signs of toxemia are common to both compartments

Etiology

Infection of parapharyngeal space can occur from:
- **Pharynx:** Acute and chronic infections of tonsil, adenoid, bursting of peritonsillar abscess.
- **Teeth:** Dental infection usually comes from lower last molar tooth.
- **Ear:** Bezold abscess and petrositis.
- **Others:** Infections of parotid, retropharyngeal, and submaxillary spaces.
- **External trauma:** Penetrating injuries of neck, injection of local anesthetic for tonsillectomy or mandibular nerve

Complications

- Laryngeal edema with respiratory obstruction.
- Jugular vein thrombophlebitis with septicemia.

- Spread of infection to retropharyngeal space.
- Spread of infection to mediastinum along with the carotid space.
- Mycotic aneurysm of carotid artery from the weakening of its wall by purulent material. It may involve the common carotid or internal carotid artery.
- Carotid blowout with massive hemorrhage.

Investigations

- CT scan of face and neck **(Fig. 6)**
- MRI of face and neck
- Fine needle aspiration cytology (FNAC)

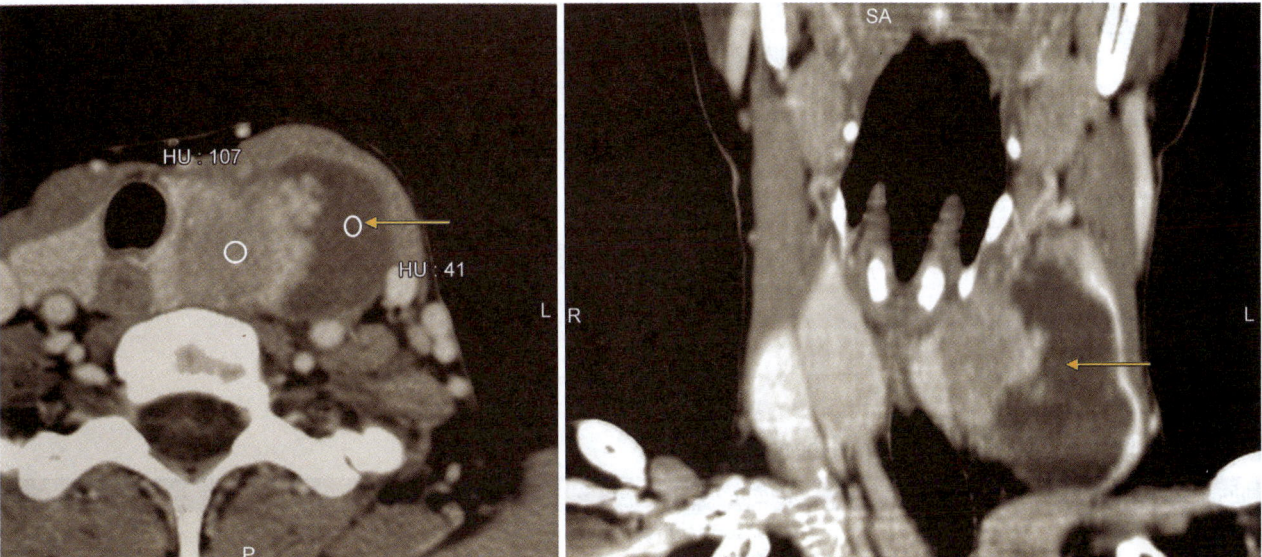

Fig. 6: Computed tomography (CT) scan of face and neck showing parapharyngeal abscess.

Treatment

- Systemic antibiotics
- **Drainage of abscess:** Done under general anesthesia.
- **If marked trismus → preoperative tracheostomy**

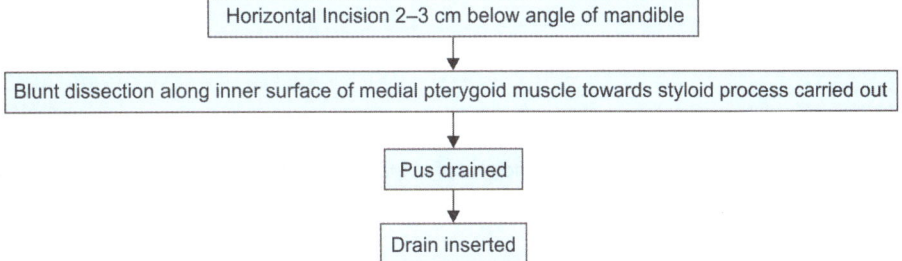

Note: Transoral drainage should never be done due to danger of injury to great vessels which pass through this space

Chapter 37

Tumors of Nasopharynx, Hypopharynx, Oropharynx and Pharyngeal Pouch

EN4.33: Describe the clinical features, investigations, and principles of management of tumors of the nasopharynx.

■ TUMORS OF NASOPHARYNX

Classification

Q. Classify the benign and malignant tumors of the nasopharynx.

Benign tumors	Malignant tumors
❖ Papilloma	❖ Nasopharyngeal carcinoma
❖ Angiofibroma	❖ Lymphoma
❖ Choanal polyp	❖ Rhabdomyosarcoma
❖ Thornwaldt's cyst	❖ Chordoma
❖ Pleomorphic adenoma	❖ Plasmacytoma
❖ Paraganglioma	❖ Hemangiopericytoma
❖ Craniopharyngioma	❖ Malignant salivary gland tumor
❖ Hamartoma	❖ Melanoma
❖ Choristoma	❖ Adenoid cystic carcinoma

Congenital Tumors of the Nasopharynx

- ❖ Teratoma
- ❖ Hairy polyp
- ❖ Epignathi

EN4.31: Describe the clinical features, investigations, and principles of management of juvenile nasopharyngeal angiofibroma (JNA).

Juvenile Nasopharyngeal Angiofibroma

Q. Write short note/essay on juvenile nasopharyngeal angiofibroma and its treatment.

Etiology

Proposed theory—based on incomplete regression of the 1st branchial arch artery.

Pathology

Juvenile nasopharyngeal angiofibromas are benign fibrovascular tumors with a characteristic—irregularly-shaped vessels, lined by endothelial cells, or showing an incomplete vascular wall architecture.

The highest density of vessels, with the characteristic irregular shape, is found below a pseudocapsule at the tumor surface, i.e., at the periphery.

Towards the center of the tumor, the amount of fibrous tissue increases, while the vessel density decreases.

Clinical Features

- ❖ Almost exclusive in young adolescent males
- ❖ Benign in nature
- ❖ Propensity to cause local destruction of tissues
- ❖ Recurrent in nature

Clinical Presentation

- ❖ **Symptoms:**
  - ➤ *Tumor in nasal cavity*—nasal mass, nasal obstruction, nasal discharge, and epistaxis
  - ➤ *Tumor in peripheral nerve tumors (PNS)*—extension to maxillary, ethmoid, or sphenoid sinuses.
  - ➤ *Tumor in orbit*—spread to orbit occurs through inferior orbital fissure giving rise to proptosis.
  - ➤ *Extension to anterior cranial fossa*—through the roof of ethmoids or cribriform plate.
  - ➤ *Extension to middle cranial fossa*—through floor of sphenoid sinus and sella turcica
- ❖ **Facial swelling:** In case tumor extends beyond the maxillary sinus.
- ❖ **Hyponasal speech:**
  - ➤ Otitis media with effusion with conductive hearing loss due to obstruction of Eustachian tube (ET) by the tumor.
  - ➤ Diagnostic nasal endoscopy (DNE)—bright red-colored nasal mass arising from the lateral wall of the posterior nasal cavity near the sphenopalatine foramen and pterygoid base/pterygoid wedge area **(Figs. 1 and 2).**
- ❖ Bony erosions of the clivus, pterygoid, and sphenoid sinus floor are the hallmarks of this tumor.

Management

- ❖ **Investigation:**
  - ➤ Contrast-enhanced computed tomography (CECT) scan is the gold standard. Computed tomography angiography to locate the blood supply of the angiofibroma, i.e., whether a tumor is receiving the blood supply from the internal carotid artery system or the external carotid artery system **(Figs. 3 and 4).**
  - ➤ Magnetic resonance imaging (MRI)—complements CT scan to see for any soft tissue extension intracranially or intraorbital.
- ❖ **Treatment:**
  - ➤ Preoperative embolization to reduce the vascularity of the tumor.
  - ➤ Blood grouping and cross-matching are done in case the need for blood transfusion arises.
  - ➤ Surgery is the mainstay of treatment. Endoscopic approach is preferred.
  - ➤ Approach used is modified Denker's (endonasal) wherein a medial side of the anterior wall of the maxillary sinus is removed to gain access to the tumor and for postoperative surveillance of the tumor **(Fig. 5).**
  - ➤ Radiotherapy is reserved for recurrent inoperable tumors with possible intracranial extension.

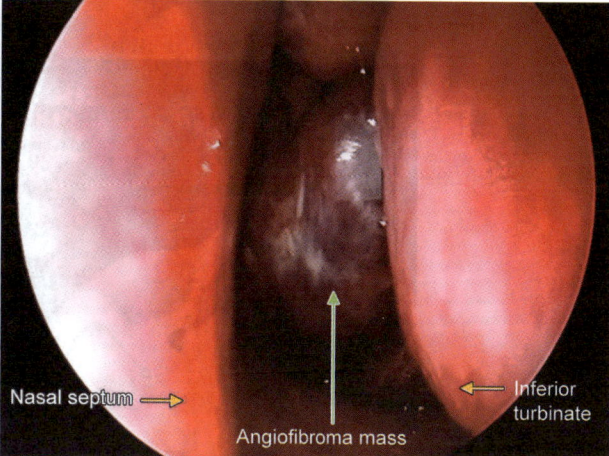

Fig. 1: Endoscopic view of nasopharyngeal angiofibroma.

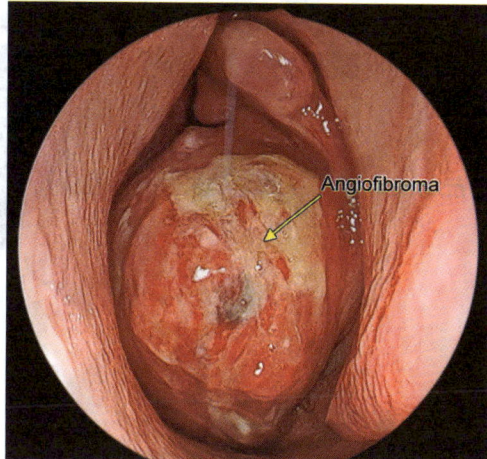

Fig. 2: Endoscopic view of extensive nasopharyngeal angiofibroma.

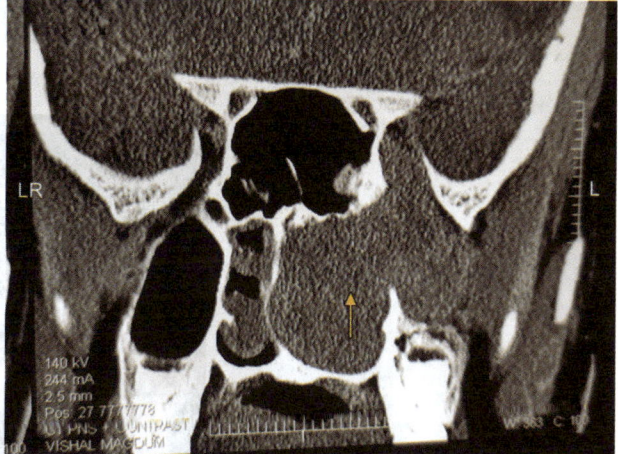

Fig. 3: Computed tomography (CT) scan showing angiofibroma mass with sphenopalatine foramen widening (arrow).

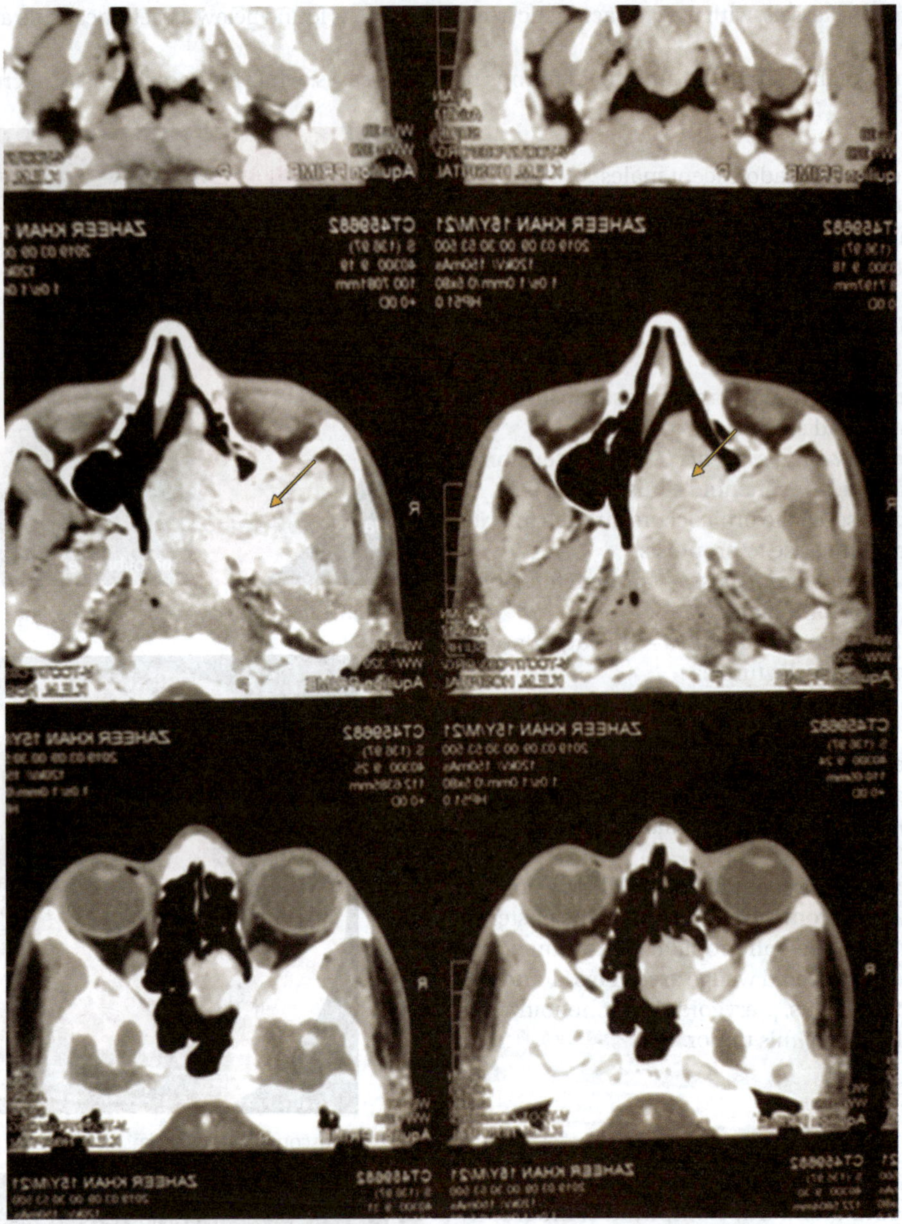

Fig. 4: Contrast-enhanced computed tomography (CECT) scan of the nose showing huge angiofibroma.

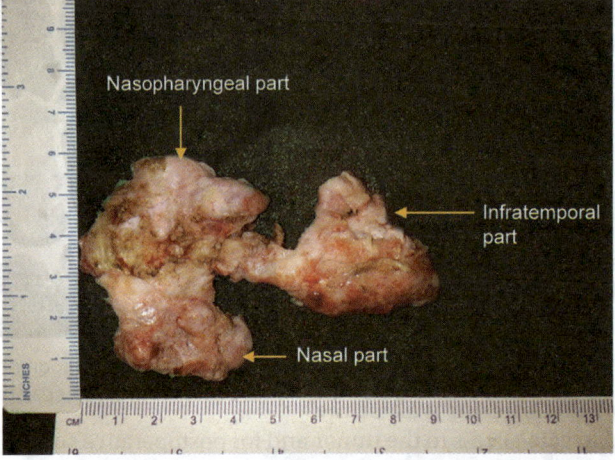

Fig. 5: Excised nasopharyngeal angiofibroma.

Theories of Etiopathogenesis of JNA

Q. What are the various theories proposed to explain the etiopathogenesis of the juvenile nasopharyngeal angiofibroma (JNA)?

- **Ringertz theory**—this theory believes that the JA always arises from the periosteum of the skull base.
- **Som and Neffson**—inequalities in the growth of bones forming the skull base led to hypertrophy of the underlying periosteum in response to hormonal influence.
- **Bensch and Ewing**—tumor arose probably from embryonic fibrocartilage between the basiocciput and basisphenoid.
- **Brunner**—origin from conjoined pharyngobasilar and buccopharyngeal fascia.
- **Marten, et al**—tumors resulted from deficiency of androgens or over-activity of estrogens.
- **Sternberg**—JNA could be a type of hemangioma seen in children which aggress with age.
- **Osborn**—swelling could be due to either a hamartoma or residual fetal erectile tissue which was under the influence of hormones.
- **Girgis and Fahmy**—observed cell of nests of undifferentiated epithelioid cells. They believed JNA to be a paraganglioma.

Surgical Approaches

Q. Enumerate surgical approaches for juvenile nasopharyngeal angiofibroma other than the endoscopic approach.

- Transpalatine
- Transpalatine + sublabial (Sardana's approach)
- Lateral rhinotomy with medial maxillectomy
- Transmaxillary (Le Fort I) approach
- Maxillary swing approach/facial translocation approach
- Infratemporal fossa approach

Nasopharyngeal Carcinoma

Q. Write a short note/essay on nasopharyngeal carcinoma.

Nasopharyngeal carcinoma (NPC) is most common in China (southern states), Hong Kong, Taiwan, Indonesia, North Africa (Tunisia and Algeria), Alaska, North Canada, and Greenland.

Etiology

- **Genetic:** Chinese have the highest susceptibility even after migration to other countries.
- **Viral:** Epstein–Barr virus (EBV) is associated with this carcinoma
- **Environmental:**
  - Air pollution
  - Smoking of tobacco and opium
  - Dry salted fish (nitrosamines)
  - Vitamin C deficient diet
  - Smoke from burning incense wood

Classification

World Health Organization (WHO) classification for nasopharyngeal carcinoma based on histopathology.
- **Type I (25%):** Keratinizing carcinoma
- **Type II (12%):** Nonkeratinizing differentiated carcinoma
- **Type III (63%):** Nonkeratinizing undifferentiated carcinoma

Clinical Presentation

- **Site:** Fossa of Rosenmüller is the most common site of origin.
- **Spread and clinical features:**
  - *Spread to nose and orbit*—cause nasal obstruction, epistaxis, and proptosis respectively
  - *Spread to ET*—cause serous otitis media
  - *Spread to foramen lacerum and ovale*—cause ophthalmic symptoms and pain due to involvement of cranial nerves III, IV, V, and VI
  - *Spread to parapharyngeal space*—cause cranial nerve palsies of cranial nerve (CN) IX, X, XI, and XII. Also, cause Horner's syndrome and trismus due to pterygoid muscle involvement.

PART 1: Diseases of ENT, Head and Neck

- *Spread to retropharyngeal nodes*—cause neck pain and stiffness
- *Spread to cervical nodes*—upper jugular and posterior triangle nodes enlargement cause multiple swellings in the neck
- *Distant metastases* form secondaries in the liver, lungs, and bones
❖ Cervical node metastases and thus neck swelling may be the only clinical manifestation in about 75% of patients.

Trotter's Triad

Nasopharyngeal carcinoma can cause:
❖ Conductive hearing loss due to ET blockage
❖ Ipsilateral temporoparietal neuralgia (CN V involvement)
❖ Palatal paralysis (CN X involvement)

Symptoms and Signs of Nasopharyngeal Carcinoma

❖ Cervical lymphadenopathy
❖ Hearing loss
❖ Nasal obstruction
❖ Epistaxis
❖ Cranial nerves palsies
❖ Headache
❖ Earache
❖ Neck pain
❖ Weight loss

Diagnosis

Nasal endoscopy examination to see the extent of the tumor, for documentation, and for taking a biopsy
❖ **Imaging:** CT scan and MRI with a contrast of neck and nasopharynx
  - CT skull base to diaphragm to look for secondaries.
  - Positron emission tomography (PET) scan—to look for secondaries in any part of the body.
❖ **Audiogram**—for diagnosing serous otitis media

Treatment

❖ **Radiotherapy**—for nasopharyngeal cancer stages I and II: External beam radiotherapy (EBRT) is used.
❖ **Chemotherapy**—for stages III and IV
❖ **Treatment of recurrent and residual disease:**
  - *Positive nodes in the neck*—radical neck dissection (RND)
  - *Recurrent/residual disease in the neck:*
    - The second course of radiation by intensity-modulated radiotherapy (IMRT)
    - Brachytherapy—high dose to the tumor with less radiation to the surrounding normal tissues
    - Nasopharyngectomy—endoscopic approach/lateral rhinotomy and medial maxillectomy/Le Fort I approach/maxillary swing

■ TUMORS OF OROPHARYNX

Types

Q. Enumerate the benign and malignant tumors of the oropharynx.

Benign tumors	Malignant tumors
❖ Papilloma	❖ Squamous cell carcinoma (most common variety)
❖ Hemangioma	❖ Lymphoepithelioma
❖ Pleomorphic adenoma	❖ Adenocarcinoma
❖ Mucous cyst	❖ Lymphomas (non-Hodgkin's mostly)
❖ Lipoma	❖ Minor salivary gland tumors
❖ Fibroma	
❖ Neuroma	

Common Sites of Malignancy in the Oropharynx

❖ Posterior one-third of the tongue
❖ Tonsil and tonsillar fossa
❖ Soft palate and anterior pillar
❖ Posterior and lateral pharyngeal wall

Gross Appearance

- Superficial spreading
- Exophytic
- Ulcerative
- Infiltrative

Etiopathogenesis

- Squamous cell carcinoma is the most common type.
- **Broad categories of oropharyngeal carcinoma:**
  - Human papilloma virus (HPV) positive oropharyngeal squamous cell carcinoma (OPSCC)
  - HPV-positive OPSCC
- HPV-16 is the most common genotype and an independent risk factor for oropharyngeal squamous cell carcinoma.

Tumors of Posterior One-third of Tongue

Presenting Symptoms

- Sore throat
- A feeling of lump in the throat
- Slight discomfort in swallowing
- Otalgia (referred pain)
- Dysphagia
- Bleeding from the mouth
- Hot potato voice

Methods of Examination

Examination under anesthesia (EUA) with digital palpation gives the best idea of the degree of infiltration of tissues.

Treatment

- T1/T2 cancers with N0/N1 neck—surgical excision with block dissection
  - Postoperative radiotherapy (RT) if surgical specimen shows stage >N1
- T3/T4 cancers—surgical excision + mandibular resection + neck dissection and postoperative radiation
- T4 lesions extending to anterior two-thirds of tongue/vallecula—total glossectomy + laryngectomy + radical neck dissection. Chemotherapy is added.
- For advanced tumors/those with poor health—palliative chemotherapy/radiotherapy

Tumors of Tonsil/Tonsillar Fossa

- Lymphomas are the tumors that present as unilateral tonsillar swellings with or without ulceration.
- Jugulodigastric group of lymph nodes is the most common group of lymph nodes involved in carcinoma of the tonsil/tonsillar fossa.

Treatment

- **Radiotherapy**—for early and radiosensitive tumors along with the irradiation of cervical nodes.
- **Excision**—tonsillectomy for superficial lesions: Larger/deep lesions—surgical excision + hemimandibulectomy and neck dissection.
- **Combination**—surgery + pre-/postoperative radiotherapy (RT), computed tomography as an adjunct can be given.

Faucial Arch Tumors

Components are soft palate, uvula, and anterior tonsillar pillar together form the faucial arch.

Characteristics of the Palatine Arch Carcinoma

- Carcinomas of palatine arch are of a squamous variety
- Superficial spreading lesions
- Well-differentiated lesions
- Late tendency for nodal metastases

Characteristics of the Carcinoma of the Posterior and Lateral Pharyngeal Wall

- Asymptomatic lesions
- Spread submucosally to the adjacent areas, such as the tonsil, soft palate, and tongue.

- May invade parapharyngeal space/anterior spinal ligament
- 60% have lymph node metastases. Bilateral lymph nodes common
- Surgical access to the lesion is through lateral pharyngotomy with/without mandibular osteotomy.

Most Common Sites for Minor Salivary Gland (MiSG) Tumors in Oropharynx

Hard palate and soft palate are the most common sites for in minor salivary gland oropharynx (**Fig. 6**).

Parapharyngeal Space Tumors

Q. Write a short note on tumors affecting parapharyngeal space.

Parapharyngeal Space (PPS) Tumors which Mimic as Oropharyngeal Tumors

- Deep lobe parotid tumors
- Neurilemmoma
- Carotid body tumor
- Lipoma
- Aneurysm of internal carotid artery

Common Tumors of Parapharyngeal Space Seen Clinically

- Salivary gland tumors, i.e., pleomorphic adenomas
- Paragangliomas
- Carotid body tumors
- Schwannomas, i.e., vagal schwannomas
- Metastases to the parapharyngeal space

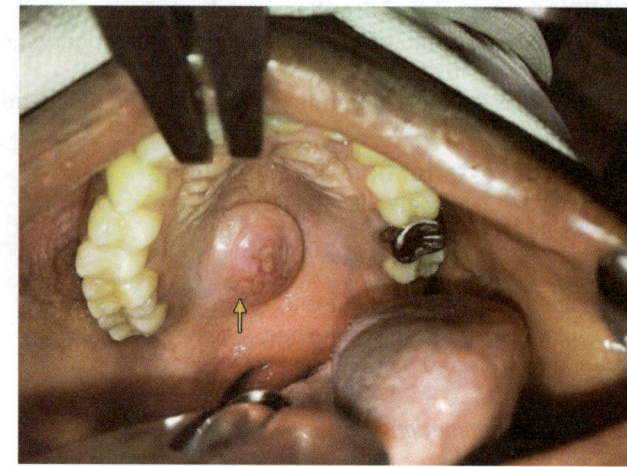

Fig. 6: Minor salivary gland tumor of hard palate (arrow).

Most Common Salivary Gland Tumors of the Parapharyngeal Space

The majority are benign lesions and pleomorphic adenomas are the most common salivary gland tumors of the parapharyngeal space (**Figs. 7 and 8**).

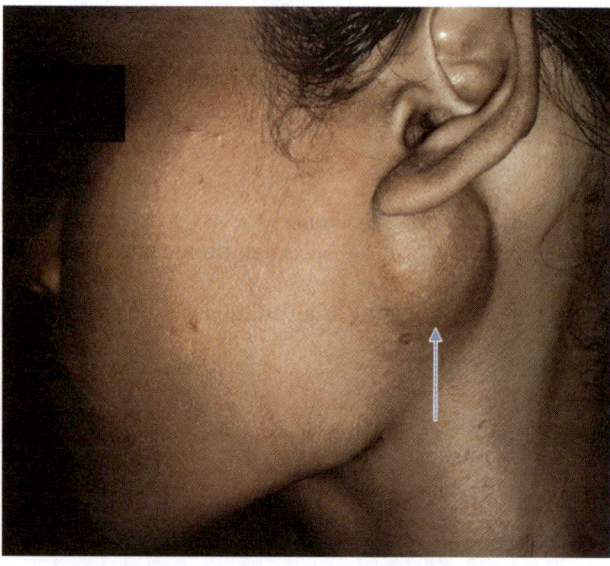

Fig. 7: Pleomorphic adenomas (arrow).

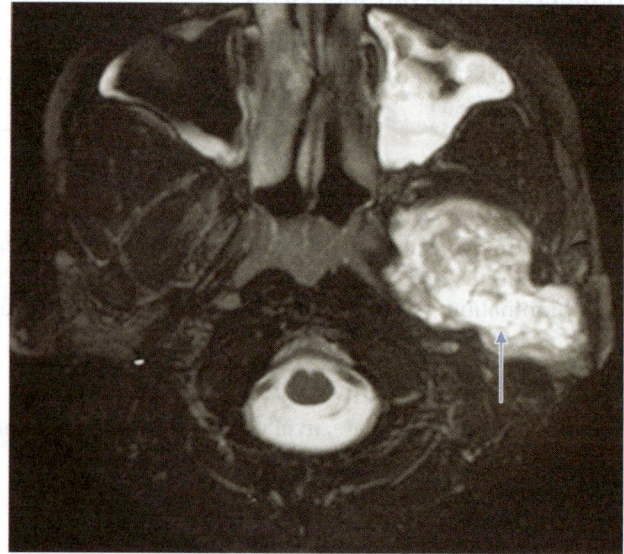

Fig. 8: Magnetic resonance imaging (MRI) of the neck showing pleomorphic adenomas (arrow).

Most Common Neurogenic Tumors of the Parapharyngeal Space

Paragangliomas are the most common neurogenic tumors of the parapharyngeal space.

CHAPTER 37: Tumors of Nasopharynx, Hypopharynx, Oropharynx and Pharyngeal Pouch

Features

- The most common metastases to the parapharyngeal space are from the nasopharyngeal cancer.
- The presence of a fat plane between the parotid and a lesion/tumor differentiates a truly PPS lesion from an extension of a deep lobe parotid lesion.

Clinical Presentation

An asymptomatic neck mass (size = 3 cm) or an intraoral mass by medial displacement of the superior pole of the palatine tonsil.

- Nasal obstruction/snoring
- Hearing loss due to ET obstruction
- Cranial nerve dysfunction—hoarseness, dysphagia, and cough
- *Paragangliomas:* Paragangliomas arise from the paraganglia along the arterial and vasculature and cranial nerves from the skull base to the aortic arch. Paragangliomas show vascularity and a "salt and paper" appearance on MRI.
- Carotid body tumors cause displacement of the angle between the internal and external carotid arteries known as Lyre's sign.
- The vagus nerve is the origin of 50% of the parapharyngeal space schwannomas and the cervical sympathetic chain is the next common source.

Surgical Approaches to Treat Parapharyngeal Space Tumors

- Transcervical
- Transcervical—transparotid
- Mandibulotomy
- Transoral robotic surgery (TORS)—used for true prestyloid benign salivary gland tumor.

> **EN4.42:** Describe the clinical features, investigations and principles of management of malignancy of the larynx and hypopharynx.

TUMORS OF THE HYPOPHARYNX AND THE PHARYNGEAL POUCH

Types

Q. Enumerate the benign and malignant lesions of the hypopharynx.

Benign lesions	Malignant lesions
❖ Papilloma ❖ Adenoma ❖ Lipoma ❖ Fibroma ❖ Leiomyoma	Squamous cell carcinoma

Various Subsites of Carcinoma of the Hypopharynx

- Pyriform sinus (PFS)
- Postcricoid region (PCR)
- Posterior pharyngeal wall (PPW)

Most Common Carcinoma of the Hypopharynx

Pyriform sinus (PFS) cancer is the most common—constitutes 60% of all hypopharyngeal cancers.

Carcinoma of Pyriform Sinus

Q. Write short note on the spread of the carcinoma of the pyriform sinus, its clinical features and management.

Spread

Local spread:

- Superiorly—vallecula and base of tongue
- Inferiorly—postcricoid region
- Medially—aryepiglottic fold and ventricle
- May infiltrate thyroid cartilage, thyroid gland
- May also present as a soft tissue mass in the neck

Lymphatic spread: Cervical lymph nodes—upper and middle group of jugular nodes

Distant metastases: Metastases to lung, liver, and bones.

Clinical Features

- ❖ **Symptoms**
  - ➢ Sticking sensation in the throat
  - ➢ Pricking sensation on swallowing
  - ➢ Dysphagia/odynophagia
  - ➢ Referred otalgia
  - ➢ Mass of lymph nodes in the neck
  - ➢ Hoarseness and laryngeal obstruction
- ❖ **Signs on clinical examination (Fig. 9):**
  - ➢ Exophytic/ulcerative and deep infiltrative growth were seen on direct laryngoscopy/endoscopy.
  - ➢ Pooling of saliva in the pyriform fossa.

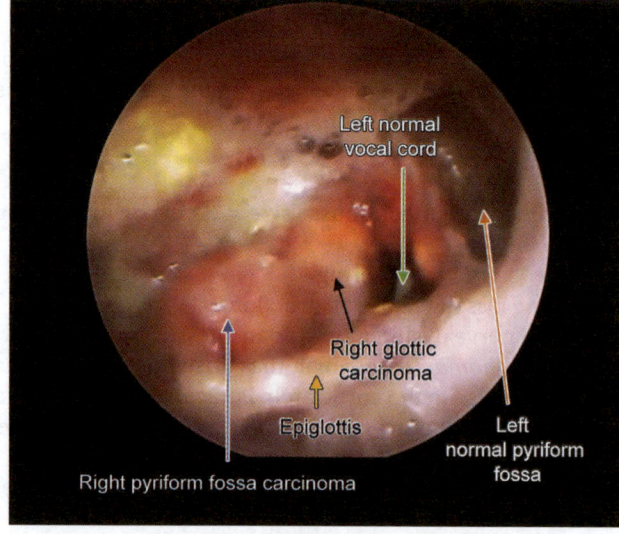

Fig. 9: Carcinoma of right pyriform fossa and right glottic carcinoma with pooling of saliva (yellow arrow).

Management

Work Up

- ❖ CT scan with contrast
- ❖ Barium swallow to evaluate the extent of the growth and status of lymph nodes.
- ❖ Direct laryngoscopy/endoscopy to take a biopsy of the lesion and send it for HPE; also, to rule out synchronous primary if any in the aerodigestive tract.

Treatment

- ❖ Early growth without nodes—radiotherapy
- ❖ Growth limited to pyriform fossa and not extending to postcricoid region—total laryngectomy (TL) + partial pharyngectomy + neck dissection (positive nodes).
  In case of N0 neck, RT can be given to the neck instead of neck dissection.
- ❖ If growth extends to pyriform sinus—total laryngectomy + total pharyngectomy + neck dissection + reconstruction of the pharyngoesophageal segment + stomach pull-up

Carcinoma of the Postcricoid Region

Q. Write a short note on carcinoma of postcricoid region.

Risk Factor

Plummer–Vinson syndrome/Paterson–Brown–Kelly syndrome **(Fig. 10)**

Spread of the Carcinoma of the Postcricoid Region

The ulcerative type of lesion spreads in an annular fashion causing dysphagia and invading the cervical esophagus, arytenoids, or recurrent laryngeal nerve (RLN).

Lymphatic spread—paratracheal lymph nodes are involved bilaterally.

Clinical Features

- ❖ Females > males. Age group affected—20–30
- ❖ Progressive dysphagia
- ❖ Progressive malnutrition and weight loss
- ❖ Voice change and aphonia—due to infiltration of RLN/postcricoarytenoid muscle.

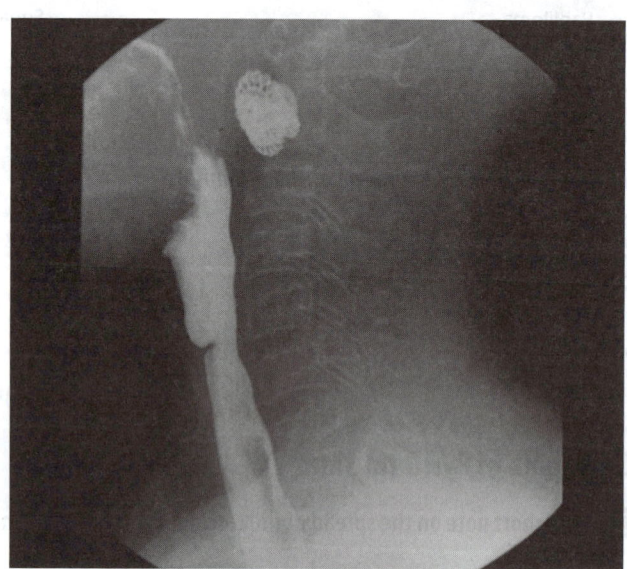

Fig. 10: Barium swallow showing cervical esophageal web in Plummer–Vinson syndrome.

Investigations and Examination

- Growth is visible on direct laryngoscopy/endoscopy
- Edema and erythema with pooling of secretions in the hypopharynx
- Laryngeal crepitus is lost
- Lateral neck soft tissue radiograph shows an increased prevertebral shadow.
- Barium swallow—to find out the lower extent of the growth
- Endoscopy—to take the biopsy and assess the extent of the growth

Treatment

- Radiotherapy (RT)—advantage of preserving the laryngeal function
- If radiotherapy fails, then—laryngo-pharyngo-esophagectomy with the stomach—pull up or colon transposition.

Carcinoma of the Posterior Pharyngeal Wall

Carcinoma of the posterior pharyngeal wall constitutes only 10% of all the laryngopharyngeal malignancies and is least common.

Treatment

- Treatment of choice—RT
- Small lesions—lateral pharyngotomy and primary repair
- Extensive lesions—laryngo-pharyngo-esophagectomy with neck dissection with the repair of esophagus.

Pharyngeal Pouch

Q. Write a short note on pharyngeal pouch.

- **Synonyms:**
  - Hypopharyngeal diverticulum
  - Zenker's diverticulum
- It is a ***pulsion diverticulum*** type diverticulum where pharyngeal mucosa herniates through the Killian's dehiscence—a potential weak area between two parts of the inferior constrictor muscle.
- **Etiology:** It is probably due to the spasm of the cricopharyngeal sphincter or due to its incoordinated contractions during the act of deglutition.
- **Age group:** >60 years of age

Clinical Features of the Pharyngeal Pouch

- Dysphagia when the pouch is filled with food presses on the esophagus
- A gurgling sound is produced on swallowing
- Undigested food may regurgitate at night
- Cough and pneumonia
- Malnourished
- Patients may have associated hiatus hernia
- Carcinoma may develop in longstanding pouch cases

Management

Diagnosis

Barium swallow or esophagography

Treatment

Options are as follows:

- Excision of the pouch **and cricopharyngeal myotomy—**done by cervical approach.
- **Dohlman's procedure**—partition wall between pouch and esophagus is divided by diathermy through an endoscope.
- Endoscopic laser treatment—the partition between the pouch and esophagus is divided with **CO_2 laser.**

Chapter 38

Laryngotracheal Trauma

EN4.30: Describe the clinical features, investigations and principles of management of trauma to the face and neck.

■ INTRODUCTION

Q. Write an essay on laryngotracheal trauma/trauma to neck. How do you classify laryngotracheal trauma? Discuss its clinical features and management.

It may be → Penetrating trauma
         → Blunt trauma

Location: Supraglottic/glottic/subglottic

■ ETIOLOGY

- Automobile accidents → most common cause
- Blow or kick on the neck
- Assault
- Strangulation
- Near hanging
- Clothesline-type injury (neck striking against a stretched wire or cable)
- Penetrating injuries with sharp objects or gunshot wounds.
- Iatrogenic injury → bronchoscopy, emergency intubation, and percutaneous tracheostomy

■ PATHOLOGY

- The degree and severity of damage vary from slight bruises externally or tear and laceration internally to a comminuted fracture of the laryngeal framework.
- Laryngeal fractures are common after 40 years of age because of the calcification of the laryngeal framework.
- In children, cartilages are more resilient and escape injury.
- **Pathological changes that may be seen:**
  - Hematoma and edema of supraglottic or subglottic region
  - Tear in the laryngeal or pharyngeal mucosa
  - Dislocation of cricoarytenoid joint
  - Dislocation of cricothyroid joint
  - Fracture of the hyoid bone
  - Fracture of thyroid cartilage
  - Fracture of the cricoid cartilage
  - Tracheal tear
  - Injury to recurrent laryngeal nerve, internal jugular vein (IJV), carotid artery, and muscles
  - Laryngotracheal separation

CHAPTER 38: Laryngotracheal Trauma

SCHAEFER CLASSIFICATION OF LARYNGOTRACHEAL TRAUMA

Group	Injury
I	Minor endolaryngeal hematoma or laceration without fracture
II	Severe edema, hematoma, nondisplaced fracture, or minor mucosal disruption without exposed cartilage
III	Massive edema, large mucosal lacerations, displaced fracture, or vocal cord immobilization with exposed cartilage
IV	Severe disruption of the anterior larynx, unstable fractures, two or more fracture lines, and extension mucosal injuries
V	Complete laryngotracheal separation

CLINICAL FEATURES

Symptoms	Signs
❖ Pain in the anterior neck ❖ Hoarseness of voice or aphonia ❖ Respiratory distress ❖ Dysphagia ❖ Odynophagia ❖ Aspiration of food ❖ Hemoptysis	❖ Bruises or abrasions or lacerations over the skin (**Figs. 1 and 2**) ❖ Tenderness on palpation of anterior larynx ❖ Subcutaneous emphysema ❖ Loss of normal thyroid prominence ❖ Distorted contour of the anterior larynx ❖ Fracture displacement of thyroid cartilage/cricoid cartilage/hyoid bone ❖ Bony crepitus ❖ Separation of cricoid cartilage from larynx/trachea (**Figs. 3A and B**)

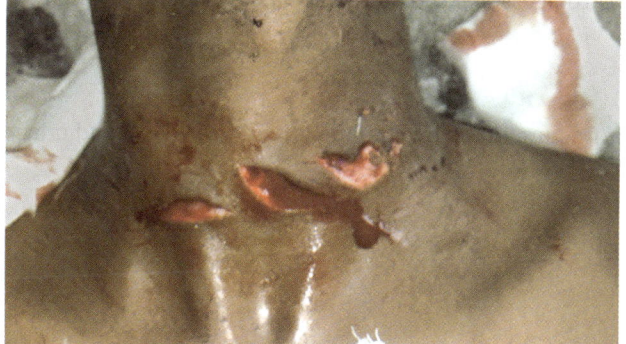

Fig. 1: Neck trauma.

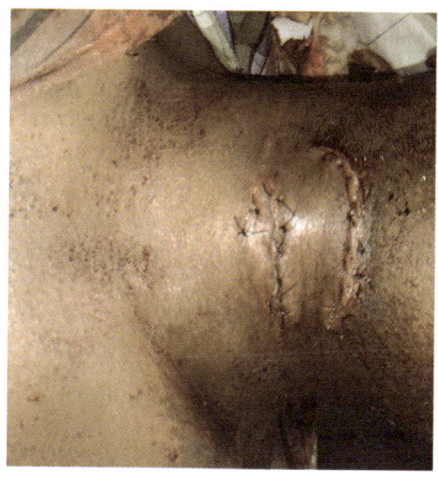

Fig. 2: Neck trauma and sutured lacerated wound.

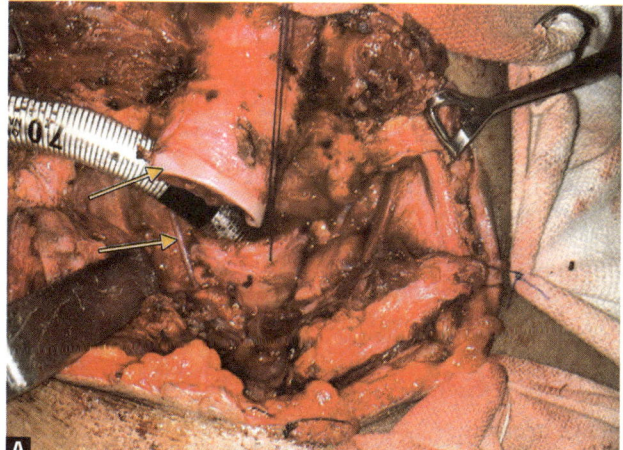
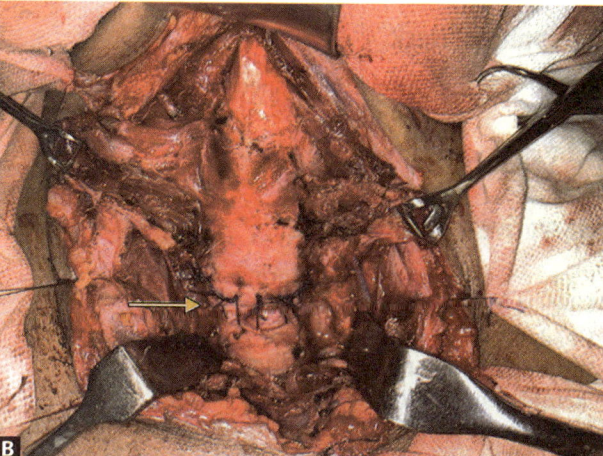

Figs. 3A and B: Tracheal resection anastomosis in complete tracheal transection.

DIAGNOSTIC EVALUATION

History
- Blunt or penetrating
- Time since injury
- What are the presenting symptoms?
- Other associated injuries, such as head, chest, cervical, abdomen, and limbs.

Examination
- Assessment of airway status/general condition
- Look for the signs (mentioned above)
- Rule out cervical spinal injuries
- In case of penetrating neck injury → look for depth of wound/soiled wound or clean. Wound/active bleeding/artery injury/muscle injury/exposed cartilage.
- If airway is stable → do indirect laryngoscopy (IDL) to rule out vocal cord palsy → flexible laryngoscopy examination to visualize larynx and pharynx.

Indirect Laryngoscopy
This can identify edema/hematoma/mucosal tears/exposed cartilage/vocal cords mobility/displacement of epiglottis/asymmetry glottis, or laryngeal inlet.

Flexible Laryngoscopy
- Give better visualization of internal mucosal structure of larynx/pharynx
- This can identify edema/hematoma/mucosal tears/exposed cartilage/vocal cords mobility/displacement of epiglottis/asymmetry glottis or laryngeal inlet.

X-ray Neck Lateral View
May show subcutaneous emphysema/displacement of epiglottis/fracture of the hyoid bone, thyroid cartilage, and cricoid cartilage.

Barium Swallow
- To rule out associated esophageal injury
- Not routinely done

Computed Tomography
Gives better visualization of bony and cartilaginous structures.

USG Doppler of Neck
It is to rule out any vessel injury especially in penetrating wounds.

TREATMENT

Conservative Measures
- Close observation and monitoring of vitals
- Voice rest
- Head end elevation
- Humidification of inspired air
- Steroid nebulization
- Intravenous (IV) antibiotic → to prevent perichondritis/cartilage necrosis.
- IV steroid → to resolve edema, hematoma, and prevent scarring and stenosis.
- Serial laryngoscopy

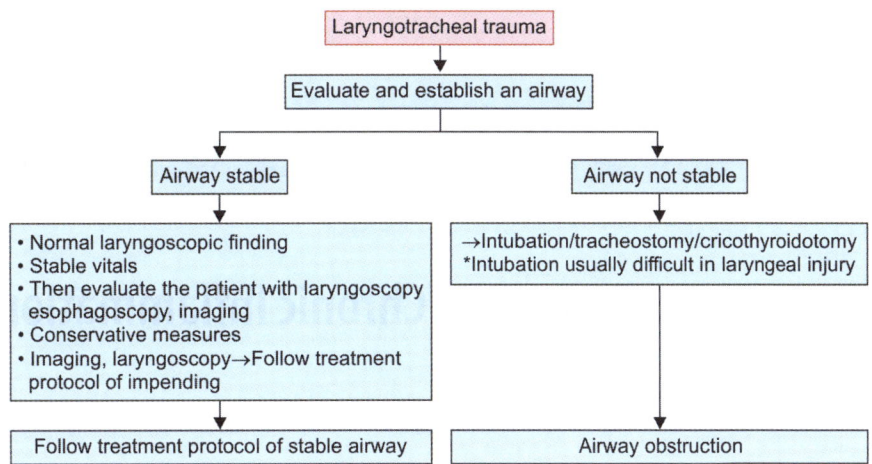

Impending Airway Obstruction Treatment Protocol

Surgery → to be done 3–5 days after injury and should not be delayed beyond 10 days.

1. Normal endolarynx or mucosal injury without fracture	→ Observation
2. Thyroid/cricoid fracture with intact endolarynx	→ Neck exploration, open reduction and internal fixation (ORIF) of laryngeal skeletal fractures with plating without thyrotomy
3. Unstable fracture or anterior commissure disrupted or major mucosal lacerations	→ ORIF of fractures, repair of mucosal lacerations, and endolaryngeal stent.
4. Stable fracture, anterior commissure intact, and minor mucosal injury	→ Neck exploration, ORIF of laryngeal fractures with plating thyrotomy with primary closure of laceration

Stable Airway Treatment Protocol

1. Normal endolarynx with/without reversible mucosal injury without fracture	→ Observation
2. Endolarynx or cartilage disruption	→ Tracheostomy or intubation, neck exploration, and repair of findings as under impending airway obstruction

Schaefer I and II injuries	Schaefer III–V
Conservative measures	Surgical intervention

■ POSTOPERATIVE

- ❖ Monitor in intensive care unit for one night
- ❖ Feeding tube until the larynx is healed
- ❖ Voice rest
- ❖ Head end elevation
- ❖ Antibiotics, analgesics, and steroids
- ❖ Regular dressing

■ REHABILITATION CARE

- ❖ Swallowing therapy
- ❖ Speech therapy
- ❖ Tracheostomy care and dressing

■ COMPLICATIONS

- ❖ Cicatrix formation
- ❖ Laryngeal stenosis (supraglottic/glottic/subglottic)
- ❖ Perichondritis and laryngeal abscess
- ❖ Vocal cord palsy
- ❖ Tracheocutaneous/laryngocutaneous fistula (rare)

Chapter 39

Acute and Chronic Inflammation of Larynx

EN4.41: Describe the clinical features, investigations and principles of management of acute and chronic inflammation of larynx.

LARYNGITIS

Q. Define and classify laryngitis.

Definition: Inflammation of the larynx.

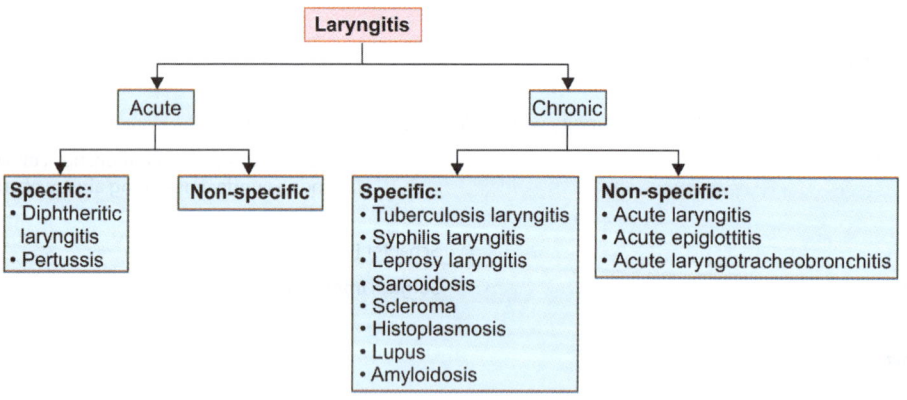

ACUTE LARYNGITIS

Q. Write a short note/essay on acute laryngitis.

It is more common in adults than children.

Infectious

- More common
- Usually follows the upper respiratory tract infection.
- **Etiology:**
  - Viral → The most common cause:
    - Examples: Rhinovirus, parainfluenza virus, respiratory syncytial virus, coronavirus, adenovirus, and influenza virus.

- Bacterial → As superinfection:
  - Examples: *Streptococcus pneumoniae, Haemophilus influenzae, Moraxella catarrhalis,* and *Staphylococcus aureus*.
    - Exanthematous febrile illnesses:
      - Measles, chickenpox, and whooping cough are also associated with acute laryngitis.
- Fungal → It is rare in immunocompetent individuals
- It more often presents as chronic laryngitis in the immunocompromised individuals or in patients using inhaled steroid medications.

Noninfectious

Etiology

- Vocal abuse
- Vocal trauma
- Vocal misuse
- Allergy
- Gastroesophageal reflux disease (GERD)
- Asthma
- Environmental pollution
- Smoking
- Inhalational injuries
- Chemical injuries

Clinical Features

- Resolves within 2 weeks
- If persistent → either due to superinfection or transition into a chronic form
- Change in voice, aphonia → later stage
- Discomfort and pain in the throat particularly after talking
- Dysphagia
- Odynophagia
- Dry cough, and throat irritation which is usually worse at night
- Frequent throat clearing
- Malaise
- Fever
- Early voice fatigue

Diagnosis

- **History**
  - Voice abuse/trauma/misuse
  - Upper respiratory illness
  - GERD
  - Sick contact
  - Immunization status
  - Allergy
  - Travel history
- **Examination of larynx**
  Indirect laryngoscopy/flexible laryngoscopy
  - Appearance varies with the severity of the disease.
  - Early stage → erythema and edema of the epiglottis/arytenoids/aryepiglottic folds/vocal cords.
  - Later → vocal cords become erythematous and edematous
  - Sticky, ropy, and secretions may also be seen between the vocal cords and in the interarytenoid region.
  - Vocal abuse/misuse history + → Reinke's edema and submucosal hemorrhage.

Treatment

- Voice rest
- Steam inhalation with tincture benzoin, menthol, or eucalyptus oil for smoothing effect and loosening viscid secretion.
- Avoidance of irritants (smoking/alcohol)
- Dietary modification
  - For a patient with GERD.
  - Avoid hot and spicy foods and fatty foods.
  - Avoid late meals.

- ❖ Medications
  - ▷ *Antibiotic:* To combat secondary infection
  - ▷ *Anti-inflammatory:* To reduce inflammation
  - ▷ *Steroid:* To reduce edema and inflammation
  - ▷ *Fungal laryngitis:* Antifungal (fluconazole)
  - ▷ Antireflux medication
  - ▷ *Cough lozenges:* To suppress irritating cough
  - ▷ Mucolytic to clear the secretion
- ❖ Tracheostomy
  - ▷ In small children, it may be a life-saving
  - ▷ It is temporary, until edema/congestion/stridor resolve

Acute Epiglottitis

Also known as supraglottic laryngitis

Q. Write short note on acute epiglottitis/supraglottic laryngitis.

Definition

- ❖ Inflammatory condition of the epiglottitis and/or nearby structures such as the arytenoids, aryepiglottic folds, and vallecula.
- ❖ Life-threatening condition → profound swelling of the upper airways → lead to asphyxia and respiratory arrest → death.

Etiology

- ❖ It is same as that of acute laryngitis.
- ❖ Affects children of 2–7 years of age but can also affect adults.
- ❖ The most commonly infectious (bacterial/viral/fungal).
- ❖ In children → *Haemophilus influenzae* type B (HiB) most common cause.
- ❖ Viruses do not cause epiglottitis, a prior viral infection may allow bacterial superinfection to develop.
- ❖ In immunocompromised patients, *Pseudomonas aeruginosa* and *Candida*.

Pathophysiology

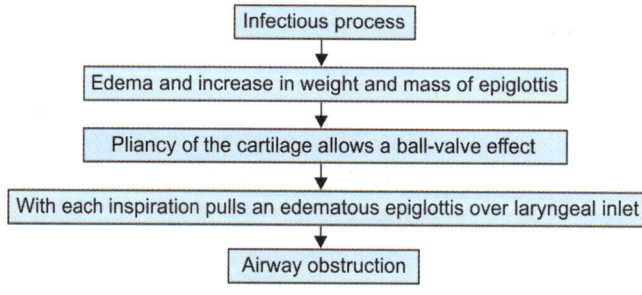

Q. Why more severe and symptomatic in pediatric age groups?

- ❖ Infant epiglottis is comprised of cartilage which is more pliant when compared to that of an adult which is more rigid.
- ❖ In a young child, the epiglottis is located more superiorly and anteriorly than in an adult.
- ❖ More oblique angle with the trachea in children.

Clinical Features

- ❖ Abrupt onset with rapid progression
- ❖ Sore throat
- ❖ 3 D's
  - ▷ Dysphagia
  - ▷ Drooling
  - ▷ Distress
- ❖ Stridor
- ❖ High fever
- ❖ Signs of septicemia

- ❖ **Tripod position** (sitting upright and leaning forward)
- ❖ **Signs**:
  - ▷ Intercostal retraction or suprasternal retraction
  - ▷ Tachypnea
  - ▷ Cyanosis
  - ▷ Nasal flaring
  - ▷ Lymphadenopathy

Diagnosis

- ❖ **Mainly clinical basis.**
- ❖ **Oropharyngeal examination:**
  - ▷ With tongue depressor → red and swollen epiglottis may be visualized
  - ▷ Indirect laryngoscopy → edema and congestion of supraglottic structures
- ❖ It is better to avoid this examination for risk of symptoms of precipitation
- ❖ Lateral soft tissue X-ray of neck → swollen epiglottis (**thumb sign**)
- ❖ **X-ray chest:** To rule out concomitant pneumonia
- ❖ **Computed tomography (CT) scan of the neck:** It is rarely needed. The supine position can precipitate disaster
- ❖ **Ultrasonography (USG) neck:** P-sign appearance in a longitudinal view.
- ❖ **Complete blood count:** Raise white blood cells (WBC) count. Raise erythrocyte sedimentation rate (ESR) level
- ❖ Blood culture
- ❖ Epiglottal culture once the airway is secured

Treatment

- ❖ Hospitalization and secure the airway (intubation or tracheostomy).
- ❖ **Intravenous (IV) antibiotic:** Ampicillin, 3rd generation cephalosporin.
- ❖ **IV steroid:** Hydrocortisone and dexamethasone
- ❖ Adequate hydration
- ❖ Humidification and oxygen
- ❖ HiB immunization
- ❖ Keep the patient in a propped-up position
- ❖ **Avoid the supine position:** Risk of precipitate of symptoms

Complications

- ❖ Cellulitis
- ❖ Cervical adenitis
- ❖ Empyema
- ❖ Epiglottic abscess
- ❖ Meningitis
- ❖ Pneumonia
- ❖ Septic shock
- ❖ Prolong intubation
- ❖ Tracheostomy
- ❖ Death

Acute Laryngotracheobronchitis

Also known as croup

Q. Write short note/essay on croup/acute laryngotracheobronchitis.

Definition

Inflammatory condition of larynx, trachea, and bronchi.

Etiology

- ❖ The most common viral infection
  - ▷ Parainfluenza type I and II virus → most common
  - ▷ *Other viruses:* Respiratory syncytial virus (RSV), rhinovirus, *Enterovirus*, influenza virus, and adenovirus.
- ❖ **Age group:** 6 months to 6 years.
- ❖ **Peak incidence:** 12 months to 2 years.
- ❖ **The most common location:** Subglottic

- Male are more often affected
- Secondary bacterial infection by gram-positive cocci

Pathophysiology

- Inhalation of the virus → First, it infects the nasal and pharyngeal areas → spread to the subglottic space (the most narrow part of the airway in children) → inflamed subglottic mucosa → edema → respiratory obstruction. This may get coupled with thick tenacious secretions and crusts which might lead to complete airway obstruction.
- When a child cries or becomes agitated, further dynamic obstruction occurs.
- Extension into the bronchi leads to wheezing, crackles, air trapping, and increased tachypnea and may get confused with acute asthma.

Clinical Features

- Barking cough or seal-like cough
- Hoarseness of voice
- Fever
- Respiratory distress
- Inspiratory stridor (high pitched)
- Signs:
    - Intercostal retraction or suprasternal retraction
    - Tachypnea
    - Cyanosis
    - Nasal flaring
    - Lymphadenopathy

Diagnosis

- Mainly clinical basis.
- Rule out other causes of stridor.
- **X-ray neck and chest: Steeple sign** (due to subglottic narrowing) on anteroposterior (AP) view of the neck.
- **Chest auscultation:** Wheezing, crackles, and decreased air movement.
- **Chest examination:** Intercostal and suprasternal retraction and tachypnea.

Treatment

- Hospitalization and securing the airway
- **IV antibiotic:** Ampicillin is effective against gram-positive cocci and *H. influenzae*
- IV or oral corticosteroids to relieve edema
- IV fluids to combat dehydration
- Oxygen supplement
- Humidification to soften crust and tenacious secretions
- **Adrenaline nebulization:** Bronchodilator
    - For moderate and severe croup.
- **Observation:** 3 hourly observations after each dose of nebulized racemic adrenaline.
- Intubation/tracheostomy for severe croup, not responding to medical treatment.

Types	Symptoms	Treatment
Mild croup	Barky cough with or without stridor, with agitation	- One dose to steroids - Discharge - Follow-up strictly
Moderate croup	Barky cough with stridor, with or without increased work of breathing	- Steroids - Nebulization with adrenaline - Observation and reassess after 3 hours
Severe croup	Barky cough, stridor at rest, and prominent increased work of breathing	- Steroids - Nebulization with adrenaline - Observation and reassess after 3 hours. - Intubation/tracheostomy

CHAPTER 39: Acute and Chronic Inflammation of Larynx

Complication: Rare

- Secondary bacterial infection
- Pneumothorax
- Dehydration
- Lymphadenitis

Difference between acute epiglottis and acute laryngotracheobronchitis

	Acute epiglottitis	Acute laryngotracheobronchitis
Age	2–7 years	6 months to 6 years
Onset	Rapid	Gradual
Causative organism	*Haemophilus influenzae* type B	Parainfluenza virus type I and II
Voice	Normal	Hoarse
Location	Supraglottic area	Subglottic area
Fever	High	Low grade
Cough	Usually absent	Barking cough
Patient's look	Toxic	Nontoxic
Chest auscultation	No wheezing	Wheezing
Odynophagia	Present with drooling	Usually absent
Radiology	Thumb sign on the lateral view	Steeple sign on AP view
Treatment	Humidified O_2, third generation cephalosporin	Humidified O_2, steroids

Diphtheritic Laryngitis

Also known as laryngeal diphtheria

Q. Write a short note/essay on laryngeal diphtheria/diphtheritic laryngitis.

Definition

- Infection of the larynx with *Corynebacterium diphtheriae (C. diphtheriae)*.
- It is usually secondary to faucial diphtheria.

Etiology

- Mostly secondary to faucial diphtheria.
- **Causative organism:** *C. diphtheriae*
- Affects children below 10 years of age.
- **Widespread immunization:** Less incidence now.

Pathology

- Formation of a tough grayish-white pseudomembrane over the larynx and trachea which may obstruct the airway.
- Exotoxins liberated by bacteria leading to myocarditis and various neurological complications.

Clinical Features

Symptoms

General Symptoms

- Low-grade fever
- Sore throat
- Malaise
- The patient is toxic with tachycardia and thready pulse

Laryngeal Symptoms

- Hoarseness of voice
- Croupy cough
- Inspiratory stridor
- Dyspnea

Signs

- A grayish-white membrane is seen on the tonsil, soft palate, pharynx, and larynx. It is adherent and removal leaves a bleeding surface
- Cervical lymphadenopathy

Diagnosis

- The diagnosis is mainly clinical.
- It is confirmed by smear and culture of *C. diphtheriae* from the laryngeal swab.

Treatment

Diphtheria antitoxin: 20,000–100,000 units IV with saline infusion after a test dose.

It neutralizes free toxins circulating in the blood.

- **Antibiotic:** Penicillin is effective against diphtheria. Erythromycin to those who are allergic to penicillin.
- **Airway maintenance and prevention of aspiration:** Intubation or tracheostomy.
- It is better to avoid intubation as it can push the membrane or its fragments into the lower respiratory tract.
- Oxygenation and IV nutrition
- Steroid to reduce laryngeal edema
- Direct laryngoscopic assisted removal of a diphtheritic membrane can be tried.
- Complete bed rest for 2–4 weeks to guard against the effects of myocarditis.
- Immunization of close contact

Complications

- Asphyxia and death
- Toxic myocarditis
- Arrhythmias
- Palatal paralysis
- Laryngeal and pharyngeal paralysis

Pertussis

Also known as whooping cough

Q. Write a short note on whooping cough/pertussis.

Definition

- Acute spasmodic cough of 3 or more week's duration.
- Notifiable communicable disease transmitted by cough and sneezing.

Etiology

- Gram negative bacillus → *Bordetella pertussis*.
- Affects all age, more severe in infants.
- Endotoxins and exotoxins produced by the bacteria induce an inflammatory response.

Clinical Features

- Prolong paroxysmal cough followed by gasping and whoop.
- Runny nose, dry cough, mild fever, similar to a common cold.

Diagnosis

- Serum serology.
- **Nasopharyngeal culture and assay:** Polymerase chain reaction (PCR).

Treatment

- Antibiotic:
  - 7–14 days course of erythromycin: Drug of choice (DOC).
  - Other: Clarithromycin and azithromycin.
  - Prophylaxis to the family members.
- Cough suppressants
- Steroids
- Immunoglobulin
- Antihistaminic or leukotriene receptor antagonists

Edema of Larynx

Also known as edema glottidis

Q. Write a short note/essay on edema of larynx/edema glottidis.

Edema of laryngeal mucosa can accompany any inflammatory condition therefore not a specific disease but rather a sign.

Common Location

- Supraglottic and subglottic → loose laryngeal mucosa.
- Edema of vocal cords occurs rarely → sparse subepithelial connective tissue.

Etiology

- **Infection**
  - Acute epiglottitis
  - Acute laryngotracheobronchitis
  - Tuberculosis of larynx
  - Syphilis of larynx
  - Infection in nearby structures—peritonsillar abscess, retropharyngeal abscess, and Ludwig's angina.
- **Trauma**
  - Surgery of tongue/floor of the mouth
  - Laryngeal trauma during intubation/**by ingested foreign body**/during laryngoscopy
  - Thermal and caustic burns
  - Inhalational burns with irritant gases/fumes
- Neoplasm of the larynx
- **Allergy:** Angioneurotic edema or anaphylaxis
- Radiation exposure
- **Systemic illness:** Heart failure/nephritis/myxedema

Clinical Features

- Airway obstruction
- Inspiratory stridor
- Laryngoscopic finding—edema of the supraglottic or subglottic region

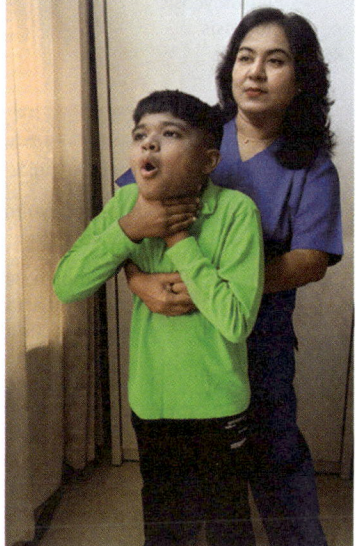

Fig. 1: Heimlich maneuver steps.

Treatment

- If stridor → **intubation/tracheostomy**
- Injection of adrenaline (1:1,000) 0.3–0.5 mL intramuscular (IM) → useful in allergic/angioneurotic edema.
- Repeat after 15 minutes if needed
- Steroids → they are useful in all the acute inflammatory conditions of larynx/trauma of larynx/allergic/postradiation.
- **Heimlich maneuver** is used for choking due to a foreign body in the airway and life is endangered. It helps in dislodging the foreign body in the throat. It is also called abdominal thrust it elevates the diaphragm and expels foreign bodies from the lungs (**Figs. 1 and 2**).
  - Get the person to stand
  - Position yourself behind the person
  - Lean the person forward and give five blows to their back with the heel of your hand
  - Place your arms around their waist
  - Make a fist and place it just above the navel, and thumb side in
  - Grab the fist with your other hand and push it inward and upward at the same time. Perform five of these abdominal thrusts
  - Repeat until the object is expelled and the person can breathe or cough on their own

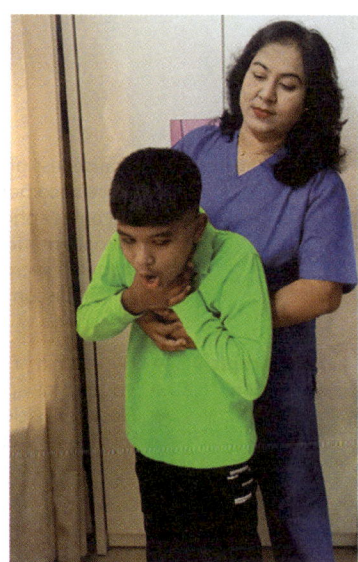

Fig 2: Choking and Heimlich maneuver steps.

CHRONIC LARYNGITIS

Q. Write an essay on chronic laryngitis and discuss its various types in brief.

Q. Write short note on (a) chronic hyperemic laryngitis/chronic laryngitis without hyperplasia, (b) Chronic hypertrophic laryngitis/chronic hyperplastic laryngitis.

Laryngitis >3 Weeks

Chronic specific laryngitis	Chronic nonspecific laryngitis

❖ Tuberculous laryngitis
❖ Syphilitic laryngitis
❖ Leprous laryngitis
❖ Lupus of the larynx
❖ Scleroma of larynx
❖ Fungal infection of the larynx
   ➢ Histoplasmosis
   ➢ Blastomycosis
❖ Amyloidosis
❖ Sarcoidosis
	❖ Chronic hyperemic laryngitis
	❖ Chronic hypertrophic laryngitis
	❖ Atrophic laryngitis (laryngitis sicca)
	❖ Pachydermia larynges
	❖ Leukoplakia or hyperkeratosis of the larynx

	Chronic hyperemic laryngitis	Chronic hypertrophic laryngitis
Also known as	Chronic laryngitis without hyperplasia	Chronic hyperplastic laryngitis
Definition	Diffuse and symmetrical inflammatory condition of the whole larynx	It may be either diffuse or localized and symmetrical, and may appear like a tumor later on
Etiology	❖ Incomplete resolution of acute laryngitis or its recurrent attacks. ❖ Septic focus in sinusitis, chronic tonsillitis, dental sepsis, and nasal catarrh may cause laryngitis. ❖ Smoking and alcohol. ❖ Vocal abuse/trauma/misuse. For example, teachers, hawkers, anchors, singers, actors, etc. ❖ Allergy to pollution, dust, chemical fumes, etc. ❖ Excessive chronic cough as seen in chronic bronchitis.	Same
Pathology		❖ Initially → hyperemia, edema, and cellular infiltration in the submucosa ❖ Ciliated respiratory mucosa changes to the squamous type and squamous epithelium of the vocal cords undergo hyperplasia and keratinization. ❖ Mucous gland becomes hypertrophy initially but then undergoes atrophy → reduced secretion and dryness of the larynx
Clinical features	❖ Hoarseness of voice ❖ Voice becomes easily tired and the patient becomes aphonic by the end of the day ❖ Throat irritation and constant clearing due to stagnant secretion ❖ Throat discomfort ❖ Dry cough	Same
Laryngoscopic examination	❖ Hyperemia of the laryngeal mucosa ❖ Vocal cords appear dull red and rounded ❖ Flecks of viscid mucus are seen on the vocal cords and interarytenoid region	❖ Dusky red and thickened laryngeal mucosa ❖ Vocal cords appear red and swollen ❖ Ventricular bands appear red and swollen ❖ Impaired vocal cords mobility due to local infiltration and edema and later due to muscular atrophy and arthritis of the cricoarytenoid joint

Contd...

Contd...

	Chronic hyperemic laryngitis	**Chronic hypertrophic laryngitis**
Treatment	Conservative measures: ❖ Elimination of septic focus ❖ Avoidance of irritants. For example, smoking, alcohol, pollutants, dust, and fumes ❖ Voice rest ❖ Speech therapy ❖ Steam inhalation to loosen secretions and give soothing effects ❖ Cough suppressants	❖ Conservative treatment is same as for chronic hyperemic laryngitis ❖ Microlaryngoscopy surgery
Example		Dysphonia plica ventricularis, vocal nodules, vocal polyp, Reinke's edema, and contact ulcer (they have been described in the relevant sections)

Reinke's Edema

Q. Write short note on Reinke's edema.

- **Reinke's space** is the subepithelial matrix of the vocal fold mucosa composed of elastin, collagen, and other extracellular proteins (also known as superficial lamina propria).
- Accumulation of fluid in this space is known as Reinke's edema.
- It is bilateral and symmetrical.
- The common condition, constitutes about 10% of benign laryngeal lesions.

Pathology

Edema develops by degrees, as a nonspecific reaction of the vocal folds to various irritative noxious agents.

Risk Factors

- Middle aged individuals
- Female >Male
- Chronic voice abuse
- Allergy
- Infection
- Smoking
- Laryngopharyngeal reflux
- Chronic sinusitis
- Hypothyroidism
- Myxedema

Clinical Features

Hoarseness of voice, low-pitched, and rough voice.

On Indirect Laryngoscopy

Edematous swelling of the vocal cords, slightly translucent, mucosa shows polypoidal changes.

Treatment

- **Elimination of risk factors:** Cessation of smoking and antireflux medication
- Microlaryngoscopy surgery → microflap technique (recent)
  - Vocal stripping (obsolete now)
- Voice rest
- Speech therapy

Pachydermia Larynges

Also known as contact ulcer

Q. Write short note on pachydermia larynges/contact ulcer.

- It is a form of chronic hypertrophic laryngitis

- Borderline/lepromatous (B/L) and symmetrical condition
- No malignant potential
- It commonly affects the posterior part of the larynx
    - Posterior part of vocal cords
    - Interarytenoid region (posterior commissure)

Etiology

- Uncertain
- It is common in males with a history of excessive alcohol and smoking
- History of GERD
- Excessive forceful talking

Clinical Feature

Hoarseness of voice (husky voice) and throat irritation.

Laryngoscopic Finding

- Heaping up of red or gray granulation tissue in the inter-arytenoid region and posterior one-third of vocal cords.
- Ulceration due to contact rubbing of vocal processes → **contact ulcer** formation.
- Biopsy is essential to differentiate the lesion from carcinoma and TB.

Treatment

- Microlaryngoscopic guided removal of granulation tissue
- Antireflux medication
- Avoidance of alcohol/smoking
- Speech therapy

Atrophic Laryngitis

Also known as laryngitis sicca

Q. Write short note on atrophic laryngitis/laryngitis sicca.

- It is seen associated with atrophic rhinitis and pharyngitis.
- It is characterized by atrophy of laryngeal mucosa and crust formation.

Clinical Features

- Hoarseness of voice
- Dry cough
- Throat irritation
- Dyspnea

Examination

- Atrophic mucosa covered with foul-smelling crusts
- When the crust is removed → mucosal excoriation and bleeding

Treatment

- Treat the causative factors
- Humidification
- Laryngeal sprays with glucose in glycerine or oil of pine—loosening of crusts.
- Expectorants containing ammonium chloride or iodides, are also helpful to loosen the crusts.

Leprous Laryngitis

Q. Write short note on leprous laryngitis.

Definition

- Infection of the larynx by the organism *Mycobacterium leprae*.
- It is a very rare condition.

Clinical Features

- It presents as diffuse nodular infiltration of supraglottic structure, it may ulcerate.
- Dyspnea and stridor.
- Later on, laryngeal deformity and stenosis may occur.
- It is associated with nasal and skin leprosy.

Diagnosis

Biopsy from the lesion.

Treatment

Antileprosy drug therapy.

Syphilitic Laryngitis

Q. Write short note on syphilitic laryngitis.

Definition

- Infection of the larynx by the organism *Treponema pallidum*.
- It is a rare condition. **Only the tertiary stage is sometimes seen**.

Types

- **Congenital syphilis**: It rarely affects the larynx.
- Acquired syphilis
  - *Secondary syphilis:* Rare, may be seen as a serpiginous ulcer on the larynx.
  - *Tertiary syphilis:* Present as gumma on the larynx.
  - *Common location:* Anterior commissure/anterior one-third vocal cord/epiglottis.

Clinical Features

Symptoms

Hoarseness of voice, dyspnea, and stridor.

Signs

On indirect laryngoscopy:
- Diffuse hypertrophy of mucosa.
- Gummatous ulcers may be seen in the anterior aspect of the glottis or on the epiglottis
- Scarring and stenosis may be seen later

Diagnosis

- Venereal disease research laboratory (VDRL) test
- Biopsy from the lesion

Treatment

- Antisyphilitic treatment
- If stridor → tracheostomy
- If stenosis → resection and anastomosis after the active infection is treated

Tuberculous Laryngitis

Q. Write short note on tuberculous laryngitis.

Definition

Infection of the larynx by *Mycobacterium tuberculosis (M. tuberculosis)*.

Etiology

- **Age:** It is common in the middle age group (20–40 years).
- It is secondary to pulmonary tuberculosis.
  - The most common cause of laryngeal TB.
  - Occurs due to stasis of sputum after bouts of coughing.
- Infection may also reach the larynx via blood-stream or lymphatic routes.
- As a part of generalized miliary tuberculosis (rare).

Location

- It affects the posterior part of the larynx more than the anterior (stagnation of sputum).
- Parts affected are:
  - Posterior commissure
  - Ventricular bands
  - Vocal cords
  - Epiglottis

Pathology

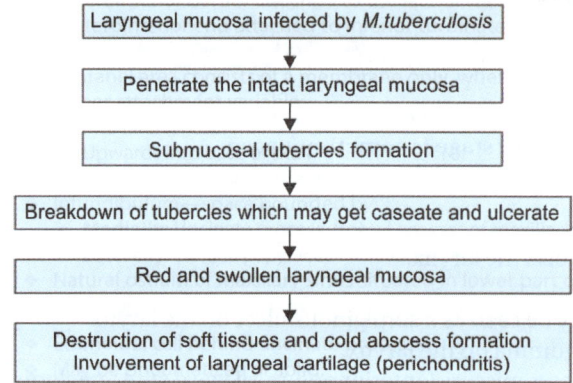

Laryngeal mucosa infected by *M.tuberculosis*
↓
Penetrate the intact laryngeal mucosa
↓
Submucosal tubercles formation
↓
Breakdown of tubercles which may get caseate and ulcerate
↓
Red and swollen laryngeal mucosa
↓
Destruction of soft tissues and cold abscess formation
Involvement of laryngeal cartilage (perichondritis)

Clinical Features

Symptoms

- Hoarseness of voice
- Intermittent weakness of voice and aphonia
- Dyspnea
- Inspiratory stridor
- Cough with expectoration
- Fever, malaise, and anorexia
- Odynophagia
- Dysphagia
- Referred otalgia
- History of pulmonary tuberculosis

Signs

Indirect laryngoscopic examination findings:
- Hyperemia of vocal cords with impaired mobility → an early sign.
- The vocal cords paresis or palsy due to local infection of muscles/recurrent laryngeal nerve (RLN)/fixation of the cricoarytenoid joint due to infection.
- A pale appearance of vocal cords with tubercles on them especially in the posterior one-third.
- Presence of granulation in the inter-arytenoid region.
- Shallow irregular ulceration over the free margins of the posterior one-third of the vocal cords extending to the inter-arytenoid region → **Mouse-nibbled appearance (Fig. 3).**
- Edema of false cords.
- Pseudoedema of the epiglottis **"turban epiglottis"**
- Perichondritis → swelling of arytenoid and epiglottis.
- Tissue necrosis with cold abscess formation is seen in the late stage.

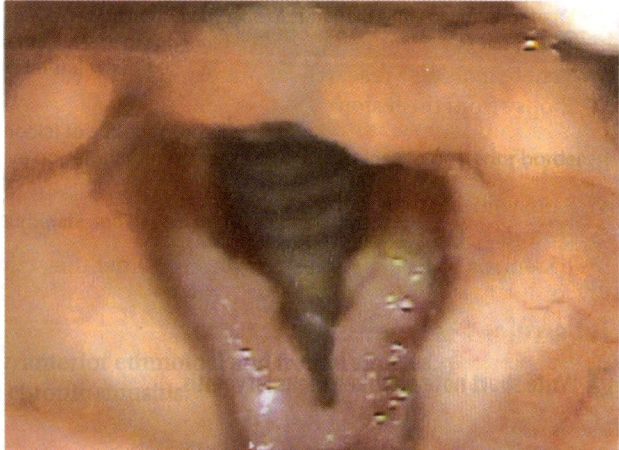

Fig. 3: Tuberculous laryngitis (mouse nibbled appearance of true vocal cords).

Diagnosis

- X-ray chest → suggestive of pulmonary tuberculosis.
- Sputum examination → it shows acid-fast bacilli.
- Mantoux skin test positive
- Biopsy from the lesion

Treatment

- Antituberculous drug therapy
- Voice rest
- Steam inhalation for a soothing effect
- Analgesic
- Anti-inflammatory
- If stridor → intubation/tracheostomy
- If cartilage necrosis → arytenoidectomy/laryngectomy

Lupus of the Larynx

Q. Write a short note on lupus of the larynx.

- Indolent tubercular infection associated with lupus of the nose and pharynx.
- **Common location:** Anterior part of larynx (unlike tuberculosis larynx).
- Painless condition
- Often remain asymptomatic for a long time
- No pulmonary tuberculosis
- **Treatment:** Antitubercular drugs therapy

Scleroma of the Larynx

Q. Write a short note on scleroma affecting larynx.

Definition

It is a chronic inflammatory condition of the larynx secondary to rhinoscleroma caused by gram-negative bacilli—***Klebsiella rhinoscleromatis*/Frisch bacilli/diplobacillus.**

Common Location

Subglottic area.

Pathogenesis

Submucosal infiltration → subglottic narrowing → dyspnea and stridor.

Clinical Features

- Associated features of rhinoscleroma
- Stridor
- Dyspnea
- Change of voice

Diagnosis

- Biopsy from the lesion
- Characteristic histological features: **Mikulicz cells** and **Russell body**

Treatment

- Steroid → to reduce fibrosis and scarring
- Antibiotic → doxycycline/tetracycline/streptomycin for 4–6 weeks.
- Oral rifampicin 400–450 mg for 4–6 weeks.
- If subglottic stenosis → reconstructive surgery/dilatation

Chapter 40: Congenital Lesions of Larynx

Q. Enumerate various congenital lesions of the larynx. Discuss them briefly.

- Laryngomalacia (congenital laryngeal stridor)
- Congenital vocal cord paralysis
- Congenital subglottic stenosis
- Laryngeal web
- Subglottic hemangioma
- Laryngoesophageal cleft
- Laryngocele
- Laryngeal cyst

LARYNGOMALACIA (CONGENITAL LARYNGEAL STRIDOR)

Q. Write a short note on most common congenital abnormality of the larynx/laryngomalacia.

Most common congenital abnormality of larynx.

Causes

Excessive flaccidity of supraglottic larynx which is sucked in during inspiration producing stridor and cyanosis.

Presentation

- **Clinical features**: Stridor increased on crying but subsides on placing a child in the prone position; normal cry.
- **Onset:** At birth or soon after, usually disappears by 2 years of age.

Investigations

- **Direct laryngoscopy**
  - Elongated epiglottis, curled upon itself (omega-shaped Ω).
  - Floppy aryepiglottic folds
  - Prominent arytenoids
- **Flexible laryngoscopy**—very useful for diagnosis

Treatment

- Conservative
- If severe respiratory obstruction—tracheostomy
- Definitive treatment—supraglottoplasty in severe laryngomalacia.

CONGENITAL VOCAL CORD PARALYSIS

- Results from:
  - Birth trauma if recurrent laryngeal nerve stretched during breech or forceps delivery
  - Anomalies of the central nervous system.

CONGENITAL SUBGLOTTIC STENOSIS (FIG. 1)

Q. Write a short note on congenital subglottic stenosis.

- Due to abnormal thickening of cricoid cartilage or fibrous tissue below vocal cords
- **Onset:** Asymptomatic till upper respiratory infection causes dyspnea and stridor.
  - Poor weight gain
- Normal cry as in laryngomalacia.

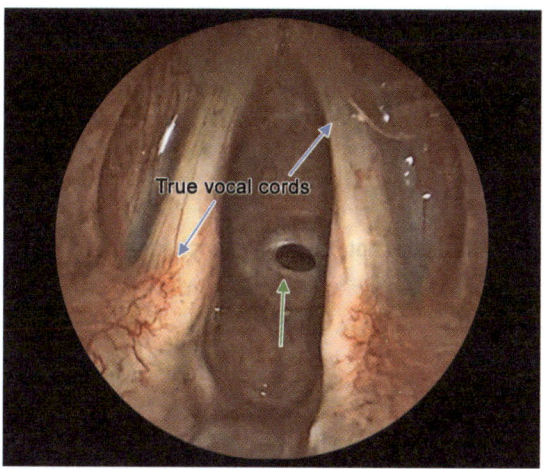

Fig. 1: Subglottic stenosis (green arrow).

Diagnosis

Full term neonate	Subglottic diameter <4 mm (Normal: 4.5–5.5 mm)
Premature neonate	3 mm in premature neonate (normal 3.5 mm)

Treatment

- **Conservative:** Many cases of congenital stenosis improve as the larynx grows
- **Surgical:** Endoscopic dilatation
  - Laryngotracheal reconstruction surgery
  - Partial cricotracheal resection anastomosis

LARYNGEAL WEB (FIG. 2)

Q. Write a short note on laryngeal web.

- Due to incomplete recanalization of larynx.
- **Site:** Web between vocal cords
  - Concave posterior margin
- **Clinical features**—at birth: Weak cry
  - Aphonia
  - Airway obstruction
- Treatment depends on thickness of web.

Thin web	Cut with a knife or CO_2 laser
Thick web	Excision via laryngofissure and placement of a silicon keel with subsequent dilatations

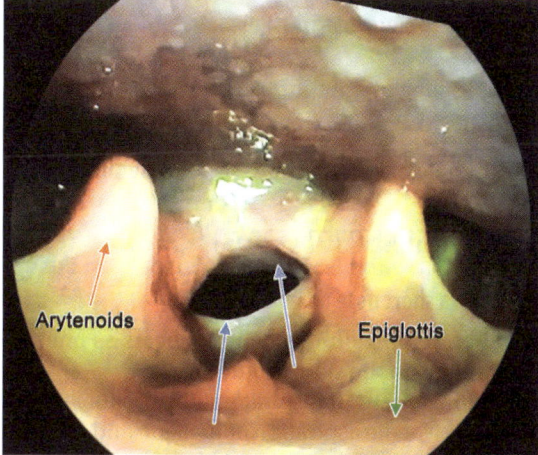

Fig. 2: Anterior and posterior laryngeal web (blue arrows).

SUBGLOTTIC HEMANGIOMA

Q. Write short note on subglottic hemangioma.

- **Onset:** Asymptomatic till 3–6 months of age when hemangioma begins to increase in size.
- 50%—associated with cutaneous hemangiomas.
- **Clinical features:** May present with stridor but normal cry.
  - Agitation of patient or crying may increase airway obstruction (due to venous filling)
- **Direct laryngoscopy: Reddish-blue mass below vocal cords**.
  - Associated mediastinal hemangioma.

Depending on the individual case, the treatment is:
- **Tracheostomy** (if the patient is in stridor) and observation, as many hemangiomas involute spontaneously.
- **Steroid therapy**: Dexamethasone 1 mg/kg/day for 1 week, then prednisolone 3 mg/kg in divided doses for 1 year
- **CO_2 laser excision** → if small lesion

LARYNGOESOPHAGEAL CLEFT

Q. Write a short note on laryngoesophageal cleft.

Abnormal posterior, sagittal communication between larynx and pharynx, extending downward between trachea and esophagus.

Etiology
- Due to failure of the fusion of cricoid lamina.
- Can be associated with vertebral anomalies, anal atresia, cardiovascular malformations, tracheoesophageal fistula, renal and limb anomalies **(VACTERL) syndrome**

Clinical Features
- The patient presents with repeated aspiration and pneumonitis.
- Coughing, choking, and cyanosis at the time of feeding.

Classification
According to Benjamin and Inglis

Types	Features
I	Cleft extends down to the vocal cords
II	Clefts extend below vocal cords and into cricoid cartilage
III	Cleft extends into the cervical trachea
IV	Cleft extend into the thoracic trachea

Treatment
Endoscopic or external surgery to close the cleft.

LARYNGEAL CYST (FIG. 3)

Q. Write a short note on laryngeal cyst.
- **Site:** Aryepiglottic fold and appears as bluish, fluid-filled smooth swelling in the supraglottic larynx.
- **Management:** If respiratory obstruction → **tracheostomy**.
  Note: Needle aspiration or incision and drainage of cyst provide an emergency airway.
- **Treatment:** Deroofing the cyst or excision with a CO_2 laser.

LARYNGOCELE

- Dilatation of laryngeal saccule and extends between the thyroid cartilage and ventricle.
- It may be **internal, external, or combined**.
- **Treatment:** Endoscopic or external excision.
  (described in detail in chapter on benign tumors of larynx)

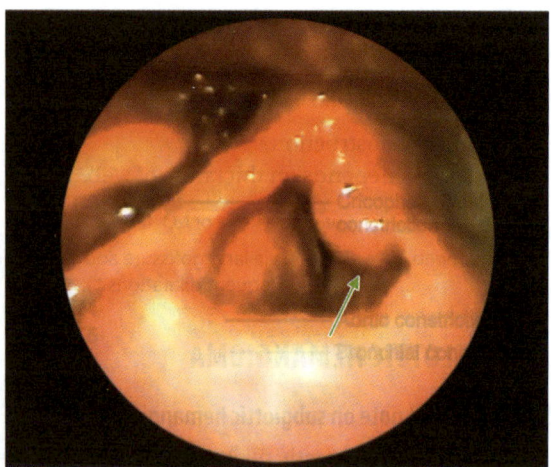

Fig. 3: Laryngeal cyst (arrow).

Chapter 41

Laryngeal Paralysis

EN4.41: Describe the clinical features, investigations and principles of management of laryngeal paralysis.

■ NERVE SUPPLY OF LARYNX

Motor Supply
- All the muscles of the larynx except cricothyroid—recurrent laryngeal nerve
- Cricothyroid—an external branch of the superior laryngeal nerve (EBSLN)

Sensory Supply
- Above the level of vocal cords—internal branch of the superior laryngeal nerve
- Below the level of vocal cords—recurrent laryngeal nerve (RLN)

Recurrent Laryngeal Nerve Injury

Differences between right and left recurrent laryngeal nerve (RLN) (Figs. 1 and 2)

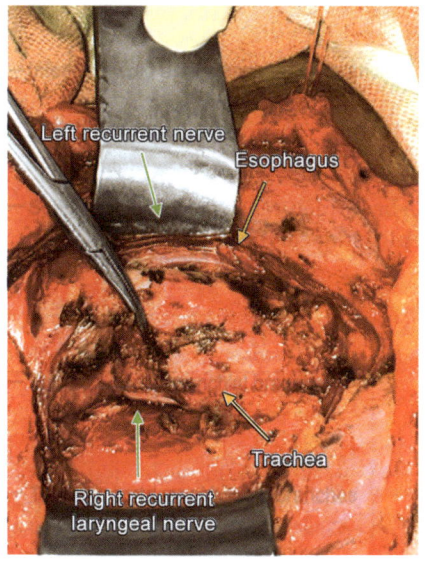

Fig. 1: Intraoperative picture showing relations and difference between right and left recurrent laryngeal nerve.

Right RLN	Left RLN
❖ Shorter in course	❖ Longer in course
❖ Intersects the subclavian and then ascends obliquely	❖ Forms a loop around the aortic arch then ascends vertically
❖ More risk of injury due to oblique course	❖ Less risk of injury

■ LARYNGEAL PARALYSIS

Q. Describe the causes of laryngeal paralysis.

Causes

Laryngeal paralysis can occur due to paralysis of RLN or superior laryngeal nerve or both.
- **Neurologic**
  - Stroke

- Wallenberg syndrome (vocal fold paralysis, dysphagia, vertigo, ataxia, Horner syndrome, hemifacial sensory deficit, and/or pain)
- Arnold Chiari malformation
- Charcot-Marie-Tooth disease
- Viral involvement—herpes simplex virus (HSV), herpes zoster virus (HZV), and Epstein–Barr virus (EBV)

❖ **Inflammatory/infectious**
- Diabetes mellitus
- Mediastinal lymphadenopathy
- Diphtheria
- Pleuritis an pleural effusion
- Pericardial effusion

❖ **Neoplastic**
- Carcinoma of the larynx
- Carcinoma of hypopharynx with laryngeal spread
- Thyroid cancer
- Large goiter
- Carcinoma esophagus
- Lung cancer
- Nodal metastasis
- Nasopharyngeal cancer
- Glomus tumors
- Vagal schwannomas
- Parapharyngeal tumors
- Lymphoma

❖ **Traumatic**
- Blunt trauma to the neck
- Penetrating neck trauma
- Skull base fractures

❖ **Iatrogenic** (surgical trauma)

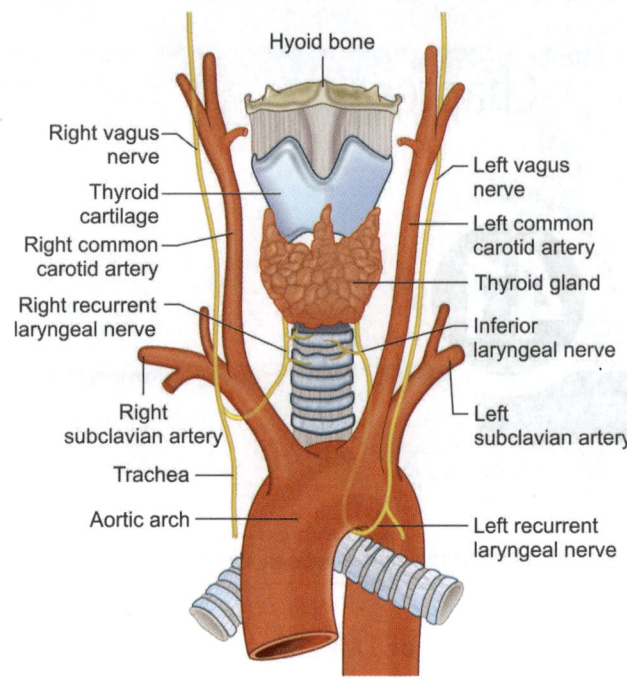

Fig. 2: Course of vagus nerve and right and left RLN.

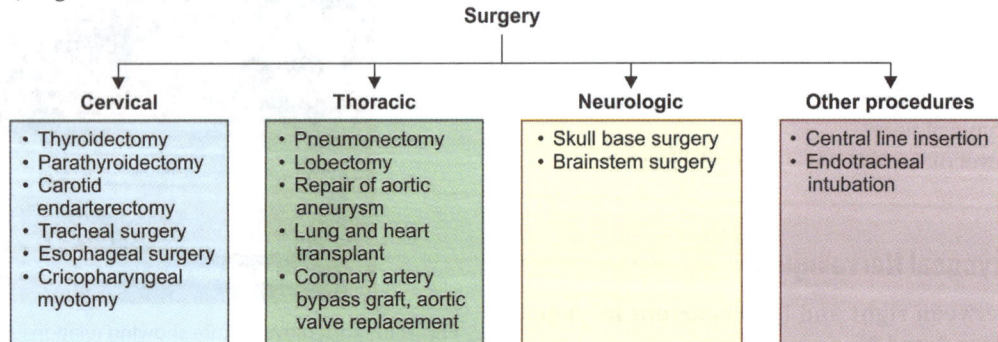

❖ **Miscellaneous**
- Enlarged left auricle
- Aneurysm of subclavian artery (right-sided RLN palsy)
- Aneurysm of the aorta (left-sided RLN palsy)
- Idiopathic

Management

Q. Discuss management of unilateral and bilateral vocal fold paralysis.

The management of vocal fold paralysis follows a detailed history, examination, and a thorough evaluation.

History and Examination

- ❖ A detailed history should be elicited, with special reference to any history of recent surgery, to rule out iatrogenic causes of laryngeal palsy. The role of preoperative laryngeal endoscopy cannot be stressed as many patients may have unilateral vocal cord paralysis with compensation of the opposite cord, which was never previously diagnosed.
- ❖ In patients presenting with laryngeal paralysis insidiously, other cranial nerves should be examined with special reference on palatal elevation, and gag reflex to look for neural involvement in neurological cases or skull base lesions.
- ❖ Chest examination should be done to look for any mediastinal mass, lymph node, tuberculosis, etc.

- A fiberoptic or rigid laryngoscopy should be done to look for the position of the vocal cords and any associated lesions of the larynx. It also allows for documenting the amount of phonatory gap and assessing the compensation of the contralateral cord, and the degree of improvement.
- Stroboscopy is particularly useful as it allows us to see the fine movements and mucosal waves.

Position of the cord (Figs. 3 and 4)	Location of the cord from the midline
Median	Midline
Paramedian	1.5 mm
Cadaveric	3.5 mm
Abduction—gentle	7 mm
Abduction—full	9 mm

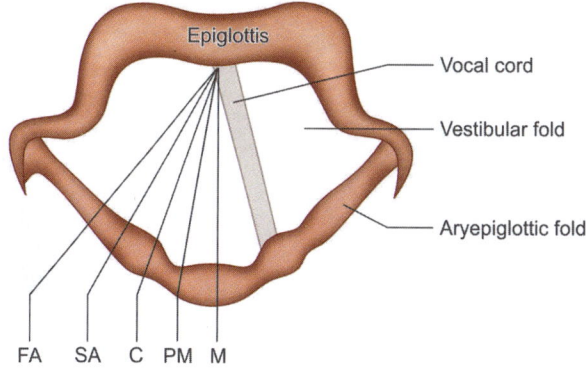

Fig. 3: Vocal cord positions.
(M: Median; PM- paramedian; C: cadaveric; SA: gentle abduction; FA: full abduction)

Investigations

- **Laryngeal electromyography:** It helps in assessing the neural integrity of the larynx, and is usually done 1 and 6 months after the onset of vocal fold paralysis, usually for unilateral vocal fold paralysis.
  If there is expected regeneration/paresis, voice therapy should be continued, and the surgery should be postponed until maximal nerve function is there.
  If the myography shows degenerating potentials, surgery is deferred until the degeneration is complete.
- **Imaging:** CT scan of the skull base and mediastinum, and magnetic resonance imaging (MRI) brain can be done to look for any identifiable etiology which is causing the paralysis. Ba swallow can be done in cases of aspiration.
  While voice is the predominant issue in cases of unilateral paralysis, in cases of bilateral paralysis, airway is the most important issue.

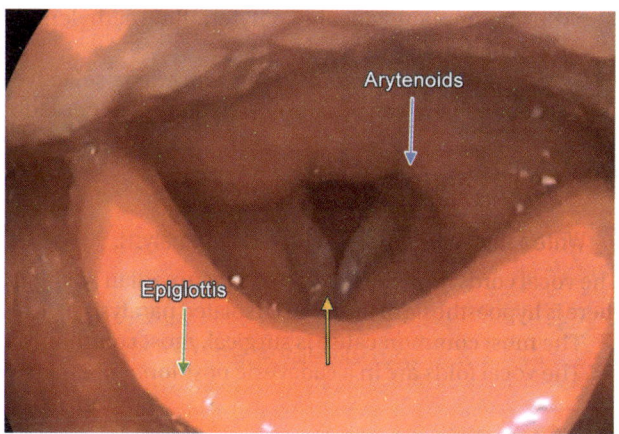

Fig. 4: True vocal cords (yellow arrow).

UNILATERAL VOCAL CORD PARALYSIS (FIGS. 5 AND 6)

Q. Write a short note/essay on unilateral vocal cord paralysis.

Isolated paralysis of the superior laryngeal nerve is rare. It is usually associated with paralysis of the RLN. It causes anesthesia above the level of vocal cords and paralysis of the cricothyroid muscle.

Isolated paralysis of the ESBLN is rare. Unilateral vocal fold paralysis may pass undetected as around one-third of the patients are asymptomatic.

The vocal folds are usually in median or paramedian position.

Theories of adducted position of vocal folds:
- **Semon's law:** This states that in all progressive organic lesions, the abductor fibers of the nerve are phylogenetically newer and thus first to be paralyzed.
- **Wagner and Grossman hypothesis:** This states that in recurrent laryngeal nerve (RLN) paralysis, the cricothyroid muscles keeps the cord in paramedian position due to its additional adductor function.

Clinical Features

- Weak voice with the inability to the raise pitch
- Aspiration is rare
- Shortening of vocal cords with loss of tension
- Flapping of the cords with respiration
- Dysphagia (in high vagal lesions)

Management

- **Conservative**
  - Speech therapy, for hoarseness of voice. Speech therapy focuses on optimizing the efficiency of voice production, minimizing counterproductive compensations, and educating them about the underlying disorder.
    The opposite vocal fold usually compensates within 6–18 months, thus a 9–12 months observation period is a must before surgical options are attempted.
  - Vocal hygiene

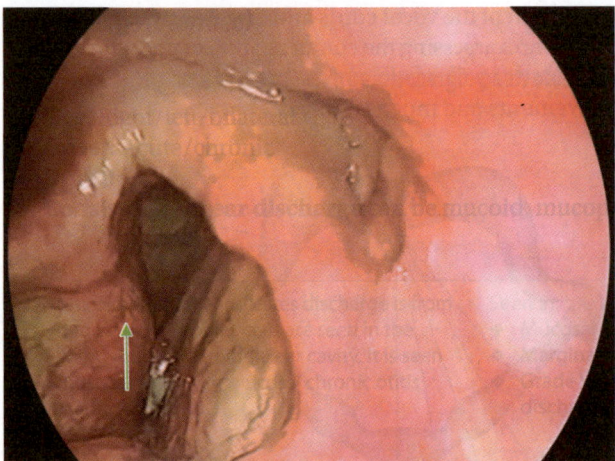

Fig. 5: Right vocal cord palsy.

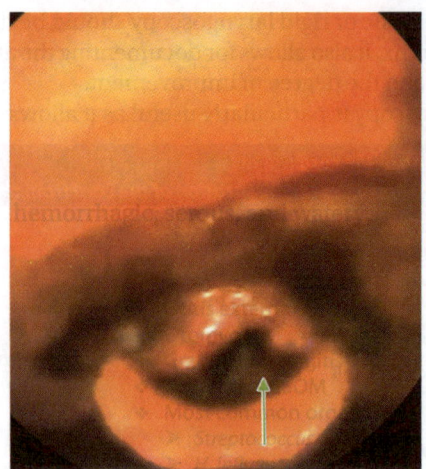

Fig. 6: Left vocal cord palsy.

- **Surgical**
  - *Injection laryngoplasty:* In this procedure, substances such as hyaluronic acid, calcium hydroxylapatite, autologous, and fat are injected to medialize the cord, percutaneously, or perorally or via direct laryngoscopy.
  - *Medialization laryngoplasty (type I):* Herein, via a window in the thyroid cartilage, the vocal folds are pushed medially using implant [silicone, polytetrafluoroethylene (PTFE), etc.]. Additionally, they can be combined with arytenoid adduction.
  - *Selective reinnervation:* In this procedure, selective reinnervation is done using the ansa cervicalis or the hypoglossal nerve. These can also be used if there is denervation during surgery, which cannot be approximated.

BILATERAL VOCAL CORD PARALYSIS

Q. Write a short note on bilateral vocal cord paralysis.

The vocal cords lie in the median or a paramedian position due to the paralysis of intrinsic muscles of the larynx. Additionally, there is hypoesthesia of the larynx. Isolated paralysis of the ESBLN is rare and usually occurs in conjunction with RLN paralysis.
- The most common cause is surgical, most commonly after thyroidectomy.
- The vocal folds are in a cadaveric position.

Clinical Features

- Dyspnea worsens with exertion
- Noisy breathing (stridor)
- Aphonia
- Aspiration—this occurs when there is ESBLN paralysis, which causes laryngeal hypoesthesia and paralysis of the cricothyroid.

Treatment

- **For airway management**
  - *Tracheostomy*—if there is a severe airway limitation, a patient might need a tracheostomy, which provides airway with minimum compromise on deglutition.
  - *Arytenoidectomy*—using laser, the medial part of the arytenoid is removed
  - *Arytenoidopexy*—using suture, the arytenoid is lateralized and fixed, and this enhances the airway
  - *Laser cordotomy (Kashima surgery)*—it is posterior cordotomy of the membranous vocal fold, anterior to the vocal process of the arytenoid. Laterally, it can be extended to the vocalis muscle and ventricle. Sometimes, it can also be combined with an arytenoidectomy. The disadvantage is that patient has a husky voice.
  - *Type II thyroplasty* (vocal fold lateralization)
  - *Laryngeal reinnervation*
- **For management of aspiration**
  - **Swallowing therapy**—the patient is taught various exercises in relation to swallowing. In the meantime, patients can be put on Ryle's tube/percutaneous endoscopic gastrostomy (PEG) tube to decrease the risk of aspiration.
  - If persistent and life-threatening aspiration, the patient may benefit from a gastrostomy or jejunostomy.

Chapter 42

Stridor and Stertor

EN4.43: Describe the clinical features, investigations and principles of management of stridor.

STERTOR

Q. Write a note on stertor and its management.

Stertor is derived from the Latin word, "stertere," which means to snore. It is a characteristically low pitch sound caused due to the turbulence due to an upper airway obstruction, above the level of the larynx, usually from a nasopharyngeal or oropharyngeal obstruction.

Causes

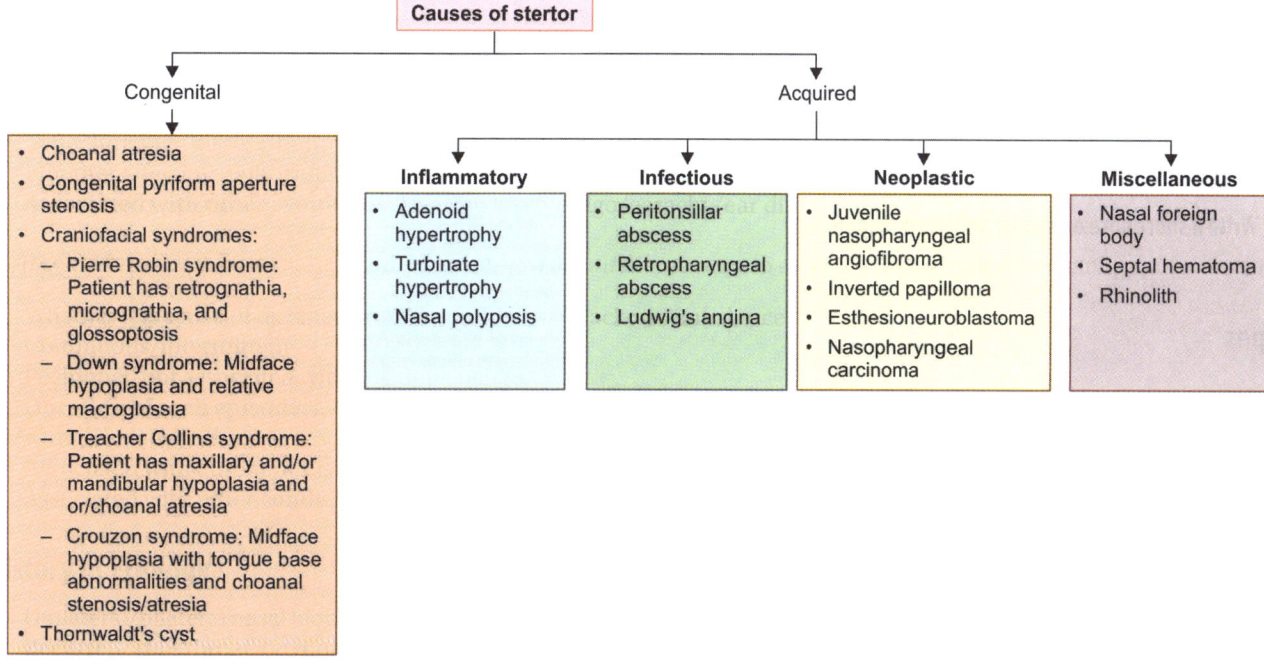

Management

- ❖ Stertor is not a disease per se. It is a manifestation of an underlying disease. The treatment is thus cause-directed.
- ❖ The role of a good history and examination is of utmost importance.

History

- A detailed history should be elicited with the patient's demographic details.
- Congenital lesions are usually picked up in the neonate period, and if the child has a syndromic association, then that might probably be the cause.
- The onset duration and progression of the stertor should be noted. If there are any associated findings like fever, dysphagia, odynophagia, and nasal obstruction then they give us some direction to think of the cause.
- Any similar complaints in the family and if any past history of similar complaints, should be duly noted.

Examination

A comprehensive examination of the ear, nose, and throat should be done.
- A general examination should be done. In children, look for any syndromic associations and features such as glossoptosis and facial hypoplasia.
- Nose should be examined to look for the presence of turbinate hypertrophy, any nasal foreign body, rhinolith, and septal hematoma. Anterior and posterior rhinoscopy should be done, if feasible to look for any mass, polyp, or adenoids.
- Detailed oral cavity, oropharynx, and neck examination should be done to look for any infective cause and for ruling out the abscess. Floor of mouth edema should be seen in case of Ludwig's angina.
- Flexible nasopharyngolaryngoscopy should be done to have a detailed look of the naso and oropharynx.

Investigations

- Complete hemogram should be done to look for leukocytosis to rule out any infection. Blood sugar levels should be noted to rule out diabetes in patients who present with abscesses. An erythrocyte sedimentation rate (ESR), Mantoux, and sputum test for GeneXpert should be done in patients suspicious of tuberculosis, especially in children presenting with retropharyngeal abscess.
- **X-ray:** X-ray of the nose and nasopharynx can be done to look for foreign body, polyps, and adenoids.
  - Neck X-ray is valuable in cases of retropharyngeal abscess.
- **Computed tomography (CT) scan:** Depending on the probable etiology, a CT scan of paranasal sinuses or that of the neck can be ordered.

Treatment

The treatment will be directed to the cause, to resolve the stertor.

STRIDOR

Q. Write a short note on stridor and its management.

Stridor is a high-pitched sound, caused due to an obstruction in the airway. It can be inspiratory, expiratory, and biphasic.

Types

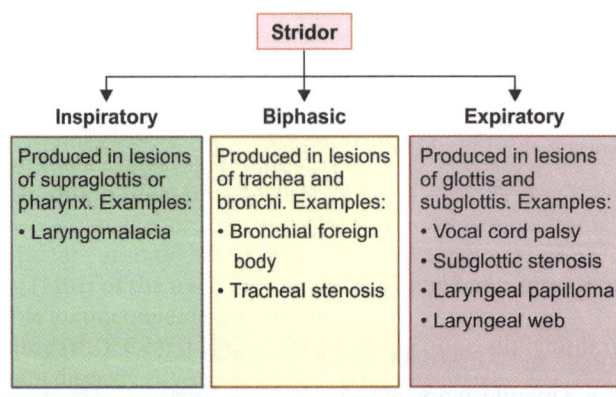

Causes

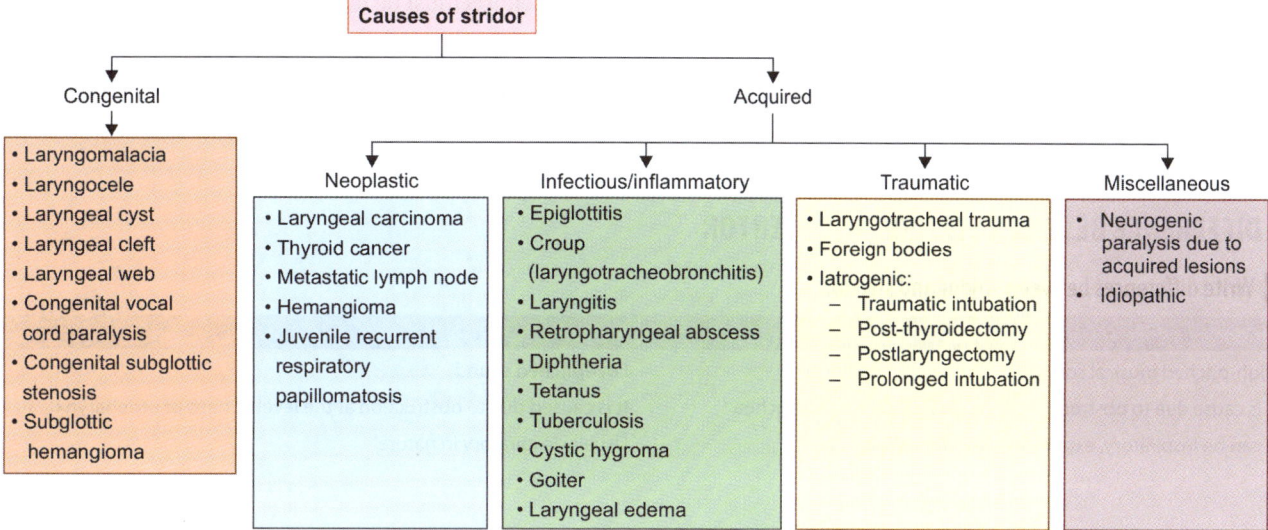

Management

- Stridor is the presentation of an underlying disease and is a symptom. The treatment depends on the cause.
- The importance of good history and examination cannot be stressed.

History

A detailed history should be elicited with the patient's demographic details. Congenital lesions usually present with stridor in the first year of:
- The onset duration and progression and relieving and aggravating factors should be noted, as laryngomalacia worsens on feeding and relieves when the baby is put in the prone position.
- Any history of recent surgery or recent admission history should be duly noted. Patients presenting with infective lesions should be asked for fever.
- If there are any associated findings such as fever, dysphagia, and odynophagia, it should be noted. If there is a history of some foreign body ingestion it should be noted.

Examination

A comprehensive examination of the ear, nose, and throat should be done.
- A general examination should be done. Any signs of flaring of alae nasi, suprasternal and substernal retractions must be noted.
- A detailed ear, nose, and throat examination should be done. The neck should be examined for any thyroid swelling, neck node, and the presence of laryngeal crepitus.
- Flexible nasopharyngolaryngoscopy or a rigid endoscopy or indirect laryngoscopy should be done to look for any lesions of the supraglottis, subglottis, and glottis. Vocal cord movement and symmetry should be duly noted.

Investigations

- Complete hemogram should be done to look for raised white blood cell (WBC) counts in patients of epiglottitis, croup, diphtheria, etc.
- Arterial blood gas analysis may show a washout of carbon dioxide and respiratory alkalosis.
- Swab for Albert's stain should be sent for diphtheria
- Radiopaque foreign bodies can be seen on chest X-rays. However radiolucent will be seen as either hyperinflation or collapse of the lung depending on the site of obstruction. If there is a large goiter there can be a shift of trachea noted on the X-ray.
- **CT scan:** CT scan of the neck can be done for abscess, laryngeal cancer, thyroid swelling, metastatic lymph node, and mediastinal lymph node to ascertain the cause of the stridor.

Treatment

- The patient's oxygen saturation (SpO$_2$) should be monitored and all efforts must be made to prevent respiratory fatigue.
- Patient should be put on high-flow oxygen.
- The cause of the stridor should be ascertained, and management must be tailor-made.
- If a patient's distress worsens, intubation should be considered, and if for any reason it is not possible, the patient can undergo a tracheostomy to secure the airway.
- The treatment will be cause specific.

DIFFERENCE BETWEEN STRIDOR AND STERTOR

Q. Write differences between stridor and stertor.

Stridor	Stertor
High-pitched musical sound	Low-pitched sound
It is cause due to obstruction at the level of larynx and trachea	It is caused due to obstruction at the level of naso or oropharynx
It can be inspiratory, expiratory, and biphasic	Usually inspiratory in nature

Chapter 43

Benign Tumors of Larynx

EN4.41: Describe the clinical features, investigations and principles of management of benign lesion of larynx.

CLASSIFICATION

Q. Classify benign tumors of larynx.

Non-neoplastic		Neoplastic
Solid	**Cystic (Figs. 2 and 3)**	

❖ Vocal nodules
❖ Vocal polyp **(Fig. 1)**
❖ Reinke's edema
❖ Contact ulcer
❖ Intubation granuloma
❖ Leukoplakia
❖ Amyloid tumors
	❖ Ductal cysts
	❖ Saccular cysts
	❖ Laryngocele
		❖ Squamous papilloma
		   ➢ Juvenile type
		   ➢ Adult-onset type
		❖ Chondroma
		❖ Hemangioma
		❖ Granular—cell tumor
		❖ Glandular tumors
		❖ Rhabdomyosarcoma
		❖ Lipoma
		❖ Fibroma

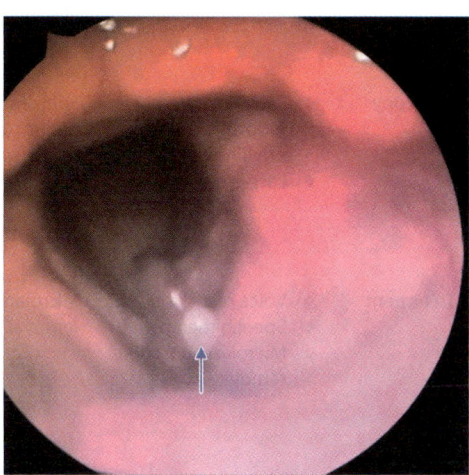

Fig. 1: Laryngoscopy (arrow) showing polyp on the left vocal cord.

SOLID NON-NEOPLASTIC LESIONS

Q. Describe salient characteristics of various solid non-neoplastic lesions.

Lesion	Vocal nodules	Vocal polyp	Reinke's edema	Contact ulcer	Intubation granuloma	Leukoplakia/ keratosis (Precancerous)
Features	Bilateral/symmetrical	Unilateral 30–50 years	Bilateral/ unilateral	Bilateral/ unilateral	Bilateral	Bilateral/ unilateral
Site	At junction of anterior one-third and post two-third (area of maximum vibration of cord, thus maximum trauma)	Same as vocal nodule	Reinke's space (potential space between vocal ligament and overlying mucosa)	Vocal processes of arytenoids	Posterior one-third of true vocal cords	Upper surface of vocal cords

Contd...

Contd...

Lesion	Vocal nodules	Vocal polyp	Reinke's edema	Contact ulcer	Intubation granuloma	Leukoplakia/ keratosis (Precancerous)
Etiology	Voice abuse (teachers, actors, singers, vendors)	Sudden shouting	❖ Voice abuse ❖ Smoking	❖ Voice abuse ❖ Gastric reflux	❖ Rough/ prolonged Intubation ❖ Large tube	❖ Chronic laryngeal ❖ Irritants (smoking/ alcohol/acid reflux)
Pathology	❖ Edema, hemorrhage in submucosal space leading to hyalinization and fibrosis ❖ Overlying hyperplastic epithelium forms nodule	Hemorrhage causing submucosal edema	Collection of edema fluid in subepithelial space	Vocal processes of arytenoids hammer against each other causing ulceration/ granuloma formation	Mucosal ulceration causing granuloma formation over exposed cartilage	Localized form of epithelial hyperplasia
Symptoms	Hoarseness and vocal fatigue	Hoarseness, diplophonia (large) dyspnea, stridor, and intermittent choking	❖ Hoarseness ❖ Deep voice	❖ Hoarseness ❖ Constant desire of throat clearing ❖ Pain in throat	❖ Hoarseness ❖ Dyspnea (large)	Hoarseness
70° scopy	❖ Early—soft, reddish, edematous swellings ❖ Late—grayish/white	Soft, smooth, and pedunculated	Sac-like appearance of vocal cords	❖ Ulcers ❖ Arytenoid Congestion	Granuloma	❖ White plaque or warty growth on cord ❖ Mobility not affected
Treatment	❖ Voice rest ❖ Speech therapy ❖ Microlaryngoscopic removal	Microlaryngoscopic removal	❖ Vocal cord stripping ❖ Speech therapy ❖ Smoking cessation	❖ Voice rest ❖ Antacids	❖ Voice rest ❖ Microlaryngo-scopic removal	❖ Vocal cord stripping and biopsy ❖ Smoking cessation

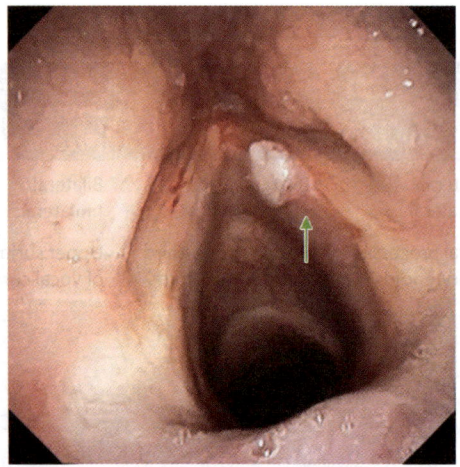

Fig. 2: Vocal cord cyst.

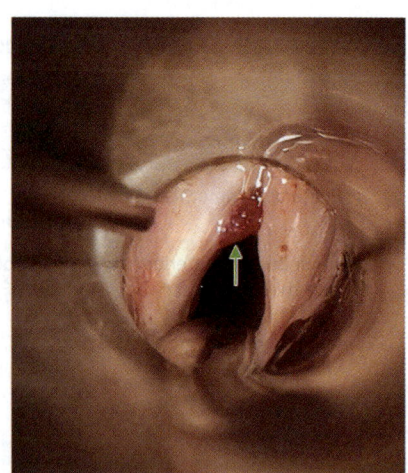

Fig. 3: Microlaryngoscopic (ML) view showing hemorrhagic cyst on the true vocal cord.

CYSTIC NON-NEOPLASTIC LESIONS OF LARYNX

Q. Discuss in brief various cystic non-neoplastic lesions of larynx.

Q. Write short note on:
  a. Ductal cysts
  b. Saccular cysts
  c. Laryngocele

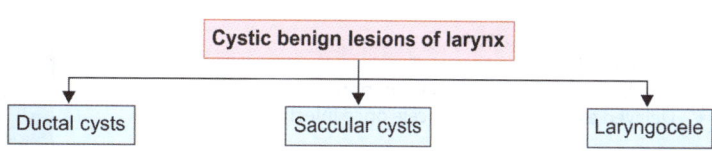

Lesion	Ductal cyst	Saccular cyst	
Definition	Retention cyst due to blockage of seromucinous glands of laryngeal mucosa	Obstruction to orifice of saccule causing secretions retention and saccule distention	
Site	Vallecula **(Fig. 4)** ❖ Aryepiglottic (AE) fold ❖ False cords ❖ Ventricles ❖ Pyriform fossa	**Anterior** Anterior part of ventricle and vocal cord	**Lateral** ❖ Larger ❖ Extends into AE fold ❖ May appear in neck through thyrohyoid membrane
Symptoms	Hoarseness, cough, throat pain, and dyspnea	Neck swelling, cough, hoarseness	
Treatment	Microlaryngoscopic excision	Excision	

Laryngocele

Definition

❖ Air-filled cystic swelling due to dilatation of saccule.
❖ Occurs because of raised transglottic pressure (trumpet players, glass blowers, and weight lifters)

Three Types

Internal, external **(Fig. 5)**, and combined

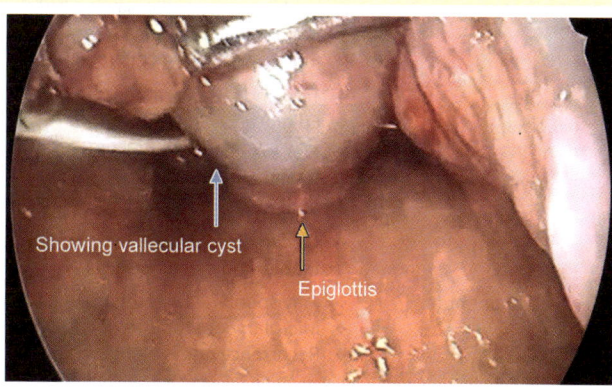

Fig. 4: Vallecular cyst.

Types	Internal	External	Combined
Definition	❖ Confined to larynx ❖ Distension of false cord and aryepiglottic (AE) fold	❖ Presents in neck ❖ Distended saccule herniates through thyrohyoid membrane	Both internal and external components seen
Clinical features	❖ Hoarseness ❖ Dysphagia	❖ Neck lump ❖ Increases on Valsalva ❖ Bryce's sign (emptying of swelling by external pressure)	

Management

Investigations

❖ Flexible nasendoscopy
❖ CT neck (with Valsalva)—to delineate laryngeal architecture **(Fig. 6)**
❖ Magnetic resonance imaging (MRI) neck

Treatment

Surgical excision of laryngocele

Two approaches:
1. Classical lateral
2. Endoscopically with CO_2

Note: A laryngocele in an adult may be associated with carcinoma.

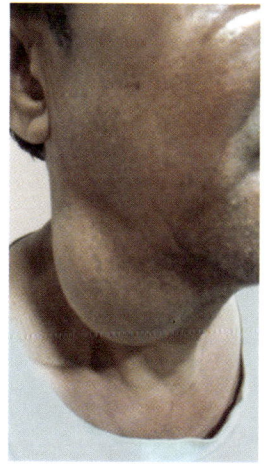

Fig. 5: External laryngocele in the neck.

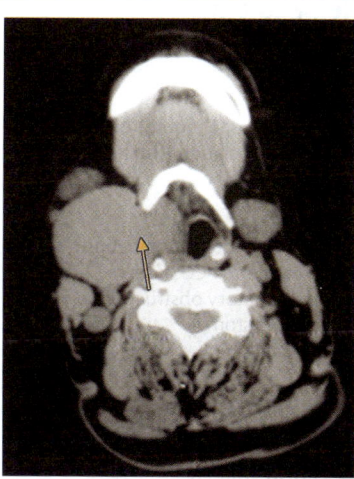

Fig. 6: Computed tomography (CT) scan of the neck showing combined (internal and external) laryngocele.

Laryngopyocele:
- Laryngocele with collection of pus.
- It can present as acute airway emergency/stridor.

Management:
- Intubation/tracheostomy
- IV antibiotics
- Needle aspiration of external component
- Delayed excision of laryngocele once infection subsides

■ NEOPLASTIC TUMORS

Q. Briefly describe various neoplastic tumors of the larynx.

Squamous Papillomas (Fig. 7)

Q. Write a short note on squamous papilloma.

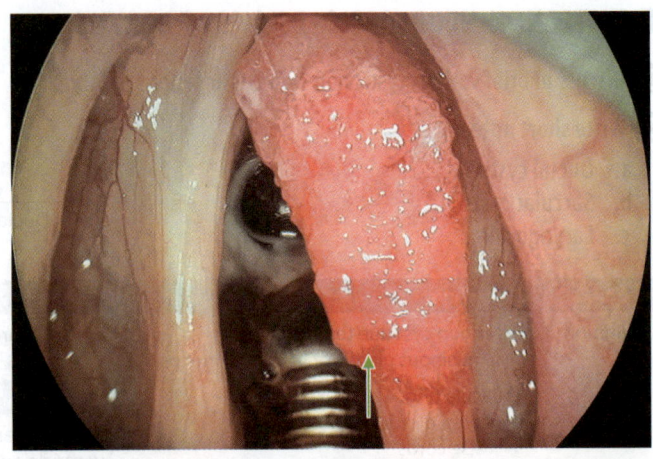

Fig. 7: Laryngeal squamous papilloma involving true vocal cords.

- ❖ 80% of the neoplastic tumors

	Juvenile	Adult-onset
❖ Features	❖ Viral [human papillomavirus (HPV)—6, 11] ❖ Multiple ❖ Infants and young children	❖ Single ❖ Smaller ❖ Males (30–50 years)
❖ Site	❖ True and false vocal cords ❖ Epiglottis ❖ May involve larynx/trachea	❖ Anterior half of vocal cord ❖ Anterior commissure
❖ Symptoms	❖ Hoarseness ❖ Stridor	❖ Similar as juvenile
❖ 70° scopy	❖ Glistening white irregular growths, pedunculated or sessile, friable, and bleeds easily	❖ Single white irregular growth, pedunculated or sessile, friable
❖ Treatment	❖ May spontaneously disappear after puberty ❖ Microlaryngoscopic removal (CO_2 laser) ❖ Recurrence rate is high	❖ Microlaryngoscopic removal ❖ Does not recur

- ❖ **Recent advances:** Interferon therapy is being tried to prevent a recurrence

Chondroma

- ❖ Arise from cricoid cartilage (anterior surface of posterior lamina)
- ❖ **Males:** 40–60 years
- ❖ **Symptoms**—dyspnea, lump in the neck, and dysphagia
- ❖ **Treatment**—surgical excision depending upon the site

Hemangioma

Infantile	Adult
Subglottic	**Glottic/supraglottic (Fig. 8)**
❖ Within first 6 months of life ❖ 50% association with head and neck hemangiomas	40–60 years
Capillary	**Cavernous**
❖ May involute spontaneously ❖ Treatment—CO_2 laser ❖ If respiratory obstruction—tracheostomy	Treatment: ❖ Steroids ❖ Radiation therapy

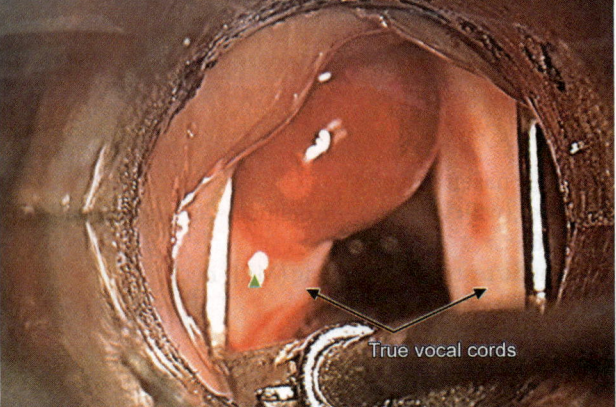

Fig. 8: Laryngeal glottic hemangioma (see arrow head).

Granular Cell Tumor

- ❖ Arises from Schwann cells:
- ❖ Submucosal
- ❖ **Histology:** Pseudoepitheliomatous hyperplasia (well-differentiated)
- ❖ **Treatment:** Complete surgical excision

Chapter 44

Carcinoma Larynx (Malignant Tumors of Larynx)

EN4.42: Describe the clinical features, investigations and principles of management of malignancy of the larynx and hypopharynx.

■ LARYNGEAL CANCER

Q. Write a short note/essay on laryngeal cancer.

- The incidence of laryngeal cancer is 3–6% in males and 0.2–1% in females.
- Males are more commonly affected than females, however, the incidence in females is increasing with more cigarette and alcohol consumption.
- The most common is squamous cell cancer (90%). Other cancers that may occur are chondrosarcoma and giant cell tumor.

Risk Factors

- Smoking
- Alcohol
- Radiation exposure
- **Genetic factors:** If there is a family history of the same, there is an added risk.
- Occupational exposure to mustard and asbestos

Types (Fig. 1)

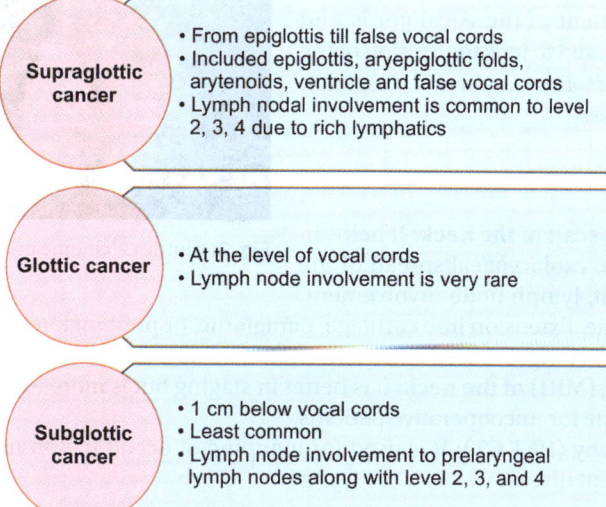

Clinical Features

❖ Hoarseness of voice is a common presentation. In subglottic tumors, there can be hoarseness due to infiltration of the recurrent laryngeal nerve or fixity of the cricothyroid joint.
❖ Dysphagia and odynophagia, are more commonly seen in supraglottic cancer.
❖ Aspiration is due to the involvement of epiglottis or neural involvement external branch of the superior laryngeal nerve (ESBLN).
❖ Stridor, if growth is occluding the lumen of the airway.
❖ Neck swelling, if lymph node metastasis is present. It is more commonly seen in supraglottic growths.
❖ Weight loss due to poor appetite, dysphagia, and odynophagia.
❖ Referred otalgia.

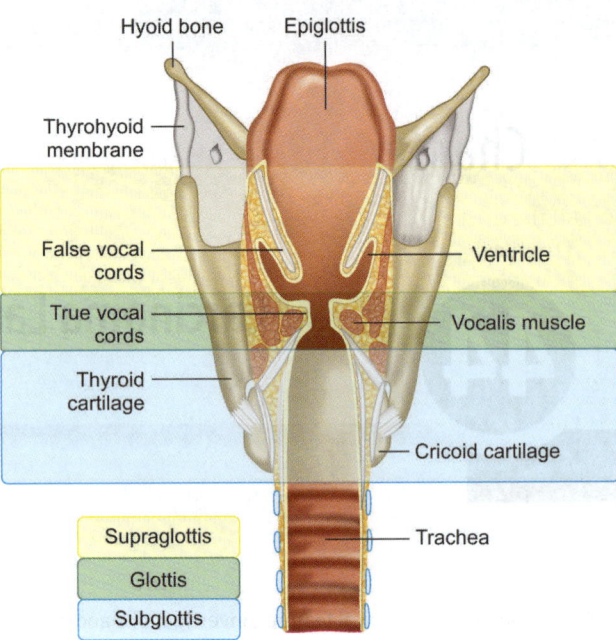

Fig. 1: The laryngeal cavity.

History

❖ Patient may present with hoarseness of voice, dysphagia, or odynophagia.
❖ Patient may have symptoms of aspiration and swelling in the neck.
❖ In the advanced stages, a patient may present with stridor as well.
❖ A proper history should be elicited, particularly of smoking and alcohol consumption.

Examination

❖ A general examination looking for pallor, icterus, cyanosis, clubbing, and lymphadenopathy should be done.
❖ A thorough ear, nose, and throat (ENT) examination should be done, with a detailed examination of the neck.
❖ Involvement of the postcricoid area should be checked by looking for the laryngeal crepitus (**scan QR code**) (Muir's crackle). Absence of the laryngeal crepitus (Muir's crackle) is called Bocca's sign.
❖ Laryngeal widening should be assessed, which is indicative of paralaryngeal involvement.
❖ Laryngeal examination—multiple methods can be used to do a detailed laryngeal examination:
  ▷ Flexible fiberoptic nasopharyngolaryngoscopy
  ▷ Rigid endoscopy using 70° endoscope
  ▷ Stroboscopy
  ▷ Indirect laryngoscopy

All the structures should be visualized with caution to look for any growth. The movement of the vocal cords and arytenoid should be carefully assessed to look for fixation of the hemilarynx **(Fig. 2)**. Any pooling of saliva should raise suspicion for extension into the pyriform fossa.

Fig. 2: Glottic carcinoma involving true vocal cord with vocal cord palsy.

Imaging

❖ **Computed tomography (CT) scan of the neck:** It helps in assessing the extent, invasion, exolaryngeal spread of the disease, cartilage involvement, lymph node involvement, and helps in staging of the same. Extension into cartilage, paraglottic, or pre-epiglottic space should be noted. Subglottis extension, hypopharyngeal, and tongue-based extension should be noted.
❖ **Magnetic resonance imaging (MRI) of the neck:** It is better in staging but is more expensive, lengthy, and has the issue of artifacts. It is also not suitable for uncooperative patients.
❖ **Positron emission tomography (PET CT):** It is used for mapping of occult lymph node metastasis and for assessing postradiation residual/recurrent disease.

Diagnosis

Suspension Microlaryngoscopy

- Patients undergo microlaryngoscopy either under general anesthesia or if the patient's airway is compromised and not in stridor can be done under local anesthesia with high flow ventilation. In patients with frank stridor, tracheostomy is preceded by microlaryngoscopy.
- All the areas within the larynx are inspected and palpated. Special care must be taken to view the anterior commissure. If there is a difficulty to visualize then 0° and 30° scopes should be used. 120° scope can be used to view the subglottis.
- A deep biopsy should be taken from the most representative area.
- Palpation of the base of a tongue and vallecula should be done to detect submucosal involvement.

Direct Laryngoscopy

- Direct laryngoscope is inserted and mapping of the lesion is done.
- Patient can be taken either in general anesthesia or under high flow jet ventilation.
- Biopsy is taken from a representative sample and then hemostasis is achieved.

Fine Needle Aspiration Cytology (FNAC) from Neck Node

If a patient is unfit for the procedure and has a palpable neck node, then FNAC can be done from the neck node.

Staging Tumor, Nodes, Metastases (TNM)

Primary Tumor (T)

Tx	Primary tumor cannot be assessed
T0	No evidence of primary tumor
Tis	Carcinoma in situ

Supraglottis

T1	Tumor limited to one subsite of supraglottis with normal vocal cord mobility
T2	Tumor invades mucosa of more than one adjacent subsite of supraglottis or glottis or region outside the supraglottic (e.g., mucosa of base of tongue, vallecula, and medial wall of pyriform sinus) without fixation of the larynx
T3	Tumor limited to larynx with vocal cord fixation and/or invades any of the following: Postcricoid area, pre-epiglottic space, paraglottic space, and/or inner cortex of thyroid cartilage
T4a	Moderately advanced local disease. Tumor invades through the thyroid cartilage and/or invades tissues beyond the larynx (e.g., trachea, soft tissues of the neck including deep extrinsic muscles of the tongue, strap muscles, thyroid, or esophagus)
T4b	Very advanced local disease. Tumor invades prevertebral space, encases carotid artery, or invades mediastinal structures

Glottis

T1	Tumor limited to the vocal cord(s) (may involve anterior or posterior commissure) with normal vocal cord mobility
T1a	Tumor limited to one vocal cord
T1b	Tumor involves both vocal cords
T2	Tumor extends to supraglottis and/or subglottis, and/or with impaired vocal cord mobility
T3	Tumor limited to larynx with vocal cord fixation and/or invasion of paraglottic space, and/or inner cortex of the thyroid cartilage
T4a	Moderately advanced local disease. Tumor invades through the outer cortex of the thyroid cartilage and/or invades tissues beyond the larynx (e.g., trachea, soft tissues of the neck including deep extrinsic muscles of the tongue, strap muscles, thyroid, or esophagus)
T4b	Very advanced local disease. Tumor invades prevertebral space, encases carotid artery, or invades mediastinal structures

Subglottis

T1	Tumor limited to the subglottis
T2	Tumor extends to vocal cord(s) with normal or impaired mobility
T3	Tumor limited to larynx with vocal cord fixation
T4a	Moderately advanced local disease. Tumor invades through the thyroid cartilage and/or invades tissues beyond the larynx (e.g., trachea, soft tissues of the neck including deep extrinsic muscles of the tongue, strap muscles, thyroid, or esophagus)
T4b	Very advanced local disease. Tumor invades prevertebral space, encases carotid artery, or invades mediastinal structures

Lymph Nodes (N)

N0	No regional lymph node metastasis
N1	Metastasis in a single ipsilateral lymph node, 3 cm or less in the greatest dimension
N2a	Metastasis in a single ipsilateral lymph node, >3 cm but not more than 6 cm in the greatest dimension
N2b	Multiple ipsilateral lymph nodes, none >6 cm in greatest dimension
N2c	Bilateral or contralateral lymph nodes none >6 cm in greatest dimension
N3	Metastasis in a lymph node, >6 cm in greatest dimension

Staging

Stage 0	Tis	N0	M0
Stage I	T1	N0	M0
Stage II	T2	N0	M0
Stage III	T3	N0	M0
	T1	N1	M0
	T2	N1	M0
	T3	N1	M0
Stage IVA	T4a	N0	M0
	T4a	N1	M0
	T1	N2	M0
	T2	N2	M0
	T3	N2	M0
	T4a	N2	M0
Stage IVB	T4b	N (any)	M0
	T (any)	N3	M0
Stage IVC	T (any)	N (any)	M1

Management

Q. Write a note on the management of laryngeal cancer.

1. Management strategies in laryngeal cancer:
   A. Surgical options
   B. Chemotherapy and radiotherapy
      - Chemotherapy
      - Radiotherapy
      - Induction chemotherapy
      - Concurrent chemoradiotherapy
2. **The management of the patient depends on the presentation, staging, and health status of the patient.**
   A. **Supraglottic cancer—T1 and T**
      - Transoral resection is suitable for cases when these lesions lie on the free border of the epiglottis, the false cords, and aryepiglottic folds.
        Disadvantage: Not suitable for lesions that are not clearly visualized on suspension, especially lesions of infrahyoid epiglottis, and in such cases,

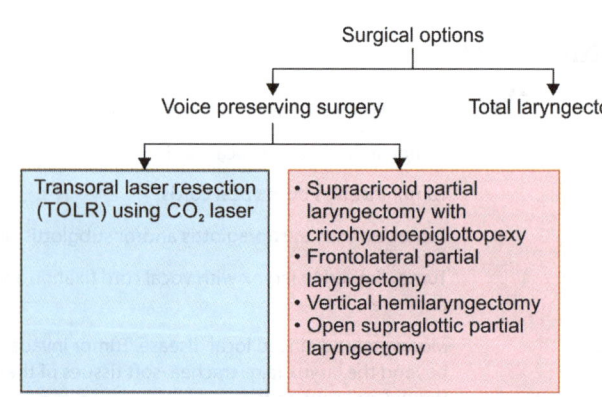

- ◊ **Open supraglottic partial laryngectomy**, for lesions that do not extend to glottis. It is suitable for lesions in the infrahyoid epiglottis which have invasion of preepiglottic space, and for young patients where radiation is being tried to be avoided
- ◊ **Supracricoid partial laryngectomy with cricohyoidopexy:** It is done when vallecula, pyriform and postcricoid are free, and both arytenoids are mobile. Vocal cord fixity is not a contraindication. It is only indicated in patients with good pulmonary reserve since there is high risk of aspiration postoperatively.
- ◊ **Radiotherapy** alone can be used for small lesions.
- ◊ **Chemoradiation** is preferred in bulkier lesions
- ◊ **Total laryngectomy:** It is the last resort and to be used in patients who are unfit for partial laryngectomy and chemoradiation.

B. **Glottic cancer—T1 and T2**
- ♦ **Laser cordectomy** using CO_2 laser can be done for T1 and T2 cancers with freely mobile vocal cords. The advantage of laser cordectomy is that it is a day care procedure. However, patient has hoarseness of voice. It is difficult for larger lesions and for anterior commissure lesions.
- ♦ If there is anterior commissure involvement or the vocal cords are not freely mobile or the exposure is inadequate, a **partial laryngectomy** is preferred. Depending on the location of the lesion, either a **vertical hemilaryngectomy** or a supracricoid partial laryngectomy (SCPL) or a **frontolateral partial laryngectomy** (safer in elderly since less risk of aspiration) can be done.
- ♦ **Radiotherapy:** There is a good voice preservation, however, patient has side effects of radiation, like radiation mucositis, and in cases of recurrence there is a difficulty in revision surgery. Chemotherapy can be added for bulkier lesions.

C. **Subglottic cancer:** There is no scope of voice conservation surgery in isolated subglottis lesions.
- ♦ Radiotherapy is the mainstay of management. It can be combined with chemotherapy in case of lymph node metastasis.

D. **Stage 3 laryngeal cancer**
- ♦ **Chemoradiotherapy: Concurrent chemoradiotherapy** has replaced surgery as the mainstay of management in stage 3 laryngeal cancer. 66–70 Gy of radiation in combination with cisplatin is given over 6–7 weeks.
  Induction chemotherapy followed by chemoradiation in responders and surgery in nonresponders is also advocated.
- ♦ Radiotherapy alone can be tried for unfit patients.
- ♦ **Supracricoid partial laryngectomy** can be tried in when vallecula, pyriform, and postcricoid are free, and both arytenoids are mobile.
  Vertical hemilaryngectomy can be done in cases where there is only preepiglottic or paraglottic space invasion with mobile arytenoids.
- ♦ **Total laryngectomy** is preferred in patients unfit for chemoradiotherapy, who have bilateral fixity of vocal cords, have stridor and aspiration, and those who have failed to respond to chemoradiotherapy.

E. **Stage 4 laryngeal cancer**
- ♦ T4a lesions are best managed by surgery followed by radiotherapy.
- ♦ Surgery is total laryngectomy with ipsilateral thyroid lobectomy and bilateral neck dissection. Level 6 is cleared if there is a subglottic extension.
- ♦ If there is an extracapsular invasion or positive/close surgical margins, chemotherapy is also added.
- ♦ T4b lesions are managed in a palliative intent with chemotherapy since it is unresectable.
- ♦ Management of the neck
  - ◊ In N0 neck, a level II to IV clearance is done. If any are positive on the frozen section, then a level V clearance is also done.
  - ◊ If there is an ipsilateral or bilateral palpable lymph node, bilateral neck dissection is done since metastasis to the contralateral side is high since the larynx is a midline organ with a bilateral lymphatic supply
  - ◊ If an extension to subglottis, level VI dissection is also done.
  - ◊ If the patient is managed by chemoradiotherapy, the neck is also included in the field. If they respond poorly, an interval neck dissection can also be done.

Chapter 45

Voice and Speech Disorders

EN4.40: Elicit, document and present a correct history, describe the clinical features, choose the correct investigations and describe the principles of management of hoarseness of voice.

■ DYSPHONIA

Q. Enumerate types of dysphonia.
- Muscle tension dysphonia
- Specific muscle tension dysphonia
  - Puberphonia/adolescent transitional voice disorder
  - Presbylaryngis
- Dysphonia plica ventricularis
- Spasmodic dysphonia
  - Abductor spasmodic dysphonia
  - Adductor spasmodic dysphonia
  - Mixed dysphonia
- Functional aphonia
- Rhinolalia clausa
- Rhinolalia aperta

■ MUSCLE TENSION DYSPHONIA

Q. Write a short note on muscle tension dysphonia.

It is the most common type of functional voice disorders. Sustained and increased tension of the laryngeal muscles leads to abnormal movement of the larynx, which causes dysphonia. Its diagnosis is based after ruling out any anatomical, psychiatric, or neurological pathology. It is an imbalance between the synergist and antagonist muscles.

It can additionally the disease can cause trauma and structural changes in the vocal fold mucosa.

Types
- **Primary**—it is seen commonly in females
- **Secondary**—when there is an associated organic defect

They are classified into four types, muscle tension dysphonia (MTD) type 1 to type 4.

Causes
Factors which may precipitate/cause this condition:
- Vocal abuse
- Stress, anxiety, and depression
- Aging
- Postural and breathing problems
- Respiratory infections

- ❖ Snoring
- ❖ Laryngopharyngeal reflux
- ❖ Dust, smoke, and fumes exposure

Clinical Features

- ❖ Reduced range of pitch
- ❖ Foreign body sensation in the throat
- ❖ Effortful voice production
- ❖ Vocal fatigue
- ❖ Discomfort with singing or speaking

Treatment

- ❖ Speech therapy
- ❖ Additionally, the cause should be found and treatment should be directed such as avoiding environmental pollutants, treatment of reflux, and psychotherapy.

■ SPECIFIC MUSCLE TENSION DYSPHONIA

Q. Write a short note on specific muscle tension dysphonia/puberphonia/adolescent transitional voice disorder/presbylaryngis.

Puberphonia/Adolescent Transitional Voice Disorder

Usually at puberty, the voice of boys becomes deeper and low-pitched. This is accompanied by a doubling of the size of the thyroid cartilage, bulking of the cricothyroid muscle, and stronger mucosal lining of the vocal cords. However, in some boys, the voice is still high-pitched at puberty.

In these patients, the vocal folds are still lax and cricothyroid muscle is still not bulky and the larynx is still high up, which causes discomfort and pain in some.

Clinical Features

- ❖ High pitched voice
- ❖ Throat discomfort
- ❖ Psychological stress due to bullying

Treatment

The treatment should proceed after ruling out endocrinological and other causes.
- ❖ Speech therapy
- ❖ Botulinum injection in cricothyroid muscle in resistant cases
- ❖ Type 3 thyroplasty (relaxation thyroplasty) in cases that failed speech therapy.

Presbylaryngis

With age, there is a change in the voice due to ossification of the larynx, loss of muscle mass, and arthritic changes in cricothyroid and cricoarytenoid joints.

Treatment

Usually patients just need reassurance, but if treatment is indicated, then:
- ❖ Speech therapy, to increase muscle bulk
- ❖ Injection medialization thyroplasty (rarely indicated)

■ DYSPHONIA PLICA VENTRICULARIS

In this condition, voice is produced by the false cords. The voice is rough, low-pitched, and unpleasant.

Causes

- ❖ **Anatomical:** This is secondary to laryngeal paralysis, vocal cord fixation, or after surgical removal of tumors.
- ❖ **Functional:** This is secondary to psychogenic causes.

Treatment

Voice therapy (better outcomes with functional case).

■ SPASMODIC DYSPHONIA

Q. Write a short note on spasmodic dysphonia and its types.

Q. Write short notes on (a) Adductor spasmodic dysphonia, (b) Abductor spasmodic dysphonia

There is a background of normal speech overlain with vocal spasms which are not under voluntary control, which causes strained and strangled speech patterns. Patients have a lot of social isolation, due to the breaks in the voice which worsens when stressed or when speaking over the phone. It can be of three types—adductor, abductor, and mixed.

Patient may have vocal tremors.

Diagnosis

- ❖ It is usually a clinical diagnosis
- ❖ Electromyography (EMG) will demonstrate bursts of involuntary spasms. It aids in the diagnosis.
- ❖ Endoscopic examination with voice recording is the gold standard.

Treatment

Botulinum toxin, which acts by binding presynaptically on cholinergic nerve terminals causing neuromuscular blockade by decreasing acetylcholine release.

The side effects are a breathy voice and aspiration, depending on dosage.

Adductor Spasmodic Dysphonia

This is more common. In this the adductor muscles of the larynx go into spasm, so the voice is strained with interrupted voice breaks. The patient has difficulty in speaking vowels.

Morphologically, the larynx is normal.

Etiology—unknown, but neurological conditions such as Parkinson's, multiple sclerosis (MS), and amyotrophic lateral sclerosis (ALS) must be ruled out.

Treatment

- ❖ **Botulinum injection** endoscopically or percutaneously (under laryngeal EMG guidance) via the cricothyroid space with dosage as per severity. Patient requires recurrent injections, depending on individual cases, ranging from 6 weeks to 6 months. Along with this, speech therapy is given, as an adjunct.
- ❖ **Section of the recurrent laryngeal nerves (RLN) to paralyze** the cord is used for intractable cases. The results are not good.
- ❖ **Selective denervation of the RLN** followed by reinnervation with ansa cervicalis, to provide a good tone.
- ❖ **Thyroarytenoid myotomy.**
- ❖ **Type 2 thyroplasty.**

Abductor Spasmodic Dysphonia

In this condition, there is a spasm of the posterior cricoarytenoid muscle, which keeps the glottis is open and hence patient has breathy breaks in the voice.

Patient has difficulty in speaking consonants.
Etiology—unknown

Treatment

- Botulinum toxin is given in the posterior cricoarytenoid muscle percutaneously or endoscopically. The results are not as good as adductor spasmodic dysphonia. Speech therapy is also given.
- In intractable cases, type I thyroplasty or a fat medialization laryngoplasty can be tried.

Mixed Dysphonia

In this condition, both adductor and abductor muscle groups are affected.

FUNCTIONAL APHONIA

This is generally seen as a part of conversion disorder, in patients who are facing mental health issues.
- Females are more commonly affected.
- Patient has a good cough.

Treatment

Psychotherapy and reassurance.

RHINOLALIA CLAUSA (HYPONASALITY OF VOICE)

It is due to the blockage of nose and nasopharynx, which causes a lack of nasal resonance.

Causes

- Rhinitis
- Nasal polyposis
- Nasal mass
- Juvenile nasopharyngeal angiofibroma (JNAF)
- Sinonasal tumors
- Nasopharyngeal cancer
- Adenoids

RHINOLALIA APERTA (HYPERNASALITY OF VOICE)

It is seen when words with little nasal resonance are resonated through the nose.

Causes

- Velopharyngeal insufficiency
- Cleft palate
- Soft palate paralysis
- Postadenoidectomy
- Oronasal fistula

Chapter 46

Snoring and Sleep Apnea

EN4.29: Describe the clinical features, choose the correct investigations and describe the principles of management of obstructive sleep apnea.

■ SNORING

Q. Define snoring. Write note on its causes.

Definition

It is the undesirable low-frequency sound produced by the vibration of upper airway walls due to partial upper airway obstruction during sleep.

Mechanism of Snoring

During sleep, relaxation of pharyngeal muscles → partial obstruction → breathing against obstruction → vibration of the soft palate, tonsillar pillars, and base of tongue → produces sound (sometimes as loud as 90dB)

Causes

Level of obstruction	Pathology
Nose	DNS, hypertrophied turbinate, polyps, nasal valve collapse, and tumors
Nasopharynx	Adenoids
Oral cavity and oropharynx	Elongated soft palate and uvula, tonsillar hypertrophy, macroglossia, retrognathia, and large tongue base
Hypopharynx and larynx	Laryngeal tumors, omega epiglottis, and laryngotracheal stenosis

Note: Site of obstruction varies from patient to patient. Also single patient can have multiple or single levels of obstruction

Congenital	Acquired	Others
❖ Nasal obstruction—choanal atresia, complete nasal agenesis, neonatal rhinitis, congenital cysts of the nasal cavity, dentigerous cysts, etc. ❖ Facial skeletal anomalies—(Crouzon's syndrome, Apert's syndrome association with narrow airway), glossoptosis, micrognathia (Treacher Collins syndrome), Pierre Robin syndrome (cleft palate) ❖ Macroglossia—(Down syndrome, Beckwith–Wiedemann syndrome), hemangioma of the floor of the mouth ❖ Pharyngeal swelling—lingual thyroid, Thornwaldt cyst, brachial cleft cyst, thyroglossal duct cyst, and hemangioma	❖ Traumatic—septal hematoma ❖ Inflammatory—tonsillitis and adenoiditis ❖ Neoplastic—juvenile angiofibroma ❖ Iatrogenic—stenosis of nasopharyngeal isthmus	❖ Pharyngeal muscle dysfunction ❖ Genetic predisposition ❖ Obesity and thick neck ❖ Endocrine disorders (hypothyroidism and acromegaly) ❖ Alcohols and sedatives ❖ Neuromuscular diseases—cerebral palsy, Duchenne muscular dystrophy ❖ Mucopolysaccharidosis

SLEEP

Q. What is sleep? Describe the physiology of sleep.

- **Definition:** Sleep is a reversible behavioral state of perceptual disengagement from and unresponsiveness to the environment. Essential as a restorative process to maintain cognitive performance and work productivity, also for physical, psychological, and emotional well-being.
- Sleep is organized into a cyclic pattern of sequential stages.
- Stages of sleep are defined using (polysomnography).

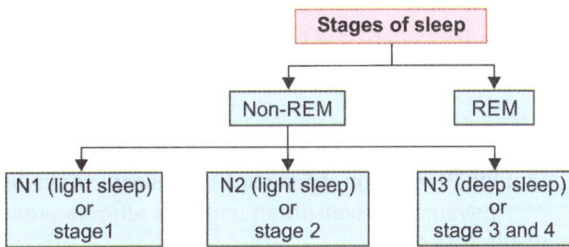

Parameters	Non-REM stage N1, N2 (stage 1 and 2)	Non-REM stage N3 (stage 3 and 4)	REM sleep
Duration	75–80% of sleep		20–25%
Pattern of breathing	Periodic	Stable	Irregular
Apneas	Short and central	Rare	Short and central
PaCO$_2$	Variable	2–8 mm Hg above wakefulness	Variable and similar to stages 3 and 4
Muscular activity	Functional but less		Muscle tone depression (tonic phase) Periods of twitchings of limbs and face—**snoring and OSA occur here**
Ribcage muscles	Active	Active	Inhibited
Diaphragm	Active	Active	Active
Upper airway muscles	Active	Active	Inhibited
Chemoresponsiveness	Decreased compared with wakefulness	Reduced compared with stages 1 and 2	Decreased compared with stages 3 and 4
Autonomic activity	Less activity—slow heart rate and low blood pressure (BP)		Increased activity—with fluctuations in BP, heart rate and respiratory rate
EEG	Passes from alpha to delta waves		Mixed frequencies, low voltage waves, may see saw-tooth waves
EMG (submental EMG)	High tonic	Slightly reduced	Atonic or lowest
EOG	No eye-rolling		Rapid conjugate eye movements
Dreaming	No		Yes (consolidation of thought and memory)
Arousibility to respiratory stimuli	Low thresholds	Low thresholds	High thresholds

(EEG: electroencephalography; EMG: electromyography; EOG: electrooculography; PaCO$_2$: partial pressure of carbon dioxide; OSA: obstructive sleep apnea)

Hypopnea, Index, and Respiratory Disturbance Index

- Cessation of respiration >10 seconds during sleep leading to arousal.
- **Hypopnea:** A decrease in airflow in association with oxyhemoglobin desaturation.
- **Index:** Number of apneas occurring per hour of sleep.
- **Respiratory disturbance index (RDI)—or/hypopnea index (AHI),** i.e., number of both apneas and hypopneas occurring per hour of sleep.
- **Arousal:** Transient awakening from sleep as a result of apnea or respiratory efforts
- **Arousal index:** It is a number of arousal events in 1 hour (<4 is normal).

Respiratory Sleep Disorders

Composed of four distinct syndromes
1. Obstructive sleep apnea/hypopnea
2. Central sleep apnea/hypopnea
3. Cheyne–Stokes breathing
4. Sleep hypoventilation

■ SLEEP APNEA/OBSTRUCTIVE SLEEP APNEA

Q. Write a short note /essay on sleep apnea/obstructive sleep apnea.

Sleep Apnea

- It is defined as cessation of ventilation for 10 seconds or longer during sleep, which leads to awakening from sleep.
- Types of sleep apnea.
  - Central sleep—impairment of respiratory drive
  - Obstructive sleep
  - Mixed—both central and obstructive

Obstructive Sleep

Defined as five or more respiratory events [hypopneas/respiratory effort-related arousals (RERAs)] per hour of sleep lasting ≥10 seconds in association with excessive daytime somnolence, waking with gasping, choking, or breath-holding spells, or witnessed spells of s, snoring or both.

Sleep Syndrome

It is defined as 30 or more apneic episodes during a 7 hours period of sleep or an index equal to or >5.

Grades of sleep syndrome

Grade	Apnea index
Mild	5–20/h
Moderate	20–40/h
Severe	>40/h

Epidemiology and Risk Factors of Sleep Apnea

- Prevalence = 5%
- Age >40 years
- **Male:** Female = 2:1
- **Obesity:** >120% of ideal body weight
- Fat in the neck plays a largest role
- About 30% of snoring males with collar size >17 inches have sleep.

Effects of Snoring on a Person's Life

- Excessive loud snoring—socially disruptive
- Disturbing to the spouse—it can be the cause of divorce—"snoring-spouse syndrome"
- Disturbed routine—the patient can have disrupted daily routine life due to: excessive daytime sleepiness, morning headaches, general fatigue, memory loss, irritability and depression, and increased risk of road accidents

Pathophysiology of Obstructive Sleep (OSA)

- **Definitive event:** Posterior movement of the tongue and palate in apposition to the posterior pharyngeal wall → occlusion of nasopharynx/oropharynx → airway obstruction, cessation of airflow → hypoxia and retention of carbon dioxide → brief arousal from sleep, restoration of airflow → patient goes back to sleep, and the cycle repeats.
- Severe repeated → retention of carbon dioxide, hypoxia → pulmonary constriction → congestive heart failure, bradycardia, cardiac hypoxia left heart failure, and arrhythmias → can be fatal

Symptoms

Night-time Symptoms

- Loud and habitual snoring
- Witnessed
- Nocturnal awakenings
- Gasping and choking episodes during sleep
- Nocturia
- Abnormal body movements

Daytime Symptoms

- Unrefreshing sleep
- General fatigue
- Morning headaches
- Excessive daytime sleepiness
- Lack of concentration, poor memory, irritability, and personality changes
- Increased risk of automobile or work-related accidents
- Decreased libido

Evaluation of Sleep Apnea

Q. How do you evaluate a case of sleep disturbances/sleep apnea/obstructive sleep clinically?

History

- Patient's bed partner gives more reliable information
- **History** includes:
  - Disruption of sleep—snoring, choking episodes, apneic events, and sweating
  - Daytime symptoms—Epworth sleepiness scale can be used to assess sleepiness, and other symptoms such as irritability, memory loss, and morning headaches.
  - History of body position during sleep
  - History of alcohol, sedatives, and caffeine intake
  - History of menopause and hormone replacement therapy
- A questionnaire for assessing daytime sleepiness can be used—called the **Epworth sleepiness scale.**

How likely are you to doze off in the following situations?	Score (0–3)
❖ Sitting and reading ❖ Watching television ❖ Sitting inactive in a public place ❖ Lying down to rest in the afternoon when circumstances permit ❖ Sitting and talking to someone ❖ Sitting quietly after a lunch without alcohol ❖ As a passenger in a car for an hour without a break ❖ In a car, while stopped for a few minutes in traffic	
0: Never dozing off, 1: Slight chance of dozing off, 2: Moderate chance of dozing off and a high chance of dozing off	Total score:

Physical Examination

- General appearance—will indicate the extent of obesity and conditions such as myxedema or acromegaly
- Height, weight, body mass index (BMI), collar size, and blood pressure should be recorded.
- Craniofacial morphology is assessed
- Complete head and neck examination—nasal, nasopharyngeal, oropharyngeal, oral, hypopharyngeal, and laryngeal examination—to define the level and cause of obstruction.
- Muller's maneuver—under endoscopic vision (using a flexible endoscope) via nose, patient is asked to inspire vigorously, with nose and mouth closed—watch for the collapse of pharyngeal wall soft tissues at the level of tongue and soft palate.

Systemic Examination

- Increased incidence of metabolic syndrome is OSA
- Associated medical conditions—hypertension, diabetes, and hypertriglyceridemia should be looked for
- Waist circumference, blood pressure, glucose levels, and triglyceride levels

Investigations

- ❖ To assess the general condition of the patient:
  - ▸ Complete blood count—look for polycythemia/anemia
  - ▸ Thyroid function tests—for hypothyroidism
  - ▸ Chest X-ray—to detect cardiomegaly or pulmonary disorders
  - ▸ ECG—if associated with cardiac disease
  - ▸ Lung function tests
- ❖ To differentiate between simple snoring and sleep apnea
  - ▸ Pulse oximetry
  - ▸ Home multichanneling
  - ▸ Overnight polysomnography
  - ▸ Multiple sleep latency tests (MSLT)
- ❖ To determine the site of obstruction
  - ▸ Nasopharyngoscopy
  - ▸ Acoustic reflection
  - ▸ Cephalometry—for craniofacial anomalies and tongue base obstruction
  - ▸ Fluoroscopy
  - ▸ Computed tomography
  - ▸ Magnetic resonance Imaging—provides excellent upper airway and soft-tissue resolution

Polysomnography

Q. What is polysomnography? What are the parameters assessed?

- ❖ **Nocturnal polysomnography**:
  - ▸ The most commonly used test
  - ▸ Gold standard investigation for OSA and other sleep-related disorders
  - ▸ Parameters assessed:
    - ◆ Sleep state:
      - ◊ Electroencephalography (EEG)—to assess nonrapid eye movement (non-REM)/rapid eye movement (REM)/stages of non-REM sleep
      - ◊ Electromyography (EMG)—submental
      - ◊ Electrooculography (EOG)—for rolling of eyes at onset of sleep, and the onset of REM
    - ◆ Respiratory variables:
      - ◊ Abdominal and chest wall movements
      - ◊ Oral and nasal airflow—to detect apnea/hypopnea
      - ◊ End-tidal CO_2
      - ◊ Arterial oxygen saturation with pulse oximetry—to detect desaturating episodes and the lowest saturation level
    - ◆ Nonrespiratory variables:
      - ◊ Blood pressure
      - ◊ Electrocardiogram (ECG)
      - ◊ Electromyogram (tibial) to detect movement and arousals
      - ◊ Sleeping position—to study the relation of positioning
      - ◊ Audio-visual recording

      Note: Other optional parameters—multilevel esophageal manometry and pH (pressure indicates breathing efforts), and penile tumescence
- ❖ **Split night polysomnography**:
  - ▸ First part of night—polysomnography
  - ▸ Second part of night—titration of pressures of continuous positive airway pressure (**CPAP**)
  - ▸ Not recommended—as apneic episodes occur more commonly in the second half of the night

Multiple Sleep Latency Test (MSLT)

Q. Write short note on multiple sleep latency test.

- ❖ To assess the degree of daytime sleepiness
- ❖ Performed after a full-night polysomnogram to ensure at least 6 hours of sleep before the test (to eliminate other causes of daytime sleepiness)
- ❖ All medications taken for 2 weeks prior to the study should be noted [selective serotonin reuptake inhibitors (SSRIs) and stimulants need to be discontinued for at least 2 weeks]
- ❖ Procedure:
  - ▸ A patient is given 20 minutes of opportunities to nap every 2 hours for 4–5 naps.

- Time taken to fall asleep is noted and mean sleep latency is calculated.
- Interpretation:
  - 10-15 minutes—mild sleepiness
  - 5-10 minutes—moderate sleepiness
  - Less than 5 minutes—severe sleepiness

Treatment

Q. Write a note on treatment of sleep apnea/obstructive sleep apnea.

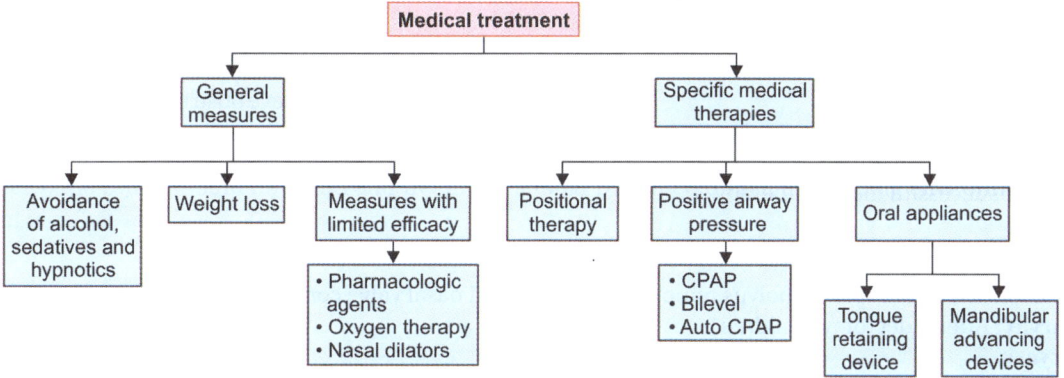

(CPAP: continuous positive airway pressure)

General Measures

- **Avoid alcohol and sedatives and hypnotics**—alcohol reduces the upper airway dilator muscle tone and increases the severity of snoring and apnea.
- Hypnotics and sedatives depress arousal mechanisms—prolonging the apneas and causing greater oxygen
- **Weight loss** causes a reduction in the severity of OSA, lessens collapsibility of the upper airway
- **Measures with limited efficacy:**
  - Pharmacological agents—protriptyline—its primary effect is by reducing the amount of REM sleep when apneas are more frequent. It has anticholinergic effects—reserved for patients with REM-related.
  - Oxygen therapy—has a limited role. It can be used in occasional patients who fail other forms of therapy—improvement in arterial oxygenation to avoid cardiovascular complications.
  - Nasal dilators—it is only for patients with obstruction in the nose, not OSA with retropalatal or retroglossal obstruction.

Specific Therapies

- **Positional therapy:** For patients with position-dependent sleep—symptoms may be alleviated by sleeping in lateral decubitus position. The devices can be used to train to sleep in lateral position. Useful only in moderate cases, not in severe OSA.
- **Positive airway pressure:**
  - Continuous positive airway pressure (CPAP):
    - Mode of action—it acts like a "pneumatic splint" where blowing air via tube and mask through the nasal or oral airway prevents the collapse of pharyngeal and palatal walls. It increases the caliber in retroglossal and retropalatal regions. It increases the lateral dimensions of the airway and thins the lateral pharyngeal wall.
    - Level of air pressure required to open the airway—varies—determined during a sleep study. Usually started with 4 cm H_2O, to increase until apneas and hypopneas eliminated
    - Noncompliance is the most common cause of failure—discomfort caused by a mask and difficulty in carrying it while traveling.
  - Bilevel systems:
    - Newer technique
    - Allows regulation of inspiratory pressure and expiratory pressure independently
  - Automatic positive airway pressure (Auto PAP):
    - Newest modification
    - These machines adjust the pressure throughout the night rather than one fixed pressure
    - Based on the detection of apneas and snoring

- **Oral appliances:**
  - Effective alternative to CPAP in mild to moderate cases
  - Two major types:
    1. Tongue retaining devices (TRD): It holds tongue in anterior position during sleep
    2. Mandible advancing devices (MAD): It keeps the mandible forward. It is useful in micrognathia and retrognathia patients.

Surgical Treatment

Q. Enumerate the surgical treatment options for sleep apnea.

Indications

- Altered daytime performance
- Specific anatomical abnormality causing OSA
- Significant cardiac arrhythmias
- Refused or unsuccessful medical therapy
- Nasal surgery to relieve obstruction can be done to facilitate the CPAP treatment
- RDI >20

Type of Surgery Depending on the Level of Obstruction

- **Nose:** Septoplasty, turbinoplasty, polyps removal, and collapsed nasal valve correction
- **Nasopharynx:** Adenoidectomy (children)
- **Oropharynx:**
  - Tonsillectomy (children)
  - Tongue base reduction—by radiofrequency or laser midline glossectomy
  - Lingual tonsillectomy
  - Uvulopalatopharyngoplasty and laser-assisted uvulopalatoplasty (LAUP)
- **Hypopharynx:**
  - Advancement pharyngoplasty
  - Genioglossus advancement with hyoid myotomy
  - Hyoid myotomy and suspension
  - Maxillomandibular advancement osteotomy
- **Tracheostomy**

Different Surgeries for Sleep Apnea

Q. Write short note on different sleep apnea surgeries.

- **Uvulopalatopharyngoplasty (UPPP):**
  - The most common surgical procedure for adult OSA
  - Removal of excessive mucosa and tissue from the palate and palatopharyngeal arch with shortening or complete removal of uvula
  - Tonsils if present are removed
  - Results in an increase in cross-sectional area at the level of the oropharynx
- **Laser midline glossectomy:**
  - Excision of midline tongue tissue by an intraoral approach
  - Results in enlargement of retrolingual airway
- **Radiofrequency volumetric tongue base reduction:**
  - A radiofrequency needle is inserted submucosally, done for 5–6 sittings
  - It causes coagulation necrosis and scarring, reducing the size of the tissue
- **Mandibular osteotomy with genioglossus advancement:**
  - Advancing the insertion of genioglossus or geniohyoid muscles without moving the entire mandible
- **Hyoid myotomy and suspension:**
  - Advances the hyoid bone anteriorly—thus advancing the epiglottis and base of tongue
  - Resulting in an increase in retrolingual space
- **Maxillomandibular osteotomy:**
  - Osteotomies are done on the maxilla and the mandible and are fixed in the anterior position with plates and screws
  - It causes esthetic facial changes.
- **Tracheotomy:**
  - Permanent tracheotomy—is done in severe OSAS
  - In patients not tolerating nasal CPAP and failing other surgical procedures

Chapter 47

Foreign Bodies in Air and Food Passages

EN2.7, 2.9, 2.10: Elicit document and present a correct history, demonstrate and describe the clinical features, choose the correct investigations and describe the principles of management of foreign bodies in the air and food passages.

■ AIR PASSAGE FOREIGN BODY

Q. Write short note on foreign bodies in air passages and briefly describe its clinical presentation and management.

Brief Anatomy of Trachea

Trachea is composed of hyaline cartilage.
- ❖ **Extension:** Lower border of cricoid cartilage till carina
- ❖ Total of 18–22 rings
- ❖ **Length:** 10–13 cm, average length = 11.8 cm
- ❖ **Diameter (inner):** 1.5–2 cm
- ❖ **Level of carina:** T5 level (posterior) or sternal angle (anterior)

Note: Most common side of foreign body (FB) lodgment is right bronchus:
- ❖ Wider
- ❖ Short
- ❖ Less angulated
- ❖ More in line with the trachea

Etiology

- ❖ The most commonly is seen in children
  - ▷ Age <4 years
  - ▷ The most common FB is peanut
- ❖ **In adults:** Foreign bodies are aspirated during deep sleep/coma/alcohol intoxication
  - ▷ The most common is denture/lose teeth (aspirated during intubation/deep sleep)
- ❖ **Location:** Bronchus (right > left) > trachea > larynx > lung (rare)

Different Types of FB

Site of lodgment	Clinical presentation
1. Larynx	❖ Death due to complete obstruction ❖ Partial obstruction—stridor, cough, hoarseness, and respiratory distress
2. Trachea	❖ Stridor, choking, wheeze, cough, audible slap, and palpatory thud
3. Bronchi	❖ Cough, wheeze, and respiratory distress ❖ Diminished air entry to the lung ❖ Lung collapse, emphysema, pneumonitis, bronchiectasis, and lung abscess are the late features

Based on composition	1. Organic	2. Inorganic
	Example: Peanut, pea, bean, gram, almond seed, wheat seed, piece of apple, or carrot, etc.	Example: A piece of plastic toy/whistle/wire, battery, safety pin, nails, pearl, broken pieces of metallic tracheostomy, marble, etc.
Based on water affinity	1. Hygroscopic	2. Nonhygroscopic
	Example: Peanut, gram, almond seed, wheat seed, rice seed, and chiku seed	Example: Same as inorganic foreign bodies
Based on nature	1. Nonirritating	2. Irritating
	Example: Plastic, glass, and metallic They remain asymptomatic for long-time	Example: All the organic foreign bodies They lead to FB reaction → congestion and edema of airway → bronchitis

Clinical Presentation

- **Initial presentation**: Choking, cyanosis, gagging, coughing, vomiting, and wheezing.
- **Symptomless interval**: Due to respiratory mucosa adapting to the presence of FB.
- **Later presentation**: Depends on the site of FB lodgment.

Different Types of Bronchial Obstructions by a FB and its Consequences (Fig. 1)

- **Partial obstruction** → air can pass in and out → **causing wheezing**
- **One-way obstruction (ball valve effect or one-way valve)** → air can enter during inspiration but cannot escape during expiration → air trapping → hyperinflation of lung → **emphysema**
- **Total obstruction** → air can neither enter nor escape → obstructive **atelectasis** → **lung collapse**
- **One-way obstruction** → reverse of type 2 → air can only escape during expiration → atelectasis → lung collapse

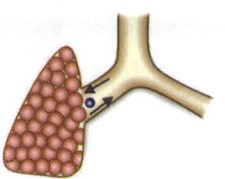
Partial obstruction presenting with wheezing. Air can pass in and out

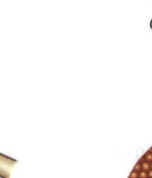
One way obstruction causing emphysema. Air can go in only

Total obstruction causing obstructive atelectasis. Air can go neither in nor out

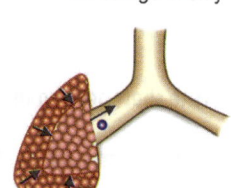
One way obstruction causing atelectasis. Air can go out only

Fig. 1: Foreign body bronchus resulting in four types of bronchial onstruction.

Management

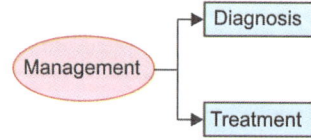

Diagnosis

History

Foreign body ingestion/increased respiratory activity.
Physical examination: Saturation/stridor/chest auscultation (wheezing, decrease air entry)/inspection (retraction of suprasternal and intercostal areas).

Imaging

- **X-ray neck:** Radiopaque, sometime radiolucent FB (size/shape/location)
- **X-ray chest:** Findings:
  - Hyperinflation of a lung on the side of FB
  - Mediastinal shift to the opposite side
  - Atelectasis/pneumonitis
  - Pneumonia/pneumothorax/pneumomediastinum/bronchiectasis (seen in prolonged retained FB)
    Disadvantages: (a) Organic FB cannot be visualized on X-ray. (b) Partial obstruction FB → no X-ray changes detected in the early phase

CHAPTER 47: Foreign Bodies in Air and Food Passages

- Computed tomography (CT) scan with or without virtual bronchoscopy: Lighly sensitive
- **CT bronchoscopy:** Done in an asymptomatic patient
- Videofluoroscopy/fluoroscopy

Treatment

Emergency surgical removal. No medical management.

Laryngeal Foreign Body

Large bolus of food obstructing the laryngeal inlet.

Tracheal and Bronchial Foreign Body

Mainstay of treatment is rigid bronchoscopic assisted FB removal.

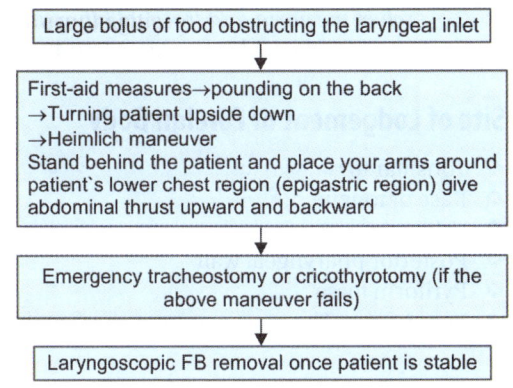

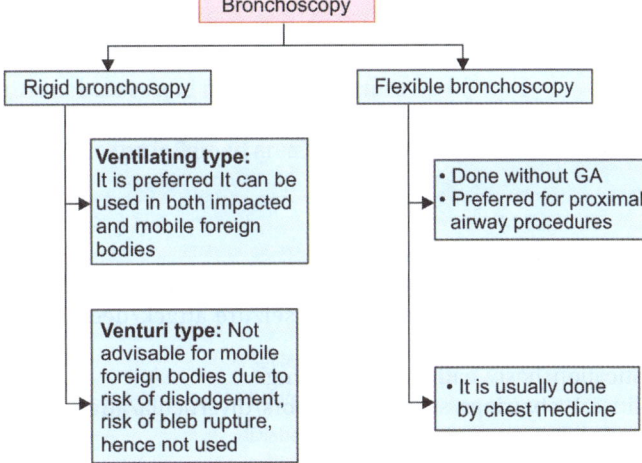

*If there is a history of suspicious FB inhalation many days back → start pt on antibiotic and steroid (to reduce edema and infection).
*Urgency of surgery depends on clinical conditions of the patient and resources available.
*Surgery can be delayed except in the following conditions:
1. Unstable vitals
2. Type of FB—peanut, button battery, and broken seeds.
*Airway foreign bodies till primary bronchus: Remove by ear, nose, and throat (ENT) surgeon.
Airway FB beyond primary bronchus: Remove by either chest medicine or cardiothoracic surgeon.

■ FOOD PASSAGE FOREIGN BODY

Q. Write short note/essay on foreign bodies in food passage. Briefly discuss its clinical presentation and management.

Brief Anatomy of Esophagus

- Muscular tube
- Extend from lower border cricoid cartilage to a cardiac orifice of the stomach (at the level of T11 vertebra)
- **Divided into:**
  - Upper one-third (proximal) → cervical part
  - Middle one-third (middle) → thoracic part
  - Lower one-third (distal) → abdominal part
- Composed of both skeletal and smooth muscular layers:
  - Upper one-third → skeletal muscle
  - Middle one-third → combination of skeletal and smooth muscles
  - Lower one-third → smooth muscle
- Length: 20–25 cm
- Three anatomical constrictions:
  1. *Upper esophageal sphincter (UES):* 15 cm from upper incisor (C6 level)

2. *Arch of the aorta and tracheal bifurcation areas:* 25–28 cm from upper incisors (T4-T5 level)
3. *Lower esophageal sphincter (LES):* 40 cm from upper incisors (T10 level)

Site of Lodgement of Foreign Body

- Tonsillar fossa
- Base of tongue
- Vallecula
- Posterior pharyngeal wall
- Pyriform fossa
- **Esophagus:** The most common site is at the level of cricopharyngeal sphincter (UES).

Common Foreign Bodies of Food Passage

- Fishbone
- Chicken bone
- Coin
- Meat bolus
- Denture
- Mutton bone
- Needle/safety pin
- Wire/nails/screws

Etiology

- Children below 5 years → most often affected (playing age/tendency to put inside the mouth)
- Accidental swallowing, example: Denture → seen during seizure attack/deep sleep/alcoholic intoxication/loss of consciousness
- **Carelessness:** Improper mastication/hasty-eating and drinking
- Anatomic or motor abnormalities: Webs/rings/strictures/tumors/diverticula/atresia/eosinophilic esophagitis/achalasia/scleroderma/esophageal spasms
- Mentally impaired
- **Psychiatric illness:** Foreign body swallowed with an attempt to commit suicide.

Clinical Features

Symptoms

Adult/older children → choking or gagging
- Hiccups/retching
- Throat discomfort
- Globus sensation
- Dysphagia
- Odynophagia
- Hypersalivation
- Regurgitation
- Retrosternal fullness
- Chest pain
- If tracheal compression present then patient presents with wheezing, cough, dyspnea and stridor
- Infant/young children/mentally impaired comes with foreign body then patient presents with drooling of saliva/gagging/irritability/poor feeding

Signs of complication: Hematemesis/tenderness in neck, chest, and abdomen/subcutaneous emphysema/odynophagia
In partial obstruction → less evidence of signs and symptoms.

Signs

- Tenderness in neck/chest regions
- Pooling of salivation in the pyriform fossa on indirect laryngoscopy
- If perforation → subcutaneous emphysema
- Unstable vitals

Complication of Esophageal Foreign Body

- ❖ Respiratory obstruction → due to tracheal compression by FB or laryngeal edema
- ❖ Periesophageal cellulitis and abscess
- ❖ Esophageal perforation
- ❖ Ulceration and stricture → overlooked FB may lead to stricture formation and ulceration
- ❖ Tracheoesophageal fistula → rare

Management/Evaluation

Diagnosis

History

Type/number of objects/location/time since ingestion/signs and symptoms.

Physical Examination

Airway patency/vitals/signs of complications.

Imaging

- ❖ X-ray neck/chest (posterior-anterior (PA) and lateral views) including abdomen
  - ▸ Mostly radio-opaque foreign bodies are detected (size/location/numbers)
  - ▸ Sometime radiolucent foreign bodies (fish bone/chicken bone/plastic denture, etc.) may also get detected
  - ▸ Esophageal foreign bodies lie in coronal plane in PA view → therefore they appear round on PA view (object such as coin and button battery)
  - ▸ It is reverse in case of tracheal foreign bodies due to orientation of vocal cords
- ❖ CT scan:
  - ▸ Highly suspicious but not detected on X-ray
  - ▸ Signs of complications
- ❖ Barium swallow: Avoided due to risk of contrast spillage if perforation + present

Treatment

Endoscopic removal using esophagoscope is the procedure of choice.

Endoscopic Removal

Based on type of foreign body, degree of obstruction and duration.

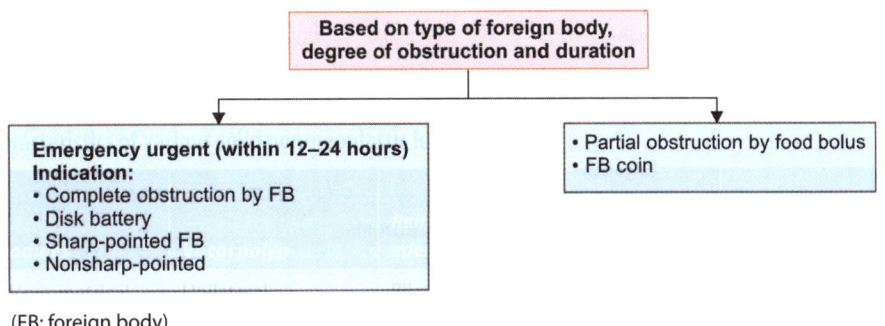

(FB: foreign body)

Cervical Esophagotomy

Impacted foreign bodies or those with sharp hooks like denture located above the thoracic inlet.

Transthoracic Esophagotomy

Impacted foreign bodies in thoracic esophagus.

Note: Special concern: Disk battery in esophagus
- ❖ Emergency removal needed.
- ❖ Most fatal complication → perforation → aortoesophageal fistula.

Chapter 48

Disorders of Esophagus and Dysphagia

EN4.45: Describe the clinical features, investigations and principles of management of diseases of oesophagus.

DISORDERS OF ESOPHAGUS

Q. Enumerate various disorders affecting esophagus. Describe them briefly.

Acute Esophagitis

Q. Write a short note on acute esophagitis.

Definition

Acute inflammation of esophageal mucosa.

Causes

- Chronic acid reflux
- Ingestion of hot liquids
- Ingestion of caustic or corrosive agents
- **Repeated instrumentation:** During esophagoscopy and upper gastrointestinal (GI) scopy
- Trauma due to swallowing foreign body
- Systemic diseases like pemphigus
- Monilial infection of the esophagus from oral thrush

Clinical Features

Dysphagia/odynophagia/retrosternal burning sensation/hematemesis

Diagnosis

- History
- Manometry studies
- Esophagoscopy

Treatment

- Ryle's tube feeding
- Soft and bland diet
- If acid reflux + → gastroesophageal reflux disease (GERD) precautionary measures
- Treat the primary causes
- **Antireflux medication:** Proton pump inhibitors (PPIs) and H_2 blockers
- Antibiotic

Perforation of Esophagus

Q. Write a short note on perforation of esophagus.

Etiology

- **Instrumental trauma (iatrogenic):**
  - During → esophagoscopy → dilatation of strictures or rings with bougies
  - Common site:
    - Just above the upper sphincter
    - Lower esophagus near hiatus

- **Spontaneous rupture:**
  - Seen after vomiting/retching
  - Common site: Lower esophagus
  - Postemetic rupture of the esophagus is known as **Boerhaave syndrome.**

Clinical Features

- **Cervical esophageal rupture:**
  - Throat pain
  - Fever
  - Dysphagia
  - Odynophagia
  - Local tenderness
  - Subcutaneous emphysema in the neck
- **Thoracic esophageal rupture:**
  - Pain in the chest area
  - Referred pain to the interscapular region
  - High fever
  - Signs of shock
  - Subcutaneous or surgical emphysema in neck and upper chest areas
  - Crunching sound over the heart (Hamman's sign): Due to the presence of air in the mediastinum
  - Pneumothorax

Most Serious Complication

Mediastinitis

Diagnosis

- History
- **Imaging:**
  - X-ray of the neck and chest → widening of the mediastinum and retrovisceral space.
  - Surgical emphysema
  - Pneumothorax
  - Pleural effusion
  - Gas under the diaphragm
  - Computed tomography (CT) scans neck to chest
  - Barium swallow → contraindicated

Treatment

Depends on the degrees of mediastinal contamination and sepsis

Non-operative
- Early perforation of cervical esophagus
- Conservative measures:→ More serious
- → Nil by mouth→If diagnosed within 6 hours
- → IV fluids
- → IV antibiotic surgical repair
- → IV PPI proton pump inhibitors (PPIs)
- → Analgesic followed by drainage and lavage
- → Parenteral nutrition (IV route) or →Delayed diagnosed Enteral nutrition (feeding jejunostomy)
- → Prophylactic low molecular weight heparin
- → All the conservative measures
- → Regular monitoring of patient
- → Intercostal chest drainage: if suppuration+

Operative
Thoracic esophageal perforation
Debridement→drainage/lavage

Corrosive Burns of Esophagus

Q. Write a short note on corrosive burn of esophagus.

Etiology

- Acids, alkalis, or other chemicals
- The most common → accidentally swallowed in children or out of curiosity
- Suicide attempts → adults

Common alkali-containing agents	Acid-containing agents
Household bleaches, drain openers, toilet bowl cleaners, detergents, dishwashing agents, etc.	Toilet bowl cleaners, antirust compound, swimming pool cleaners, vinegar, formic acid, etc.

Pathophysiology

- Substances with extremes PH <2 or >12 → very corrosive → severe injury
- **Most affected locations:** Esophagus and stomach → due to longer contact time
- **Other areas:** Oral cavity, pharynx, upper airways, and duodenum
- Alkaline substances ingested → react with proteins and fat → liquefactive necrosis → which leads to deeper tissue penetration → more destructive → mediastinitis and peritonitis
- Acidic substance ingested → react with tissue protein and convert it into acid protein → coagulation necrosis
- Three stages of corrosive burns of esophagus:
    1. Stage of acute necrosis
    2. Stage of granulation
    3. Stage of stricture formation

Clinical Presentation

Site involvement	Presentation
Epiglottis and larynx	Hoarseness of voice and stridor
Upper gastrointestinal tract (GIT)	Dysphagia and odynophagia
Gastric	Hematemesis and epigastric pain

Complications

Early	Late
Perforation → mediastinitis → peritonitis → shock → death	- Stricture formation - Gastric outlet obstruction - Malignant transformation

Paterson–Brown–Kelly Syndrome

Also known as Plummer-Vinson syndrome.

Q. Write short note on Plummer–Vinson Syndrome/Paterson–Brown–Kelly syndrome.

- Precancerous lesion
- About 10% cases → risk development of postcricoid carcinoma

Etiology

- **Sex:** It is common in female.
- **Age:** It is common in the fourth decade of life.
- Iron deficiency anemia
- Immunodeficiency
- Vitamin deficiency
- Autoimmune disease

Clinical Features

- Dysphagia to solid > liquid
- Feeling of lump in the throat
- Glossitis
- Angular stomatitis
- Koilonychia
- Iron deficiency anemia
- Pallor
- Achlorhydria

Diagnosis

- **Indirect laryngoscopy:** Normal
- **Barium swallow:** Web in the postcricoid region **(Fig. 1)** (it is due to subepithelial fibrosis in this region)
- **Cricopharyngoscopy and esophagoscopy:** Web formation at the postcricoid region
- **Complete blood count:** Serum iron profile and hemoglobin level

Treatment

- Ferrous sulfate and folic acid
- Multivitamins
- Dilatation of web with esophageal bougies
- Regular follow-up is needed as this is a precancerous condition

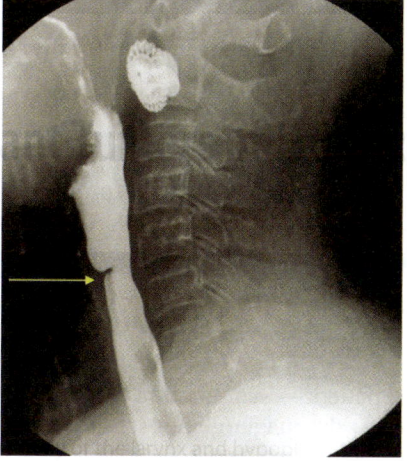

Fig. 1: Barium swallow showing esophageal web.

Hiatus Hernia

Q. Write a short note on hiatus hernia.

Definition

- It is a condition in which the upper part of the stomach or other internal organ bulges through an opening (hiatus) in the diaphragm into the chest.
- Stomach pushes through that opening and into the chest and compromises the lower esophageal sphincter (LES).
- This laxity of the LES → allows gastric content and acid to reflux into the esophagus → GERD → reflux esophagitis.

Types

- **Type I (sliding type):** The most common type (90%). Gastroesophageal junction (GEJ) displaced upward toward the hiatus. Gastroesophageal reflux disease present.
- **Type II (paraesophageal type):** Part of the stomach migrates into the chest.
- **Type III (combination of type I and II)**
- **Type IV:** Stomach as well as additional organs such as colon, small intestine or spleen, and also herniate into the chest.

Diagnosis

- Barium swallow
- Endoscopy (esophagogastroduodenoscopy)
- Manometry
- pH monitoring
- **CT scan:** Not routinely done

Treatment

Types of hiatal hernia	First line treatment
1. Type I	- Proton pump inhibitors for 3 months - Avoid smoking, alcohol, and spicy foods - Weight reduction - Avoid straining
2. Type II, III, and IV	Laparoscopic fundoplication

Barrett Esophagus

Q. Write a short note on Barrett's esophagus.

- Premalignant condition
- Normal esophageal squamous epithelium → metaplastic columnar epithelium
- There is a presence of columnar mucosa extending at least 3 cm into the esophagus
- High risk of adenocarcinoma of the esophagus.

Etiology

- GERD → it is most common
- **Risk factors:** Hiatal hernia, pregnancy, obesity, asthma, diabetes, peptic ulcers, connective tissue disorder, and smoking.
- Male predominance
- Inheritance → autosomal dominant
- White ethnicity

Clinical Features

Most patient → symptoms of GERD
Other → dysphagia/globus sensation

Screening for Barrett Esophagus

- Male gender
- At least 5 years of chronic GERD symptoms
- Age >50 years
- History of smoking
- White ethnicity
- Central obesity
- Family history

Diagnosis

- Endoscopy → salmon-pink colored extensions of mucosa or tongues of mucosa that grow into the esophagus above the gastroesophageal junction (GEJ).
- Biopsy → columnar metaplasia, goblet cells, and dysplastic changes
- pH monitoring
- Immunohistochemistry
- CT scan

Treatment

- **Nondysplastic Barrett** → endoscopic surveillance every 2–3 years.
- **Low-grade dysplasia** → endoscopic radiofrequency ablative therapy or endoscopic surveillance every 1 year.
- **High-grade dysplasia** → endoscopic mucosal resection (EMR) followed by ablation of remaining mucosa.
- **Adenocarcinoma** → esophagectomy or EMR with ablation (early-stage Ca)
- Proton pump inhibitors
- Postablation → regular follow-up

Benign Stricture of Esophagus

Q. Write a short note on benign strictures of esophagus.

Definition

An abnormal narrowing of the esophageal lumen.

- Malignant stricture
- Esophageal adenocarcinoma
- Esophageal squamous cell carcinoma
- Metastatic

Etiology

- Burns due to corrosive substances or hot fluids
- Trauma postinstrumentation
- Trauma due to impacted foreign bodies
- Ulceration due to reflux esophagitis
- Ulceration due to diphtheria or typhoid
- Sites of surgical anastomosis
- Congenital
- Radiation injury

- ❖ Chemotherapy-induced stricture
- ❖ Infectious esophagitis
- ❖ Eosinophilic esophagitis

Clinical Features

- ❖ Progressive dysphagia, first to solid then to liquid
- ❖ Regurgitation and cough → if a complete obstruction
- ❖ Malnourished patient

Diagnosis

- ❖ Barium swallow
- ❖ Esophagoscopy → to exclude malignancy

Treatment

- ❖ Dilatation with bougies
- ❖ Stricturoplasty
- ❖ Intralesional injection of steroid
- ❖ Esophageal stents → for recurrence cases and malignant stricture
- ❖ Surgical resection → for recalcitrant benign condition and malignant case
- ❖ Feeding gastrostomy → to give rest to the inflamed area above the stricture

Motility Disorders

Q. Enumerate motility disorders affecting esophagus. Describe them briefly.

Primary disorders	Secondary disorders
Achalasia cardia	Severe esophagitis
Diffuse esophageal spasm	Scleroderma
Nutcracker esophagus	Diabetes
Nonspecific esophageal dysmotility	Parkinson's disease
	Stroke

Hypermotility disorders	Hypomotility disorders
Cricopharyngeal spasm	Achalasia cardiac
Diffuse esophageal spasm	Gastroesophageal reflux disease (GERD)
Nut cracker esophagus	Scleroderma
Hypertensive lower esophageal sphincter	Amyotrophic lateral sclerosis
	Presbyoesophagus

Cricopharyngeal Spasm

Q. Write short note on cricopharyngeal spasm.

Definition

- ❖ Failure of relaxation of the upper esophageal sphincter (UES).
- ❖ Characterized by incoordination between the relaxation of UES and simultaneous contraction of the pharynx.

Etiology

- ❖ Cardiovascular accidents
- ❖ Parkinson's disease
- ❖ Bulbar polio
- ❖ Multiple sclerosis
- ❖ Muscular dystrophies

Clinical Features

Dysphagia

Diagnosis

Based on etiologies

Treatment

Treat the etiologies

Diffuse Esophageal Spasm

Q. Write short note on diffuse esophageal spasm.

- Unknown etiology
- Characterized by strong nonperistaltic contractions with normal relaxation of the sphincter

Clinical Features

- Nonprogressive dysphagia to both solids and liquids foods
- Odynophagia
- Substernal chest pain
- May stimulate angina

Diagnosis

- Manometry → periodic occurrence of simultaneous high-amplitude contractions with intervening periods of normal peristalsis
- Barium swallow → corkscrew or rosary beads appearance

Treatment

- Rule out coronary artery disease (CAD)
- Reassurance/nitrates/calcium channel blocker
- If gastroesophageal reflux disease present → proton pump inhibitors
- Botulinum toxin injection
- Dilatation of lower esophagus
- Surgery (myotomy) has no established role

Nutcracker Esophagus

Also known as Jackhammer esophagus.

Q. Write a short note on nutcracker esophagus/Jackhammer esophagus.

Definition

- Hypercontractile esophagus (strong and high amplitude contractions)
- Peristaltic contractions present unlike DES
- Unknown etiology

Clinical Features

- Dysphagia and substernal chest pain
- Women > men

Diagnosis

- Manometry → peristaltic waves with significantly elevated amplitude
- Endoscope → normal finding/GERD finding may be seen

Treatment

- Reassurance
- Calcium channel blockers → to relax LES and palliate the dysphagia symptoms
- Nitrate → help relax the LES and improve symptoms
- If gastroesophageal reflux disease present → proton pump inhibitors
- Botulinum toxin injection
- Surgery → myotomy

Achalasia Cardiac

Also known as cardiospam.

Q. Write short note on achalasia cardiac/cardiospasm.

Definition

An esophageal smooth muscle motility disorder that occurs due to a failure of relaxation of the lower esophageal sphincter characterized by the absence of peristalsis in the body of the esophagus and high-resting pressure in the lower esophageal sphincter.

Risk of squamous cell cancer development.

Etiopathogenesis

- Degeneration of the myenteric plexus and vagus nerve fibers of the lower esophageal sphincter
- There is a loss of inhibitory neurons containing vasoactive intestinal peptide (VIP) and nitric oxide synthase at the esophageal myenteric plexus.
- In severe case → cholinergic neurons also involve
- Exact reason of nerve degeneration is not known
- Many theories have been proposed
  - Autoimmune
  - Viral infection
  - Genetic predisposition
  - Idiopathic
  - Chagas disease → *Trypanosoma cruzi*
  - Infiltration by gastric carcinoma
  - Neurodegenerative disorders

Clinical Features

- Dysphagia is more to liquid than solid
- Regurgitation of food
- Chest pain
- Nocturnal cough
- Heartburn
- Weight loss → emaciated person
- Severe dilatation → tracheal compression and stridor
  - Bullfrog neck appearance

Diagnosis

- Barium swallows → tapering of the lower esophagus (bird's beak appearance) with dilatation of proximal esophagus.
  - Sigmoid-like appearance in severe cases
- Manometric studies → are the most sensitive test (gold standard).
  - Low pressure in the body of the esophagus and high pressure at LES and failure of the sphincter to relax.
- Endoscopy → to exclude benign strictures or malignancy.
- Esophageal pH monitoring to rule out GERD.

Treatment

- **Nonsurgical options:**
  - *Pharmacotherapy:* Nitrate/calcium channel blockers/phosphodiesterase-5 inhibitors. (They are smooth muscle relaxant → reduces lower esophageal sphincter pressure)
  - If gastroesophageal reflux disease present → proton pump inhibitors
  - Botulinum toxin injection
  - Pneumatic dilatation
- **Surgical options:**
  - *Laparoscopic Heller myotomy:* A preferred one
  - Peroral endoscopic myotomy
  - Esophagectomy (last resort)

Gastroesophageal Reflux Disease

Q. Write short note on GERD/reflux disorder of esophagus.

Definition
- Regurgitation of gastric contents into the esophagus due to reduced LES action.
- Risk of development of adenocarcinoma of the esophagus.

Risk Factors
- Pregnancy
- Hiatus hernia
- Scleroderma
- Excessive use of tobacco and alcohol
- Drugs such as anticholinergic, β-adrenergic, and calcium channel blockers
- Overweight
- Overeating
- Short interval between meals and sleeping
- Spicy foods

Mechanism
- The presence of sliding hiatus hernia
- The reduced LES pressure
- An increase in the number of LES relaxation
- Abnormal esophageal peristalsis that fails to clear any refluxate
- Poor gastric motility and excessive gastric acid production

Clinical Features

Typical symptoms	Atypical symptoms
Retrosternal pain	It is due to proximal reflux
Heartburn	Voice change
Regurgitation	Coughing
Dyspepsia	Sore throat
Vomiting	Globus sensation in the throat
Dysphagia	Throat irritation/itching
These symptoms become apparent after meals or when lying supine	Throat clearing
	Sinusitis
	Asthma
	Worsening of respiratory symptoms due to reflux and microaspirations

Diagnosis
- Endoscopy → any mucosal damage, hernia, and strictures
- 24-hour pH and bile monitoring → pH <4 for >5% of the 24-hour period.
- Manometry → to identify any underlying motility disorders
- Barium swallow → to exclude underlying motility disorders and may also demonstrate reflux

Treatment
- Lifestyle modification
- Elevation of the head end of the bed at night
- Sleep on left lateral position
- Avoiding food at least 3 hours before bedtime
- Avoid smoking, alcohol, caffeine, carbonated drinks, chocolates, and spicy foods
- Antacids
- **H_2 blockers:** Ranitidine and cimetidine
- **PPIs:** Pantoprazole, rabeprazole, esomeprazole, and lansoprazole
- **Drugs that increase the tone of LES:** Metoclopramide
- **Antireflux surgery:** Nissen's fundoplication

Complications of GERD

Esophageal	Extraesophageal
Esophagitis	Laryngitis
Stricture	Pachydermia larynges
Barrett's esophagus	Aspiration pneumonia
Adenocarcinoma	Asthma
	Bronchiectasis
	Posterior glottic stenosis
	Otitis media with effusion

Scleroderma

Q. Write short note on scleroderma of esophagus.

- Systemic collagen disorder
- Weakening of smooth muscles of lower two-thirds of esophagus and LES.
- Dysphagia may precede cutaneous lesions.
- Many patients have hiatus hernia or reflux esophagitis or stricture.
- Barium swallow: Absence of peristalsis in lower two-thirds of esophagus.
- **Treatment:** Dilatation/antireflux surgery/PPIs/H_2 blockers.

Globus Hystericus

Also known as globus pharyngeus.

Q. Write short note on globus hystericus/globus pharyngeus.

- **Definition:** It is a functional disorder characterized by the feeling of a lump in the throat.
- No true dysphagia
- **Etiology:** Due to psychological imbalance or cancerphobia.
- It is commonly seen in adult females.
- There is a normal clinical examination.
- **Treatment:** Reassurance and psychiatric treatment.

NEOPLASMS OF ESOPHAGUS

Q. Enumerate benign and malignant neoplasms affecting esophagus.

Benign Neoplasm

Q. Enumerate benign neoplasms affecting esophagus. Write a short note on it.

- Rare compared to malignant.
- Leiomyoma is the most common type (smooth muscle tumor).

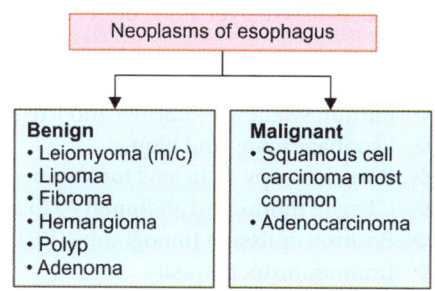

Clinical Feature

Dysphagia, globus sensation, pain, and bleeding.

Diagnosis

- Barium swallow → ovoid filling defect
- Endoscopy and biopsy → submucosal swelling
- CT scan with contrast

Treatment

- Endoscopic enucleation
- Endoscopic mucosal resection

Carcinoma of Esophagus

Q. Write short note on carcinoma of esophagus.

Incidence
High in China, Japan, USSR, and South Africa.

Etiology
- Smoking, alcohol, tobacco, poor nutritional intake, and human papillomavirus
- **Premalignant condition:** Benign stricture, hiatus hernia, achalasia cardiac, diverticula, Plummer–Vinson syndrome, and Barrett's esophagus.

Pathology
- Squamous cell carcinoma → most common (90%)
- Adenocarcinoma (3%) → second common
- Other types are rare

Spread of Cancer
- Direct → infiltration of esophageal wall and adjoining structure such as trachea, bronchus, aorta, pericardium, and recurrent laryngeal nerve.
- Lymphatic → depending on the site involved. Cervical, mediastinal, or celiac nodes may be involved. Supraclavicular node in both cervical and thoracic lesions.
- Bloodborne → liver, lungs, bone, and brain.

Clinical Features
- **Early symptoms:** Substernal discomfort, foreign body sensation in the throat.
- Progressive dysphagia, first to solid then to liquid.
- Pain
- Hematemesis/melena
- Loss of appetite
- Aspiration/hoarseness of voice → due to recurrent laryngeal nerve involvement.
- Emaciation
- Metastasis to liver, lung, bone, and brain → jaundice/shortness of breath, bone, pain, delirium, and confusion.

Diagnosis
- Barium swallow → narrow and irregular lumen (**Fig. 2**)
- Esophagoscopy and biopsy
- Bronchoscopy → to look for lesion extension into trachea and bronchi
- CT scan thorax and abdomen → to assess extent of lesion and nodal involvement.
- Positron emission tomography (PET) scan à to rule out distant metastasis.
- Immunohistochemistry

Treatment
- A superficial lesion, limited to mucosa → endoscopic resection
- Lesion penetrating the submucosa with negative lymph nodes → direct surgical resection with lymphadenectomy
- Lesion penetrating muscularis propria with positive nodes → chemoradiation
- Advanced unresectable or metastasis → palliative therapy
  - Advanced stage → palliative therapy

Prognosis
5 years survival is not >20%.

CHAPTER 48: Disorders of Esophagus and Dysphagia

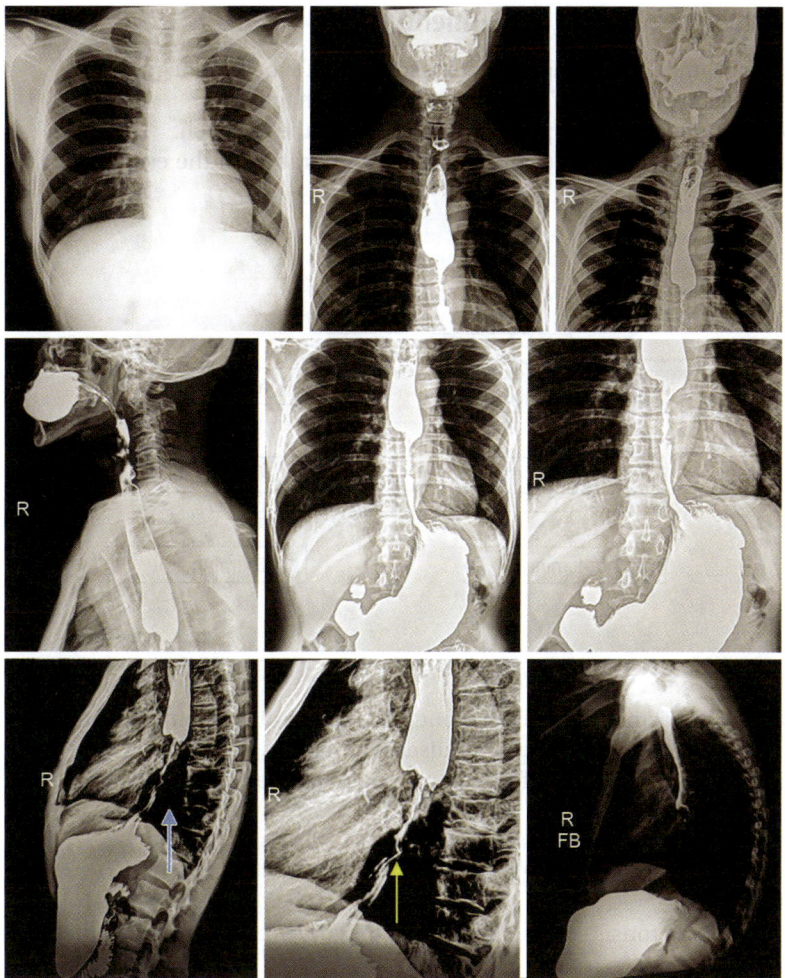

Fig. 2: Barium swallow showing a filling defect in esophagus (blue arrow), rat tail appearance (yellow arrow), and shouldering effect in carcinoma of the esophagus.

EN4.37: Elicit document and present a correct history demonstrate and describe the clinical features, choose the correct investigations and describe the principles of management of type of dysphagia.

■ DYSPHAGIA

Q. Define dysphagia. Describe briefly its types, etiology, clinical features and management.

Definition

- **Dysphagia:** Difficulty in swallowing. It is a symptom and not a disease.
- **Odynophagia:** Pain during swallowing
- Dysphagia solid >liquid → physical obstruction
- Dysphagia liquid > solid → motor disorders

Phases of Swallowing

- Oral/buccal phase
- Pharyngeal phase
- Esophageal phase

Type Based on the Location of Swallowing Impairment

- ❖ **Oropharyngeal dysphagia**: Difficulty moving food bolus from oral to the esophagus.
- ❖ **Esophageal dysphagia**: Difficulty passage of food through the esophagus.
- ❖ **Esophagogastric dysphagia**: Impaired food passage from LES into the stomach.
- ❖ **Paraesophageal dysphagia**: Due to extrinsic compression or infiltration of the esophagus that results in narrowing of the lumen

Etiology

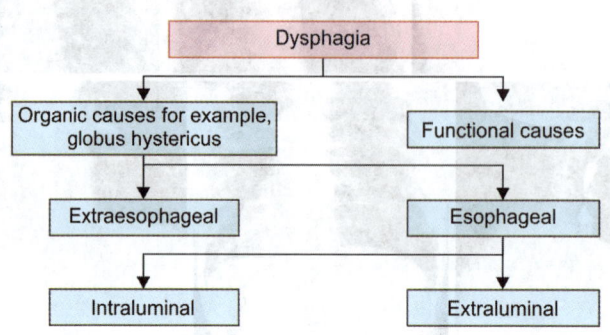

Pre-esophageal Causes

- ❖ **Oral phase:**
  - ▷ *Disturbance in mastication:* Trismus, fracture of mandible, tumors of jaw, temporomandibular joints disorder.
  - ▷ *Disturbance in lubrication:* Xerostomia, Mikulicz's disease, and sicca syndrome.
  - ▷ *Disturbance in tongue mobility:* Paralysis of the tongue, painful ulcer, carcinoma tongue, lingual abscess, and total glossectomy.
  - ▷ *Defects of the palate:* Cleft palate and oronasal fistula.
  - ▷ *Lesions of the oral cavity:* Stomatitis, Ludwig's angina, and ulcerative lesions.
- ❖ **Pharyngeal phase:**
  - ▷ *Obstructive lesions:* Tumors of tonsil/soft palate/base of tongue, pharynx, supraglottic, or obstructive hypertrophic tonsils.
  - ▷ *Inflammatory conditions:* Acute tonsillitis, peritonsillar abscess, retropharyngeal, or parapharyngeal abscess, and acute epiglottitis.
  - ▷ *Spasmodic conditions:* Tetanus and rabies
  - ▷ Paralytic conditions: Paralysis of soft palate due to diphtheria, bulbar palsy, and stroke.

Esophageal Causes

- ❖ **Intraluminal causes (in the lumen and the wall)**
  - ▷ *Congenital*
    - ♦ Atresia
    - ♦ Stricture
    - ♦ Web
    - ♦ Tracheoesophageal fistula (TEF)
  - ▷ *Neoplastic*
    - ♦ Carcinoma
    - ♦ Benign neoplasm
  - ▷ *Infective*
    - ♦ Esophagitis
  - ▷ *Traumatic*
    - ♦ Postcorrosive injury
    - ♦ Iatrogenic injury resulting in perforation and fistula formation, e.g., bronchoscopy, thyroidectomy, and tracheostomy
  - ▷ *Neurological*
    - ♦ Spasm of the upper esophageal sphincter (UES)
    - ♦ Diffuse esophageal spasm
    - ♦ Amyotrophic lateral sclerosis
    - ♦ Stroke
    - ♦ Myasthenia gravis
    - ♦ Tetanus
    - ♦ Parkinson's disease
    - ♦ Multiple sclerosis
  - ▷ *Miscellaneous*
    - ♦ Achalasia cardia
    - ♦ Hiatus hernia
    - ♦ Esophageal diverticulum
    - ♦ Plummer–Vinson syndrome

- Scleroderma
- Foreign body
- **Extraluminal causes (outside esophagus)**
  - *Compression of the cervical esophagus*
    - Goiter
    - Neoplasms of thyroid
    - Parathyroid adenoma
    - Carotid body tumor
  - *Compression of the thoracic esophagus*
    - Retrosternal goiter
    - Mediastinal neoplasm
    - Left atrial enlargement
    - Aortic aneurysm
  - *Compression of the abdominal esophagus*
    - Hepatomegaly
- Globus hystericus
- Presbydysphagia
- Pharyngeal pouch/diverticulum
- Enlarged cervical lymph nodes
- Cervical spondylosis (pressure on the esophagus due to osteophytes)
- Pressure by aberrant blood vessels (dysphagia lusoria)
- Pericardial effusion/cardiomegaly

Evaluation of Dysphagia

History

- Age → certain diseases occur more in certain age groups.
  - *Fourth to the sixth decade:* Malignancy of esophagus
  - *Fourth decade:* Plummer–Vinson syndrome
  - *Second to the fourth decade:* Achalasia cardia
- Sex → Plummer–Vinson syndrome is seen commonly in females.
- Onset
  - *Sudden:* Foreign bodies (FB) ingestion/ingestion of corrosive
  - *Insidious:* Stricture/malignancy
- Duration
- Progressive → malignancy
- Intermittent → spasmodic episodes
- Dysphagia more to solid or liquid
  - More to solid → malignant or stricture
  - More to liquid → paralytic lesions
- Intolerance to acidic foods/spicy foods
- Level of sensation of dysphagia
- **Any associated symptoms:**
  - Regurgitation
  - Aspiration
  - Heart burn
  - Cough at night
  - Odynophagia
  - Referred otalgia
  - Hoarseness of voice
  - Hematemesis
  - Cachexia
  - Weight loss
- Previous corrosive ingestion, trauma, and foreign body ingestion
- Previous surgery → bronchoscopy, neck surgery, glossectomy, etc.
- Systemic illness → neuromuscular disorders, autoimmune disease, diabetes, TB, diphtheria, anemia, etc.
- Addiction → alcohol, smoking, and tobacco

Examination

- **General physical examination**
  - Malnutrition
  - Pallor
  - Jaundice
  - Koilonychia
  - Voice quality
- **Examination of oral cavity, oropharynx, hypopharynx, and larynx**
  - To exclude pre-esophageal causes
  - Mouth opening adequate or not
  - Check for gag reflex and palatal palsy also
  - IDL → vocal cord status, pooling of secretion, any growth

- Examination of neck (thyroid swelling, lymph node, and abnormal pulsation)
- Examination of chest, abdomen, and cardiovascular
- Examination of CNS with cranial nerves (to rule out neurological causes)

Blood Investigation

- **Hemoglobin level:** Low in Plummer–Vinson syndrome/chronic dysphagia
- **Complete blood count:** ESR, C-reactive protein, WBC counts → may be raised in infective/inflammatory conditions
- Liver and kidney function test
- Thyroid function test
- Blood sugar → to rule out DM
- VDRL to rule out syphilis
- Autoimmune profile → to rule out autoimmune diseases

Radiography

- **X-ray neck lateral view:** To exclude cervical osteophytes, any soft tissue lesions of postcricoid or retropharyngeal space
- **X-ray chest:** To exclude CVS, pulmonary, mediastinal lesions, and FB
- **Barium swallow:**
  - Useful in the diagnosis of malignancy, achalasia, stricture, diverticula, hiatus hernia, and esophageal spasm.
  - When combined with videofluoroscopy → motility disorders can be diagnosed
- **CT scan:**
  - To exclude any extrinsic compression
  - To rule out any brain/chest pathology
- MRI → when neurological causes are suspected.

Manometry

It helps in diagnosis of—motility disorders, whether esophageal spasm is spontaneous or acid induced.

24-Hour Esophageal pH Monitoring

To rule out GERD

Esophagoscopy

Direct examination of esophageal mucosa and permits biopsy.

Other Investigations

- FEES → reduced or absent endolaryngeal sensation and aspiration can be detected.
- Nasolaryngoscopy → to rule out local causes
- Bronchoscopy
- Cardiac catheterization → vascular anomalies
- Thyroid scan → malignant thyroid

(CNS: central nervous system; CVS: cardiovascular system; DM: diabetes mellitus; ESR: erythrocyte sedimentation rate; IDL: indirect laryngoscopy; FEES: fiberoptic endoscopic evaluation of swallowing; MRI: magnetic resonance imaging; TB: tuberculosis; VDRL: venereal disease research laboratory; WBC: white blood cells)

Treatment

- **Treat the cause.**
  Example:
  - Correction of anemia in Plummer–Vinson syndrome.
  - Removal of foreign body
  - Dilatation of web/stricture
- **Nutritional supplements (especially in patient with chronic dysphagia)**
  - Ryle's tube feeding or feeding gastrostomy
  - High protein diet
  - Multivitamins

Chapter 49

Human Immunodeficiency Virus in Ear, Nose, and Throat

EN4.46: Describe the clinical features, investigations and principles of management of HIV manifestations of the ENT.

ACQUIRED IMMUNODEFICIENCY SYNDROME (AIDS)

Q. Discuss briefly the modes of transmission, structure of HIV and its pathogenesis.

Acquired immunodeficiency syndrome is caused by retroviruses.
- **HIV type I**—the most common and very pathogenic
- **HIV type II**—which is less common and less pathogenic

It has been well documented that 70–90% of patients with HIV will at some stage present with an ear, nose, and throat (ENT) manifestation of the disease.

MODES OF TRANSMISSION

- **Blood and blood products:**
  - Via transfusions
  - Sharing infected needles, e.g., intravenous (IV) drug abuse
  - Use of non-sterile needles and skin-piercing instruments
- **Sexual transmission:**
  - Homosexual (42%)
  - Heterosexual (~33%)
- **Maternal-fetal transmission:** During pregnancy, during or after birth and via breast milk.
- **Through body fluids:** Saliva, sweat, tears, and urine.

STRUCTURE OF HIV (FIG. 1)

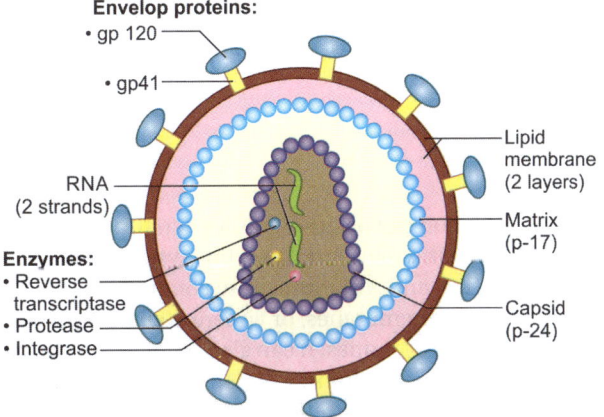

Fig. 1: Structure of human immunodeficiency virus (HIV)-1 virion.

PART 1: Diseases of ENT, Head and Neck

■ PATHOGENESIS

> Once the virus enters the body, it attacks T-lymphocytes and other cells which have CD4 surface markers. CD4 T-lymphocytes are associated with a helper-inducer function of the immune system

> Fusion of virus to the cell membrane allows the viral core to be injected into the host cell. Reverse transcriptase, an enzyme present in the viral core, changes viral ribonucleic acid (RNA) to deoxyribonucleic acid (DNA) and migrates to the host genome

> Viral integrase helps viral DNA to integrate into the host's genome and the latter is then called a provirus

> Provirus directs the synthesis of new HIV particles.
> If a fall in CD4 lymphocytes below 500 cells/mm$_3$, (normal 600–1,500 cells/mm$_3$), the immune system starts breaking down and opportunistic infections and malignancies occur, then it is called AIDS

When CD4-cell count falls below 200 cells/mm^3, death occurs within 2–3 years.

Stage 1: Primary—Acute infection

- Short, flu-like illness—occurs 1–6 weeks after the infection
- No symptoms at all
- Infected person can infect other people
- Earliest marker—gp24; no antibodies detected
- Seroconversion illness occur

Stage 2: Asymptomatic

- Lasts for an average of 10 years
- This stage is free from symptoms
- There may be lymphadenopathy
- The level of **HIV** in the blood drops to very low levels
- **HIV** antibodies are detectable in the blood

Stage 3: Symptomatic

- The symptoms are mild and constitutional
- The immune system deteriorates
- Emergence of opportunistic infections and cancers
- ↓CD4 count 500–200/μL

Stage 4: (HIV) AIDS

- The immune system weakens further
- Severe life-threatening infections CD4 <200/μL leading to an AIDS diagnosis.

■ LESIONS OF HIV MANIFESTATIONS

Q. What are the types of HIV lesions?

Three types of lesions are:

1. **Opportunistic infections:** All types of infection can occur—viral, bacterial, protozoal, or mycobacterial. They can involve any area of the ear, nose, throat, head, neck, and the central nervous system (CNS).
2. **Unusual malignancies:** Kaposi sarcoma (KS) and lymphomas are common.
   - Kaposi sarcoma can involve skin, mucous membranes, or viscera. Kaposi sarcoma may be seen in the skin of the face (nose, ear, or external ear canal), neck, or extremities. It can also occur in oral, nasal, nasopharyngeal, oropharyngeal, or laryngeal mucosa. KS causes obstructive symptoms.
   - Non-Hodgkin lymphoma can involve nodal and extranodal sites.
   - Hodgkin lymphoma is less common.

CHAPTER 49: Human Immunodeficiency Virus in Ear, Nose, and Throat

3. **Neurological disorders:** They can be due to primary HIV infection or opportunistic organisms.
    - Primary HIV infection of the CNS can cause encephalopathy (AIDS dementia complex), myelopathy, peripheral neuropathy, and cranial nerve involvement, most often VIIth but occasionally Vth and VIIIth.

HIV MANIFESTATIONS IN ENT

Q. What are various ENT manifestations in HIV?

Human immunodeficiency virus manifestations in different areas in ENT and head and neck:

Ear	Nose and paranasal sinuses	Oral cavity and oropharynx	Others
❖ Kaposi sarcoma ❖ Seborrheic dermatitis of the external canal ❖ Malignant otitis externa ❖ Serous otitis media ❖ Acute otitis media ❖ *Pseudomonas* and *Candida* infection of the external and middle ear ❖ Mycobacterial infections ❖ Sensorineural hearing loss—due to viral infection of the auditory nerve or cochlea ❖ Herpes zoster (Ramsay–Hunt syndrome) ❖ Facial paralysis	❖ Herpetic lesions of the nose ❖ Recurrent sinusitis ❖ Chronic sinus infection ❖ Fungal sinusitis ❖ Kaposi sarcoma ❖ Lymphomas–B-cell type ❖ Burkitt lymphoma	❖ Candidal infection ❖ Herpetic lesions of the palate, buccal mucosa, lips, or gums. ❖ Giant aphthous ulcers ❖ Adenotonsillar hypertrophy ❖ Kaposi sarcoma of the palate ❖ Non-Hodgkin lymphoma of tonsil or tongue ❖ Hairy leukoplakia ❖ Gingivitis ❖ Laryngitis—fungal, viral (herpes simplex, cytomegalovirus), or tubercular	❖ Parotitis ❖ Xerostomia ❖ Diffuse parotid enlargement ❖ Lymphoepithelial cysts of parotid ❖ Lymphadenopathy

ORAL MANIFESTATIONS OBSERVED IN HIV+ INDIVIDUALS

Q. Discuss briefly various oral manifestations in HIV patients.

- Fungal
- Neoplastic
- Viral
- Bacterial
- Others

Fungal Manifestations

Oral Candidiasis (Fig. 2)

Q. Write a note on oral candidiasis.

- It is the earliest and most common findings suggesting HIV infection in >95% of HIV infected persons.
- Established as a precursor to AIDS within 1–2 years of its appearance.
- Frequency and type are usually indicative of disease progression.
- It is characterized by a typical cottage cheese inflammatory appearance.
- It can manifest in four different ways:
    1. *Pseudomembranous candidiasis:* Classic form identified by a white plaque, can be scraped off, leaving an erythematous, and bleeding base **(Figs. 3A and 4)**.
    2. *Hyperplastic candidiasis:* Thick white plaques that cannot be scraped off **(Figs. 2 and 5)**.
    3. *Atrophic candidiasis:* Flat atrophic lesions involving oral and oropharyngeal mucosa **(Figs. 3B and C)**.
    4. *Angular cheilitis:* These are oral commissure erythematous lesions that can involve the adjacent skin **(Fig. 6)**.
- **Diagnosis:** Clinical, culture, and examination of hyphae in 10% of potassium, oxygen, and hydrogen (KOH) mount.
- **Treatment:**
    - Topical—clotrimazole 1%. Nystatin
    - Oral—fluconazole tablet, 100 mg/day; Itraconazole solution, 200 mg/day
    - Resistant patient:
        - Intravenous (IV) amphotericin (0.3–0.5 mg/kg) for 2 weeks.
        - IV caspofungin 70 mg → 50 mg for 2 weeks.

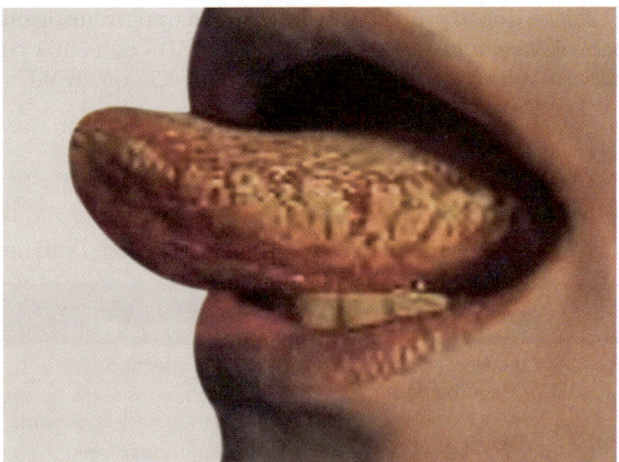

Fig. 2: Candidiasis.

Pseudomembraneous Candidiasis (Thrush)

❖ Removable whitish plaque that can appear on any oral mucosal surface.
❖ When wiped away, it will leave a red or bleeding underlying surface.

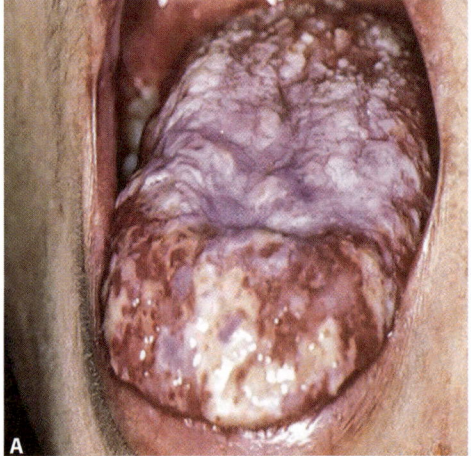

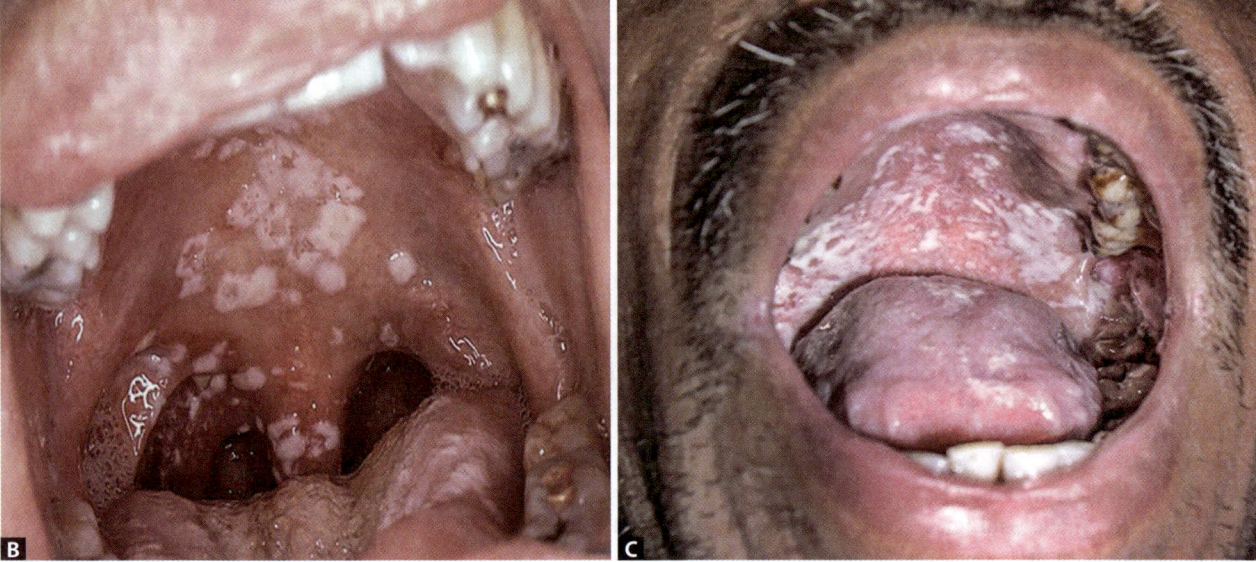

Figs. 3A to C: (A) Pseudomembranous candidiasis of tongue; (B) Atrophic candidiasis involving oropharynx; (C) Atrophic candidiasis involving oral cavity.

Erythematous Candidiasis

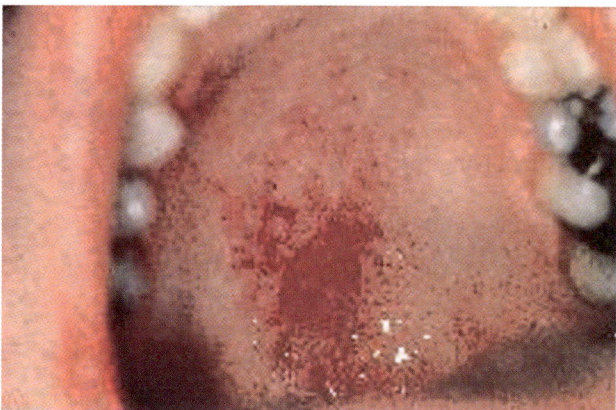

Fig. 4: Erythematous candidiasis of tongue.

Hyperplastic Candidiasis

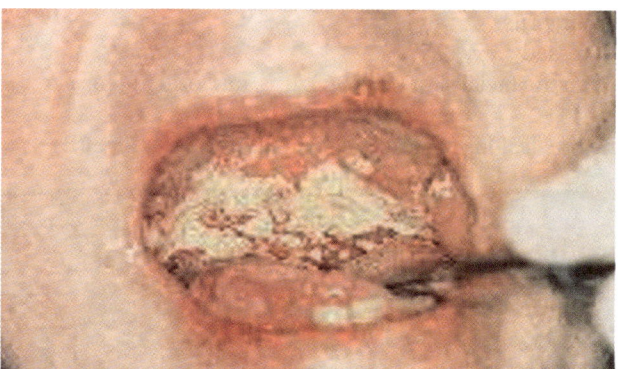

Fig. 5: Hyperplastic candidiasis involving oral cavity and soft palate.

Angular Cheilitis

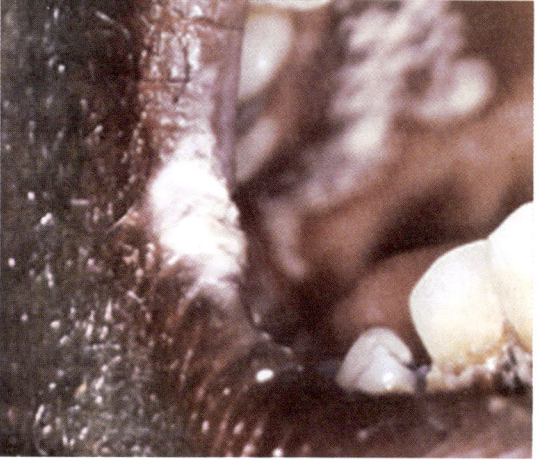

Fig. 6: Angular cheilitis involving oral cavity and angle of mouth.

Viral Manifestations

- Herpes zoster
- Oral hairy leukoplakia
- *Cytomegalovirus* (CMV) ulcers

- Human papilloma virus (HPV) lesions
- Herpes simplex virus (HSV) lesions

Herpes Simplex Ulcer

Q. Write short note on herpes simplex ulcer.

It involves the oral mucosa, periorally, involving the lips and skin.
- Painful, solitary, or multiple and vesicular; and they might coalesce **(Fig. 7)**.
- **Treatment:**
    - Acyclovir (400 mg QID)
    - IV acyclovir [5 mg/kg three times a day (TDS)]
    - Famciclovir (500 mg tds) —for 7–14 days

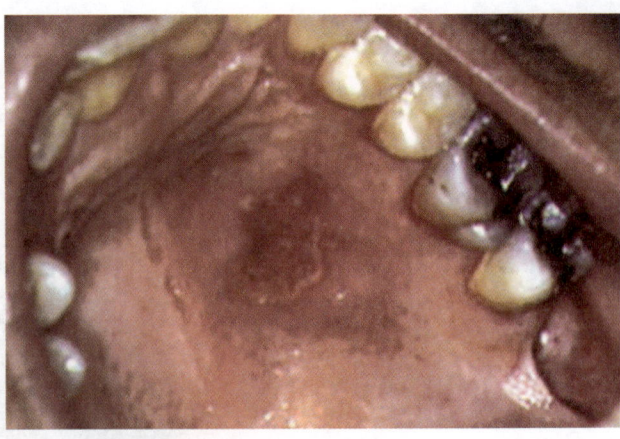

Fig. 7: Herpes simplex ulcer involving palate.

Herpes Zoster (Shingles)

Q. Write short note on herpes zoster.

- Reactivation of the varicella-zoster virus
- In the elderly and immunosuppressed
- Following pain, vesicles appear on the facial skin **(Fig. 8A)**, lips, and oral mucosa
- Frequently unilateral
- Skin lesions form crusts and the oral lesions coalesce to form large ulcers **(Fig. 8B)**

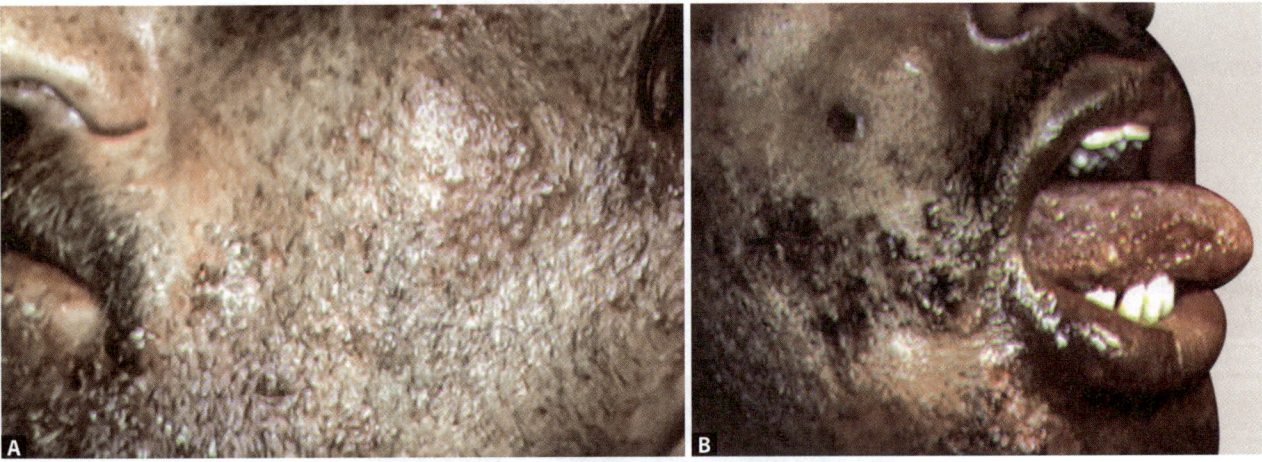

Figs. 8A and B: Vesicles of herpes zoster involving facial skin; (B) Skin crust and oral ulcers of herpes zoster.

Treatment:
- Acyclovir (800 mg 5 times a day) limits the duration of the lesions for 7–10 days.
- Famciclovir (500 mg tds) for 7 days.

Hairy Leukoplakia

Q. Write a short note on hairy leukoplakia.

- Occurs in male homosexual patients
- Associated with the Epstein–Barr (EBV) virus
- As the CD4 count increases
- Pathognomonic of HIV infection and often indicates progression to AIDS
- Lesion most frequently appears on the lateral aspect of the tongue **(Figs. 9A to C)** with a thick, vertically correlated (hairy) whitish plaque

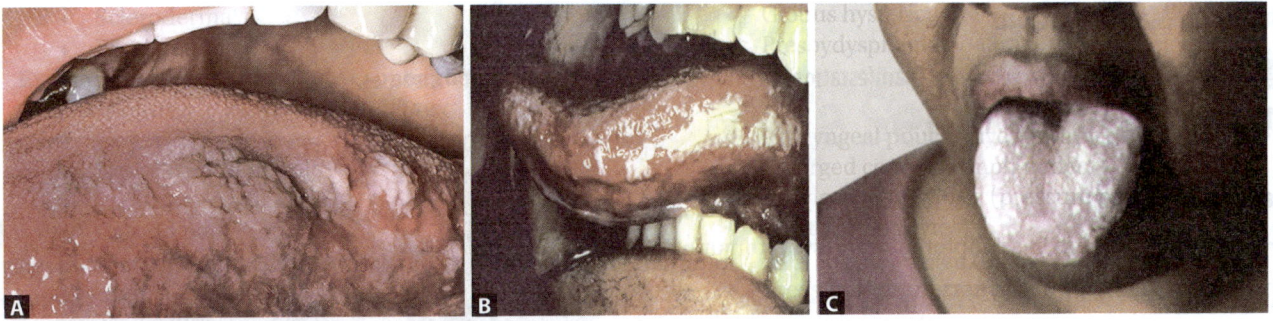

Figs. 9A to C: Whitish nonremovable lesions of hairy leukoplakia.

- Whitish, nonremovable, vertically corrugated patches found on the lateral region of the tongue.
- **Diagnosis:** Clinical appearance and biopsy.
- **Treatment:** Palliative, if the lesion is symptomatic.
  Treated with acyclovir (2 g/day), sulfa drugs, zidovudine, or topical retinoic acid.

Cytomegalovirus (CMV) Ulcers

- Painful, with punched-out, nonindurated borders
- Appear necrotic with a white halo
- **Diagnosis:**
  - Biopsy
- **Treatment:**
  - Acyclovir or ganciclovir

Human Papillomavirus (HPV) Lesions

Q. Write a short note on HPV lesions in AIDS/HIV patient.

- Human papillomavirus is associated with oral warts, papillomas, skin warts, and genital warts.
- May appear as solitary or multiple nodules (**Fig. 10A**).
- Or as multiple, smooth-surfaced raised masses (**Fig. 10B**).

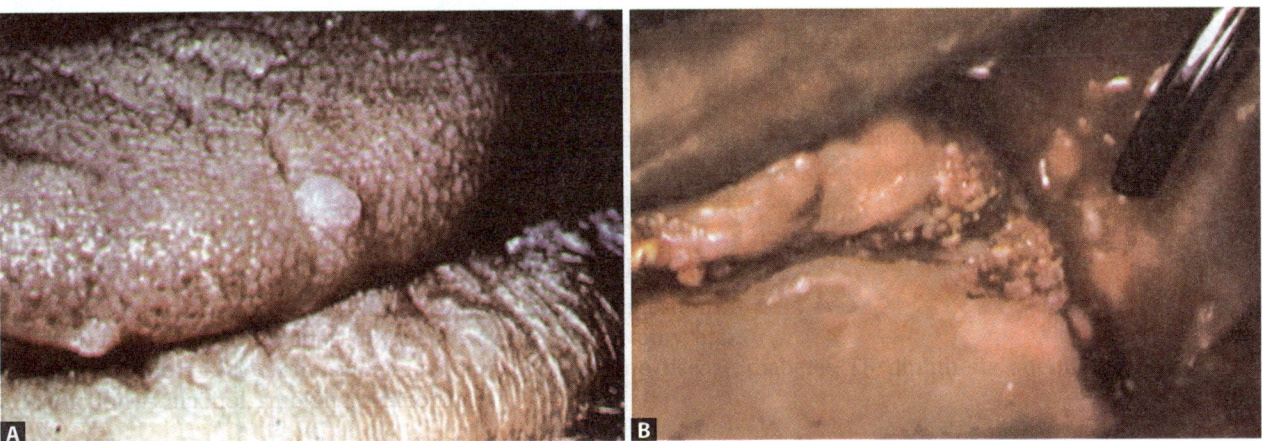

Figs. 10A and B: (A) Oral warts over tongue in HPV; (B) HPV lesions over oral mucosa.

- It may be cauliflower-like, spiked, or raised with a flat surface.
- **Diagnosis:**
  - Biopsy
- **Treatment:**
  - Surgical removal
  - Laser surgery
  - Cryotherapy

Bacterial Manifestations

Q. What are the various bacterial oral manifestations in HIV? Write a note on periodontal diseases.

Q. Write short note on aphthous ulcer.

Periodontal Disease

- It is fairly common in asymptomatic and symptomatic HIV-infected individuals.
- Two forms:
    1. Linear gingival erythema (LGE)
    2. Necrotizing ulcerative periodontitis (NUP)

Linear Gingival Erythema (Red-Band Gingivitis)

- 2–3 mm erythematous band on the gingiva **(Fig. 11)**
- Mild pain and spontaneous bleeding. It responds poorly to conventional therapy. It might be a precursor to necrotizing ulcerative periodontitis.

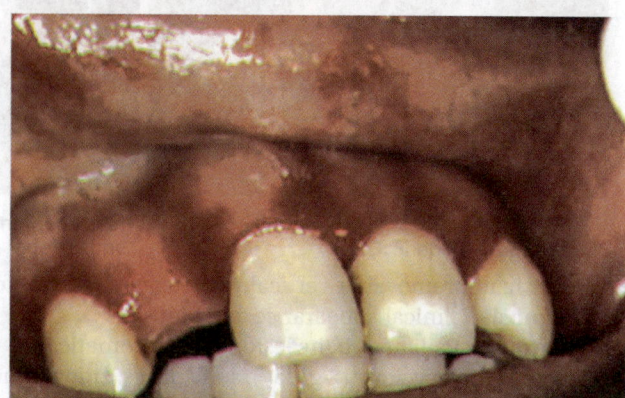

Fig. 11: Erythematous band on gingiva in red band gingivitis of periodontal disease.

Necrotizing Ulcerative Periodontitis

Q. Write short note on acute nectrotizing periodontitis.

- Rapidly progressive, extensive destruction, and loss of bone and periodontal tissue **(Figs. 12A and B)**.
- Painful, with bleeding and halitosis
- Distinguished from conventional periodontitis by its accelerated rate of progression and its deep-seated nongingival pain
- Associated with severe immune deterioration.
- **Diagnosis:** History and clinical appearance.
- **Biopsy:** It differentiates from other lesions such as non-Hodgkin's lymphoma (NHL) and CMV infection.
- **Treatment:** Antibiotics—metronidazole, mouth rinses, and irrigation with povidone iodine, debridement, and mechanical cleaning.
- Frequent dental visits

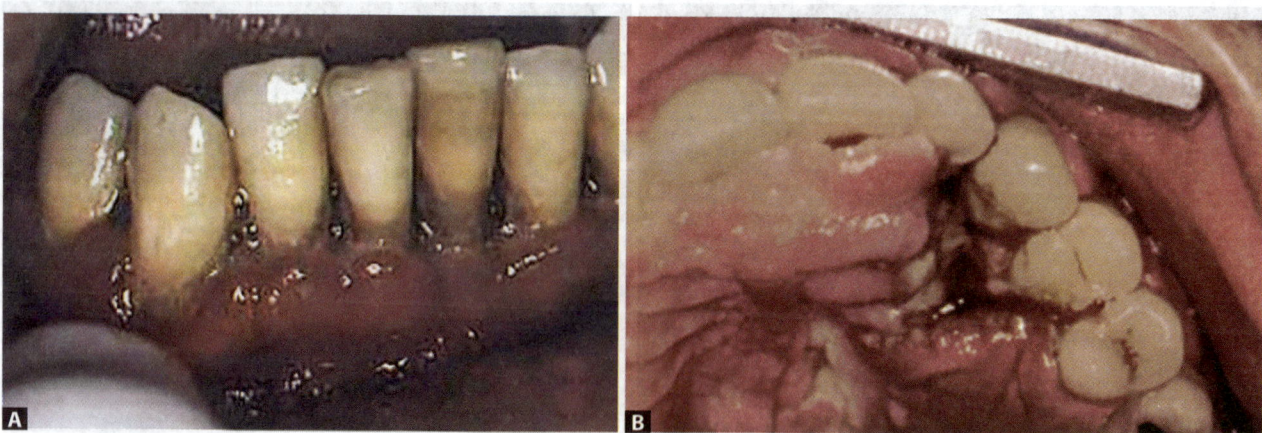

Figs. 12A and B: Extensive destruction and loss of bone and periodontal tissue in necrotizing ulcerative periodontitis.

Aphthous Ulcerations (Canker Sores)—Minor

- 2–5 mm in diameter, covered by a pseudomembrane and surrounded by an erythematous halo **(Fig.13)**.
- No known cause for recurrent ulcers.
- Stress, acidic foods, and tissue-barrier breakdown.

Aphthous Ulcerations—Major

- >10 mm in diameter, painful **(Fig. 14)**, persist for months and can cause impairment of speech and swallowing.

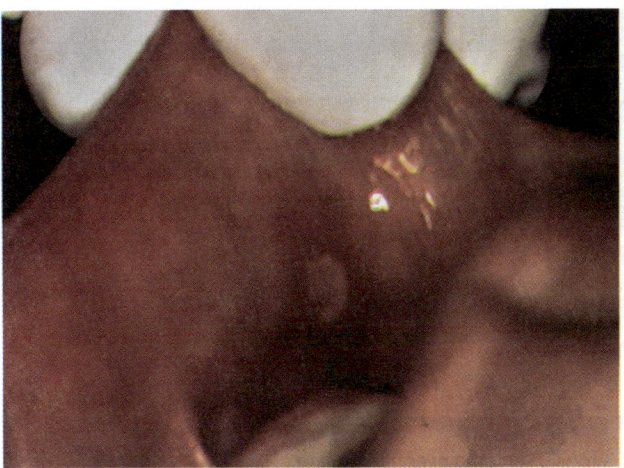

Fig. 13: Apthous ulcer involving mucosa of lower Lip.

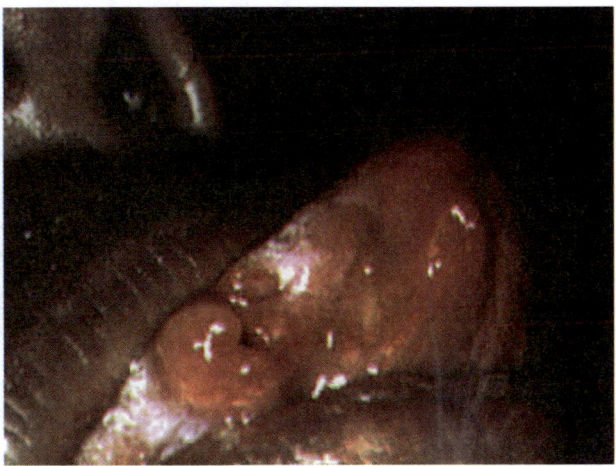

Fig. 14: Apthous ulcer major lesion involving tongue.

- ❖ **Diagnosis:**
  - ▷ Clinically
  - ▷ Biopsy rules out other causes
- ❖ **Treatment:**
  - ▷ Palliative, oral and topical rinse.
  - ▷ Miles "mixture"—liquid tetracycline, hydrocortisone, linocain, and nystatin.
  - ▷ Topical tetracycline—analgesic

Neoplastic Oral Manifestations

Q. Write a note/essay on neoplastic manifestations of HIV in oral cavity.

There are two types of neoplasms associated with oral manifestations in HIV individuals
1. Kaposi's sarcoma (KS)
2. Non-Hodgkin's lymphoma

Kaposi's Sarcoma

Q. Write a short note/essay on Kaposi's sarcoma.

- ❖ The most common oral tumor in AIDS patients
- ❖ **Risk:** 1% via blood transfusion; 21% via homosexual contact
- ❖ **HHV-8:** Causative agent

Clinical Presentation

- ❖ It can be found anywhere in the gastrointestinal tract, lungs, and skin; commonly seen on the hard or soft palate and gums.
- ❖ Dark, purple/pink macular lesions can be found on any oral mucosal surface but palate is involved in 95% of cases (**Figs. 15 to 18**).
- ❖ About 90% of the patients have multiple lesions, visceral more common, 63% in head and neck.
- ❖ Three forms:
  1. Classic—elderly men and Jewish descent.
  2. Endemic—in Africa—black young men and children.
  3. Epidemic—in AIDS and immune-compromised individuals
- ❖ It can enlarge, ulcerate, or get infected
- ❖ Pain and bleeding are common

Diagnosis

- ❖ An excisional biopsy is indicated, preferably from a cutaneous lesion, as these lesions are vascular and can bleed.
- ❖ Mesenchymal cell tumor involving blood and lymphatic vessels.
- ❖ **Haptoglobin-related protein (Hpr) report:** Interweaving bundles of spindle-shaped cells with vascular slits and red blood cells (RBC) and extravasations.

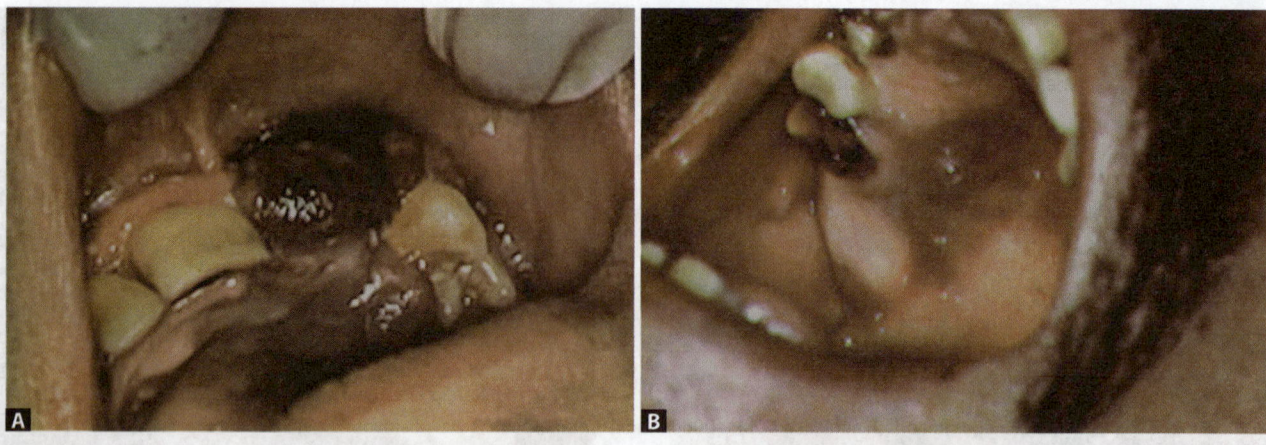

Figs. 15A and B: Purple macular lesions of Kaposi's sarcoma over hard palate.

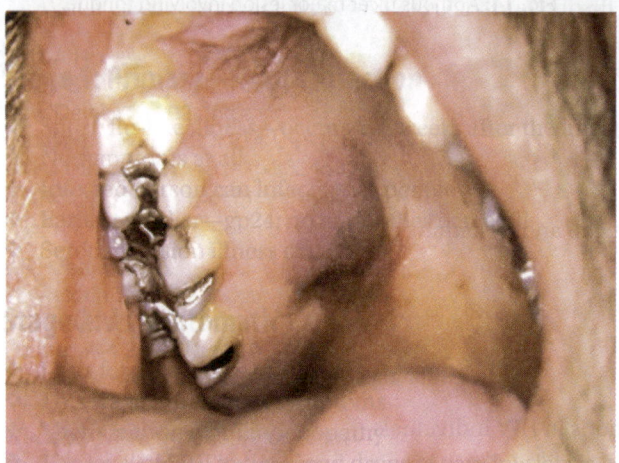

Fig. 16: Pink macular lesions of Kaposi's sarcoma over hard palate.

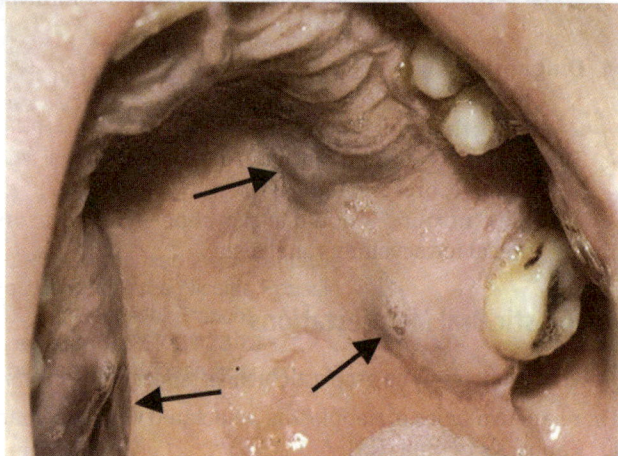

Fig. 17: Ulcerative lesions of Kaposi's sarcoma over hard palate.

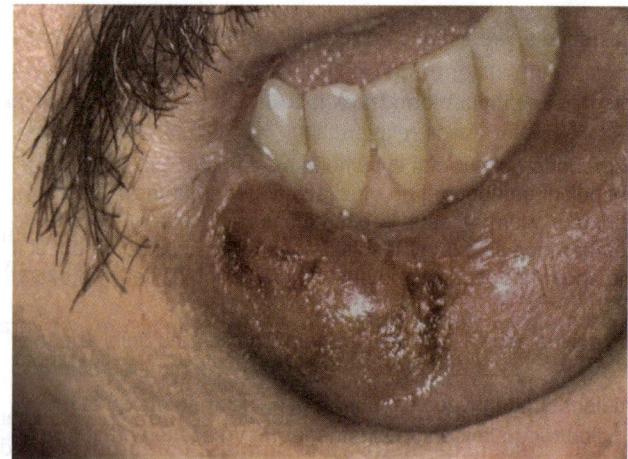

Fig. 18: Purple macular lesions of Kaposi's sarcoma over lower lip.

Differential Diagnosis

- Non-Hodgkin lymphoma (ulcerative)
- Bacillary angiomatosis
- Physiologic pigmentation
- Indications of treatment:
    - Symptomatic oral or visceral lesions
    - Pain or edema in lymphadenopathy
    - Cosmetic disfigurement

Treatment

Aim is palliative; not curative.
- **Local:**
    - Alitretinoin topical gel—35–50% local response
    - Radiation—15 Gy in 10 divided doses; 90% response.
    - Intralesional vinblastine or vincristine
    - Cryotherapy—liquid nitrogen
    - Laser therapy
    - Surgical excision
- **Intensification of highly active antiretroviral therapy (HAART):** Improved immunity, antiviral effect against HHV 8.
- **Chemotherapy:**
    - Reserved for visceral disease.
    - **Agents**—vincristine, vinblastine, anthracycline, bleomycin, and paclitaxel.

- Liposomal anthracyclines as a single agent-first line of treatment.
- Antiangiogenic compounds—thalidomide and retinoids
  - Antivirals—ganciclovir and cidofovir

Non-Hodgkin's Lymphoma

Q. Write a short note on Non-Hodgkin's lymphoma in HIV patients.

- Diffuse undifferentiated NHL
- B cell in origin
- Agent: Epstein–Barr virus (40–60%)
- It occurs in 10–30% of AIDS patients
- Nodal/extranodal can occur **(Figs. 19A and B)**
- Occurs in the late stage of disease when CD4 count <200/mm^3

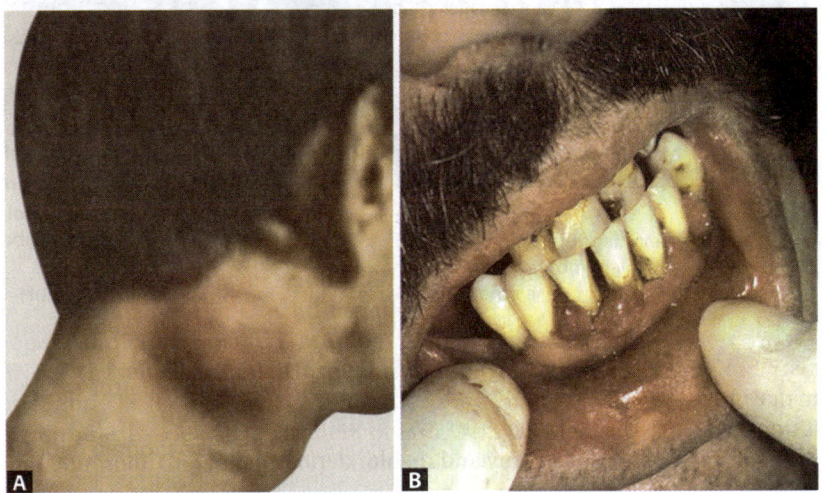

Figs. 19A and B: (A) Non-Hodgkin's lymphoma involving neck node; (B) Non-Hodgkin's lymphoma involving oral cavity.

- **Extranodal sites:** Oral cavity, sinonasal region, pharynx, orbit, parotid, and CNS.
- **Symptoms:** Fever, night sweats, weight loss.
- Epistaxis, nasal obstruction, proptosis, mass in the oral cavity, loose teeth, hoarseness of voice, and dysphagia.
- **Diagnosis:** Fine needle aspiration cytology (FNAC), open biopsy, and immunohistochemistry (IHC).
- Computed tomography (CT)/magnetic resonance imaging (MRI) of the brain, chest, abdomen, head, and neck.
- Lumbar puncture—60% have asymptomatic leptomeningeal lymphoma
- **Prognosis**—60% high-grade tumors, 33% medium-grade tumors
- Significantly worse course.
- Factors for ↓life expectancy
  - Extranodal involvement
  - Previous AIDS diagnosis
  - CD4 count <200/µL

Treatment:

- Multiagent chemotherapy
- HAART
- Radiotherapy—of localized disease or symptomatic lesions.

Other Manifestations

Xerostomia (Dry Mouth)

Q. Write short note on dry mouth/xerostomia in HIV patients.

- Reduced salivary flow
- Major contributing factor in dental decay in HIV-infected individuals
- Many medications lead to xerostomia **(Figs. 20A and B)**

- Didanosine (DDI), zidovudine, and foscarnet
- Antidepressants
- Antihistamines
- Antianxiety drugs

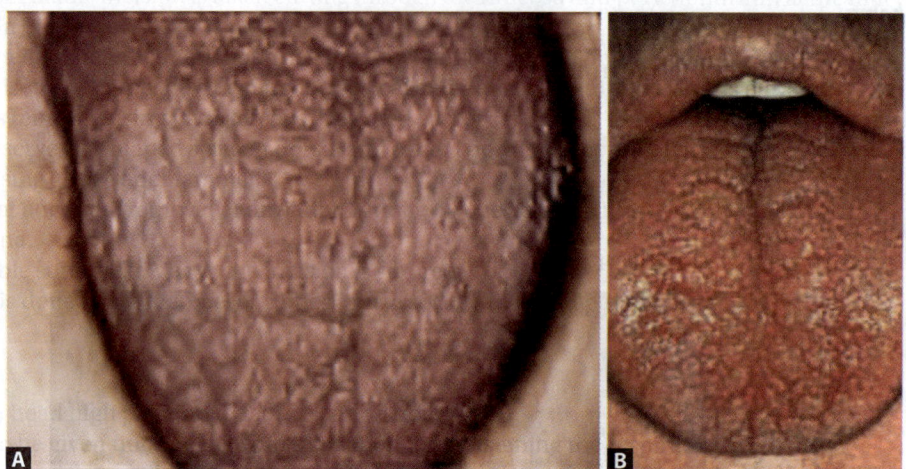

Figs. 20A and B: Dry tongue.

- ❖ **Other factors:**
  - Salivary gland disease
  - Smoking
- ❖ **Treatment:**
  - Salivary stimulants:
    - Sugarless gum or candy
    - Salivary substitutes
    - Caries can occur, so rinse with fluoride daily and regular dentist visits (2–3 times/year)

HIV-Esophagus

- ❖ Odynophagia and dysphagia esophagitis—*Candida*, CMV.
- ❖ Lymphoma and Kaposi's sarcoma can present as dysphagia.

CERVICAL LYMPHADENOPATHY IN HIV

Q. What are the causes of lymphadenopathy in HIV? Discuss in brief.

HIV lymphadenopathy	
HIV- related	Persistent generalized lymphadenopathy (PGL)
Opportunistic infections	Tuberculous lymphadenitis, CMV, toxoplasmosis, infections with *Nocardia* species, fungal infections (histoplasmosis, penicilliosis, *Cryptococcus*, etc.)
Reactive lymphadenopathy	Pyomyositis, pyogenic skin infections, ear, nose, and throat (ENT) infections
STIs	Syphilis, inguinal lymphadenopathy due to donovanosis, chancroid or lymphogranuloma venereum (LGV)
Malignancies	Lymphoma, Kaposi's sarcoma

Evaluation of HIV Lymphadenopathy

- ❖ History—tuberculosis (TB) contact, exposure to pets, alcohol, and tobacco consumption.
- ❖ Weight loss, night sweats, and fever.
- ❖ Fine needle aspiration cytology (FNAC)—initial investigation; if possible, cell block created from the sample.
- ❖ Sample sent for cytology, culture, and stains for aerobic-anaerobic bacteria, mycobacteria, and fungi; flow cytometry.
- ❖ Open biopsy is done in inconclusive FNAC and lymphoma.

Persistent Generalized Lymphadenopathy (PGL)

Presenting Signs and Symptoms

- Lymph nodes **larger than 1.5 cm** in diameter in **two or more extra inguinal** sites of **three or more months duration.**
- Nodes are nontender, symmetrical, and often involve the posterior cervical, axillary, occipital, and epitrochlear nodes

Histologic Patterns in PGL

- Follicular hyperplasia
- Follicular involution
- Lymphoid depletion
  Lymph node (LN) architecture is of prognostic value in disease progression to AIDS.
  Life expectancy decreases as the patient progresses through the above stages.

Tuberculosis Lymphadenopathy

Presenting Signs and Symptoms

- The cervical nodes are most commonly involved
- Usual course of lymph node disease is as follows:

$$\text{Firm, discrete nodes}$$
$$\downarrow$$
$$\text{Fluctuant nodes matted together}$$
$$\downarrow$$
$$\text{Skin breakdown, abscesses, and chronic sinuses}$$
$$\downarrow$$
$$\text{Healing and scarring}$$

- Fluctuant cervical nodes that develop over weeks to months without significant inflammation or tenderness, suggest infection with *Mycobacterium tuberculosis (M. tuberculosis)*, atypical mycobacteria, or scratch disease *(Bartonella henselae)*.
  - In severe immune compromised patients, tuberculosis lymphadenopathy may be acute and resemble acute pyogenic lymphadenitis.
  - Miliary TB is an important consideration in patients with generalized lymphadenopathy
  - Nocardiosis: **Clinical Symptoms may evolve:**
    - Chronic lymphadenopathy
    - Abscesses (skin, pulmonary, etc.)

Diagnosis

- Fine-needle aspiration of the involved lymph node.
- Organism may stain weakly on acid-fast staining. The organisms are different from the Koch's bacilli because of their thread-like filaments.
- Nocardia organisms are easily recognized on gram-stain.

Management and Treatment

- Trimethoprim/sulfamethoxazole (TMP/SMX) 10/50 mg/kg bid or minocycline 100 mg bid combined with amikacin 15–25 mg/kg daily.

Or

- Ceftriaxone 2 g daily combined with amikacin.
- The use of aminoglysides should be limited to 2 weeks.

Fungal Infections (Histoplasmosis, Penicilliosis, Cryptococcosis)

- Fever
- Lymphadenopathy
- Often skin lesions or lung lesions

Diagnosis

Biopsy for histology and culture of skin lesions or lymph nodes often reveals the diagnosis.

Management and Treatment

- Initial treatment for histoplasmosis and penicillinosis:
  - Amphotericin B for moderate to severe cases.
  - Itraconazole 200 mg daily is the preferred lifelong maintenance therapy.
  - If itraconazole is not available, use ketoconazole 400 mg daily.
- For *cryptococcosis* give:
  - Amphotericin B (IV) 0.7 mg/kg daily for 14 days, followed by fluconazole 400 mg daily for 8–10 weeks.
  - After that, maintenance therapy consists of fluconazole 200 mg once a day.

Hodgkin's Lymphoma

- 10 times more risk; aggressive clinical course
- Type—mixed cellularity and lymphoid depletion.
- 80–100% association with EBV
- Symptoms—mass in head and neck, constitutional
- Diagnosis—FNAC and biopsy
- Treatment—chemotherapy and HAART

Parotid Swellings

- Higher incidence in HIV patients
- 30% HIV + children have bilateral/persistent parotid swelling
- Benign lymphoepithelial cysts (BLC) **(Fig. 21B)**
- The most common cause of bilateral/persistent parotid swelling **(Fig. 21A)**
- Associated with ductal metaplasia; always seen in associated with paraganglioma (PGL)

Minimal symptoms

Diagnosis: FNAC

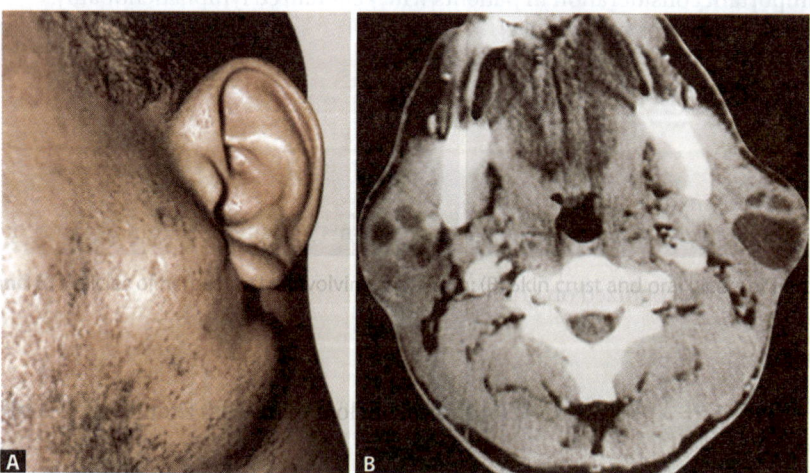

Figs. 21A and B: (A) Parotid swelling; (B) MRI neck showing benign lymphoepithelial cyst in both the parotid gland.

- **Differential diagnosis:**
  - Sjogren's syndrome
  - Cystic Warthin's tumor
  - Branchial cleft cysts
  - NHL
  - Metastatic Kaposi sarcoma
- **Treatment of benign lymphoepithelial cyst:**
  - Low dose radiation
  - Repeated needle aspirations and doxycycline injection.

SINONASAL INFECTIONS

Q. Write a note/essay on sinonasal infections/nasal manifestations in HIV.

- It is the most common symptom in HIV+
- Up to 70% of patients manifest nasal symptoms
- Nasal obstruction—adenoid hypertrophy
- Neoplasms—NHL, Kaposi sarcoma
- It can present as nasal mass, epistaxis, and diplopia.

Sinusitis

- Maxillary and ethmoid most common.
- **Symptoms**—fever, facial pain, nasal congestion, purulent discharge, and headache
- **Organisms**—*Streptococcus pneumoniae* (*S. pneumoniae*), *S. viridance*, *Staphylococcus aureus* (*S. aureus*), *Haemophilus influenzae* (*H. influenzae*).
- **Other**—*Legionella pneumophila* (*L. pneumophila*), *Cryptococcus neoformans* (*C. neoformans*), *Acanthamoeba*, CMV.
- *Pseudomonas aeruginosa* (*P. aeruginosa*): CD4 <200.

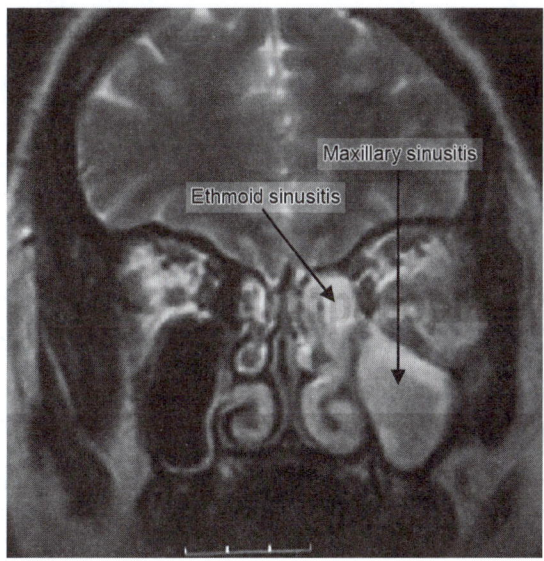

Fig. 22: MRI showing sinustis involving etmoid and maxillary sinus.

Management

- **CT scan**—to know the extent of disease, bony erosion, and orbital involvement **(Fig. 22)**.
- *Broad-spectrum antibiotics*: Amoxyclav and cefuroxime
- *Decongestants*—Pseudoephedrine
- *Mucolytics*—Guaifenesin
- **Pseudomonas**—antipseudomonal penicillin or cephalosporin and aminoglycoside for 4–6 weeks, aggressive treatment, and surgical drainage.

Invasive Fungal Sinusitis

- In late-stage AIDS
- Life-threatening condition.
- *Pathogen*—*Aspergillus fumigatus* (**A. Fumigatus**), *Candida albicans* (*C. albicans*), and *Rhizopus*
- **Symptoms**—facial swelling, paresthesias, pain, fever, proptosis, ↓vision, diplopia, and meningeal signs.
- **Endoscopy**—pale ischemic mucosa and necrotic plaques
- **Diagnosis:**
  - CT-bony erosion and orbital invasion **(Fig. 23)**
  - MRI—low-intensity T2 image
  - Biopsy from middle meatus; sent for histopathology reporting and fungal culture
- **Treatment:**
  - ***Surgical debridement***—to minimize fungal load; via endoscopy, and orbital exenteration.
  - ***Systemic antifungals***—Amphotericin B; poor renal function—liposomal amphotericin B, Triazoles, and caspofungin, as an alternative therapy.
  - **HAART**—improve immune status.

OTOLOGIC MANIFESTATIONS OF HIV

Q. Write short note/essay on otologic manifestations of HIV.

External Ear

Seborrheic Dermatitis

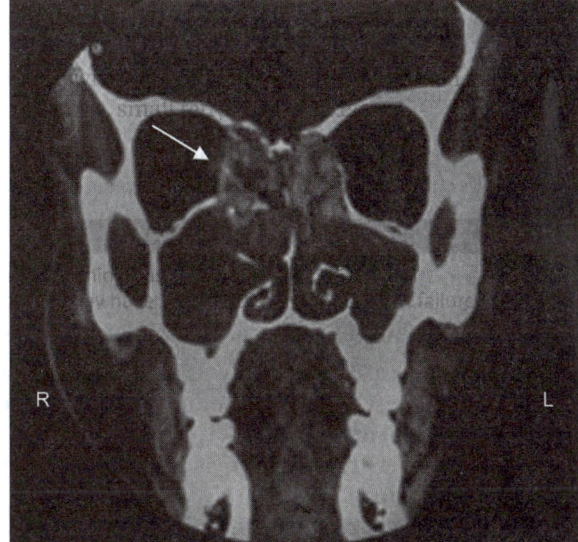

Fig. 23: CT PNS showing involvement of ethmoid sinuses with bony erosion.

- Scaly patches involving the external auditory canal (EAC), face, and scalp.
- **Treatment:** Zinc-pyrithione shampoo, coal tar, selenium sulfide, and ketoconazole.

PART 1: Diseases of ENT, Head and Neck

Kaposi's Sarcoma

- Involves pinna and EAC
- It causes conductive hearing loss

Otitis Externa

- Severe infection of EAC
- Agent: *P. aeruginosa*.
- Symptoms: Severe otalgia, otorrhea, and fever.
- Treatment: Topical antibiotic drops with acetic acid and steroid.
- Canal debridement and oral fluoroquinolones in resistant cases.

Skull Base Osteomyelitis

Q. Write short note on skull base osteomyelitis.

- Complication of otitis externa (OE), low CD4 count, and neutropenia.
- Symptoms: Otalgia, otorrhea, fever, facial nerve palsy, and cranial nerve involvement.
- **Otoscopy**—granulation tissue at the bony-cartilaginous junction. Debris in EAC.
- Diagnosis:
  - *Tc-99 scan*: ↑ uptake in the temporal bone
- **Gallium-67 bone scans:** Monitor response to the treatment.
- **Treatment:** 6 weeks IV antibiotics—antipseudomonal penicillins/third generation cephalosporin and aminoglycosides or quinolones.
- *A. fumigatus*: Otitis externa/malignant OE in patients with AIDS.
  - Diagnosis: Send debris from external auditory canal for fungal culture and histopathological reporting
  - Treatment: Amphotericin B; debridement of soft tissue and bone
- *Pneumocystis carinii (P. carini)*—cyst/polyp in EAC
  - Diagnosis: Biopsy and staining with Gomori's methenamine silver stain.
  - Treatment: Trimethoprim—sulfamethoxazole

Middle Ear

Serous Otitis Media

Etiology: Eustachian tube obstruction by adenoid hypertrophy or sinonasal disease.

Acute Otitis Media (Fig. 24)

- More frequent in children.
- Etiology—*S. pneumoniae, H. influenzae, Moraxella catarrhalis (M. catarrhalis), A. fumigatus,* and *P. carini*
- Complications—intracranial extension, facial palsy, and petrous apicitis ↑ with immunocompromised individuals.

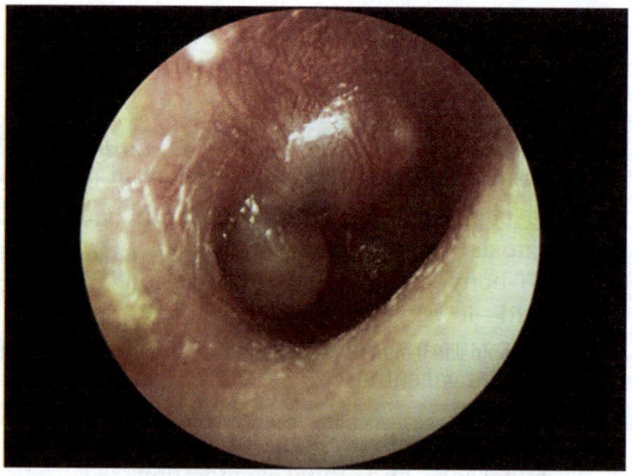

Fig. 24: Congested and bulging tympanic membrane In acute otitis media.

Sensorineural Hearing Loss

Q. Write short note on sensorineural hearing loss in HIV patients.

- Approximately 49% of the patients suffer from various degrees of sensorineural hearing loss (SNHL).
  - Aural fullness, vertigo, and tinnitus may be present.
  - **Differential diagnosis:**
    - Ototoxic drugs—acyclovir, zidovudine (AZT), ganciclovir, and isoniazid.
    - Otosyphilis
    - Cryptococcal meningitis, CNS toxoplasmosis
    - Tuberculous meningitis
    - Central effects of HIV—autoimmune demyelination of VIIIth nerve, subacute encephalitis, aseptic meningitis
    - NHL, hearing loss (HL) involving CNS, progressive multifocal leukoencephalopathy (PML)
    - Cerebrovascular accidents
    - Idiopathic

- ❖ **Evaluation of SNHL:**
  - ▷ Rule out potentially life-threatening diseases.
  - ▷ History—headache, fever, neck stiffness, disequilibrium, and neurological symptoms. List of all medications.
  - ▷ Pure tone audiogram, speech discrimination test.
  - ▷ Serology—venereal disease research laboratory (VDR), fluorescent treponemal antibody absorption (FTA-ABS), erythrocyte sedimentation rate (ESR), antineutrophil cytoplasmic antibody (ANCA), rheumatoid factor (RF); SR, cryptococcal antigen (CrAg).
  - ▷ Lumbar puncture—fungal, bacterial culture; cytology.
  - ▷ CT/MRI brain.
- ❖ **Management**:
  - ▷ Stop ototoxic drugs, if possible.
  - ▷ **Otosyphilis**—higher doses of penicillin; cautious use of steroids.
  - ▷ Penicillin G up to 24 MU/day for 3 weeks.
  - ▷ **Cryptococcal meningitis:** Amphotericin B (0.7 mg/kg/day) for 2 weeks, followed by fluconazole (400 mg/day) for 6 weeks with lifelong suppression with fluconazole (200 mg/day).
  - ▷ Important to **avoid indiscriminate use of steroids** in sudden SNHL; **for the risk of precipitating life-threatening infections** like cryptococcal meningitis.
  - ▷ Rehabilitation with hearing aids can be considered.

Facial Palsy

Q. Write short note on facial palsy in HIV patients.

- ❖ Human immunodeficiency virus patient has 100 times more risk of facial palsy
- ❖ It can occur in up to 7.2% patients of HIV.
- ❖ Isolated facial palsy may be the first symptom of HIV infection with acute infection in the early stage.
- ❖ **Ramsay–Hunt syndrome:** (Herpes zoster oticus) in late HIV infection.
- ❖ **Symptoms:** Facial palsy, herpetic vesicles along the VIIth nerve. dermatome, and on concha, severe pain.
- ❖ **Treatment:** High dose of acyclovir and steroids.
- ❖ Differential diagnosis of facial palsy in HIV infection:
  - ▷ *Isolated facial palsy:*
    - ♦ Geniculate ganglionitis—herpes simplex, herpes zoster, CMV, EBV, and HIV.
    - ♦ Malignant otitis externa
    - ♦ Complicated otomastoiditis
    - ♦ Malignancy of parotid.
    - ♦ Autoimmune demyelination
    - ♦ Idiopathic (Bell's) palsy
  - ▷ *Associated with other neurologic abnormalities:*
    - ♦ Effects of HIV—autoimmune demyelination, mononeuritis multiplex, and encephalitis.
    - ♦ CNS infection—toxoplasmosis, cryptococcal meningitis, PML, TB meningitis.
    - ♦ Neoplasms—NHL, metastatic Kaposi sarcoma.

■ EVALUATION OF HIV PATIENT

- ❖ History—otorrhea, fever, headache, meningeal signs, and flu-like illness.
- ❖ Examine—the ear, vesicles in the concha, and parotid masses
- ❖ Audiometry
- ❖ Serology—VDRL, FTA-ABS, ESR, ANCA, RF; SR, cryptococcal Ag.
- ❖ Lumbar puncture—fungal, bacterial culture; and cytology
- ❖ CT/MRI brain
- ❖ HIV testing to be done in all cases of facial palsy

■ MANAGEMENT OF HIV PATIENT

- ❖ Corticosteroids—benefits weighed against the risk of further immunocompromised.
- ❖ Should be given in early HIV, bilateral facial palsy.
- ❖ High dose acyclovir—effects not proven
- ❖ Eye care—artificial tears and tarsorrhaphy
- ❖ Plasmapheresis—multiple cranial nerve palsy due to autoimmune origin, where steroids are risky.

ANTIRETROVIRAL THERAPY

Q. Classify antiretroviral drugs. Briefly discuss antiretroviral therapy.

Four Major Classes of Drugs

- **Nucleotide reverse transcriptase inhibitors (NRTI)**—prevent the formation of proviral DNA from RNA.
  - *Mechanism:* Inhibit reverse transcriptase enzyme.
  - Example:
    - Zidovudine (AZT)
    - Didanosine (ddI)
    - Zalcitabine (ddC)
    - Stavudine (d4T)
    - Lamivudine (3TC)
- **NNRTI**—prevent the formation of proviral DNA
  - *Mechanism:* Inhibit reverse transcriptase enzyme by binding to them.
  - Example:
    - Delavirdine
    - Nevirapine
    - Efavirenz
    - Tenofovir (nucleotide analog)
- **Protease inhibitors (PI)**— prevent cleavage of viral proteins into their functional forms by binding to viral protease enzyme.
  - Mechanism: Interrupt the protein processing and virus assembly.
  - Example:
    - Saquinavir
    - Ritonavir
    - Indinavir
- **Fusion inhibitors**—interfere with the entry of the virus into the target cells.
  - *Mechanism:* They bind to HIV-gp41
  - Example:
    - Enfuvirtide

Highly Active Antiretroviral Therapy

- Combination of three drugs
  - 2 NRTI +1 PI
  - 2 NRTI + 1 NNRTI
  - 1 NRTI + 1 NNRTI + 1 PI
- Reduced chances of drug resistance
- Effectively ↓es viral load.

Criteria for Starting HAART

- CD4 <200/μL irrespective of WHO stage—or
- WHO stage 4 AIDS-defining illness irrespective of CD4 count.
- Viral load above 5,000–10,000 copies/mL.

First-line Therapy (Regimen 1)

- Stavudine 40 mg BD + lamivudine 150 mg BD
- Efavirenz 600 mg HS
- Nevirapine 200 mg BD
- Monitor—CD4 count, viral load, and liver function tests (LFTs) every 6 months.
- **Failure on ART 1:** ↓ CD4 count, ↑ viral load and disease progression, opportunistic infections.

Second-line Therapy (Regimen 2)

- Zidovudine 300 mg BD + didanosine 400 mg OD and lopinavir (400 mg)/ritonavir (100 mg) BD.
- Prophylaxis for opportunistic infections:

➢ Co-trimoxazole for *Pneumocystis carinii* pneumonia (PCP)
➢ Fluconazole for cryptococcal meningitis

Postexposure Prophylaxis (PEP)

❖ About 0.3% risk after needle prick injury.
❖ **High-risk factors**—deep injury, visible blood on the device, large inoculum, a source in the terminal stage.
❖ Commence treatment at the earliest.
❖ Check serostatus of the source patient.
   ➢ Exposure on intact skin—no PEP
   ➢ Mucosal splash or nonintact skin—two-drug therapy.
   ➢ Percutaneous sharps—two drug or three drug (if high risk).
   ➢ Percutaneous (deep, IV cannula)—three drug or two drug (if source status is unknown).

PEP Drugs

❖ Zidovudine 300 mg BD + lamivudine 150 mg BD for 28 days +/-
❖ Lopinavir (400 mg)/ritonavir (100 mg) BD for 28 days.

Adverse drug reaction (Figs. 25A and B):

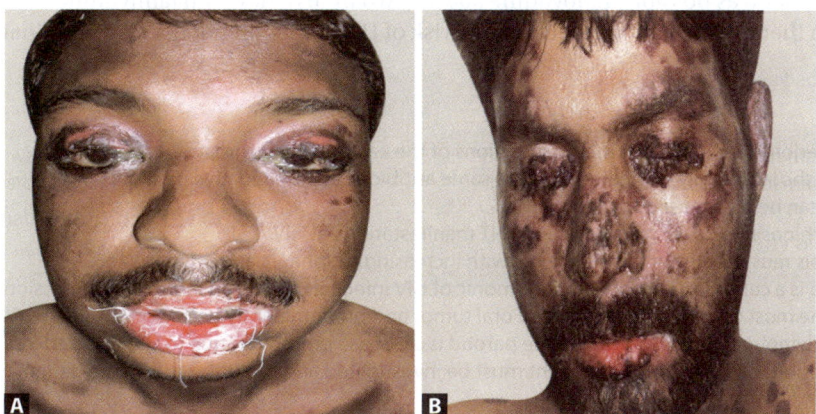

Figs. 25A and B: Facial edema, necrotic lesions due to side effect of antiretroviral drugs.

■ UNIVERSAL PRECAUTIONS ARE THE BEST DEFENSE

Pediatric AIDS is becoming increasingly frequent. Most cases are due to transmission from the mother. Intrapartum trauma is the most frequent (70%) mode of transmission. Transplacental and breast milk transmission are less frequent. Positive Elisa or Western Bolt tests do not indicate HIV infection in a child <18 months. The tests for HIV antigens like p24 antigenemia or qualitative PCR for HIV are needed to diagnose HIV infection in infants. The standard immunization schedule is recommended also for the HIV-infected children. Health is unaffected in the first 6 months of life. However, life expectancy is only about 5 years as a minor, recurrent upper and lower respiratory tract infections begin in the 1st year in some and by the 3rd year in most. Failure to thrive, diarrhea, and lymphadenopathy are other common indicators. Cutaneous viral, fungal, bacterial, and parasitic infections are common. Hepatosplenomegaly, lymphoid interstitial pneumonia, sicca syndrome, HIV encephalopathy, cardiomyopathy, and lymphomas are all more common in children than adults. The principles of management are similar to those in adults. Antiretroviral drugs that can be administered in children include azidothymidine, dideoxynosine DDL, 3 TC, nelfinavir, and nevirapine.

When the AIDS epidemic broke out in the USA in the year 1981, and even a few years later, AIDS was believed to affect only the homosexual population. Today the dominant mode of HIV transmission is by heterosexual intercourse. This has, therefore, made it very difficult to control, and hence the infection has become endemic in many parts of the world including India. The prevalence was homosexuality in India is popularly believed to be very low (<5%).

■ PREVENTION OF AIDS OR HIV INFECTION

Following are the guidelines for operation theaters—the minimum necessary staff and equipment should be present in the operating theater (OT) during surgery. The operating table should be covered with a disposable plastic sheet. Staff with a wound or abrasion or skin disease should stay out. Staff should wear sterile disposable plastic gowns, double gloves, goggles, and overshoes. Cutting electrocautery is preferred over scalpel. The clips are preferred over suturing with needles. This reduces the chances of accidental cutting or penetrating trauma. Sharp instruments should never be handed down from one person to another. They should always be carried on a tray. Disposal of needles and blades to be done as per the guidelines. Reusable instruments should be double autoclaved. Resuscitation by the ventilator is preferred to mouth-to-mouth resuscitation.

Following are the guidelines for examining or treating patients in an out-patient department—use gloves and goggles during endoscopy. Videoendoscopy is preferred. Fluid and tissue specimens should be put in a bottle with a stopper and be carried by the gloved hands. Whenever possible, use disposable instruments. Reusable instruments should be washed with gloved hands with soap and water and then put in 2% glutaraldehyde for 20 minutes or autoclave. The needles need to be destroyed by a needle cutter and then disposed off in a thick plastic container with a tight cap. Alternatively, they can be sterilized in a plastic tray containing 1% of sodium hypochlorite before being disposed off in a plastic container. Needle should never be recapped as this increases the chance of needle stick injury. Surgical blades should be disposed of in a way similar to needles. Large equipment and furniture or floor-stained with tissue fluid can be disinfected by wiping with sodium hypochlorite 1% (prepared fresh by 1:10 dilution of common household bleach).

Postexposure prophylaxis refers to the measures taken to reduce the chance of infection with HIV after a person has been exposed to the risk of acquiring HIV, e.g., in a health worker or after transfusion with infected blood or after risky sexual exposure. The risk of transmission is highest if the infected fluid is blood or semen. It is delivered into the body by penetrating the wound. The amount of fluid was large, if the patient was in the late stage of HIV infection and in case of nonpenetrating wounds if the area of contact was large or mucosal. In such cases, begin a two or three drug antiretroviral prophylaxis within 2 hours of exposure or as soon as possible. Zidovudine 300 mg two times a day with lamivudine 300 mg/day for 4–6 weeks is the basic regimen. Such therapy substantially reduces the risk of HIV infection but does not eliminate the risk.

■ SUMMARY

1. Routine infections predominate when it comes to infections of the ear, nose, and throat.
2. HIV-positive patients should initially be treated with the same antibiotic as HIV-negative patients.
3. Multiple oral lesions can be present simultaneously.
4. Oral candidiasis and rhinosinusitis are most common ENT manifestations of HIV.
5. Esophageal candidiasis must be suspected in patients with increasing dysphagia and odynophagia.
6. Oral hairy leukoplakia is a condition almost pathognomonic of HIV infection and often indicates progression to AIDS.
7. Kaposi's sarcoma is the most common HIV-associated oral tumor and predominantly occurs on the palate.
8. HIV-associated cystic lymphoepithelial disease of the parotid is a disease process unique to HIV-infected individuals.
9. Otitis media with effusion (OME) in the adult patient must be investigated and the HIV status of the patient ascertained.

PART 2

Operative Procedures

Outline

Section 1: Ear
50. Tympanoplasty
51. Mastoidectomy
52. Myringotomy
53. Wax Removal

Section 2: Nose
54. Septoplasty and Submucous Resection of Septum
55. Polypectomy
56. Functional Endoscopic Sinus Surgery
57. Endoscopic Septoplasty
58. Nasal Packing

Section 3: Throat
59. Tonsillectomy
60. Adenoidectomy
61. Thyroidectomy

62. Tracheostomy
63. Cricothyroidotomy

Section 4: Various Scopy
64. Laryngoscopy
65. Microlaryngoscopy
66. Esophagoscopy
67. Bronchoscopy

Section 5: Recent Advances
68. Laser in ENT
69. Coblation
70. Radiofrequency
71. Cryosurgery
72. Robotics in ENT
73. Chemotherapy in ENT
74. Radiotherapy in ENT

PART 2

Operative Procedures

Outline

Section One
50. Tymponoplasty
51. Mastoidectomy
52. Myringotomy
53. Wax Removal

Section Two
54. Septoplasty and Submucous Resection of Septum
55. Polypectomy
56. Functional Endoscopic Sinus Surgery
57. Eustachian Tuboplasty
58. Nasal Polyps
59. Septal Abscess
60. Tonsillectomy

61. Adenoidectomy
62. Tracheostomy
63. Chronic Otitis Media
64. Laryngoscopy
65. Microlaryngoscopy with integral ...
66. Esophagoscopy
67. Bronchoscopy

Section Three
68. Laser in ENT
69. Cryosurgery
70. Radiofrequency surgery in otorhinolaryngology
71. Robotics in ENT
72. Radiotherapy in ENT

Section 1: Ear

Chapter 50: Tympanoplasty

EN4.10: Observe and describe the indications for and steps involved in myringotomy and tympanoplasty.

■ INTRODUCTION

Q. What is tympanoplasty/myringoplasty? Write a note/essay on its indications and contraindications and procedure.

Tympanoplasty: It is a surgical procedure to eradicate disease in the middle ear and to reconstruct the hearing mechanism, with or without tympanic membrane grafting.

Myringoplasty: It is a surgical to reconstruct the tympanic membrane without examining/repairing ossicular chain for hearing in middle ear.

Total perforation tympanic membrane results in 40 to 45 dB of conductive hearing loss.

Goals of tympanoplasty:
- To achieve dry ear by eradicating middle ear disease.
- Improvement in hearing by closure of tympanic membrane by grafting and/ or ossicular reconstruction.

■ INDICATIONS

Tympanic membrane perforations and associated hearing loss with or without middle ear pathology such as chronic suppurative otitis media, non-healed traumatic perforation, tympanosclerosis, small retraction pockets.

■ CONTRAINDICATIONS

Absolute	Relative
❖ Poor health ❖ Acute middle ear infection ❖ Malignant tumors of the outer ear/ middle ear ❖ Uncontrolled cholesteatoma ❖ Malignant otitis externa ❖ Complications of chronic ear diseases like—meningitis, brain abscess, lateral sinus thrombosis ❖ Only/significantly better hearing ear to avoid postoperative sensorineural hearing loss (SNHL)	❖ Non-functioning Eustachian tube ❖ Smokers: They have 3 fold increased risk of graft failure

PROCEDURE

Anesthesia

- **Local anesthesia** with intravenous injection is most commonly used.
- For anxious, uncooperative and revision surgeries, general anesthesia may be used.

Steps of Surgery

- Various incisions for the surgery are shown in **Figures 1 to 3**.
- Patient is made to lie in supine position with the head turned to the opposite side. Intravenous sedation is given.
- Using 2% lignocaine with adrenaline (1:200000) solution, local infiltration is given in the post aural region and the external auditory canal.
- Aseptic painting and draping is done.
- William Wilde's incision is taken 5 mm behind the postauricular region from the zygoma above, parallel to the sulcus to the mastoid tip below.
- The incision is deepened to reach the level of the temporalis fascia.
- Mollisons self-retaining hemostatic retractor is applied to retract the soft tissues and temporalis fascia is exposed adequately and is then harvested.
- The incision is deepened till the periosteum is reached and the periosteal flap is elevated using a Farabeuf periosteal elevator to expose the spine of Henle.
- A posterior meatotomy is done just below the level of spine of Henle.
- Mollisons retractor is applied for better exposure.
- Now using a microscope, the external auditory canal and the tympanic membrane are inspected.
- Using a sickle knife, margin of the perforation is freshened, undersurface of the tympanic membrane is undermined using a circular knife.
- Then two incisions are taken at 6 o'clock and 12 o'clock on the meatal wall.
- Using a circular knife, posterior tympanomeatal flap is elevated till the fibrous annulus.
- The annulus is elevated using curved picked and middle ear is entered.
- The middle ear mucosa is inspected, the ossicular status is and mobility of ossicular chain is checked.
- After finding the ossicular chain to be mobile, the harvested temporalis fascia graft is introduced into the middle ear under the tympanomeatal flap.
- The temporalis fascia graft is adjusted properly and tympanomeatal flap is reposited back.
- Medicated gelfoam pieces are kept at the edge of the graft and the external auditory canal.
- Mollisons retractor is removed and the incision is closed in layers.
- Mastoid dressing is given.

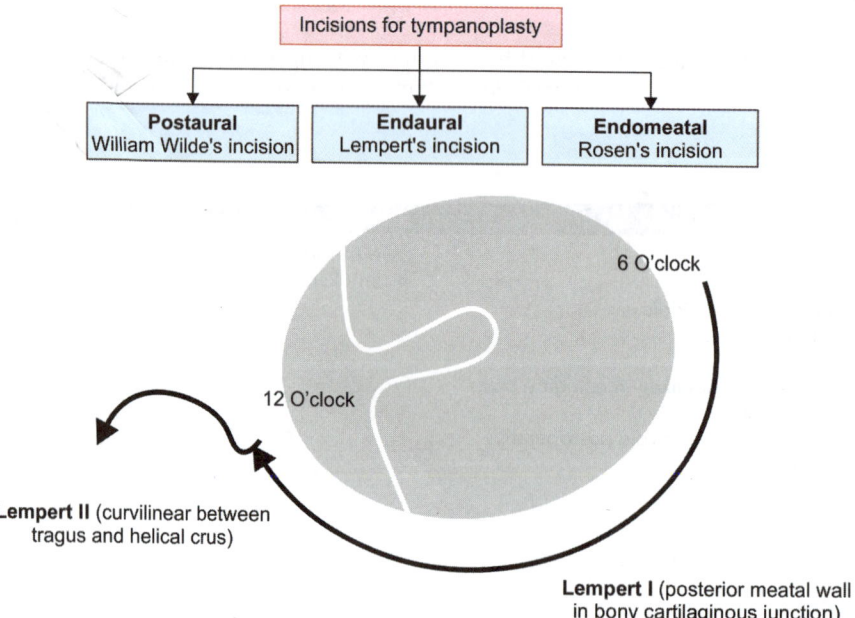

Fig. 1: Lempert's endaural incision.

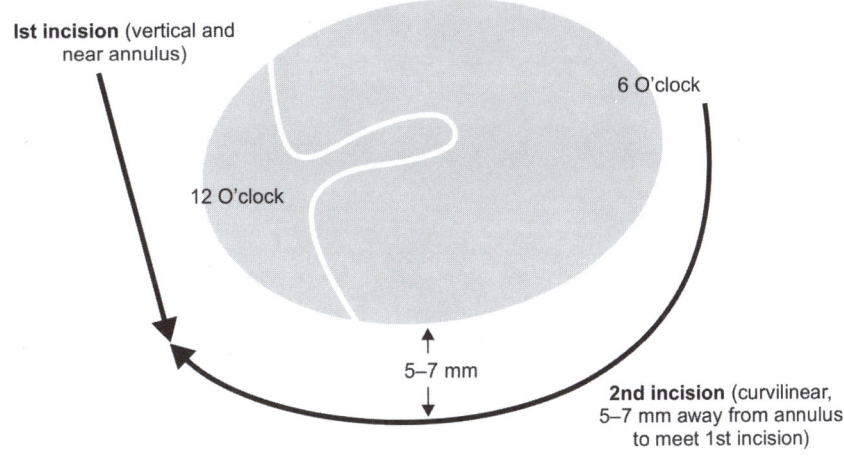

Fig. 2: Rosen's endomeatal incision.

Postoperative

- Postoperatively antibiotics and analgesics are given.
- Check dressing is done after 24 hours to look for bleed, soak or hematoma.

COMPLICATIONS OF TYMPANOPLASTY

Intraoperative	Postoperative
- Bleeding - Facial palsy due to local infiltration - Tear of tympanomeatal flap - Damage to the chorda tympani - Injury to dehiscent facial nerve	- Hematoma of temporalis muscle - Giddiness and nystagmus due to iatrogenic vestibular injury - Failure of graft uptake - Wound infection - Perichondritis - Sensorineural hearing loss due to avulsion of the stapes

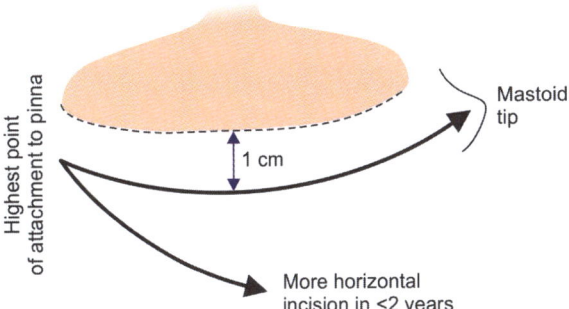

Fig. 3: William Wilde's postaural incision.

GRAFTING MATERIALS USED IN TYMPANOPLASTY

- Temporalis fascia
- Cartilage—most commonly tragal cartilage and conchal cartilage are used.
- Perichondrium
- Fat
- Acellular dermal homografts like alloderm, life cell corporation, etc.
- Tutopatch
- Xenograft–bovine pericardium.

WULLSTEIN'S CLASSIFICATION OF TYMPANOPLASTY

Q. Write a short note on Wullstein's classification of tympanoplasty.

Type I: Repair of tympanic membrane perforation; Ossicular chain is intact and hence there is no need for ossicular chain repair.
Type II: Ossicular chain is partially eroded (manubrium of malleus) but preserved. It is repaired by draping the tympanic membrane onto the remaining malleus and the long process of incus.
Type IIIA: Reconstructive material is interposed between the capitulum and the undersurface of the tympanic membrane.
Type IIIB: Reconstructive material is placed from the stapes footplate to the undersurface of the tympanic membrane.
Type IV: Graft is directly placed onto the round window, leaving the stapes footplate exposed.
Type V: Middle ear is covered to protect the window and to allow sound transmission to pass to a fenestrated lateral semicircular canal.

Prerequisites for tympanoplasty:
- Dry ear
- Middle ear space should be there
- Patent Eustachian tube
- Absence of infection in ear, nose or throat
- Choose larger perforation
- Choose ear with more hearing loss (the side where weber's lateralises)

Chapter 51

Mastoidectomy

EN4.11: Enumerate the indications, describe the steps and observe mastoidectomy.

MIDDLE EAR SURGERIES

Q. What are the various middle ear surgeries? Enumerate and describe in a sentence each.

- **Myringoplasty:** Repair of tympanic membrane with a graft
- **Tympanoplasty:** Removal of disease from middle ear
  - Repair hearing mechanism by ossiculoplasty +/- myringoplasty
  - No mastoid surgery
- **Mastoidectomy:** Drilling out mastoid air cells to eradicate disease
- Tympanomastoidectomy = Removal of disease from middle ear and mastoid and restore hearing (ossiculoplasty +/- myringoplasty)

MASTOIDECTOMY

Q. What is mastoidectomy? Enumerate its types.

It is a surgical procedure involving removal of mastoid air cells to eradicate the middle ear cleft disease and restore its function or as an approach to other surgeries **(Figs. 1 to 3)**.

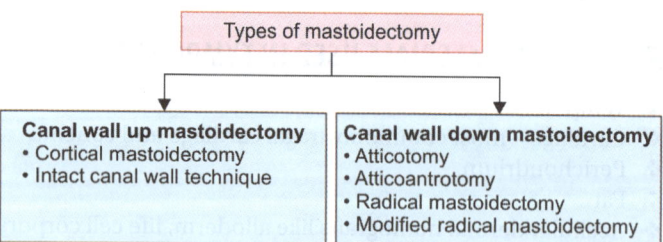

Types of mastoidectomy

Canal wall up mastoidectomy
- Cortical mastoidectomy
- Intact canal wall technique

Canal wall down mastoidectomy
- Atticotomy
- Atticoantrotomy
- Radical mastoidectomy
- Modified radical mastoidectomy

SURGICAL APPROACHES

Q. What are the various surgical approaches for mastoid and ear surgery?

	Approach	Incision	Steps	Uses	Comments
1.	Postaural	William Wilde's	❖ 5–10 mm behind and parallel to postaural sulcus ❖ Starts from highest attachment of pinna above to mastoid tip below	❖ Mastoidectomy ❖ Tympanoplasty ❖ Facial nerve decompression ❖ Endolymphatic sac surgery	In childern: Incision is taken more posteriorly and away from mastoid tip, as the facial nerve is more superficial
2.	Endaural	Lempert's	Two parts: 1. Lempert 1: On posterior meatal wall, at bony cartilaginous junction from 6 o'clock to 12 o'clock 2. Lempert 2: Starts from 1st incision at 12 o'clock, passes upwards through incisura terminalis and upward	❖ Large tympanic membrane perforations ❖ Excision of osteomas or exostosis of ear canal ❖ Limited disease: Modified radical mastoidectomy	Incisura is devoid of cartilage, thus incision through it prevents cartilage injury

Contd...

Contd...

	Approach	Incision	Steps	Uses	Comments
3.	Transcanal/ Endomeatal	Rosen's	Two parts: Vertical: At 12 o'clock, 5-7 mm outwards Curvilinear: At 6 o'clock to meet first incision in posterosuperior region	❖ Inlay myringoplasty ❖ Stapes surgery ❖ Exploratory tympanotomy	Requires external ear canal to be wide enough

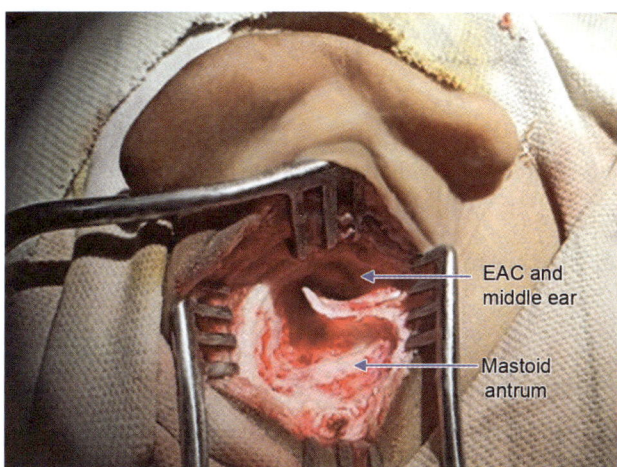

Fig. 1: Showing canal wall down mastoidectomy surgery intraoperative (atticoantrostomy).
(EAC: external auditory canal)

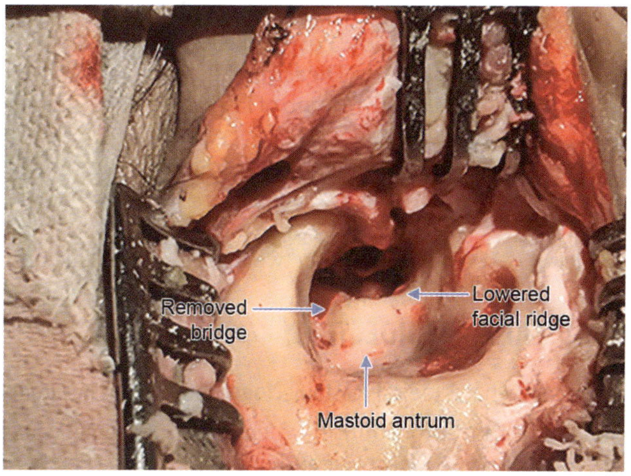

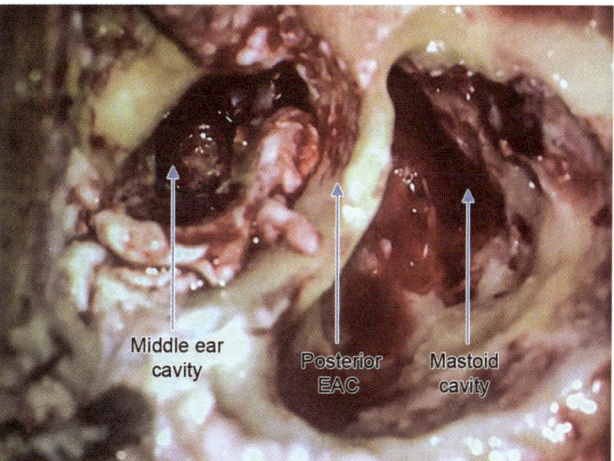

Fig. 2: Showing canal wall down mastoidectomy surgery intraoperative [Modified radical mastoidectomy (MRM)].

Fig. 3: Showing canal wall up mastoidectomy surgery intraoperative (cortical mastoidectomy).

CORTICAL MASTOIDECTOMY

Q. Write short note/essay on cortical mastoidectomy.

- Cortical/simple/complete/schwartz mastoidectomy
- **Definition:** Complete exenteration of all accessible mastoid air cells and converting them into a single cavity with intact posterior meatal wall.
- **Steps in cortical mastoidectomy:**
  Incision: Postaural curved incision, 5-10 mm behind and parallel to postauricular groove, cutting upto the periosteum.
  Note: In children–incision is more short and horizontal, to avoid injury to facial nerve which is superficial at mastoid
  ↓

Exposure of the mastoid cortex: Periosteum incised and elevated using Farabeuf's elevator. Mollison's self-retaining hemostatic mastoid retractor is applied to retract the soft tissue.

↓

Exposure of antrum: Drilling of cortex over suprameatal/ Mac Evan's triangle to expose mastoid antrum 1.5cm deep to the cortex in an adult.

↓

Mastoid air cells exenteration: All accessible air cells are removed, keeping the boundaries intact.
Boundaries : Superiorly: Tegmen tympani
Posteriorly: Dural sinus plate
Anteriorly: Posterior EAC wall
Inferiorly: Digastric ridge
Medially: Dome of lateral semicircular canal

↓

Smoothening: Cavity is smoothened using diamond burr and edges are kept bevelled to facilitate keeping soft tissue for obliteration of the cavity.

↓

Closure: Wound is closed in two layers—soft tissue and the skin. Tight mastoid dressing applied.

RADICAL MASTOIDECTOMY

Q. Describe what is radical mastoidectomy and its steps in surgery.

A mastoidectomy procedure in which posterior meatal wall, tympanic membrane remnants, ossicles except footplate of stapes, and mucosa are all removed and entire middle ear cleft, i.e., middle ear proper, mastoid antrum and the air cells are made into a single cavity with blocking of eustachian tube by a muscle piece or cartilage. This procedure is rarely done nowadays.

Steps in surgery:

- Incision—postaural
- Mastoid antrum and air cells are opened similar to cortical mastoidectomy.
- Removing bridge, lowering the ridge—meatal wall that bridges over the attic region at notch of Rivinus superiorly is removed. Posterior meatal wall over lying the vertical segment of facial nerve "ridge' is lowered.
- Removal of anterior and posterior buttresses
- Ossicles—malleus and incus are removed
- Cavity is completely exteriorised and cleared of the disease. Bony overhangs are removed and cavity smoothened with diamond burr. Saline wash is give to clear the cavity
- Meatoplasty—a meatal flap based on concha is raised and reflected into mastoid to cover the facial ridge. Widening of the meatus by removing small piece of cartilage is done to facilitate inspection and access to the cavity.
- Obliteration of cavity—done for the large cavities using temporalis muscle
- Closure of the wound—ribbon pack soaked in antiseptic solution is packed in cavity and out through the meatus. Wound is sutured in layers and mastoid dressing applied.

MODIFIED RADICAL MASTOIDECTOMY

Q. Describe modified radical mastoidectomy and its steps in sugery.

A mastoidectomy procedure involving removal of mastoid air cells, the disease from attic and antrum region, the posterior meatal and lateral attic wall with maximum preservation of hearing.

Steps in Modified Radical Mastoidectomy

- Postaural incision
- Exposure of mastoid area and drilling of cortical bone
- Lateral attic wall is removed and cholesteatoma/granulation tisse/unhealthy mucosa is removed completely. Diseased ossicles are removed and the normal ones preserved.
- Facial ridge is lowered
- Cavity is smoothened with diamond burr and saline wash given to remove all the bone dust.
- Reconstruction of hearing mechanism is done—ossicular and tympanic membrane reconstruction using grafts or prosthesis
- Meatoplasty—similar to that in radical mastoidectomy
- Closure—wound sutured in layers and mastoid dressing applied.

CHAPTER 51: Mastoidectomy

Q. Describe and compare indications, postoperative care and complications in different surgical approaches in mastoid surgery.

Mastoidectomy type	Indications	Postoperative care	Complications

Cortical	❖ Acute coalescent mastoiditis
	❖ Masked mastoiditis
	❖ As an initial stage of transmastoid surgery for:
	  ➢ Facial nerve decompression
	  ➢ Middle ear
	  ➢ Inner ear—acoustic neuroma
	  ➢ Endolymphatic sac surgery
	  ➢ Skull base
		❖ Antibiotics, decongestants
		❖ To avoid straining, coughing, sneeze with mouth open to prevent middle ear pressure changes
		❖ Suture removal after 7th day
			❖ Damage to structures:
			  ➢ Dural plate
			  ➢ Dura
			  ➢ Sigmoid sinus
			  ➢ Lateral semicircular canal
			  ➢ Facial nerve
			❖ Dislocation of incus
			❖ Postoperative wound infection and gapping
			❖ Persistence of discharge

Modified radical	❖ Disease: Cholesteatoma/granulations restricted to the attic and antrum ❖ Localised chronic otitis media	❖ Mastoid dressing removed on day 3 and check for signs of perichondritis or infection of ear pack. ❖ Sutures removed after 7th day and ear pack changed ❖ Suctioning of cavity and cleaning till epithelialization of cavity is complete ❖ Rest same as above	❖ Perichondritis of pinna ❖ Cavity problems – some cavities do not heal and continue to discharge, thus requiring regular suctioning and cleaning ❖ Same as in cortical mastoidectomy
Radical	❖ Cholesteatoma involving structures like eustachian tube, round window niche, peri labyrinthine air cells or hypotympanic cells ❖ Revision mastoid surgery for residual disease ❖ As an approach to petrous apex	❖ Same as above	❖ Severe conductive deafness due to removal of ossicles and tympanic membrane ❖ Rest same as modified radical procedure

Chapter 52

Myringotomy

EN4.10: Observe and describe the indications for and steps involved in myringotomy and tympanoplasty.

■ INTRODUCTION

Q. Write a short note/essay on myringotomy.

It is the incision of the tympanic membrane to:
- Confirm the diagnosis of serous otitis media
- To aspirate fluid from middle ear
- To insert a ventilation tube when necessary

■ INDICATIONS

- Acute suppurative otitis media (ASOM)
    - Severe earache with impending rupture of tympanic membrane
    - Failure of medical treatment
    - Complications of ASOM like facial palsy, labyrinthitis or meningitis
- Serous otitis media
- Atelectatic tympanic membrane—to improve middle ear ventilation. Ventilation tube/grommet may be inserted.
- In suspected cases of nasopharyngeal malignancy, fluid aspirated can be sent for cytology.

■ CONTRAINDICATIONS

It is contraindicated in suspected intratympanic glomus tumor as myringotomy can cause excessive bleeding.

■ PROCEDURE

Q. Describe steps involved in myringotomy.

Anasthesia

- **General anesthesia:** It is required in patients with acute suppurative otitis media irrespective of the age of the patient as ASOM is a very painful condition. It is also used in infants and children.
- **Local anesthesia:** Can be used in older children and adults. 2% lignocaine is injected at four points in the external auditory canal in the subcutaneous plane just deep to the hair bearing area.

CHAPTER 52: Myringotomy

Steps of Operation

- The patient is in supine position with the head turned to one side resting on a head ring.
- The pinna and adjacent skin are thoroughly cleansed using any suitable agent. Sterile towels are applied leaving only the pinna uncovered. The ear canal is cleaned of wax and debris.
- Local anesthesia is injected in the ear canal.
- Under operating microscope, aural speculum is inserted and the tympanic membrane is incised using a sharp myringotome.
- In serous otitis media, a radial incision is taken in the antero-inferior or antero-superior quadrant. It splits the tympanic membrane fibers and hence it foe short-term drainage of middle ear fluid. This incision is away from incudostapedial joint, chorda tympani nerve, facial nerve hence there are less chances of damage to these structures and less postoperative complications.
- A circumferential incision is taken in the postero-inferior quadrant in acute suppurative otitis media. This incision cuts the fibres of Tympanic membrane hence it is for long term drainage.
- Ventilation tube/grommet is inserted through the incision **(Fig. 1)**.

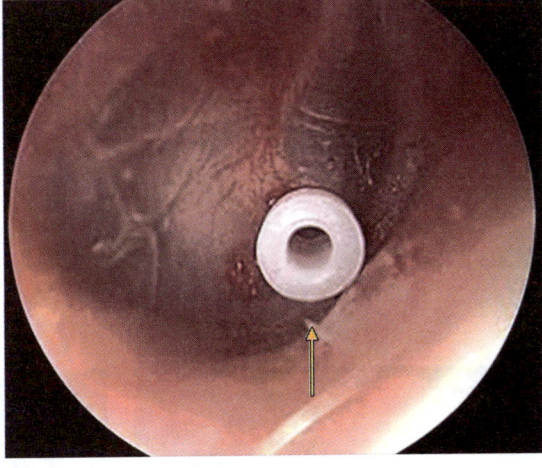

Fig. 1: Showing myringotomy with grommet insertion.

Postoperative Care

Acute otitis media: Antibiotic treatment is continued and aural toilet by dry mopping with cotton wool is done as often as discharge reappears in the canal.

Secretory otitis media: Follow up audiometry and periodic review until grommet is extruded. Patients are advised to avoid water entering the ears.

COMPLICATIONS

- Damage to the incus, stapes, incudostapedial joint, facial nerve or chorda tympani.
- Injury to jugular bulb
- Scarring and hyaline degeneration.

GROMMET

Q. Write a short note on grommet and its types.

Material:
- Fleuroplstic
- Silicon
- Titanium
- Silver coated
- Stainless steel

Extrusion of grommet: Tympanic membrane epitheliazation is towards periphery and hence the grommet automatically gets extruded within a period of 6 months to 2 years.

Types of Grommet

Short-term grommet (extrudes in < 6 months)	Long-term grommet (stays for 6 months to 2 years)
Shah, Shephard, Sheehy, Baxter, Donaldson, Bobbin **(Figs. 1, 3 to 7)**	Goode's T tube, Armstrong **(Figs. 2 and 8)**

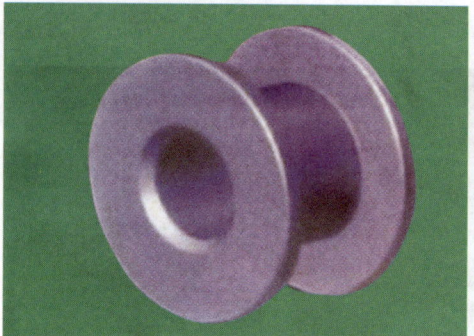

Fig 1: Sheehy grommet.

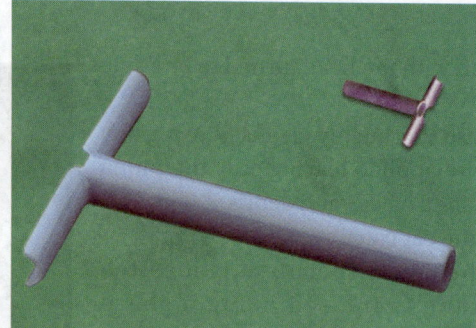

Fig 2: Goode's T tube.

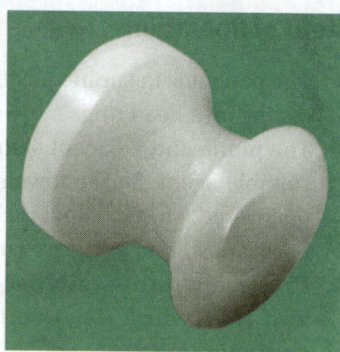

Fig. 3: Shepard grommet.

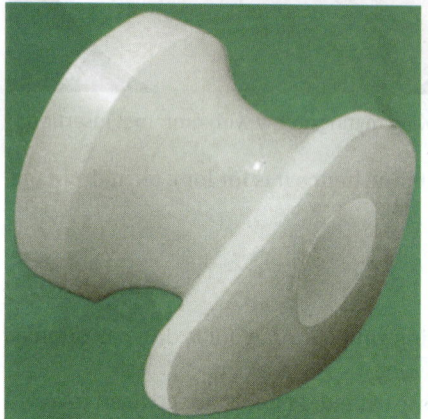

Fig. 4: Shah grommet.

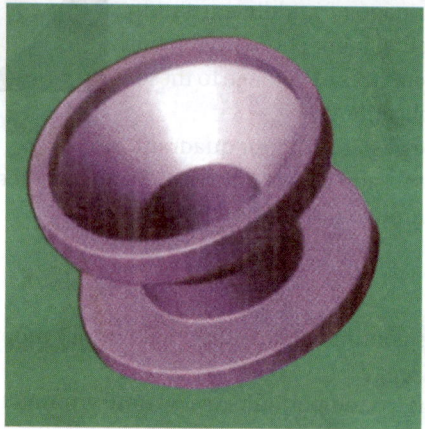

Fig 5: Reuter Bobbin grommet.

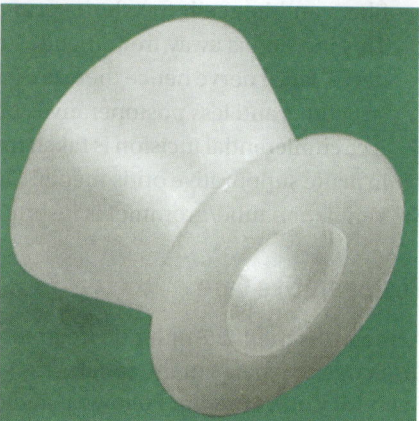

Fig. 6: Baxter grommet.

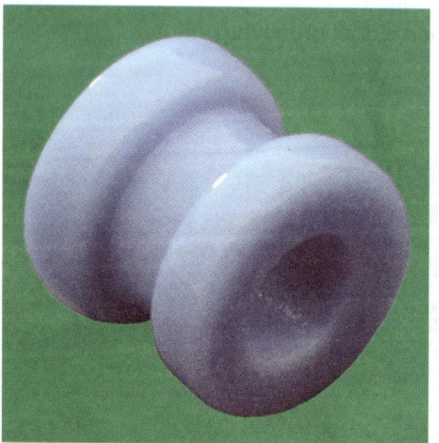

Fig. 7: Donaldson grommet.

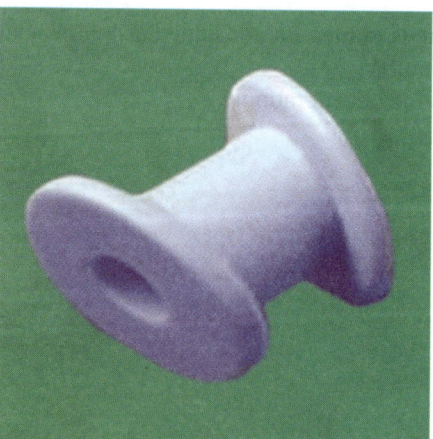

Fig. 8: Armstrong grommet.

Chapter 53

Wax Removal

EN4.9: Demonstrate the correct technique for syringing wax from the ear in a simulated environment.

COMPOSITION OF WAX

Q. Write a short note/essay on impacted wax and its removal by syringing.

Wax is composed of:
- Secretions of Sebaceous glands
- Ceruminous glands
- Hair
- Desquamated epithelial debris
- Keratin
- Dirt

ROLE OF WAX

Wax has a protective function:
- As it lubricates the ear canal and entraps any foreign material that happens to enter the canal
- Has an acidic pH and is bacteriostatic and fungistatic.

SYMPTOMATOLOGY

Patient usually present with:
- Impairment of hearing
- Sense of blocked ear
- Tinnitus and giddiness may result from impaction of was against tympanic membrane (TM)
- Long standing impacted wax may ulcerate the meatal skin and result in wax granuloma.

TECHNIQUE OF WAX REMOVAL

- Removal by syringing
- Instrumental manipulation by ear bud or wax hook
- Hard impacted wax may require prior softening with wax solvents.

■ REMOVAL OF WAX BY SYRINGING (SCAN QR CODE)

❖ Boiled water cooled to room temperature is used.
❖ Pinna is pulled upwards and backwards and water from syringe is to be directed on the posterio-superior wall of external auditory canal (EAC).
❖ Pressure of water built up deeper to wax, expels the wax out.
❖ In an impacted wax it is necessary to create a space between the wax and meatal wall for the jet of water to pass.

■ INSTRUMENTAL MANIPULATION

❖ Cerumen hook
❖ Jobson Horne probe

Technique of Instrumental Manipulation

A space is created between the wax and meatal wall, the instrument is passed beyond the wax and whole plug then dragged out in a single piece.

■ WAX SOLVENTS

❖ 5% sodium bicarbonate in equal parts of glycerine and water
❖ 2% paradichlorobenzene

■ COMPLICATIONS

❖ Giddiness (vagal nerve stimulation)
❖ Otomycosis
❖ Trauma to EAC

Section 2: Nose

Chapter 54

Septoplasty and Submucous Resection of Septum

EN4.22: Enumerate the indications, observe and describe steps in the septoplasty.

SUBMUCOUS RESECTION OF SEPTUM

Q. Write a short note/essay on submucous resection (SMR) of septum.

Submucous resection of the septum involves removal of the deviated parts of the bony and cartilaginous septum. It is a more radical procedure and these days it has been replaced by septoplasty.

Indications

- Deviated nasal septum causing nasal obstruction.
- Recurrent otitis media due to deviation of the nasal septum.
- Septal spur causing recurrent epistaxis.
- As a part of other procedures if it compromises surgical approach in functional endoscopic sinus surgery (FESS), dacryocystorhinostomy (DCR), cerebrospinal fluid (CSF) leak repair, juvenile nasopharyngeal angiofibroma (JNA) removal, orbital decompression, pituitary surgery.
- In conjunction with septorhinoplasty.

Contraindications

- Bleeding disorders
- Acute rhinosinusitis
- Patients below 18 years of age since facial skeleton develops until 18 years of age.

Procedure

Q. Write a note on the operative steps, preoperative and postoperative care of SMR. Write a note on its complications.

Preoperative Care

- If patient has active rhinosinusitis, it needs to be treated with a course of antibiotics (amoxicillin-clavulanic acid), antihistaminics and nasal decongestants.
- **Investigations:** Complete hemogram, coagulation profile, liver and kidney function tests, serology for hepatitis B, C and HIV, chest X-ray and ECG. These are needed to see patient's fitness for anesthesia.
- **Consent for surgery:** Written informed consent has to be taken. If patient has concomitant symptoms of allergic rhinitis patient must be explained that after surgery, the symptoms of allergic rhinitis will persist.
- Patients are usually operated under local anesthesia and intravenous sedation, with general anesthesia reserved for apprehensive adults.

Steps of Surgery

- Patient is sedated with dexmedetomidine/midazolam/ketamine and then local infiltration of lignocaine 2% with one in 2 lakh adrenaline is given in both sides of the septum in subperichondrial plane.
- Using 11 number blade, incision is taken cutting through the mucosa and perichondrium at the mucocutaneous junction (Freer's incision).
- Flaps are elevated in the mucoperichondrial and mucoperiosteal flap on one side.
- Cartilage is incised and opposite side mucoperiosteal and mucoperichondrial flap is elevated.
- Bony septum is removed using Luc's forceps. Deviated part of cartilage is removed using Ballenger swivel knife. Care must be taken to preserve 'L'- shaped strut on dorsal and caudal border of septum. If there is a deviation at the maxillary crest, it is removed using gouge and hammer.
- Confirmation of adequate removal of deviation is done by checking air blast on the table or if instrument easily reaches posterior choana.
- Using absorbable suture like Vicryl, the incision is sutured.
- Nasal packing is done using merocel or ribbon gauze soaked in liquid paraffin.

Postoperative Care

- Patient is given head high position to reduce congestion.
- Patient can also be given tincture benzoin inhalation for moistening the respiratory mucosa.
- Patient is placed under antibiotic cover till discharge and then given one week of oral antibiotics, painkillers and antihistaminics.
- Nasal pack is removed after 24 to 48 hour and patient is started on nasal douching.

Complications

- **Bleeding**: It usually is managed by compression and tranexamic acid.
- **Septal hematoma** and **septal abscess**: If untreated it can cause cartilage necrosis. It is treated by draining of the hematoma/abscess followed by compression nasal packing and systemic antibiotics.
- **Septal perforation**: If bilateral mucoperiosteal and mucoperichondrial flaps tear.
- **Nasal deformity**: Extensive removal can cause **saddle nose, tip collapse, supratip** depression and columellar retraction.

■ SEPTOPLASTY

Q. Write a short note/essay on septoplasty and its procedure.

Septoplasty is a more conservative surgery for the septal framework where maximum effort is taken to preserve the septal framework.

Indications

- Deviated nasal septum causing nasal obstruction.
- Recurrent otitis media due to deviation of the nasal septum.
- Septal spur causing recurrent epistaxis.
- As a part of other procedures if it compromises surgical approach in FESS, dacrocystorhinostomy (DCR), CSF leak repair, juvenile nasopharyngeal angiofibroma (JNAF) removal, orbital decompression, pituitary surgery.
- In conjunction with septorhinoplasty.
- As a part of surgery for obstructive sleep apnea.
- Recurrent headache due to spur impinging on lateral nasal wall.

Contraindications

- Bleeding disorders
- Acute rhinosinusitis
- Patients below 18 years of age; in these patients usually limited septoplasty is done.
- Uncontrolled diabetes mellitus and hypertension

Procedure

Q. Write a note on the operative steps, preoperative and postoperative care of septoplasty.

Preoperative Care

- If patient has active rhinosinusitis, it needs to be treated with a course of antibiotics (Amoxicillin-clavulanic acid), antihistaminics and nasal decongestants.
- **Investigations:** Complete hemogram, coagulation profile (bleeding time, clotting time, platelet count), liver and kidney function tests, serology for hepatitis B, C and HIV, chest X-ray and ECG. These are needed to see patient's fitness for anesthesia.
- **Consent for surgery:** Written informed valid consent has to be taken. If patient has concomitant symptoms of allergic rhinitis patient must be explained that after surgery, the symptoms of allergic rhinitis will persist.
Patients are usually operated under local anesthesia and intravenous sedation, with general anesthesia reserved for apprehensive adults.

Steps of Surgery

- Patient is sedated with dexmedetomidine/midazolam/ketamine and then local infiltration of lignocaine 2% with one in 2 lakh adrenaline is given in both sides of the septum in subperichondrial plane using 25 number 1.5" needle.
- Using 11 number blade, incision is taken 2–3 mm superior to the mucoutaneous junction on the concave side (Killian's incision).
- Flap is elevated in the mucoperichondrial and mucoperiosteal flap.
- Bony cartilage junction is dislocated using freer's elevator and opposite side mucoperiosteal and mucoperichondrial flap is elevated.
- Bony septum is removed using Luc's forceps. If there is a deviation at the maxillary crest, it is removed using gouge and hammer. Deviated cartilage is corrected by crosshatching, shaving, scoring or excision.
- Confirmation of adequate removal of deviation is done by checking air blast on the table or if instrument easily reaches posterior choana.
- Using absorbable suture like Vicryl, the incision is sutured.
- Anterior nasal packing is done using Merocel/Netcell or ribbon gauze soaked in liquid paraffin. Absence of anterior and postnasal bleeding confirmed. Anterior nasal dressing given.

Postoperative Care

- Patient is given head high position to reduce congestion.
- Patient can also be given tincture benzoin inhalation for moistening the respiratory mucosa and prevent dryness of throat. Oral antiseptic gargles given.
- Patient is placed under antibiotic cover till discharge and then given one week of oral antibiotics, painkillers (analgesics) and antihistaminics.
- Nasal pack is removed after 24 to 48 hour and patient is started on nasal douching.

Complications

Q. What are the complications of the septoplasty?

- **Bleeding:** It usually is managed by compression and tranexamic acid.
- **Septal hematoma and septal abscess:** If untreated it can cause cartilage necrosis. It is treated by draining of the hematoma/abscess followed by compression nasal packing and systemic antibiotics.
- Nasal synechiae formation **(Fig. 1)**
- **Septal perforation:** If bilateral mucoperiosteal and mucoperichondrial flaps tear **(Fig. 2)**.
- **Nasal deformity:** Extensive removal can cause saddle nose, tip collapse, and columellar retraction, supratip depression.

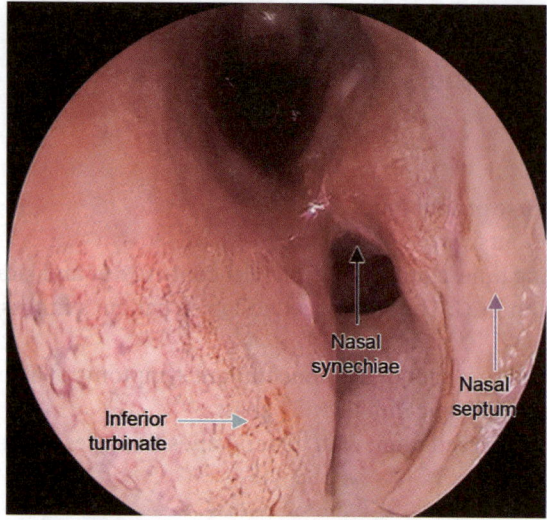

Fig. 1: Endoscopic view of nasal synechiae.

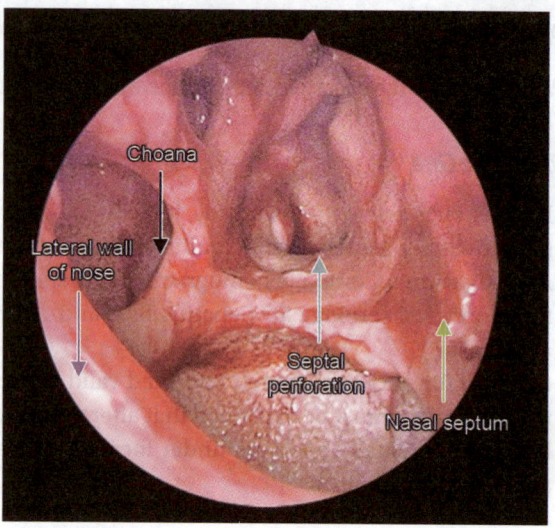

Fig. 2: Endoscopic view of septal perforation.

■ SUBMUCOSAL RESECTION VERSUS SEPTOPLASTY

Q. Enumerate the differences between septoplasty and SMR.

	Submucosal resection (SMR)	Septoplasty
1.	More radical procedure	More conservative procedure
2.	Flaps raised on both sides	Flaps raised on one side
3.	Deviated cartilage and bone removed	Deviated cartilage is removed
4.	Not done in less than 18 years	Not done in less than 18 years
5.	Killian's incision	Freer's incision
6.	More chances of postoperative complications like: ❖ Supratip deformity ❖ Nasal tip drop ❖ Saddle nose deformity ❖ Septal hematoma ❖ Septal abscess ❖ Septal perforation ❖ Nasal synechiae formation	Less chances of postoperative complications like: ❖ Supratip deformity ❖ Nasal tip drop ❖ Saddle nose deformity ❖ Septal hematoma ❖ Septal abscess ❖ Septal perforation ❖ Nasal Synichiae formation
7.	Indicated for posterior DNS	Indicated for anterior DNS
8.	Cannot be combined with rhinoplasty	Can be combined with rhinoplasty by extending the Freer's incision
9.	Not preferred	One of treatment modality in management of epistaxis
10.	Not preferred	As approach to hypophysectomy and anterior skull base surgery

Chapter 55

Polypectomy

■ INTRODUCTION

Q. Define polyp and its various sites in ENT.

Polyp
- Polyp is a smooth mass of edematous and inflamed prolapsed mucosa.
- Polyp can be sessile or pedunculated.

Site of Polyp in ENT
- **Ear:** External auditory canal, middle ear
- **Paranasal sinuses:** Antrochoanal polyp, ethmoidal polyp
- **Laryngx:** Vocal cords, epiglottis, vallecula

■ POLYPECTOMY

Q. Define polypectomy. Write a short note on different polypectomy procedures.

Polypectomy is the surgical procedure for removal of polyp.

Different Methods of Polyp Removal

Aural polyp	Nasal polyp	Vocal polyp
❖ Snaring method using aural snare ❖ With forcep under microscopic examination	❖ Snaring method using nasal snare ❖ With forcep/debrider/coblator under endoscopic examination	❖ Laser excision ❖ Microlaryngoscopic scissor/forcep ❖ Coblator

```
        Wire gauge diameters for various snares
         ↓              ↓              ↓
    Aural snare    Nasal snare    Laryngeal snare
         ↓              ↓              ↓
    28 Gauge       30 Gauge       32 Gauge
```

Aural Polypectomy

Origin → External auditory canal and middle ear.

Etiology:

- **External auditory canal polyp:** External auditory canal polyp, external auditory canal haemangioma
- **Middle ear polyp:** Aural polyp due to chronic suppurative otitis media (CSOM)/glomus tumor/adenoma/facial nerve neurinoma.

Procedure:

- Previously → it was done using aural snare which is obsolete now.
- It is done under local anesthesia under microscopic vision.
- Patient in supine position with head turned to opposite side.
- External auditory canal (EAC) infiltrate with lox 2%+adrenaline.
- Using ball probe, polyp is palpated and origin of polyp is delineated.
- Using Balluchi microscissor, the stalk of polyp cut and sent for biopsy.
- Adrenaline soaked cottonoid kept in EAC.

Nasal Polypectomy

- Snaring method → obsolete now. But nasal snare was used to remove nasal polyps.
- Now, nasal polyp is being removed using Blekesley forcep/debrider blade/coblator.

Laryngeal Polypectomy

- Snaring method → obsolete now
- Now, vocal cord polyp is being removed under microlaryngoscopic guided using Jackson microlaryngoscope with chest piece and microlaryngoscopy forcep/scissor/laser/coblator (laryngeal wand) under general anesthesia.

Note: Never avulsed a polyp to prevent recurrence.

Chapter 56

Functional Endoscopic Sinus Surgery

■ INTRODUCTION

Q. Write a short note/essay on functional endoscopic sinus surgery (FESS).

Functional endoscopic surgery is a procedure to re-establish the drainage of the natural ostia and to restore ventilation and mucociliary clearance.

Principle of FESS

It is based on the principle that clearing the blocked ostium will restore the mucociliary clearance and the diseased mucosa normalizes.

■ EQUIPMENT FOR FESS

- 4 mm 0° endoscope
- Angled endoscopes: 30°, 45°, 70° **(Fig. 1)**.
- Camera
- Display screen
- Light source

■ INDICATIONS OF FESS

Q. What are indications and contraindications of FESS?

- Chronic bacterial sinusitis
- Nasal polyposis
- Recurrent sinusitis
- Fungal ball
- Allergic fungal rhinosinusitis (AFRS)
- Invasive fungal sinusitis
- Rhinolith removal
- Mucocoele removal
- Surgery for epistaxis
- Rhinosporidosis removal
- Antrochoanal polyp

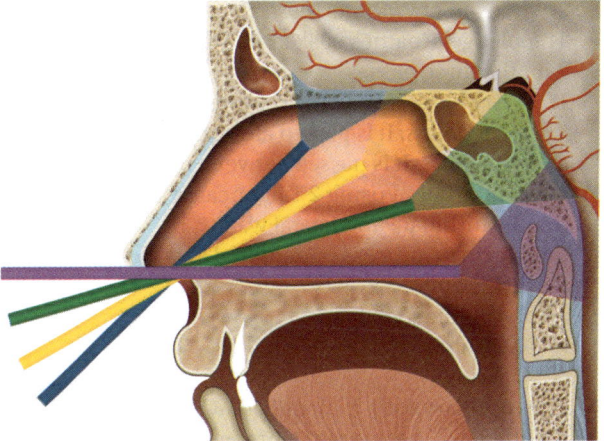

Fig. 1: Various scopes used for FESS.

Endoscopic versus open approach to sinuses
- Improved visualization and better access
- Avoids need for brain retraction; less damage to brain tissue
- Less neurovascular manipulation in well selected cases
- Pediatric cases; preservation of facial skeleton
- Improved cosmesis, improved outcomes

■ EXTENDED INDICATIONS OF FESS

- Dacrocystorhinostomy
- Juvenile nasopharyngeal angiofibroma (JNA) excision

PART 2: Operative Procedures

- Sinonasal mass excision
- Cerebrospinal fluid (CSF) rhinorrhea repair
- Optic nerve decompression
- Orbital decompression
- Pituitary tumor excision
- Hypophysectomy

CONTRAINDICATIONS

- Medically unfit patient
- Disease inaccessible by endoscopy
- Osteomyelitis of sinus
- Sinusitis with intracranial complications

PROCEDURE

Q. Describe the process/steps of procedure of functional endoscopic sinus surgery.

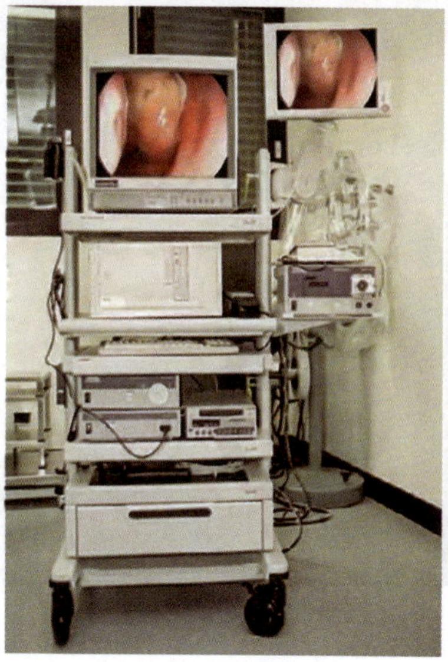

- First stack system positioned infront of surgeon **(Fig 2)**. It is usually done **under general anesthesia (GA)**, some surgeons prefer local anesthesia (LA) especially in unfit patients. Decongestion is done in the observation room with pledgets or nasal patties.
- Patient lies in **supine position** with head on a ring, and head end can be elevated to 15–30°.
- The two techniques are:
  1. *Stammberger's technique (anterior to posterior):* Surgery is done from uncinate process towards sphenoid sinus.
  2. *Wigand's technique (posterior to anterior):* Surgery starts from sphenoid sinus and proceeds anteriorly.
- The pledgets/patties soaked in 4% xylocaine adrenaline are removed and a thorough endoscopic examination is done with the three passes.
  1. *First pass:* Between the septum and inferior turbinate up to choana to visualize the nasopharynx and Eustachian tube
  2. *Second pass:* It is passed along the middle meatus.
  3. *Third pass:* It is passed between the superior turbinate and the septum up to the visualization of sphenoid ostia.
- Local infiltration using 2% lignocaine adrenaline given on the axilla of the middle turbinate, septum, uncinate process, middle turbinate and lateral wall.
- The uncinate process is identified and the uncinectomy is done. It can be done using:
  - Sickle knife
  - Backbiting forceps
  - Rostrum
  - Debrider
- The maxillary ostia is identified, widened and the maxillary sinus is cleared.
- Clearance of the anterior ethmoids, beginning with the bulla ethmoidalis is then done.
- Posterior ethmoids are then cleared after removal of the basal lamella (ground lamella) and cleared.
- If there is involvement of the frontal sinus, then the frontal recess is cleared. If there is isolated frontal sinus involvement, it can be accessed without removing the bulla, called as the 'intact bulla technique'.
- The sphenoid sinus can then be approached via the inferomedial aspect of the most posterior ethmoid cell. Alternatively, it can also be approached medically by identifying its ostium around 1.5 cm above the roof of the nasopharynx.
  Care should be taken not to damage the optic nerve and the internal carotid artery that lies in its wall. Care should be taken in case of presence of Haller cell and Onodi cell.
- After completion of surgery and achieving hemostasis, nasal packing is done.

Fig. 2: Stack system positioned in front of surgeon.

Postoperative Care

- Nasal pack removed after 24–48 hours. Patient kept in head high position to relieve nasal congestion.
- Antibiotics given postoperatively for one week.
- After pack removal, patient is started on nasal douching for optimal healing and crust removal.
- Antihistaminics
- Pain killers
- Steroid sprays—for cases of polyposis, AFRS
- Oral steroids—for pan polyposis cases may be given or in revision cases.
- **Endoscopic toileting:** Under Local Anaesthesia (LA), patient is examined and clots, crusts, debris are removed. It also allows to remove synechiae and adhesions, with evaluation of the healing of the cavity.

COMPLICATIONS OF FESS

Q. Write a short note on complications of FESS.

- ❖ **Local complications:**
  - ➢ Bleeding
  - ➢ Adhesions and stenosis
  - ➢ Anosmia
  - ➢ Injury to nasolacrimal duct
  - ➢ Dental pain
- ❖ **Orbital complications:**
  - ➢ Orbital fat prolapse **(Fig. 3)** into nose (Stankiewicz sign) due to injury to Lamina Papyracea
  - ➢ Periorbital ecchymosis
  - ➢ Periorbital emphysema
  - ➢ Orbital hemorrhage
  - ➢ Loss of vision
  - ➢ Diplopia
- ❖ **Intracranial complications:**
  - ➢ CSF leak
  - ➢ Meningitis
  - ➢ Brain abscess
  - ➢ Intracranial hemorrhage
  - ➢ Stroke
  - ➢ Death

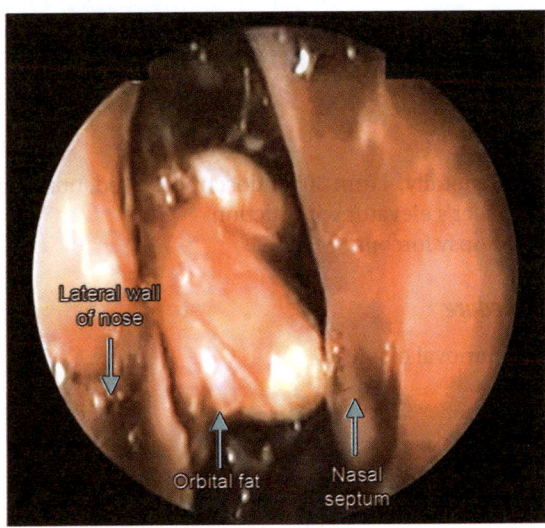

Fig. 3: Prolapse of obital fat.

EN3.2: Observe and describe the indications for and steps involved in the performance of diagnostic nasal endoscopy.

DIAGNOSTIC NASAL ENDOSCOPY

Definition

Q. Write a short note/essay on diagnostic nasal endoscopy.

- ❖ It is a direct visualization of nasal and sinus passages using a magnified high-quality view.
- ❖ Generally, OPD procedure as an adjunctive diagnostic tool to evaluate nasal and sinonasal anatomy and pathology.

Advantages

- ❖ Better visualization with illumination
- ❖ Preoperative, postoperative and medical management of patients
- ❖ Detect pathologies which can be missed on anterior rhinoscopy

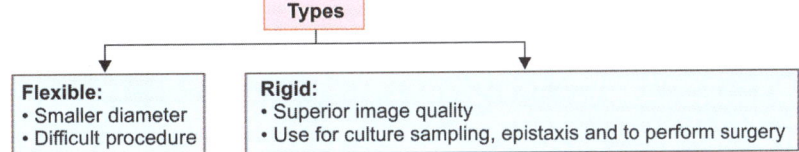

Indications

- ❖ Sinonasal complaints not detected on anterior rhinoscopy
- ❖ Diagnosis of epistaxis, anosmia, nasal obstruction
- ❖ To evaluate response to treatment
- ❖ Removal of foreign bodies
- ❖ Biopsy from nose and nasopharynx

Anesthesia

- ❖ Topical spray: 4% xylocaine
- ❖ Oxymetazoline as vasoconstrictor pack

PART 2: Operative Procedures

Position
Supine or sitting

Instruments
- Generally, 4 mm 30° endoscope is used, but if narrow nasal passage 2.7 mm 30°/70° endoscope
- Freer's elevator with suction
- Biopsy forceps

Procedure
- Removal of packs

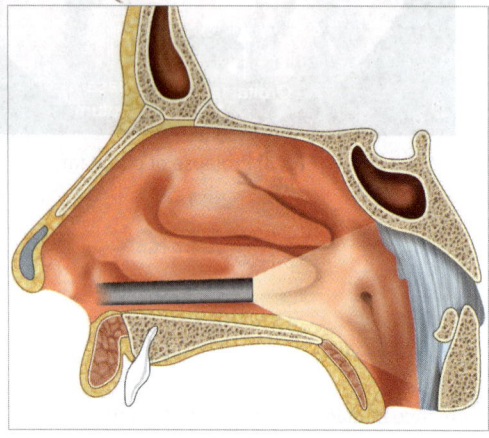

Fig. 4: Structures seen on first pass.

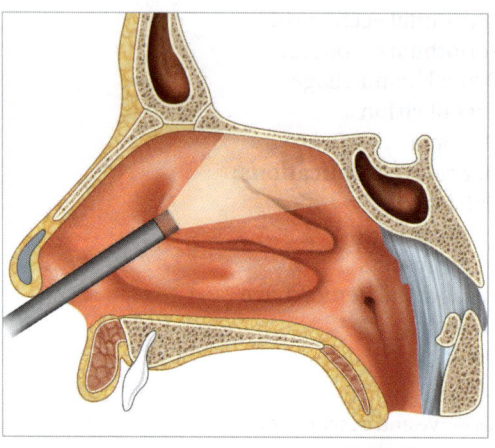

Fig. 5: Structures seen on second pass.

- **First pass (Fig. 4)**
    - Examination of nasopharynx and inferior meatus
    - Pass endoscope along the nasal floor
    - Examine opening of eustachian tube, choana, posterior ends of turbinates
- **Second pass (Fig. 5)**
    - Examination of sphenoethmoidal recess, superior meatus, opening of sphenoid sinus and posterior ethmoid cells.
    - Pass endoscope medial to middle turbinate
- **Third pass (Fig. 6)**
    - Examination of middle meatus
    - Pass endoscope from front to middle meatus
    - Examine structures of middle meatus

Complications
- Bleeding
- Discomfort

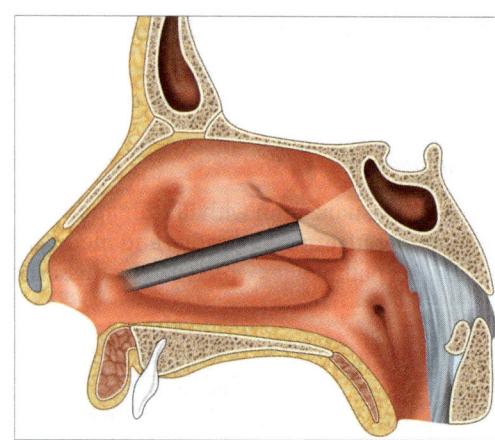

Fig. 6: Structures seen on third pass.

Chapter 57: Endoscopic Septoplasty

■ DEFINITION

Q. Write a short note/essay on endoscopic septoplasty.

Minimally invasive technique that helps to correct septal deformity under excellent visualization or as adjunct to other nasal surgeries.

■ INDICATIONS

- Same as conventional septoplasty
- Additional indications (as an adjunct):
  - Vidian neurectomy
  - Cerebrospinal fluid (CSF) leak closure
  - Trans-septal hypophysectomy
  - Internal maxillary artery ligation
  - Extensive angiofibroma
  - Dacryocystorhinostomy (DCR)

■ CONTRAINDICATIONS

Same as conventional septoplasty (*refer* to Chapter 54).

■ ANESTHESIA

Same as conventional septoplasty (*refer* to Chapter 54).

■ POSITION

Same as conventional septoplasty (*refer* to Chapter 54).

■ PROCEDURE

Q. Write a short note on procedure of endoscopic septoplasty.

Patient in supine position. Parts are painted and draped under strict aseptic condition. Nasal decongestion done with lox 4% + adrenaline solution (surface anesthesia). Local infiltration 2% lignocaine adrenaline given for local anesthesia, can be done under general anesthesia

↓

Freer's incision taken on the same side of deviated nasal septum

↓

Using suction elevator instruments, mucoperichondrial and mucoperiosteal flaps elevated. Anterior and inferior tunnels created

↓

Bony-cartilaginous junction identified and dislocated

↓

Opposite side mucoperiosteal flap elevated

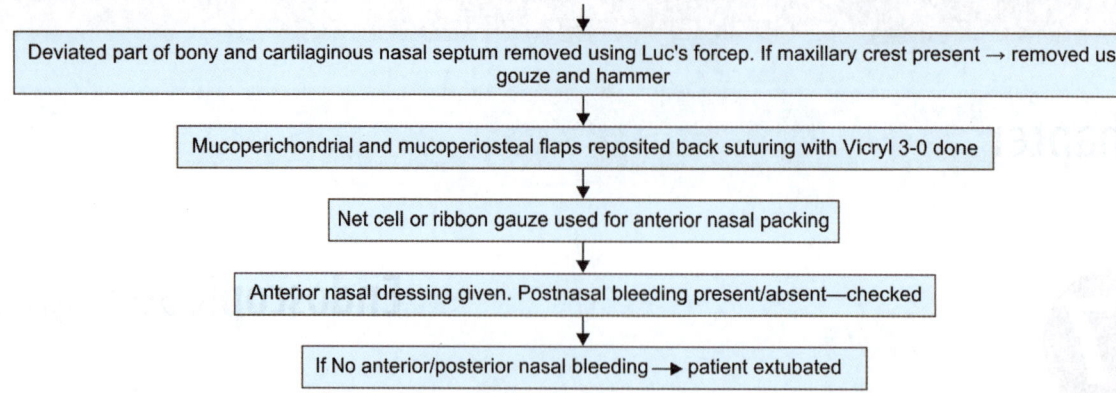

POSTOPERATIVE CARE

Same as conventional septoplasty (*refer* to Chapter 54).

COMPLICATIONS

Same as conventional septoplasty (*refer* to Chapter 54).

ADVANTAGES OF ENDOSCOPIC SEPTOPLASTY OVER CONVENTIONAL SEPTOPLASTY

Q. What are the advantages of endoscopic septoplasty over conventional septoplasty?

- Improved visualization.
- Magnification of the surgical field.
- Endoscope can be passed easily under septal mucosal flaps hence minimal lifting of flap.
- Incision can be performed more posterior in the nose immediately anterior to the area of deviation → extent of mucosal elevation anteriorly is minimized → reduced postoperative edema.
- It allows improved evaluation of the posterior nasal septal deformities.
- Concomitant assessment of the middle meatus.
- As an adjunct to endoscopic dacryocystorhinostomy (DCR) and extended indications of functional endoscopic sinus surgery (FESS) surgeries.
- Video imaging is helpful for education of residents and staff.
- It is easier to correct posterior deviation and isolated spurs.
- Complications are lesser.
- Minimal manipulation → minimal tissue damage.
- Minimal removal of septum and hence precise reconstruction.
- In case of isolated spurs it is easier to avoid mucosal tears as the vision is better.

Chapter 58

Nasal Packing

EN2.10: Identify, resuscitate and manage ENT emergencies in a simulated environment (including tracheostomy, anterior nasal packing, removal of foreign bodies in ear, nose, throat and upper respiratory tract).

ANTERIOR NASAL PACKING (FIGS. 1A TO C)

Q. Write a short note/essay on anterior nasal packing.

Indication
Anterior epistaxis

Methods
- Packing in vertical layers
- Packing in horizontal layers

```
Preferably done under general anesthesia
           ↓
Make patient lie down in supine position
           ↓
A ribbon gauge of 1 m (2.5 cm in adult and 1.2 cm in children) soaked in liquid paraffin/petroleum is required for each nasal cavity
           ↓
Few centimeters of gauge are folded upon itself and inserted along the floor of the nasal cavity using bayonet nasal packing forcep
           ↓
Then the whole nasal cavity is packed tightly by layering the gauge from floor to the roof (horizontal fashion) or from back to the front (vertical fashion)
           ↓
Anterior nasal dressing given
```

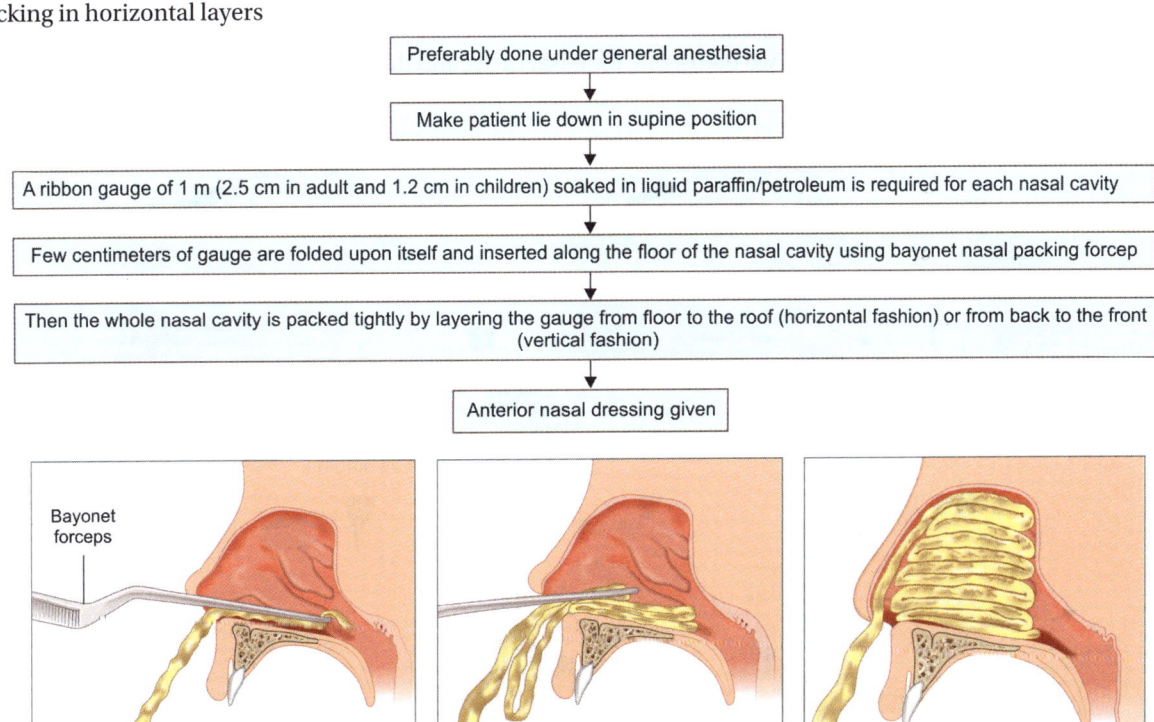

Figs.1A to C: Anterior nasal packing.

Advice

- Nasal pack to be remove after 24–48 hours
- If keep for >48 hours → risk of infection → toxic shock syndrome
- Must give antibiotic coverage

Contraindications

- Significant facial/nasal bone fracture
- Basilar skull fracture
- Hemodynamic instability or airway compromise

Complications

- Rebleeding after removal of pack
- Necrosis of nasal mucosa
- Infection, particularly sinusitis
- Toxic shock syndrome
- Packing migration
- Aspiration

POSTERIOR NASAL PACKING (FIGS. 2A TO F)

Q. Write a short note/essay on posterior nasal packing.

Indication

Posterior epistaxis

Material Used for Packing

- Gauze piece folded into the shape of a square/cone.
- Foley's catheter size 12–14 F can also be used.
- **Dual nasal balloon catheter(recent):** Two bulbs, one for nasal cavity and the other for the postnasal packing.

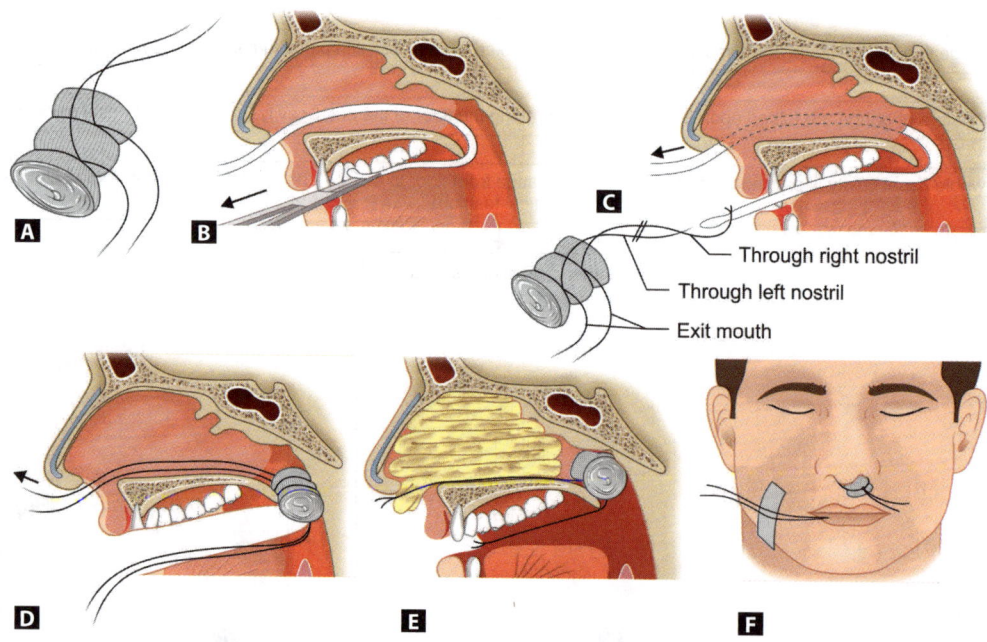

Figs. 2A to F: Anterior and posterior nasal packing procedure.

Method

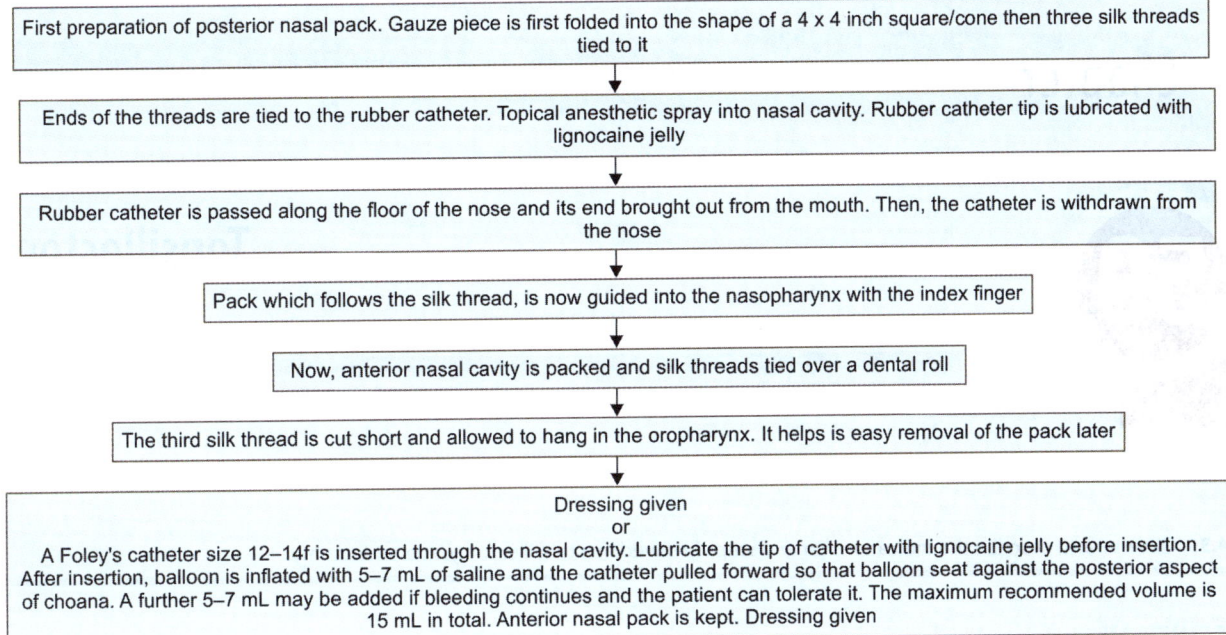

Advice

- Hospitalization
- Antibiotic coverage
- Removal after 48 hours

Contraindications

- Skull base fracture
- Significant nasal bone or maxillofacial trauma
- Airway compromise or hemodynamic instability
- Cardiopulmonary instability (risk of increase morbidity and mortality with posterior nasal packing) → Relative contraindication

Complications

- Rebleeding on removal
- Otitis media due to Eustachian tube obstruction
- Sinusitis
- Toxic shock syndrome
- Pressure necrosis of nasal mucosa
- Dislodgement and airway obstruction
- Cardiopulmonary complication → due to nasopulmonary reflex

Section 3: Throat

Chapter 59: Tonsillectomy

EN4.39: Observe and describe the indications for and steps involved in a tonsillectomy/adenoidectomy.

■ DEFINITION

Q. Write a short note/essay on tonsillectomy.

It is an operation performed for removal of the palatine (faucial) tonsils.

■ INDICATION

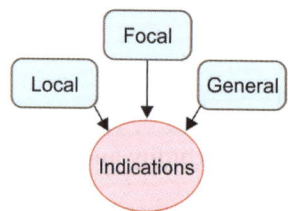

I. Local (tonsillar pathology): Indications	❖ Chronic tonsillitis (> 4–6 attacks of acute tonsillitis/year) ❖ Peritonsillar abscess (quinsy) (interval tonsillectomy—4–6 weeks after drainage of abscess) ❖ Diphtheria carriers not responding to antibiotics ❖ Sleep apnea syndrome (enlarged tonsils causing respiratory obstruction) ❖ Tonsillar cyst and benign tumors ❖ Tonsillitis causing febrile seizures ❖ Tonsillolith (symptomatic) ❖ Suspected foreign body ❖ Malignancy of the tonsil (presenting as an ulcer) ❖ Approach for styloidectomy, glossopharyngeal neurectomy and palatopharyngoplasty
II. Focal (adjacent structures infected by recurrent tonsillitis): Indications	❖ Persistent non-specific jugulodiagstric lymphadenitis ❖ Tuberculous cervical lymphadenitis (tonsil—the portal of infection) ❖ Eustachian tube (ET) catarrh due to recurrent tonsillitis resulting in otitis media with effusion (OME) or chronic suppurative otitis media (CSOM)
III. General (recurrent tonsillitis-focus of infection for other systems of the body): Indications	❖ Subacute bacterial endocarditis or rheumatic heart disease ❖ Acute glomerulonephritis ❖ Asthma or chronic bronchitis (exacerbation) ❖ Rheumatic fever or rheumatic arthritis ❖ Urticaria, erythema multiformae (exacerbation) ❖ Conjunctivitis, choroiditis ❖ Failure to thrive in children

CONTRAINDICATIONS

- Acute tonsillitis
- Upper respiratory tract infection (URTI)
- < 5 years of age
- Blood dyscrasias and bleeding disorder
- Granular pharyngitis
- Uncontrolled systemic disease: Diabetes mellitus, cardiac disease, hypertension, allergy, asthma, etc.
- Submucous cleft palate
- Pregnancy and during the menses
- Polio epidemic

METHODS

Q. What are the different methods of tonsillectomy?

Cold methods	Hot methods
Dissection and snare	Laser
Guillotine	Electrocautery
Microdebrider	Radiofrequency
Harmonic scalpel	
Coblation	
Cryosurgery	

Guillotine Surgery

Q. Why is guillotine method of tonsillectomy not practiced nowadays?

- It can only be done for patients with large, mobile tonsils and not for small, non-mobile and fibrotic tonsils.
- Damage/injury to the surrounding soft tissues is common.
- There are chances of incomplete excision of tonsillar tissue.
- It cannot be performed under local anaesthesia.

Cryosurgery

Q. What are the advantages and disadvantages of the cryosurgery method for tonsillectomy?

Advantages

- Bleeding is less due to thrombosis of vessels caused by thawing, so can be used in patients with blood coagulation disorders
- Pain is negligible

Disadvantages

- Need for separate cryosurgery instrument; cost of which can be a constraint.
- Tonsillar tissue cannot be sent for histopathology examination as there is destruction of tissue by thawing.
- Can leave an uglydepigmented scar
- May not be possible to remove entire tonsillar tissue in one sitting.

Coblation Method

Q. What are the merits and demerits of the coblation method for tonsillectomy?

Merits

- Coblation tonsillectomy significantly reduces the operation time and intraoperative blood loss.
- Tonsillar capsule can be preserved which leads to less postoperative pain
- Every area of the tonsillar fossa is accessible to the wand tip, so less chance of left-over residual tissue
- It is associated with early recovery of dietary routine.
- Tonsillar reduction surgery can be performed in young children without compromising the immunological function of lymphoid tissue.

PART 2: Operative Procedures

Demerits
- Cost of the equipment, i.e., coblator wand is high
- Steep learning curve
- Coblator wand cannot be reused for next surgery as it can lead to infection.
- Postoperative secondary bleeding is common as compared to conventional cold steel technique.

Anesthesia
General anesthesia (GA) with endotracheal intubation using a cuffed endotracheal tube with a throat pack of roller gauze.

Position of Patient
Rose's position (Fig. 1): Patient lies in supine position with neck extended by placing a sand bag under the shoulders. Flexion of the cervical spine and extension of the atlanto-occipital joint.

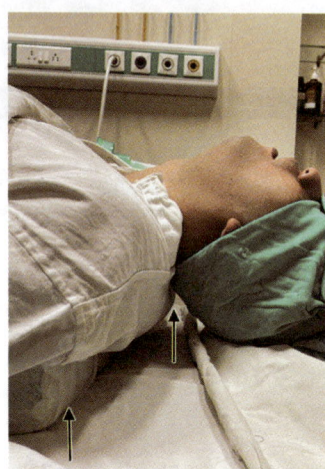

Fig. 1: Showing Rose's position during tonsillectomy surgery.

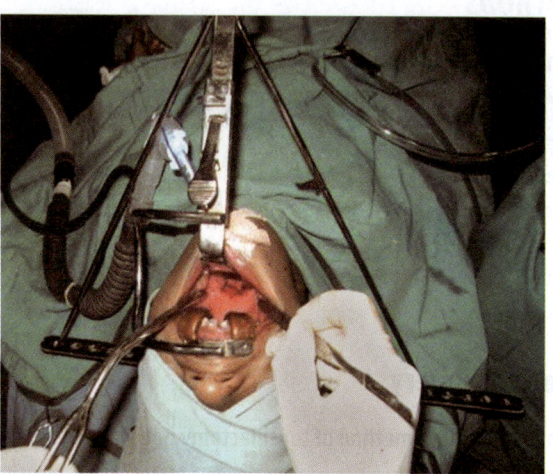

Fig. 2: Showing Boyle Devis mouth gag and intraoperative procedure of tonsillectomy surgery.

■ COLD DISSECTION AND SNARE METHOD (FIG. 2)

Q. Describe the steps of tonsillectomy surgery by dissection and snare method.

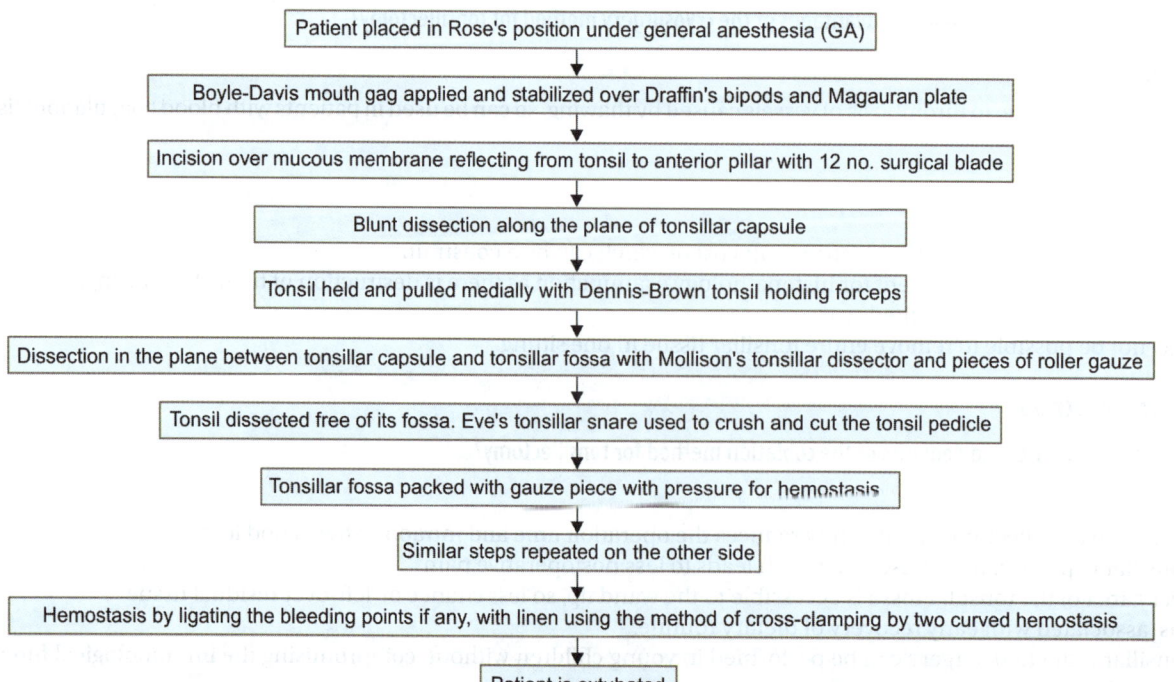

POSTOPERATIVE CARE

Q. How to manage postoperative patient of tonsillectomy?

- Patient position—left lateral position preferably
- Nil by mouth for 6 hours
- Vitals—pulse, temperature, respiratory rate charting
- IV antibiotics and analgesics for 24 hours.
- Cold saline with dilute hydrogen peroxide gargles every 4 hourly for 48 hours.
- Cold liquids after 6 hours, e.g., ice-cream, cold milk, or coconut water
- Antibiotics, anti-inflammatory and analgesics syrups after discharge for 7 days.
- Condy's gargles (1: 4000 $KMnO_4$) for 7–10 days
- Plenty of clear fluids orally.
- Semi-solid diet after 2nd postoperative day.
- Semi-solid diet converted to solid diet once the patient is able to swallow.

COMPLICATIONS

Q. Enumerate the complications of tonsillectomy surgery.

Immediate (during surgery/within 6 hours of surgery)	Delayed (after 6 hours of surgery)
❖ **Anesthesia related** Causes:- ➢ Hypotension/hypertension ➢ Arrhythmia ➢ Syncope ➢ Vasovagal shock ❖ **Primary hemorrhage**—intraoperative hemorrhage controlled by pressure followed by ligation of bleeding vessel ❖ **Trauma** to surrounding structures—anterior/posterior pillar, lips, uvula, teeth, or soft palate ❖ **Aspiration** of blood ❖ Facial edema ❖ Surgical emphysema	❖ **Reactionary hemorrhage**—occurs up to 48 hours after surgery Causes: ➢ Slippage of tied knot ➢ Dislodgement of blood clot ➢ Rise in BP during extubation ➢ Failure to secure all the bleeding vessels ❖ **Secondary hemorrhage**—seen commonly on 6th–8th postoperative day ❖ Due to infection resulting in sloughing off of the walls of the ligated vessels ❖ Infection ❖ Recurrent/residual tonsillitis ❖ Exacerbation of granular pharyngitis ❖ Change of voice ❖ Lingual quinsy ❖ Aspiration of a fragment of tonsillar tissue

Reactionary Hemorrhage

Q. Write the clinical features and management of reactionary hemorrhage following tonsillectomy.

Clinical Features

Symptoms

- Child may be seen to spit out blood or vomit large amount of altered blood
- Child is seen to swallow despite the sedative effect
- Child may swallow blood and thus may lead to aspiration

Signs

- Child looks pale
- **Pulse:** tachycardia—fast but weak, thready pulse
- **Temperature:** Raised temperature
- **Respiratory rate:** Raised

Management

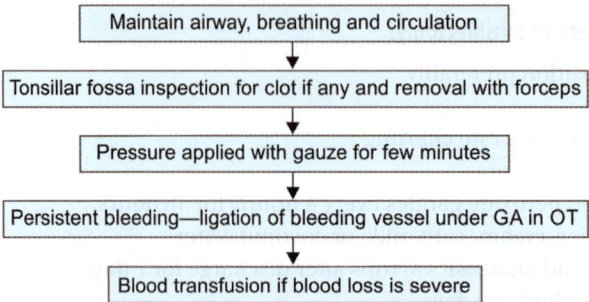

Secondary Hemorrhage

Q. Write the clinical features and management of secondary hemorrhage following tonsillectomy.

Clinical Features

- **Symptoms**: Patient spits out blood or blood clots, pain
- **Signs**: Rise in temperature.

Tonsillar fossa shows slough and blood clots.

Management

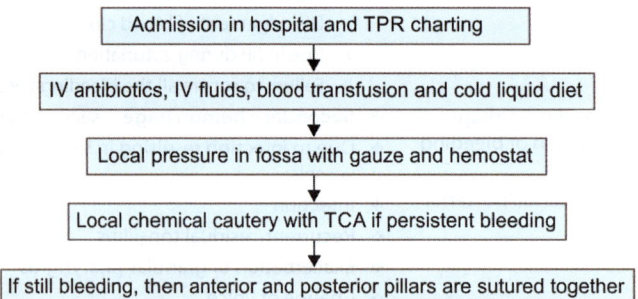

Q. What is the final option if post-tonsillectomy bleeding is not controlled despite ligating bleeding vessel and suturing the pillars together?

External carotid artery ligation in the neck just above the origin of superior thyroid artery branching off from the external carotid artery.

Other option is MRI angiography with embolization.

Chapter 60

Adenoidectomy

EN4.39: Observe and describe the indications for and steps involved in a tonsillectomy/adenoidectomy.

DEFINITION

Q. Write a short note on adenoidectomy/adenoid surgery. What are the indications and contraindications of adenoidectomy?

It is an operation performed for removal of the nasopharyngeal lymphoid tissue (adenoids).

INDICATIONS

- Adenoid tissue hypertrophy with adenoid facies.
- Adenoid hypertrophy causing snoring, mouth breathing, sleep apnea
- Enlarged adenoids causing recurrent upper respiratory tract infection
- Enlarged adenoids causing secretory otitis media by obstructing Eustachian tube opening
- Recurrent ear discharge in benign chronic otitis media associated with adenoiditis
- Recurrent adenoid tissue infection causing failure to thrive in children

CONTRAINDICATION

- Active infection, i.e., acute respiratory tract infection
- Submucous cleft palate
- Bleeding diathesis

METHODS

Q. What are the different methods used for adenoidectomy surgery?

- Using the St. Clair Thompson adenoid curette
- Using the La-Force Adenotome
- Finger dissection
- With 0° endoscope and microdebrider simultaneously

Anesthesia
General anesthesia with oral endotracheal tube.

Position
Same as tonsillectomy surgery—Rose's position.

Procedure

Q. Describe in brief the procedure for adenoidectomy surgery.

PART 2: Operative Procedures

```
Boyle's-Davis mouth gag applied and adenoids palpated digitally
   ↓
Adenoid curette is introduced with blade towards the tongue
   ↓
Blade of adenoid curette introduced just beyond the soft palate
   ↓
Curette is rotated through 180 degree and introduced in the nasopharynx
   ↓
Curette is held like a dagger and brought in contact with bony posterior septum
   ↓
With firm downwards strokes (sweeping motion) adenoid tissue is shaved off
   ↓
Hemostasis achieved by pressure with gauze and nasopharyngeal pack
   ↓
Gauze and pack removed followed by palpation for adenoid tags if any
   ↓
Adenoid tags removed with small adenoid curette/Luc's forceps
   ↓
Nasopharyngeal pack kept and completed hemostasis achieved
   ↓
Patient is extubated
```

■ COMPLICATIONS

Q. Enumerate the complications of adenoidectomy.

Postnasal Bleeding

Q. What is the source of postnasal bleeding after adenoidectomy surgery? How will you mange it?

Basisphenoid artery which supplies the bed of the adenoids and ascending pharyngeal artery which supply the substance of the adenoid tissue.

Immediate (during surgery/within 6 hours of surgery)	Delayed (after 6 hours of surgery)
❖ **anesthesia related** **Causes:** ➢ Hypotension/hypertension ➢ Arrhythmias ➢ Vasovagal shock ❖ **Primary hemorrhage:** ➢ Intraoperative hemorrhage controlled by pressure pack ➢ Removal of adenoid tags if any ➢ Repacking for 10–12 minutes ➢ Rarely postnasal pack for 24 hours required ❖ **Trauma** to soft palate, uvula, tongue or ET opening ❖ **Trauma to atlanto-occipital joint** if neck is kept in extended position	❖ **Reactionary hemorrhage:** Controlled by pressure packing for 3-5 minutes or even up to 10 minutes ❖ **Secondary hemorrhage:** Controlled by postnasal pack under GA and higher antibiotics ❖ **Secretory otitis media** due to stenosis of the ET orifice following trauma and fibrosis ❖ **Rhinolalia aperta** (nasal twang) if surgery performed in a patient with submucous cleft palate

Management

```
Adenoid pack made up of gauze pieces and ribbon gauze placed in the adenoid bed and pressure applied for 15-20 min–if still bleeding then
   ↓
Posterior nasal packing under general anesthesia (GA) with anterior nasal packing by roller gauze or nasal tampons—kept for 48 hours
   ↓
IV antibiotics started to avoid infection and blood arranged in case of need for transfusion
   ↓
If bleeding still not controlled, then external carotid artery ligation or MRI angiography with embolization
```

Postnasal Packing

Q. What are the different methods of postnasal packing?

- Postnasal pack made up of roller gauze soaked in antibiotic ointment to which 2 linen tapes and one thread are tied and passed over 2 red rubber catheters
- Foley's catheter
- Double lumen catheter with single inflatable balloon
- Double lumen catheter with two inflatable balloons
- Absorbable gelatin (gelfoam)
- Oxidized cellulose (surgicel).

Chapter 61

Thyroidectomy

■ INDICATIONS

- ❖ Large thyroid swellings causing cosmetic deformities, mulinodular goiters **(Fig. 1)**
- ❖ Malignant thyroid swellings.
- ❖ Thyroid swellings suspicious of malignancy on fine needle aspiration cytology (FNAC).
- ❖ Thyroid swelling causing compression symptoms like dyspnea, dysphagia, hoarseness of voice.
- ❖ Thyroid swelling with retrosternal extension

■ PREOPERATIVE

- ❖ All routine blood investigations
- ❖ Blood grouping and cross matching
- ❖ Written consent for scar, post-operative need for calcium and thyroxine supplementation, hoarseness of voice
- ❖ Euthyroid status

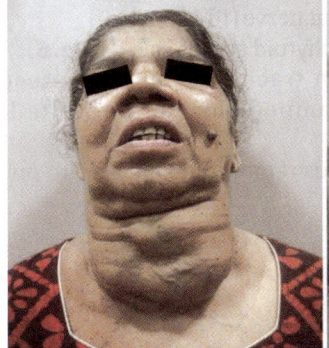
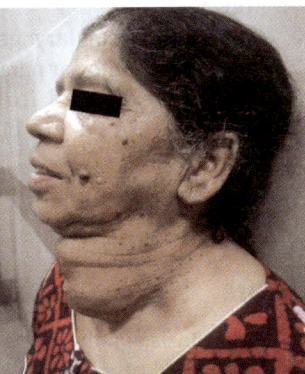

Fig. 1: Patient with goiter anterior and lateral view.

Anesthesia

General anesthesia.

Position

Supine, neck extended, pillow below shoulders, ring under head and sand bags by side of neck.

■ STEPS OF SURGERY

Q. What are the steps of thyroidectomy surgery?

1. Infiltration
2. Incision
3. Exposure
4. Dissection
5. Devascularization
6. Identification of recurrent laryngeal nerve (RLN)
7. Delivery of specimen
8. Hemostasis
9. Closure

Infiltration

Saline adrenaline along line of incision and in the anterior neck in subcutaneous plane.

Incision

Kocher's skin crease incision **(Fig. 2)** (curvilinear 2 cm above suprasternal notch and from one sternocleidomastoid to other).

Exposure

- Subcutaneous tissue and platysma incised in one layer **(Fig. 3)**. Subplatysmal flaps are raised. Upper flap raised till hyoid bone and lower till suprasternal notch **(Fig. 4)**.
- Deep fascia is incised vertically avoiding anterior and external jugular veins and strap muscles.
- Strap muscles are retracted.
- Thyroid gland is exposed laterally upto the sternocleidomastoids.

Dissection and Devascularization

- Dissection is carried onto superior pole. Superior thyroid artery, vein ligated and divided **as close to superior pole as possible (Fig. 5) to avoid injury into nerve.**
- Dissection carried to inferior pole and inferior thyroid artery ligated and divided close to inferior pole and away from tracheoesophageal groove.
- Look for recurrent laryngeal nerve (RLN) **(Fig. 8)**.
- Superior and inferior parathyroid glands saved **(Fig. 6)**.
- Isthmus separated from trachea by blunt dissection and isthmus hooked up, clamped close to opposite lobe and divided.
- Diseasesd lobe and isthmus removed taking care to protect RLN **(Figs. 7 and 9)**.

Closure

- Hemostasis achieved.
- Corrugated rubber drain or suction drain kept, brought out through a separate stab incision.
- Deep fascia sutured vertically with 3-0 vicryl.
- Platysma sutured with 3-0 vicryl interrupted sutures.
- Skin approximated with 4-0 proline subcuticular stiches/skin clips.
- Thyroid dressing given.

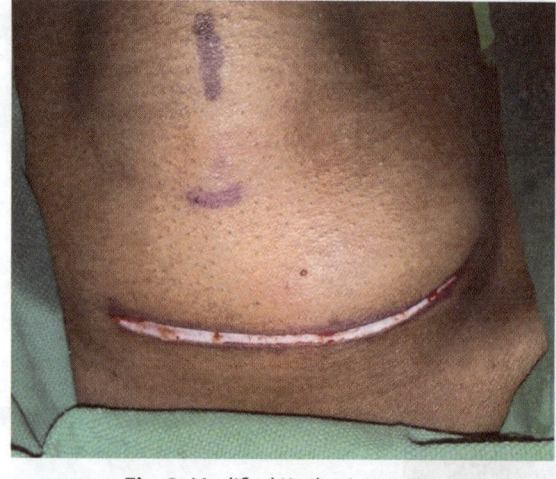

Fig. 2: Modified Kocher's incision.

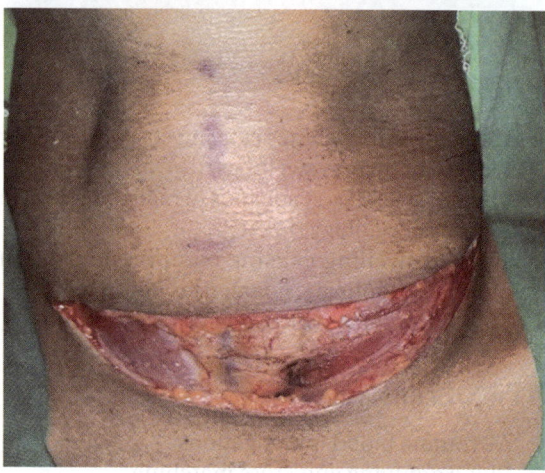

Fig. 3: Raising of subplatysmal flap.

IMP: During extubation, vocal cords movements checked to rule out RLN damage.

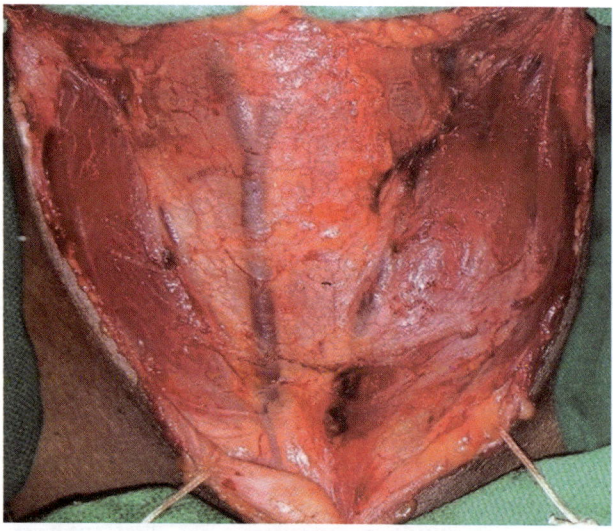

Fig. 4: Achieving adequate exposure.

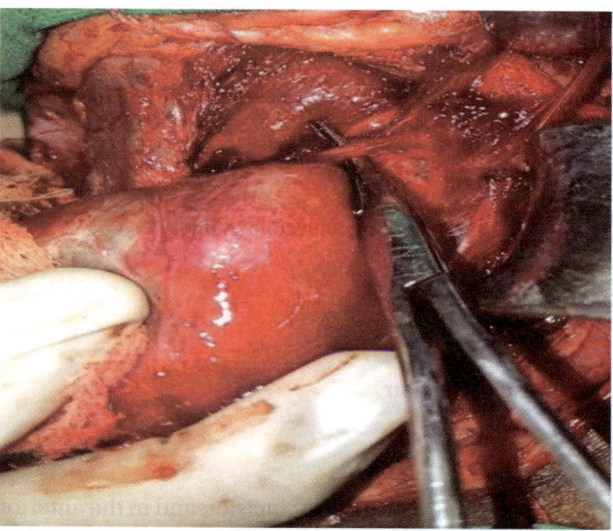

Fig. 5: Superior thyroid vessels ligated.

CHAPTER 61: Thyroidectomy

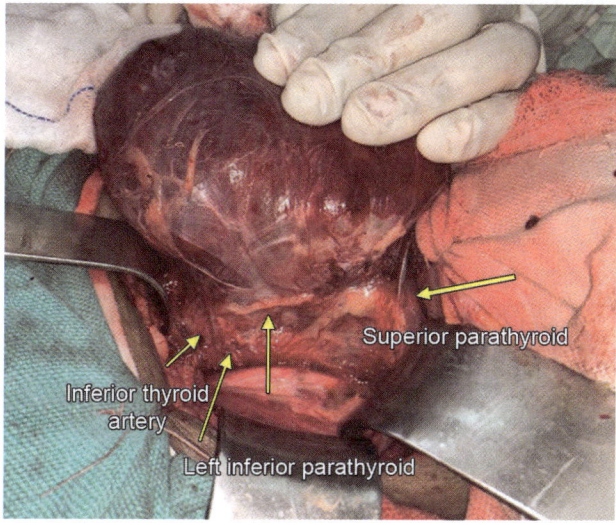

Fig. 6: Intraoperative picture showing enlarged thyroid gland, recurrent laryngeal nerve, inferior thyroid artery, superior and inferior parathyroid glands.

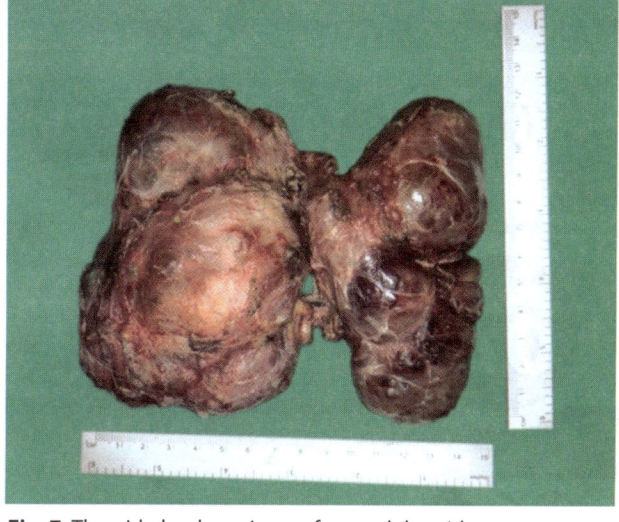

Fig. 7: Thyroid gland specimen after total thyroidectomy surgery.

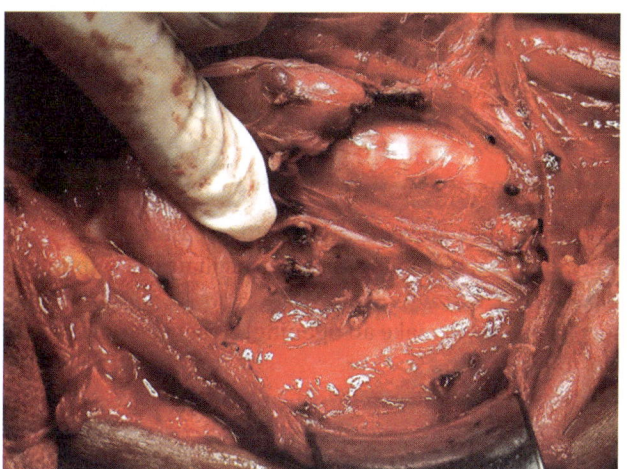

Fig. 8: Left recurrent laryngeal nerve identified.

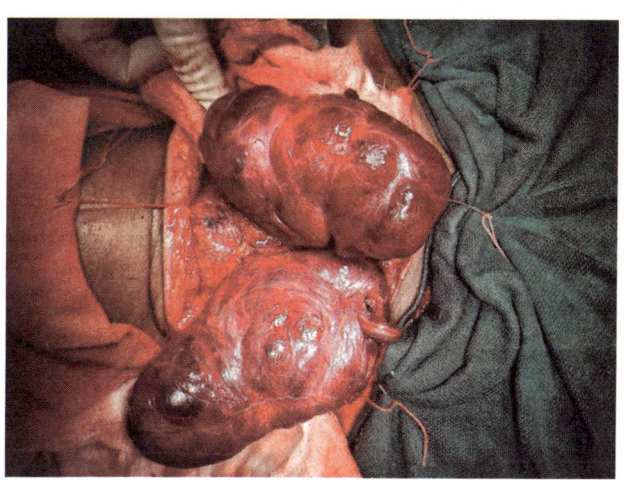

Fig. 9: Huge thyroid B/L lobes delivered from its retrosternal extent.

POSTOPERATIVE CARE

- Nil by mouth (NBM) for 6 hours
- Removal of drain after 48–72 hours
- Suture removal by 10th day
- Serum calcium monitoring

COMPLICATIONS

Q. Enumerate the complications of thyroidectomy surgery.

Intraoperative	Postoperative	

- Primary hemorrhage
- Damage to trachea
- Damage to external/recurrent laryngeal nerve
- Thyroid crisis/storm
	IMMEDIATE
	- **Breathlessness**
	  Causes:
	  - Tracheomalacia
	  - Vocal cord palsy
	  - Large hematoma compressing trachea
	  - Damage to pleura in large/retrosternal goiter
	- **Reactionary hemorrhage**
	- **Hoarseness of voice**
	- **Wound complications**
	  - Flap edema/necrosis
	  - Infection/stitch abscess
		DELAYED
		- Hypothyroidism
		- Hypoparathyroidism
		- Hypocalcemic tetany
		- Hypertrophied scar/keloid formation

Chapter 62

Tracheostomy

EN2.10: Identify, resuscitate and manage ENT emergencies in a simulated environment (including tracheostomy, anterior nasal packing, removal of foreign bodies in ear, nose, throat and upper respiratory tract).
EN4.44: Observe and describe the indications for and steps involved in tracheostomy and the care of the patient with a tracheostomy.

INTRODUCTION

Q. Define tracheostomy. Discuss briefly its types, procedure, indications and complications.

- Tracheostomy is defined as making an opening in the anterior wall of trachea and converting into an stoma.
- Life saving procedure where is an opening is made in the anterior wall of trachea so to assist and facilitate the respiration by bypassing obstruction.
- The word "tracheostomy" is derived from the Latin "trachea" and "tomein" (to make an opening). Tracheostomy means opening in the anterior wall of trachea, which is a step in tracheostomy.

HISTORY

- One of the oldest surgical procedures
- 100 BC: Asclepiades of Persia is credited as the first person to perform tracheostomy
- 1546: The first successful tracheostomy was performed by Italian physician Brasavola for laryngeal abscess
- 1718: Heister coined the term *Tracheostomy*
- *Caron:* 1st successful pediatric tracheostomy (1766)
- Antonio M. Brasavola: First successful tracheostomy
- Tracheostomy for diphtheria: Chevalier Jackson
- Good postoperative care: Pierre Bretonneau
- 1909: Chevalier Jackson codified indications and techniques for modern tracheostomy and warned of complications of high tracheostomy (cricothyrotomy)
- 19th century: Bretonnear and troussear, treatment of diphtheria
- Loreiz and Hiester coined the term '*Tracheostomy*'
- Fabricius first used the vertical incision
- Moure first used supine position, until then sitting position was used
- Early tubes were made of bone, rubber, silver, etc.

CHAPTER 62: Tracheostomy

ANATOMY OF TRACHEA
- **Tracheal length:** 10–14 cm
- **Tracheal diameter:** 15–20 mm
- **Extent:** C_6 (Larynx) to T_5 (carina)
- 15–20 'C' shaped cartilages
- Mucosa lined by ciliated pseudostratified columnar epithelium

SURGICAL ANATOMY OF TRACHEOSTOMY
- **Landmark:** Anterior triangle of neck
  - *Superior:* Cricoid cartilage
  - *Inferior:* Suprasternal notch
  - *Lateral:* SCM
- Skin and subcutaneous tissue
- Superficial cervical fascia
- Strap muscle
- Cervical fascia
- Thyroid gland
- Pretracheal fascia
  - *Blood supply:* Inferior thyroid veins

FUNCTIONS

Q. Enumerate functions of tracheostomy.

- Relieves upper airway obstruction
- Decreased dead space by > 1/3rd almost 50%
- Intermittent positive pressure ventilation
- To administer anesthesia
- To deliver medications
- Provides humidifications
- Protects against aspiration
- Reduces air flow resistance
- Provide access for tracheobronchial toilet

ADVANTAGES OF TRACHEOSTOMY
- It can be kept for a longer time
- Patient can swallow
- It decreases dead space by 50%
- It decreases respiratory resistance
- Tracheal stenosis is not very common
- Tracheal toilet is easier
- No risk of main stem bronchus intubation

INDICATIONS

Q. Enumerate indications of tracheostomy.

Absolute Indications
- Respiratory obstruction
- Respiratory failure
- Respiratory paralysis
- Removal of retained secretions
- Reduction of dead spaces
- **Prolonged ventilation:** Most common indication today.

Encountered in:
- Severe brain injury
- Acute respiratory distress syndrome (ARDS)
- Multiple organ dysfunction syndrome (MODS)
- Severe chronic obstructive pulmonary disease (COPD)
- Pneumonia refractory to treatment

Congenital
- **Intrinsic**
  - Laryngeal web
  - Laryngomalacia
  - Subglottic stenosis
  - Hemangioma
  - Cysts
- **Extrinsic**
  - Bilateral choanal atresia
  - Pierre Robin syndrome
  - Cystic hygroma
  - Lymphangioma

Inflammatory
- Acute laryngotracheobronchitis
- **Acute epiglottitis:** TB, syphilis, scleroma
- **Extrinsic:** Ludwig's angina, parapharyngeal/retropharyngeal abscess

PART 2: Operative Procedures

Neoplastic

- Benign: RRP, adenoma
- Malignant
- Ca larynx
- Ca thyroid
- Ca esophagus
- Bronchogenic ca
- Mediastinal masses
- Lymphoma
- Secondary metastatic lymphadenopathy

Traumatic

- Accidental
- Laryngeal cut throat injuries
- Strangulation
- Corrosive poisoning
- Extralaryngeal—faciomaxillary injuries
- Hematoma base tongue

Surgical

- Thyroidectomy
- Cardiac surgeries

Miscellaneous

- FB in air passages
- Angioneurotic edema

Retained Secretions

- **Inability to cough:**
  - Coma
  - Respiratory muscle spasm
  - Respiratory muscle weakness
- **Painful cough:**
  - Chest injury
  - Flail chest
  - Pneumonia
- **Aspiration:**
  - Bulbar polio
  - Polyneuritis
  - B/L adductor cord palsy

Respiratory Insufficiency

- Central
- Coma—uremia, head injury, cerebrovascular accidents, diabetic ketoacidosis, hepatic dysfunctions
- Respiratory centre depression base skull, barbiturate poisoning, bulbar poliomyelitis
- Peripheral/neuromuscular
- Guillain-Barre syndrome (GBS), tetanus
- Pulmonary
- Pneumothorax, pneumomediastinum, flail chest

Common Indications

- Long-term intubated patient in cases of head injury
- Ca larynx
- Tetanus
- Laryngeal trauma

Indications for Permanent Tracheostomy

- Carcinoma larynx
- Carcinoma hypopharynx
- Bilateral abductor vocal cord palsy

CONTRAINDICATION

Q. Enumerate contraindications of tracheostomy.

- An emergency tracheostomy is a life saving procedure, and there is no absolute contraindications to it

CHAPTER 62: Tracheostomy

- Relative contraindications to a planned tracheostomy:
  - Bleeding disorders
  - Anticoagulant therapy
  - Tracheal neoplasms
  - Enlarged thyroid
  - Patient not willing for surgery

TYPES

Q. What are types of tracheostomy?

- **According to timing:**
  - Emergency/slash tracheostomy
  - Elective/orderly/routine/tranquil tracheostomy
    - Therapeutic
    - Prophylactic
- **According to position:**
  - *High:* Above isthmus. Done in cases of Ca larynx and cases of severe stridor
    Disadvantage:
    - Perichondritis of cricoid cartilage
    - Subglottic stenosis
  - *Mid:* At level of 2nd and 3rd tracheal rings. Most preferred
  - *Low:* Below level of isthmus
    Disadvantage: Trachea is deep at this level and is close to several large vessels and pleura
- **According to duration:**
  - Temporary tracheostomy
  - Permanent tracheostomy

PROCEDURES

Q. Describe tracheostomy procedure.

Preoperative Work up

- Assessment of patient clinical condition
- Platelet count, Hb
- PT/INR
- Informed consent is taken for procedure and complications
- Inj. TT, atropine

OT Room Set Up

- **Surgeon:** Right side of patient
- **Assistant:** Left side of patient
- **Scrub nurse:** Right side of surgeon
- **Anesthetist:** Head end of patient

Patient's Position

- Supine position
- Arms by the side
- Neck stabilized and fixed in midline
- Sandbag under the shoulder to place neck in hyperextension

Anesthesia

Local anesthetic (2% lignocaine with Adr 1:200,000) is used
- Provides analgesia
- Elevates tissue planes for easy dissection
- Decreases bleeding
- Decreases tracheal reflexes during introduction of tube

Skin Incision

- Taken one finger breadth below cricoid cartilage and two fingers above suprasternal notch.
- Very easy, quick to make
- Can be extended in a difficult neck
- Not as cosmetic as horizontal incision

- Done in a horizontal skin crease
- More cosmetic
- However, it is difficult to adjust level of tracheostomy tube and difficult to close incision after tube removal

Tracheal Exposure

- Done in a horizontal skin crease
- More cosmetic
- However, it is difficult to adjust level of tracheostomy tube and difficult to close incision after tube removal

Tracheal Incision

- After intratracheal injection of 1-2 cc of lignocaine, tracheal incision is done
- Inverted 'U' shaped incision is preferred (Bjork flap)

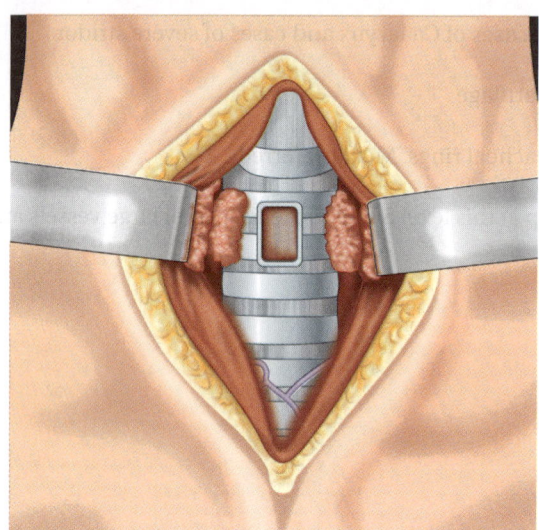

Inserting Tracheostomy Tube

- Tube with obturator is introduced
- Obturator is removed
- Cuff is inflated and tube secured by fixation
- The 2 flanges can also be sutured to skin

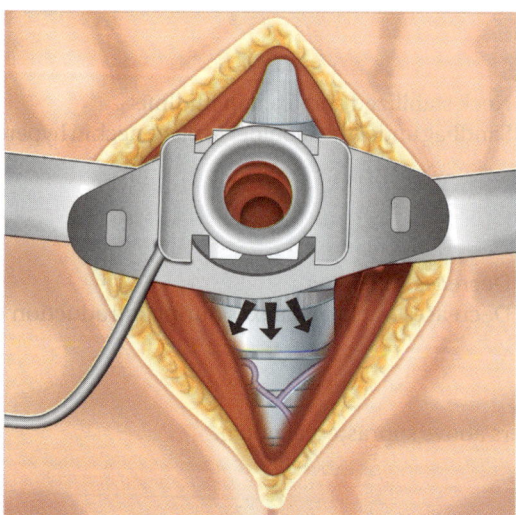
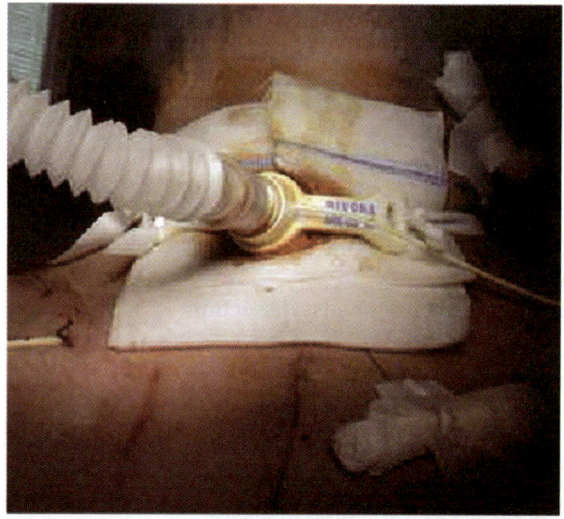

Dressing

Highly absorbent
- ❖ Open porous dressing
- ❖ Prevents leakage
- ❖ Zig zag opening

Post Tracheostomy Care

- ❖ CXR PA after 4 hrs
- ❖ Daily dressing
- ❖ Suctioning every ½ hrly or sos
- ❖ Deflate the cuff every 2 hrly for 10 min then reinflate by 4–6 cc air (keep deflated if patient is off ventilator)
- ❖ Mycolytics
- ❖ Nebulization—saline, mucolytic
- ❖ Chest physiotherapy

Changing Tracheostomy Tube

- ❖ Changed on 6–7 postoperative day
- ❖ Pressure dressing placed
- ❖ Tracheotomy tract closes spontaneously in 2–3 days

Tube Exchange: Difficult Situations

- ❖ When the stoma is scarred, calcified, distorted or obscured by granulation tissue
- ❖ When the trachea is deviated or rotated
- ❖ When the trachea is narrowed or smaller than normal
- ❖ When the patient is a child
- ❖ When the patient is obese
- ❖ If the tube must be placed quickly in an emergency
- ❖ If it is a new or recent tracheostomy
- ❖ If the person performing the change is not well-trained

COMPLICATIONS

Q. Describe complications of tracheostomy and its management.

- ❖ Immediate
- ❖ Early
- ❖ Late

Complications	Causes	Management
1. Apnea	CO_2 washout Loss of hypoxic drive	Carbogen, blockade, ventilation
2. Bleeding	Thyroid vessels, anterior jugular vein, tracheal vessels, aberrants	Suction, ligation, cauterization
3. Pneumothorax	Low tracheostomy with injury to pleura-clinical features **Clinical features:** Subcut emphysema Hamman's sign, high RR	Investigation: Oblique lateral CXR Treatment: Chest tap with under seal drain, O_2, antibiotics
4. Subcutaneous emphysema	Tight packing around tube, false passage, pretracheal fascia not opened, large stoma	Trial of high flow O_2, compression dressing, releasing incision
5. Injury to surrounding structures	Injury to recurrent laryngeal nerve (RLN) Tracheoesophageal (T-E) due to a stab incision	Injury to RLN T-E fistula due to a stab incision
6. Early bleed	Sepsis, coagulopathy Stomal granulation	Packing antibiotic gauze, antibiotics
7. Obstruction	Mucus, crusts (tracheitis sicca)	Suction, humidification
8. Chest infection	Especially in pre-existing lung pathology	Antibiotics, tracheal swab

Complications	Causes	Management
9. Granulations		Excise, cautery, laser
10. Aerophagia	Esp. in infants due to swallowing. Clinical features: Abdominal distention, vomit, dyspnea, hypotension	Decannulation, Different shaped tube to decrease irritation, NG tube
11. Atelectasis	Overly long tube	Reposition, smaller tube
12. Dislocation of tube	During change of position, loose tie, excessive coughing, excessive movements of patients	Reinsertion in experienced hands Tying tube flanges to skin, Securing tapes with neck in flexion
13. Blocked tube	Improper suctioning	Regular suction, change the tube
14. Non-closure of fistula	Tract lined with skin	Elliptical incision around fistula and excision of tract
15. Tracheoesophageal fistula	Trauma to post tracheal wall or in stab type trach	Definitive surgical repair
16. Difficult decannulation	Decreased resp effort—dependency, granulation, edema, stenosis	Gradual weaning
17. Keloid	Infection of wound	Triamcinolone injection, Z-plasty
18. Tracheal stenosis	Long-standing tube, incorrect pressure, not deflating the tube	Immediate exploration, secure airway, finger tamponade through stoma, median sternotomy with ligation of vessel

■ TRACHEOSTOMY TUBES

Q. Describe different types of tracheostomy tubes.

- **Metal:** *German silver—alloy of Cu (65%), Ni (18%) and Zn (17%)*
- **Synthetic:**
  - PVC
  - Silicon
    - Cuffed
    - Uncuffed
    - Fenestrated
    - Unfenestrated

Metal Tracheostomy Tubes

- Chevalier Jackson
- Negus
- Alder Hey
- Sheffield

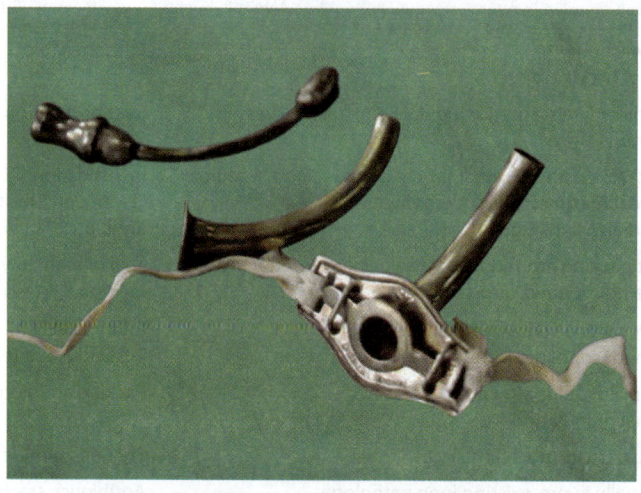

Metal tracheostomy tubes: Chevalier Jackson

CHAPTER 62: Tracheostomy

Synthetic Tubes

- Shiley
- Great Ormond Street
- Portex
- Bivona

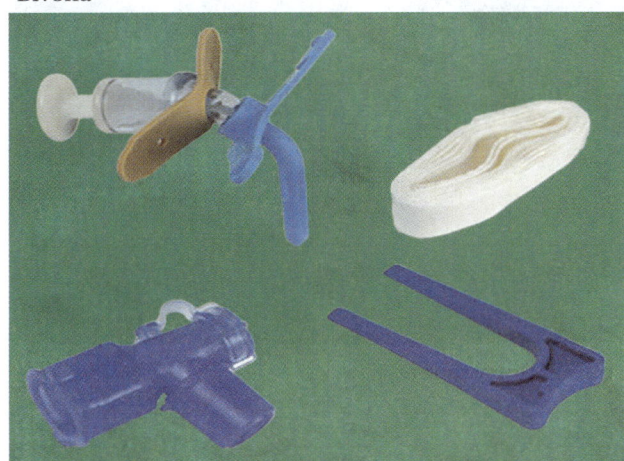

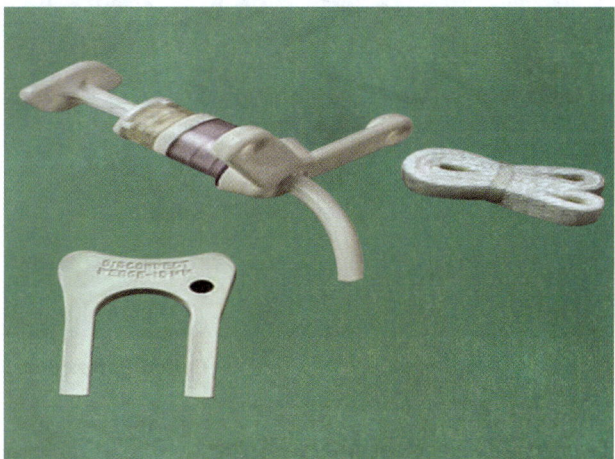

Bivona uncuffed

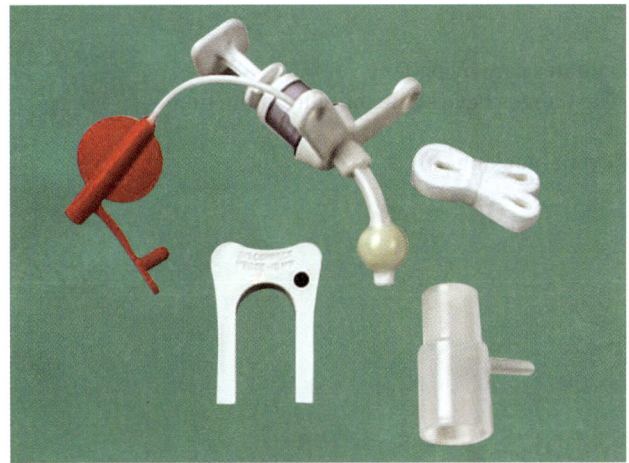

Bivona cuffed

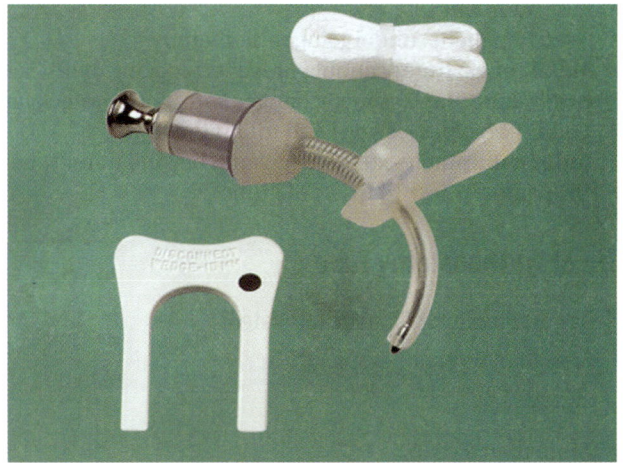

Bivona cuffed flexible tube

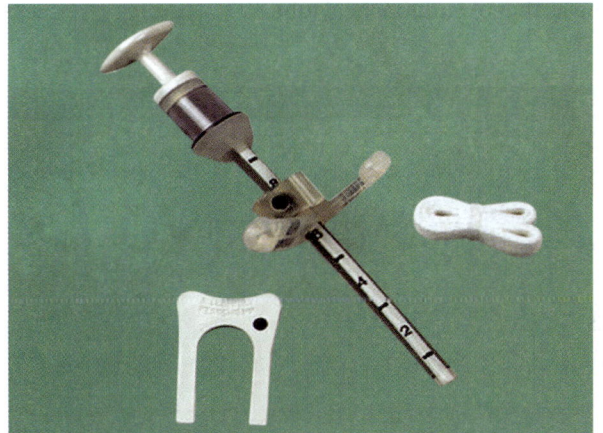

Bivona hyperflex uncuffed tube with adjustable neck flanges

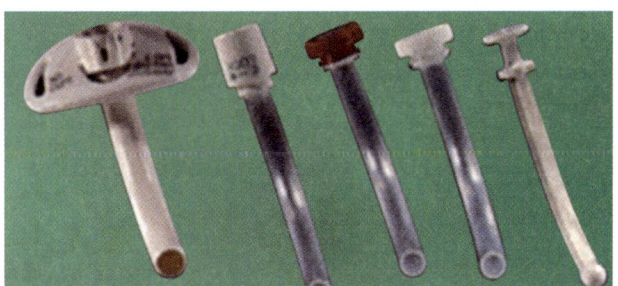

Uncuffed tubes

Cuffed Tubes

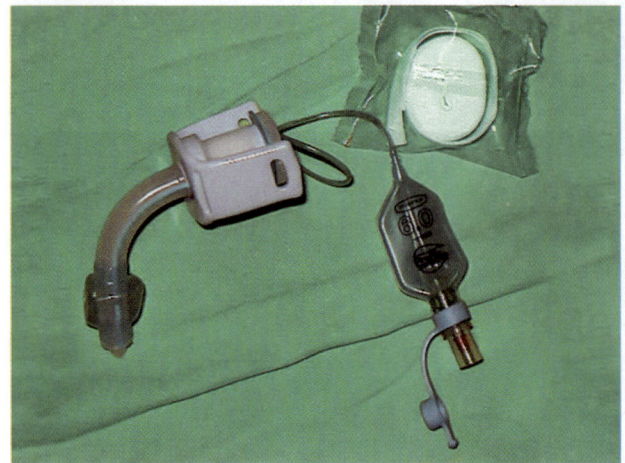
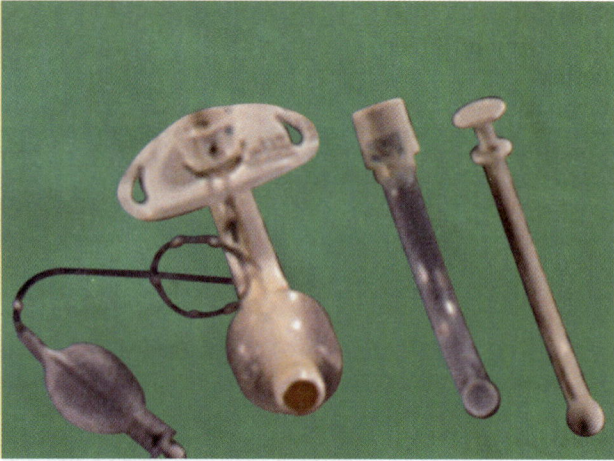

Cuffed Portex Blue line tracheostomy tube

Q. Enumerate differences of metal vs. synthetic.

- **Synthetic:** Thermolabile and conform to patients tracheal anatomy
- **Cuffed:** Permit PPV and prevent aspiration
- **Fenestrated:** Allow phonation
- Less traumatic
- Used in patients undergoing radiotherapy
- **Metal tubes:** Inner cannula prevents blocking of tube and facilitates care by patient
- **Outer cannula:** Has metal flanges with slots for neck tapes. The flanges have some mobility at the tube
- **Lock:** Two types—swivel and rotating
- **Inner cannula:** It extends a few mm beyond outer tube to prevent blocking
- **Obturator/pilot:** To insert the tube

Size of Tracheostomy Tube

Q. How tracheostomy tube size calculated?

- Less than 6 years:
  $$\frac{\text{Age in years} + 3.5}{3}$$
- More than 6 years:
  $$\frac{\text{Age in years} + 4.5}{4}$$
- For an intubated patient number of tracheostomy tube is same as that of endotracheal tube.
- *Size of pediatric tubes according to age*

Age	Size
Preterm–1 month	2.5–3
1–6 months	3.5
6–18 months	4
18 moths–3 years	4.5
3–6 years	5
6–9 years	5.5
9–12 years	6
12–14 years	7

Special Purpose Tubes

Speaking Valves (Montgomery)

- Allow patient to vocalize without occlusion
- Provides one way airflow to redirect air through larynx
- Thin silicone diaphragm for low resistance and cough release mechanism

TRACOE® Comfort

- Flexible, transparent, more pliable at body temp
- Low profile neck plate—more cosmetic
- Widest size range, custom fits and fenestrations

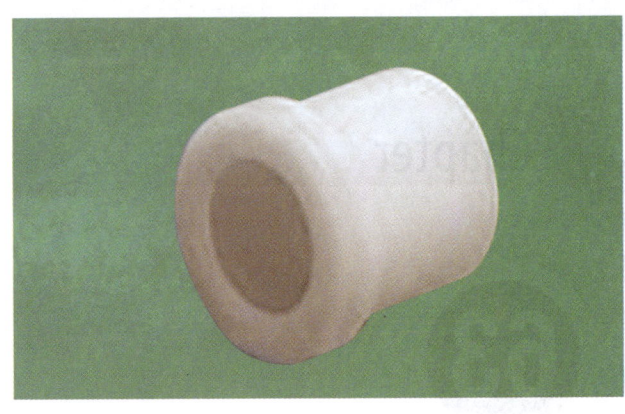

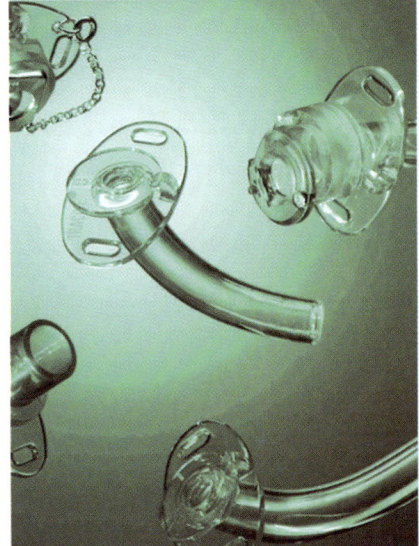

DECANNULATION

Pre-decannulation Assessment

- Clinical assessment
- **Physiological assessment:** Patency of airway through tube is compared with that through mouth CT/MRI/endoscopic examination

Methods

- Sequential downsizing of tube
- Surgical decannulation

One Step Decannulation

- Patient admitted for decannulation
- Bronchoscopic examination in a spontaneously breathing patient for patency of airway
- If airway is patent and cords are mobile, decannulation is done

Intubation Period Before Tracheostomy

- Before 1970's: >8 days
- Now this period is fixed individually based on clinical and endoscopic findings. Average period in a large series—34 days.

Chapter 63: Cricothyroidotomy

■ INDICATIONS

- ❖ Severe bleeding in maxillofacial injuries
- ❖ Foreign bodies
- ❖ Repeated failed intubation
- ❖ Cervical spine injuries
- ❖ Smoke inhalations
- ❖ Burns

■ CONTRAINDICATIONS

- ❖ Infant and children as they do not have cricothyroid membrane
- ❖ Inflammation and malignancy of larynx

■ EMERGENCY TRACHEOSTOMY

Q. Write short note on emergency tracheostomy.

- ❖ Tube inserted through cricothyroid membrane
- ❖ Position: Neck extension
- ❖ Vertical midline skin incision
- ❖ Finger dissection
- ❖ Horizontal incision over cricothyroid membrane
- ❖ Space widened, cannula inserted
- ❖ Formal tracheostomy done as soon as possible
- ❖ Cannula can cause stenosis, dysphonia
  - ➢ Time: 15–30 seconds

Fig. 1: Showing Incision for cricothyrotomy procedure.

Percutaneous Dilatational Tracheostomy (Ciaglia et al. Technique) (Fig. 2)

Prerequisites for Percutaneous Dilatational Tracheostomy

- Procedure can be performed only in intubated patients with long neck admitted in ICU
- In those patient who have ability to hyperextend the neck
- Easy intubation in case accidental intubation

Q. Write short note on percutaneous dilatational tracheostomy.

- Short incision
- Large bore needle inserted between 2 tracheal rings
- Guidewire introduced
- Serial dilatation over guidewire
- **Rapitrach:** 1 step dilatation
- **Complications:** Tracheal collapse, tracheoesophageal fistula can occur post puncture procedure
- **Contraindications:** <16 years, large goiter, neck tumors
- **Procedure:**
  - Guidewire introduction, with removal of sheath
  - Guidewire and catheter are advanced together into the trachea as far as the skin positioning marks on the guide catheter to the skin.
  - Guidewire, guide catheter, and dilator unit are advanced together into the trachea to the skin positioning mark.
  - The tracheotomy tube is loaded onto a dilator and advanced into the trachea over the guidewire and catheter. The guidewire and catheter are removed, leaving only the tracheostomy tube in the trachea.

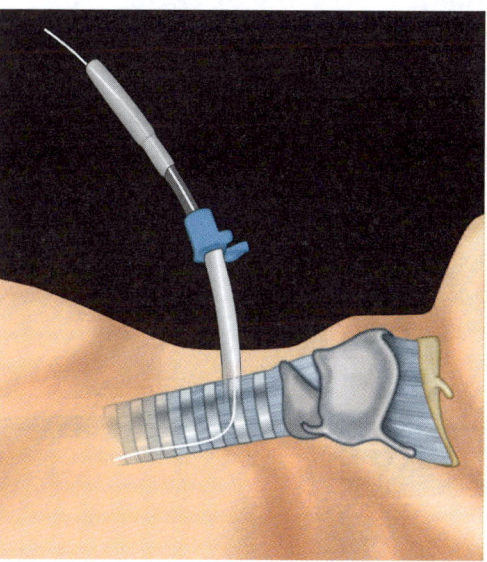

Fig. 2: Percutaneous dilatational tracheotomy.

Section 4: Various Scopy

Chapter 64: Laryngoscopy

EN3.3: Observe and describe the indications for and steps involved in the performance of rigid/flexible laryngoscopy.

■ DIRECT LARYNGOSCOPY

Q. Write a short note on direct laryngoscopy and discuss the steps of procedure.

Definition

It is direct visualization of larynx and hypopharynx using laryngoscope.

Indications

Diagnostic	Therapeutic
❖ When indirect laryngoscopy not possible: 　➢ Infants 　➢ Children 　➢ Uncooperative individuals 　➢ Mentally retarded individuals ❖ Unexplained symptoms like hoarseness of voice, dyspnea, stridor, dysphagia, odynophagia, aspiration, chronic cough, hemoptysis, globus sensation. ❖ When a lesion on indirect laryngoscopy needs further evaluation. ❖ When indirect laryngoscopy is difficult to perform due to excessive gag reflex. ❖ When it is difficult to visualized structures due to overhanging epiglottis. ❖ To examine hidden areas of: 　➢ *Hypopharynx:* Base of tongue, valleculae, apex of pyriform fossa. 　➢ *Larynx:* Infrahyoid epiglottis, anterior commissure, ventricles, and subglottic region. ❖ To find the extent of growth and take a biopsy. ❖ As a part of panendoscopy.	❖ Removal of benign lesions of larynx, e.g., papilloma, fibroma, vocal nodule/polyp/cyst. ❖ Removal of foreign body from larynx and hypopharynx. ❖ Removal of thickened secretion and crust. ❖ For endotracheal intubation ❖ To inject Teflon paste in unilateral vocal cord palsy. ❖ Dilatation of laryngeal strictures.

Contraindications

Absolute	Relative
❖ Pott's spine ❖ Cervical spine injuries ❖ Cervical spondylosis ❖ Fracture of maxilla/mandible	❖ Trismus ❖ Ankylosis of temporomandibular joint ❖ Short neck ❖ Micrognathia ❖ Systemic diseases 　➢ Diabetes mellitus/hypertension (DM/HTN) 　➢ Cardiac problem

Preoperative Preparation

- General anesthesia (GA) fitness
- Consent
- Mallampati score
- I/V antibiotic shot
- Inj. TT 0.5 mL I/M
- Preoxygenation

Position

- Patient in supine position.
- Head elevated by placing a pillow underneath.
- **Sniffing position/barking dog position/Boyce's position:** Flexion of neck at thorax and extension at atlanto-occipital joint.
- This particular position brings the larynx in direct axis with the oral cavity.

Anesthesia

- GA is preferred.
- Can be performed under local anesthesia (LA): LOX 4% xylocaine spray

Procedure

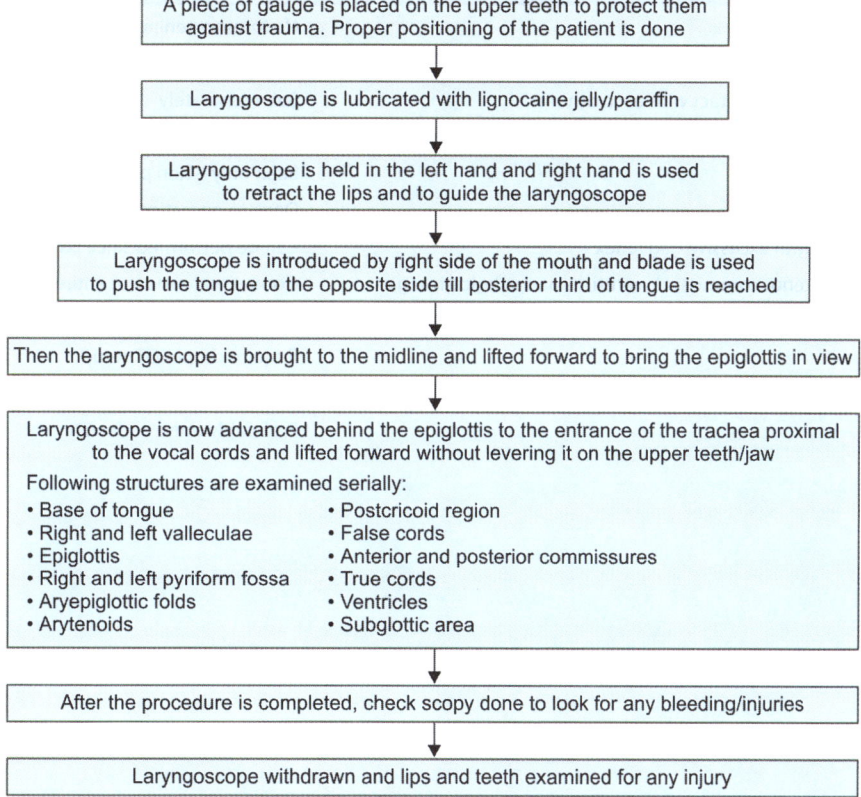

Postoperative Care

- Left lateral decubitus position to prevent aspiration of blood/secretions
- Monitor respiration → laryngeal spasm/cyanosis
- Watch for respiratory distress
- Trauma to larynx → laryngeal edema → respiratory distress
- Antibiotic
- Analgesic

Complications

- Injury to lips/gum/teeth/tongue/palate
- Stimulation of posterior pharyngeal wall may cause vasovagal attack leading to hypoxia and bradycardia
- Cervical spine injury due to hyperextension
- Laryngeal edema
- Laryngospasm
- Anesthetic complication

Hidden areas
- Hypopharynx
  - Base of tongue
  - Valleculae
  - Apex of pyriform fossa
- Larynx
  - Laryngeal surface of epiglottis
  - Anterior commissure
  - Ventricle
  - Subglottic area

DIFFERENCES BETWEEN INDIRECT LARYNGOSCOPY AND DIRECT LARYNGOSCOPY

Q. Write difference between direct and indirect laryngoscopy.

Indirect laryngoscopy	Direct laryngoscopy
Foreshortening of AP diameter	No foreshortening
Two-dimensional image	Three-dimensional image
True and false cords appear to be in contact with each other	Seen separately
Inverted mirror image	Direct visualization
Movement of vocal cords seen better	Seen only when performed under LA
OPD procedure	Done in operation theater (OT)
Difficult to perform in patient with excessive gag reflex	Can be performed since patient is under GA
Inadequate visualization of anterior commissure, ventricle, and subglottic region.	Good visualization of entire larynx and its hidden area
Free of complication	Complication present
Easily available	Require proper OT setup
Hidden areas difficult to see	Good visualization of hidden areas
No anesthesia required	Preferably done under GA

Chapter 65: Microlaryngoscopy

■ DEFINITION

Q. What is microlaryngoscopy? Discuss in brief its indications, contraindications and procedure.

Microlaryngoscopy is the procedure to view the larynx with the aid of a microscope, with special focus on the vocal cords.

■ INDICATIONS

Diagnostic	Therapeutic
❖ To take biopsy from suspicious lesions to rule out malignancy ❖ To evaluate the endolaryngeal spread of any malignancy ❖ In cases of hoarseness of voice, with no identifiable pathology on laryngoscopy	❖ Removal of vocal cord polyp, nodules, and cysts ❖ For excision of tumors using transoral laser resection ❖ For fat implantation in case of sulcus vocalis ❖ For removal of recurrent respiratory papillomatosis ❖ For endolaryngeal botulinum injection ❖ For vocal cord stripping in Reinke's edema ❖ For injection thyroplasty

■ CONTRAINDICATIONS

Absolute	Relative

❖ Pott's spine
❖ Cervical spine injuries
❖ Cervical spondylosis
❖ Fracture of maxilla/mandible
	❖ Trismus
	❖ Ankylosis of temporomandibular joint
	❖ Short neck
	❖ Micrognathia
	❖ Systemic diseases
	   ➤ Diabetes mellitus/hypertension (DM/HTN)
	   ➤ Cardiac problem as the chest piece can cause cardiac tamponade effect

■ EQUIPMENT

- ❖ Microlaryngoscope
- ❖ Chest piece
- ❖ Light source
- ❖ Instruments (microlaryngoscopy forceps, scissors, vocal cord spreader, injection needle, sickle knife, suction cannula)

■ ADVANTAGES OF MICROLARYNGOSCOPY OVER DIRECT LARYNGOSCOPY

- ❖ Binocular vision
- ❖ Bimanual handling as surgeon's both hands are free

- High resolution magnification
- Better illumination
- Use of CO_2 laser possible
- Teaching is possible through side tube of microscope or camera with monitor
- Medicolegal documentation in the form of intraoperative pictures or video recording

DISADVANTAGE OF MICROLARYNGOSCOPY OVER DIRECT LARYNGOSCOPY

Considerable force needed; thus high risk of tissue injury, injury to teeth as the scope rests on incisor teeth, fracture rib may occur, cardiac tamponade effect.

PROCEDURE (STEPS) (FIGS. 1 AND 2)

- Patient is intubated with a special microlaryngoscopy tube, which occupies the posterior glottis, giving the surgeon ample space to operate.
- Patient is in supine position with flexion of the neck and extension of the shoulder (optional).
- The teeth are protected with gauze before introducing the scope.
- The largest caliber laryngoscope with the light source is introduced and the endotracheal tube is followed from uvula to epiglottis and finally positioned when the vocal cords and anterior commissure are in view. Supracricoid pressure might be needed which is given by the assistant.
- It is then secured in position with the chest piece. A soft towel is kept between the patient and the chest piece to avoid trauma and tamponade to the chest.
- The whole assembly is then secured using dynaplast/micropore which is stuck from one side of the bed to the neck to the other side of bed.
- The light source is now removed and the **microscope is now used**, at a **focal length of 350–400 mm,** with a **distance of 20 cm from the laryngoscope**.
- Magnifying telescopes (0, 30, 70°) can be used to aid visualization.
- After this, the true vocal cords, false cords, ventricle, arytenoid, and subglottis are assessed.
- Depending on the indication, the procedure is complicated.
- Hemostasis is achieved.
- Patient extubated.

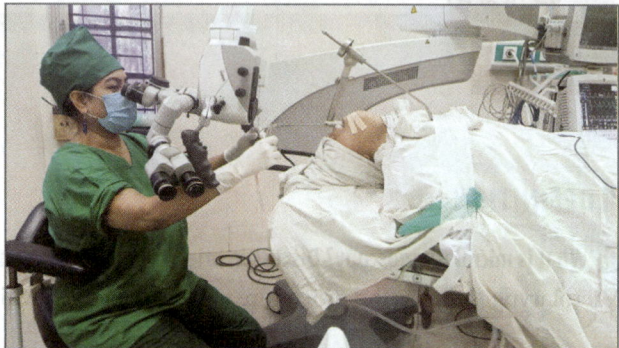

Fig. 1: Microlaryngoscopy surgery procedure.

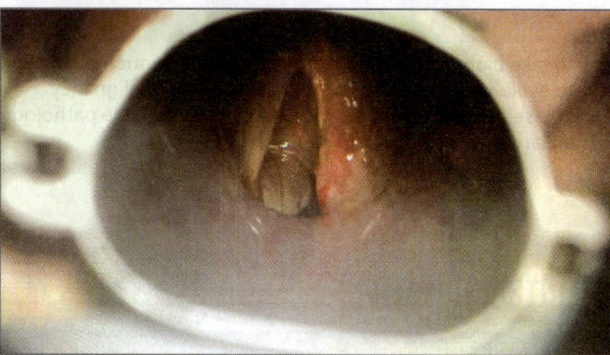

Fig. 2: Microlaryngoscopy view of true vocal cord lesion.

Chapter 66

Esophagoscopy

EN2.9: Observe and describe the indications for and steps involved in the removal of foreign bodies from ear, nose and throat.
EN2.10: Observe and describe the indications for and steps involved in the skills of emergency procedures in ear, nose and throat.

■ TYPES

Q. Write a short note on esophagoscopy and discuss briefly its types and procedure.

It is of two types:
1. Rigid esophagoscopy
2. Flexible fiber optic esophagoscopy

Rigid esophagoscopy	Flexible fiber optic esophagoscopy
Done for removal of foreign bodies	May be used for removal of small foreign bodies
Done in cases of esopharyngeal dilatation	Used for taking biopsies, dilatation of strictures, and injection of esopharyngeal strictures
More effective for management of upper esophageal lesions	Used for examination of the mid and lower esophagus
More difficult to perform than flexible scopy especially in presence of dental and spinal abnormalities	Easier to use than rigid esophagoscope and be used in patients with dental or spinal deformities
Requires general anesthesia	Can be done under local anesthesia and photography can be performed

■ INDICATIONS

Therapeutic

- Removal of foreign body
- Dilatation of esophageal stricture
- Endoscopic removal of benign lesions, e.g., fibroma, papilloma, cysts, etc.
- Insertion of Soutar's or Mousseau-Barbin tube in cases of esophageal carcinoma.
- Injection of esophageal varices.

Diagnostic

- To take punch biopsies.
- To investigate cause for dysphagia, e.g., carcinoma esophagus, cardiac achalasia, strictures, etc.
- To find cause for retrosternal burning, e.g., reflux esophagitis or hiatus hernia
- To find cause for hematemesis, e.g., esophageal varices
- As part of panendoscopy

ANESTHESIA

An endotracheal general anesthetic appropriate for age and weight administered either by relaxant or spontaneous respiration technique.

Local anesthesia can be used with 2% lignocaine spray. Using a Jackson applicator, 2 mL of anesthetic agent is sprayed between the vocal cords with a laryngeal cannula.

Superior laryngeal nerve block may also be used.

PROCEDURE

- **Position: The patient lies supine with the head and neck flexed upon the chest.** This position helps to attain the axes of mouth, pharynx, and esophagus in a straight line so rigid tube can pass easily.
- Esophagoscope is lubricated using jelly and held between the fingers and thumb of the right (for right-handed surgeon) while the lips are retracted with the left fingers and thumb. A piece of gauze is kept over upper teeth to prevent trauma.
- The tip of the esophagus is introduced into the right side of the mouth under the upper surface of the tongue until the right side of the larynx or endotracheal tube is visualized.
- **Identification of arytenoids**: The scope is then gently advanced using the left thumb and index finger. Arytenoids are seen after identifying epiglottis.
- **Passage through cricopharyngeus**: The head is extended at the atlanto-occipital joint. The scope is passed from the right pyriform fossa toward the midline, and it is then advanced downward applying a forward tilt of the tip using the left thumb.
- **Crossing the aortic arch and left bronchus**: This narrowing usually lies about 25 cm from the incisors. Aortic pulsation can be seen. Gradually the neck is extended as the scope in further advanced downward.
- **Passing the cardia**: Cardia is identified by the redder and more velvety mucosa.
- After the procedure, check scopy is done to inspect the esophageal wall.

POSTOPERATIVE CARE

- Patient is kept in semiprone position.
- Sips of plain water followed by normal diet after an uneventful esophagoscopy.
- They are observed for signs and symptoms of esopharyngeal perforation like—interscapular pain, marked dysphagia with fever and subcutaneous emphysema.

COMPLICATIONS

- Injury to the lips and teeth.
- Trauma to the posterior pharyngeal wall.
- **Perforation of the esophagus:** The most common site is at Killian's dehiscence near the cricopharyngeal sphincter. Signs of esophageal perforation during surgery are sudden give way sensation while introducing the esophagoscope, sudden blackening sensation during scopy, tachycardia, and hypotension.
- Compression of trachea by the instrument during the procedure causing obstruction of respiration, and cyanosis.

Chapter 67

Bronchoscopy

EN2.9: Observe and describe the indications for and steps involved in the removal of foreign bodies from ear, nose and throat.
EN2.10: Observe and describe the indications for and steps involved in the skills of emergency procedures in ear, nose and throat.

■ DEFINITION

Q. What is bronchoscopy? Discuss briefly its types, indications, procedure and complications.

Definition: It is a direct inspection and examination of the larynx, trachea, and bronchi for diagnostic or therapeutic purposes, using a rigid or a flexible bronchoscope.

Rigid bronchoscopy: Removal of foreign body under direct vision with protected airway

Flexible fiberoptic bronchoscopy can be performed easily under sedation and local anesthesia. Causes less discomfort for the patient than rigid bronchoscopy.

■ INDICATIONS

Diagnostic	Therapeutic
❖ Suspected foreign body	❖ Removal of tracheobronchial foreign bodies **(Figs. 1 to 3)**
❖ Vocal cord palsy	❖ Removal of broncholith
❖ Cases of recurrent laryngeal nerve palsy	❖ Removal of retained bronchial secretions in unconscious or head injury patients
❖ Biopsy of malignancy or suspected mass in tracheobronchial tree	❖ Dilatation in case of tracheal stenosis
❖ Bronchial lavage and cytological examination of bronchial secretions, e.g., TB, malignancy	❖ Aspiration of lung abscess if it bursts into a bronchus
❖ Persistent unexplained cough or hemoptysis for more than 5–6 weeks	❖ Removal of benign tumors like papillomas or granulations
❖ To detect spread of carcinoma from esophagus or thyroid	❖ Bronchoscopically implanted radium seeds in bronchus for malignancies
❖ Atelectasis of the lung	❖ In case of difficult endotracheal intubation
❖ Unexplained obstructive emphysema to rule out a foreign body	
❖ Fungal infections of the tracheobronchial tree such as, actinomycosis, blastomycosis, and histoplasmosis	
❖ To know the effect of radiation on bronchial tumors	

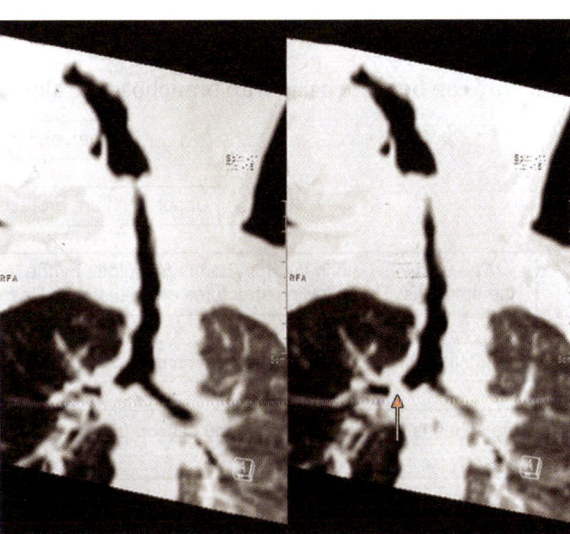

Fig. 1: Computed tomography (CT) virtual bronchoscopy showing foreign body in right main bronchus.

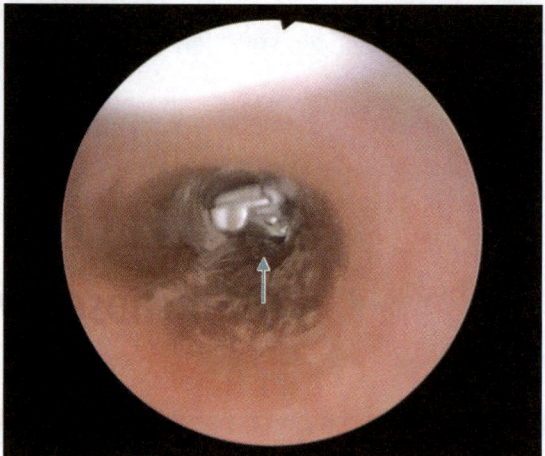

Fig. 2: Bronchoscopic view of foreign body in bronchus.

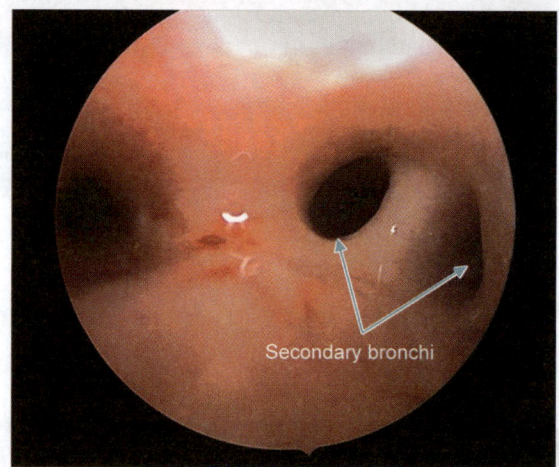

Fig. 3: Bronchoscopy view after removal of foreign body from bronchus.

CONTRAINDICATIONS OF BRONCHOSCOPY

- Rigid bronchoscopy has to be performed by an experienced surgeon in a well-equipped operation theater.
- **Relative indication:** Cervical vertebral column diseases like cervical spondylosis to avoid dislocation of spine
- Aortic aneurysm
- Presence of active hemoptysis or recent episode of massive hemoptysis is a temporary contraindication
- Bleeding disorders
- Any medical contraindications such as active pulmonary tuberculosis (Kochs) or diabetes or hypertension
- **Trismus:** Flexible bronchoscope can be used.

PROCEDURE

Anesthesia

- **General anesthesia:** Using ventilating bronchoscope connected with the Boyle's apparatus or a jet ventilation by a Venturi which supplies oxygen under high pressure in jets and intravenous anesthetic agents are used.
- Local anesthesia of the nose and throat is required for a flexible fiberoptic bronchoscope.

Position

Supine position with extension of the head and flexion of the neck (Boyce's position)

Procedure

Procedure can be done using with bronchoscope alone or direct laryngoscope with detachable blade and bronchoscope.

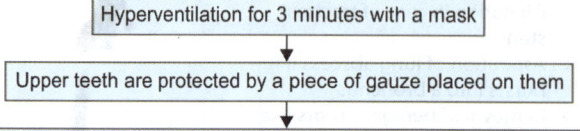

Hyperventilation for 3 minutes with a mask
↓
Upper teeth are protected by a piece of gauze placed on them
↓
The scope is held in the right hand and guided by the left hand from the right corner of the mouth along the tongue gradually till the epiglottis. The following structures are visualized: Base tongue, right vallecula, right tonsillar pillars and right tonsil, and epiglottis
↓
The epiglottis is lifted up with the tip of the bronchoscope and the glottis is visualized as an anteroposterior chink between the two vocal cords
↓
Now the scope is turned through 90° and passed under vision through the glottis into the trachea till the carina, visualizing the openings of right and left primary bronchi
↓
To enter the right primary bronchus, the patient's head is turned toward the left so as to align the trachea and the bronchus. Similarly, the patient's head is turned to the right to enter the left bronchus

Contd....

Contd....

> The primary bronchi are inspected and the openings of the secondary bronchi are visualized. During removal of the scope, care is taken to turn the scope through 90° at the glottis so that the bevel faces the right vocal cord. Hence, both cords are also inspected. The scope is always removed under vision

> *Note:* Endotracheal intubation, as done for other endoscopies, cannot be used in a bronchoscopy as the scope passes through the same passage (trachea). Hence, the surgeon and anesthetist share the same passage and hence have to work in coordination

Precautions During Bronchoscopy

- Use appropriate size of bronchoscope according to age of the patient
- Do not introduce and remove bronchoscope repeatedly
- Do not force the bronchoscope through the closed glottis
- Procedure should not be prolonged in infants and children to avoid subglottic edema in postoperative period.

Postoperative Care

- Keep the patient in humid room
- Watch for respiratory distress due to laryngeal spasm or subglottic edema due to prolonged or repeated procedure.

COMPLICATIONS

- **Complications of anesthesia:**
    - Cardiac arrhythmias
    - Hypertension
    - Hypotension
    - Vasovagal arrest
- Cardiac arrest or respiratory arrest due to bronchoscope touching the carina resulting in vagal stimulation
- Damage to lips, teeth, tongue, or vocal cords
- Dislocation of the arytenoid from the cricoarytenoid joint resulting in fixation of vocal cord
- Subglottic edema and dyspnea
- Dislocation of cervical vertebra with resultant quadriplegia if done in a patient with diseased cervical spine
- Tracheal or bronchial tear
- **Difficulty in removing a foreign body due to:**
    - Difficulty in catching it, e.g., small marble
    - Foreign body slipping deeper into the tracheobronchial tree
    - Disintegration of the foreign body on catching, e.g., long standing peanut
    - Mucosal edema and impaction of the foreign body
    - Foreign body embedded in the wall of the tracheobronchial tree, e.g., denture with wires

RIGID BRONCHOSCOPY VERSUS FLEXIBLE BRONCHOSCOPY

Advantages of Rigid Bronchoscopy over Flexible Bronchoscopy

- Ventilation can be done through the scope.
- Better control of ventilation in children
- Foreign body removal is easier especially in children.
- Large piece of biopsy can be taken.
- Better control of hemorrhage
- Useful in massive hemoptysis
- Tip of bronchoscope can be pressed over the bleeding area.

Disadvantages

- Nasal cavity is not seen.
- Supraglottic area difficult to evaluate

- ❖ Only segmental bronchi can be reached.
- ❖ Bedside examination is not possible.
- ❖ Technically difficult procedure especially in jaw and neck abnormalities or injuries
- ❖ Requires operation theater facilities. Expenses for operation theater and anesthesia increase the total cost.

FLEXIBLE FIBEROPTIC BRONCHOSCOPY

Q. Write short note on flexible fiberoptic bronchoscopy.

These days flexible fiberoptic bronchoscopy has replaced rigid bronchoscopy for diagnostic procedures particularly in adults.

Anesthesia: Topical

Route: Through endotracheal tube or nose

Structures Seen

- ❖ Nasal cavity
- ❖ Undistorted view of supraglottic and glottis areas
- ❖ Segmental and even subsegmental bronchi

Advantages over Rigid Bronchoscopy

- ❖ The smaller size of scope permits examination of subsegmental bronchi.
- ❖ It provides magnification and better illumination.
- ❖ Easier to use in patients with neck or jaw abnormalities and injuries where rigid bronchoscopy may almost be impossible technically.
- ❖ This procedure can be performed under topical anesthesia and is very useful for bedside examination of the critically ill patients.
- ❖ The suction/biopsy channel provided in the fiberscope helps to remove secretions, inspissated plugs of mucus or even small foreign bodies.
- ❖ Flexible bronchoscope can also be easily passed through endotracheal tube or the tracheostomy opening.

Disadvantages

- ❖ It has limited utility in children because of poor control over ventilation as airway is compromised by scope.
- ❖ Foreign body removal is difficult. Contraindicated in children.
- ❖ Only small piece of biopsy can be taken.
- ❖ Control of hemorrhage is difficult.
- ❖ Cost of procedure is less.

Section 5: Recent Advances

Chapter 68

Laser in ENT

■ INTRODUCTION

Q. Define laser. Discuss briefly the component, types and uses of lasers in ENT.

Light amplification by stimulated emission of radiation (Laser) is an electro-optical device that emits organized light in a narrow intense beam.

- **Maiman** built first laser in **1960** with use of synthetic ruby.
- **Carbon dioxide laser** was developed in **1965.**
- **Polanyi** developed the articulated arm to deliver the infrared radiation from the CO_2 laser to remote target.
- **Strong and Jako** introduced CO_2 laser excision for treatment of laryngeal disease in **1972.**

■ COMPONENT OF LASER

- Optical resonating chamber
- Two reflecting mirrors
- Space between two mirrors filled with lasing medium

■ PRINCIPLE OF LASER

An external energy source (electric current) excites the lasing medium within the optical cavity. This causes many atoms of lasing medium to be raised to a higher energy state and resulted into emission of stored energy in the form of photons.

Zones of Tissue Damage

- **Vaporizes the tissue**: The center of the wound is an area of tissue vaporization that makes crater and carbon flakes
- **Middle area of thermal necrosis:** Cuts and coagulates blood vessels
- **Outer areas of thermal conductivities and repair:** This is the outermost area that heals with passage of time

■ ADVANTAGES

- Precise treatment of specific area of disease
- Preservation of normal tissue
- Minimal surrounding tissue damage
- Precise control, minimal bleeding, and minimal postoperative edema
- Treatment delivery to area those are difficult to access (tongue base, trachea, larynx, and middle ear)
- Reduces local tumor recurrence
- Reduces operative time
- Less postoperative pain and less recovery time, hospital stay

TYPES OF LASERS

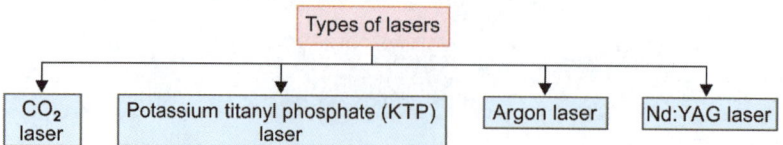

Type	Wavelength	Application
Potassium titanyl phosphate (KTP)	❖ 532 nm ❖ Visible wavelength ❖ Penetration 0.9–1 mm ❖ Absorption: Skin pigmentation and hemoglobin	❖ **Ear** ➤ Middle ear surgery ➤ Cholesteatoma excision ➤ Stapes surgery ❖ **Nose** ➤ Sinus surgery ➤ Inferior turbinate excision ➤ Nasal papilloma excision ➤ Nasopharyngeal stenosis release ❖ **Larynx** ➤ Supraglottoplasty ➤ Laryngeal cyst excision ➤ Laryngeal stenosis release ➤ Tracheal stenosis release
CO_2 laser **(Fig. 1)** **Fig. 1:** Laser machine.	❖ 10,600 nm ❖ Infrared wavelength penetration: 0.2–0.3 mm ❖ Absorption: Tissue with higher water content	❖ **Ear**—stapedotomy ❖ **Oral cavity** ➤ Oral leukoplakia ➤ Verrucous carcinoma ➤ Oral cancer ➤ Tonsillectomy ➤ Uvulopalatopharyngoplasty ❖ **Nose** ➤ Nasopharyngeal angiofibroma ➤ Choanal atresia ➤ Familial hemorrhagic telangiectasia ❖ **Larynx** ➤ Recurrent respiratory papillomatosis ➤ Supraglottic laryngectomy ➤ Subglottic hemangioma ➤ Laryngeal web ➤ Subglottic stenosis ➤ Tracheal stenosis ➤ Uvulopalatopharyngoplasty ➤ Cordotomy
Neodymium:Yttrium – Aluminum–Garnet (Nd-YAG) Laser	❖ Wavelength 1064 nm ❖ Infrared wavelength ❖ Penetration 4 mm ❖ Absorption—increases absorption in pigmented tissues, charred debris	❖ **Vascular lesion** ➤ Arteriovenous (AV) malformations. Hereditary telangiectasia ➤ Hemangioma ➤ Angiofibroma ❖ **Esophageal lesion** ❖ Tracheobronchial lesion
Argon laser	❖ Wavelength: 485–5151 nm ❖ Infrared wavelength ❖ Penetration 0.8–1 nm ❖ Absorbed by pigmented tissue and hemoglobin	❖ Stapedotomy ❖ Treatment for skin lesion

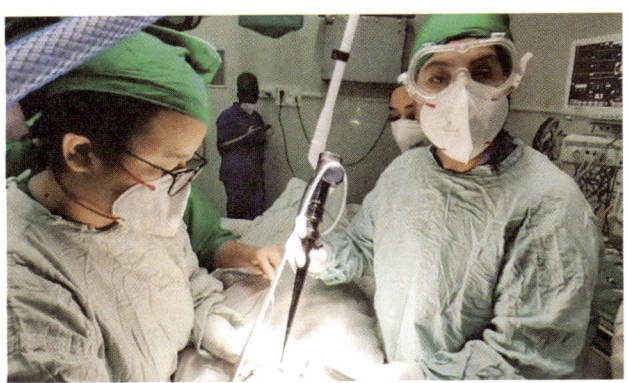

Fig. 2: Laser surgery being done with CO_2 laser.

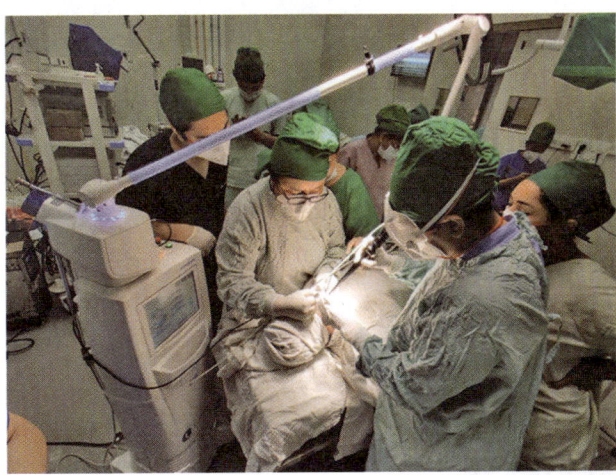

Fig. 3: Intraoperative set up while laser surgery is being done.

LASER SAFETY PRECAUTIONS (FIGS. 2 AND 3)

- Nonflammable endotracheal tube to be used
- Fill the cuff of the endotracheal tube with saline colored and methylene blue
- Maintain low inspired O_2 (<30% FiO_2)
- Avoid nitrous oxide
- **Education:** Qualified trained physician, nurse to be involved in surgery
- Develop education policies for surgeon, anesthesiologist
- Eye protection goggles to be worn by surgeon and staff
- Eye protection of patient undergoing surgery
- **Board mentioning safety precautions of laser to be displayed in surgery operation theater (OT) room**
- **In case of laser fire of airway:**
  - 50 cc saline bulb syringe and basin of saline should be ready.
  - Stop ventilation immediately
  - Withdraw tube flush saline
  - Re-establish airway immediately
  - Bronchoscopy to assess degree of injury
  - IV steroids
  - Keep patient intubated

Chapter 69

Coblation

INTRODUCTION

Q. Write short note/essay on coblation technique.

- The term coblation is derived from "controlled ablation."
- First discovered by Hira V Thapliyal and Philip E Eggers.

MECHANISM OF ACTION

- This procedure involves nonheat driven process of soft tissue dissolution using radiofrequency energy under conductive medium like normal saline.
- When current from radiofrequency probe passes through saline medium it breaks saline into sodium and chloride ions. These highly energized ions form a plasma field which break organic molecular bonds within soft tissue causing its dissolution.

EFFECT OF PLASMA ON TISSUE

- It is purely chemical and not thermal.
- Plasma generates H and OH ions.
- These ions make plasma destructive. OH radical causes protein degradation.
- When coblation is being used the interface plasma and dissected tissue acts as a gate for charged particles.
- Collateral tissue damage is low.
- The thickness of plasma is only 100–200 μm thick around the active electrode.

STAGES OF PLASMA GENERATION

1st stage (vapor gas piston formation)	Characterized by transition from bubble to film boiling. This decreases heat emission and causes increase in surface temperature
2nd stage	Stage of vapor film pulsation. Tissue ablation occurs during this stage
3rd stage	Reduction of amplitude of current across the electrodes
4th stage	Dissipation of electron energy at the metal electrode surface
5th stage (stage of thermal dissipation of energy)	This stage is due to recombination of plasma ions, active atoms, and molecules

COMPONENTS

Radiofrequency (RF) Generator
- Generates RF signals. It is controlled by microprocessor.
- This generator is capable of adjusting the setting as per the type of wand inserted.
- Two settings are set, i.e., coblation (plasma setting) and cauterization (nonplasma setting).

Example:

For tonsil wand, the recommended setting would be.
- Coblation → 7 (plasma setting)
- Cauterization → 3 (nonplasma setting)

Irrigation System
Wand
- It has two electrodes, i.e., base electrode and active electrode.
- These electrodes are separated by ceramic.
- These suction wands simultaneously dissect, ablate, and remove the tissue.
- Saline flows between these two electrodes.
- Current generated flows between these two electrodes via the saline medium.

Examples:
- Tonsil and adenoid wands are the commonly used wand for all oropharyngeal surgeries.
- Laryngeal wand is of two types:
  1. Normal laryngeal wand used for ablating laryngeal mass lesions.
  2. Mini laryngeal wand used to remove small vocal cord polyps.
- Nasal wand is commonly used for turbinate reduction.
- Separate tunneling wands are available for tongue base reduction.

Foot Pedal Control
It has two color-coded pedals.
- Yellow → For coblation
- Blue → Radiofrequency (RF) cautery

EQUIPMENT SPECIFICATION
- Modes of operation → Dissection, ablation, and coagulation.
- Operating frequency → 100 kHz.
- Power consumption →110/240 v, 50/60 kHz.

Efficiency of Ablation can be Improved by
- Intermittent application of ablation mode
- Copious irrigation of normal saline
- By using cold saline plasma generated becomes more efficient in ablating tissue.

Coblation Wand can work in Two Settings

Plasma power setting 6–9	Nonplasma power setting 1–5
Plasma layer is formed	No plasma layer is formed.
Tissue is removed	Tissue is not removed
Shallow depth of penetration	Deeper depth of penetration
Higher voltage is used	Lower voltage is used
Temperature generated is less	Temperature generated is more
Molecular dissociation	Cellular vibration/oscillation

PART 2: Operative Procedures

■ OTOLARYNGOLOGICAL SURGERIES WHERE COBLATION IS USEFUL

- Adenoidectomy
- Tonsillectomy
- Tongue base reduction for obstructive sleep apnea (OSA)
- Tongue channeling
- Uvulopalatopharyngoplasty (UPPP)
- Lingual tonsillectomy
- Cordectomy
- Nasal polypectomy
- Turbinate reduction
- Kashima's operation
- Removal of benign lesions of larynx including papilloma
- Rhinophyma excision
- Vallecular cyst excision
- Thyroidectomy
- Benign oral, palatal tumor excision
- Juvenile nasal angiofibroma excision along with nasal endoscope

■ ADVANTAGES OF COBLATION OVER CONVENTIONAL PROCEDURES

- Bloodless surgery
- Less postoperative pain
- Decreased incidence of postoperative nausea and dehydration
- Faster recovery
- Less postoperative discomfort
- Minimal instrumentation
- No toxic byproducts of ablation
- Less operative duration
- Less intraoperative blood loss

■ DIFFERENCES BETWEEN COBLATION AND CONVENTIONAL ELECTROSURGICAL DEVICES

	Coblation device	Conventional electrosurgical devices
Temperature	40–70°C	400–600°C
Effects on target tissue	Gentle removal/dissolution	Rapid heating, charring, burning, and cutting
Thermal penetration	Minimal	Deep

Chapter 70

Radiofrequency

■ DEFINITION

Q. Write a short note/essay on radiofrequency use in ENT.

Radiofrequency (RF) is high frequency alternating current used to ablate tissues (cut/coagulate).

■ PRINCIPLE

It entails giving high-frequency energy to structures causing ablation, inflammation, and subsequent healing with fibrosis.

The temperature-controlled RF technique operates by inserting an electrode placed submucosally causing ionic agitation, heating up of tissues which result in protein coagulation and tissue necrosis but no charring. Scar formation occurs after 3 weeks which is then gradually reabsorbed by the body, thus shrinking tissue volume while leaving overlying mucus membrane intact.

The RF generator regulates energy flow to form a precise lesion **(Fig. 1)**. It generates electromagnetic waves of very high frequency between 350 kHz and 4 MHz.

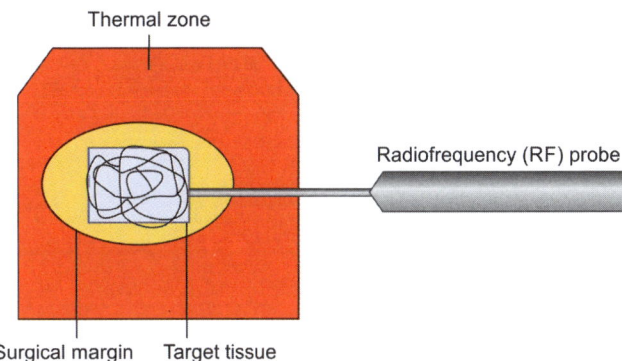

Fig. 1: Mechanism of action for using radiofrequency.

■ USES

- Obstructive sleep apnea
- Nasal masses/polyp
- Tonsilloadenoid resection
- Oral cavity lesions
- Benign head and neck lesions
- Turbinate reduction
- Lingual thyroid reduction
- Microlaryngeal lesions (to remove granulomas, papillomas, and cyst)
- Correction of rhinophyma
- Cosmetic removal of skin lesions

■ ADVANTAGES

- Relative incision in precision making
- Bloodless field
- Decrease postoperative pain
- Excellent healing with fibrosis
- Minimally invasive
- It can be performed as an outdoor procedure
- Cost-effective procedure

PART 2: Operative Procedures

■ DIFFERENT PROCEDURES

Radiofrequency Assisted Adenoidectomy Surgery

Performed after retracting lower edge of palate with tongue depressors or tourniquets and then coagulation of adenoid can be done with bipolar forceps.

Dissection of lower edge of adenoid can be done using RF needle.

Radiofrequency Assisted Somnoplasty Surgery

- Done for obstructive sleep apnea (OSA)
- Volumetric tissue reduction of palate to stiffen or scar soft palate due to temperature-controlled RF by using RF bipolar probe.

Radiofrequency Assisted Tonsillectomy Surgery

- RF needle is used to incise/open plane for tonsillar dissection.
- Tonsils are exposed on either side.
- Tissue dissection is done using RF probe.

Radiofrequency Assisted Tongue Base Reduction Surgery

Temperature-controlled volumetric reduction of tongue base achieved by giving RF energy to multiple sites of posterior tongue base with bipolar probe.

Radiofrequency Assisted Uvulopalatopharyngoplasty/Uvulopalatoplasty

Uvular and lateral cuts with RF in cutting mode with redefining posterior pillars or tonsillectomy with suturing of pillars.

Chapter 71

Cryosurgery

■ INTRODUCTION

Q. What is cryosurgery? Discuss in brief its procedure, advantages, disadvantages and use in ENT.

Cryosurgery is a technique that uses rapid freezing of tissues to temperature of –30°C or below, causing destruction of the tissue by slow thawing.
- Agents used to freeze the tissue
  - *Open method:* Liquid nitrogen spray, carbon dioxide snow, nitrous oxide
  - *Closed system:* Cryoprobe
    - Based on Joule-Thomson effect—rapid expansion of compressed gas through a small hole produces cooling
    - Probes in current use—tip temperature of –70° or below
    - Probes are available in different sizes and shapes for different areas of application
    - Attached thermocouples can be inserted into the tissue to monitor temperature

Method

- Local or general anesthesia (sometimes no anesthesia as freezing itself cause numbness)
- Area to be frozen—insulated
- Cryoprobe applied to the tissue → frozen quickly for 3–8 minutes → allowed to thaw slowly (implant a thermocouple to ensure depth of freezing be adequate)
- Area frozen should include a margin of normal tissue
- The area is allowed to heal by secondary intention, necrotic slough falls off in 3–6 weeks
- Repeat procedure may be required for the desired result.

■ MECHANISM OF TISSUE DESTRUCTION

Freezing of tissue causes cell death through following mechanisms.

Dehydration	• Water in and outside the cell freezes, causing electrolyte excess • pH of the medium also changes • Dissolved gases and urea reach toxic concentrations causing cell death
Denaturation	• Lipoprotein-rich membranes become permeable to cations • Thawing of cations-rich cells undergo lysis
Thermal shock	• Arrests the respiratory function of cell
Vascular stasis	• Both arterial and venous—ischemic infarct • Microthrombosis—seen within few hours of procedure • Hence useful to treat vascular tumors
Cryoimmunization	• Autoantibodies to frozen tissues • Provides subsequent immunity specific to the tumor

USES OF CRYOTHERAPY IN ENT PROCEDURES

	Uses of cryosurgery	
1.	Benign vascular tumors	❖ Hemangiomas involving skin, oral cavity, or oropharynx ❖ As an adjunct to treat vascular tumors, e.g., angiofibroma and glomus tumor
2.	Premalignant lesions	❖ Leukoplakia—involving the cheek, tongue, and floor of mouth ❖ To treat solar keratosis
3.	Malignant lesions	❖ Skin cancers––Bowen's disease (intraepithelial carcinoma) and basal cell carcinoma (94–97% cure rate) ❖ Skin cancers at multiple sites ❖ Useful for tumor overlying the cartilage as the latter does not undergo necrosis with freezing ❖ Palliation of advanced cancers or residual or recurrent tumors––mainly to debulk the tumor mass or to reduce the tendency of tumor to bleed, and to relieve pain ❖ Recurrent skin cancer or lesions with ill-defined margins should not be treated by this method ❖ Use in primary malignant lesion of the oral cavity and oropharynx is limited to early lesions (T1 N0) involving floor of mouth, tongue, and palate (used very selectively, in patients who are otherwise high-risk groups and have a short expectancy of life due to other concurrent disease)
4.	Other uses	❖ Turbinoplasty—to reduce nasal turbinate size to improve the airway ❖ Allergic rhinitis—to control sneezing and rhinorrhea ❖ Tonsil reduction—in poor-risk patients

ADVANTAGES AND DISADVANTAGES

	Advantages	Disadvantages
1.	Used in poor risk patients can be applied without anesthesia or under local anesthesia	No tissue is available for biopsy in case of small lesions
2.	To treat bleeding disorders or coagulopathies	Not possible to assess margins of tumor to know whether free of malignant cells
3.	Used in multiple cancers, palliation of recurrent cancers where second course of radiation is not advisable	No control on depth of freezing.
4.	Minimal post-treatment discomfort or pain	When used for skin lesions, cryotherapy causes depigmentation and loss of hair due to destruction of hair follicles.
5.	Preferred to electrosurgery as it causes minimal scarring. Can be used at sites, notorious for keloid formation, e.g., presternal region. It is an out-patient procedure	Anesthesia of the part is required when lesion is near the nerve, e.g., ulnar or digital.
6.	Early recovery, outpatient procedure	Laser therapy is preferred over this except in cost-effective areas
7.	Cost-effective procedure	

Chapter 72

Robotics in ENT

INTRODUCTION

Q. Write a short note/essay on robotics and robotic surgeries in ENT.

Robotic surgery was first performed in 1985 which was **stereotactic brain biopsy**. The first ENT robotic surgery was done in 2005 which was **vallecular cyst marsupialization**. The United States Food and Drug Administration (US-FDA) approval was given for transoral robotic surgery (TORS) in 2009 **(Fig. 1).** Robotic cochlear implantation has also been recently developed and successfully performed.

ADVANTAGES OF ROBOTIC SURGERY

- Higher level of precision
- Multiplanar tissue dissection
- Three-dimensional anatomical visualization
- Superior instrumentation control
- Better instrument manipulation
- Absence of surgical field visualization limitations
- Motion scaling
- Wristed instrumentation eliminates hand tremors of surgeon
- Less hemorrhage
- Better outcomes
- Fewer complications
- Less morbidity
- Shorter hospital stay
- Easier to learn, train, and master

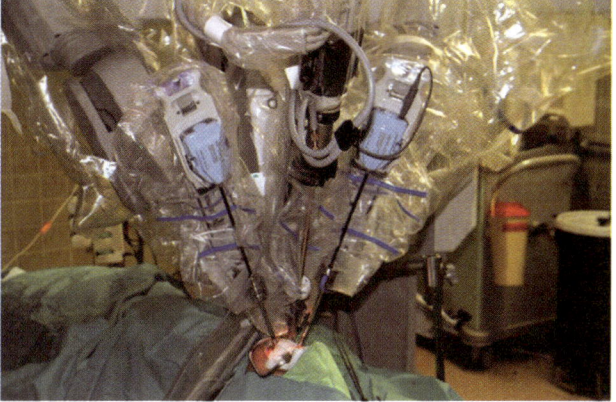

Fig. 1: Transoral robotic surgery (TORS).

DISADVANTAGES OF ROBOTIC SURGERY

- Expensive
- Higher cost of maintenance
- Larger instruments for small surgical field
- Bulky
- Needs more space in operation theater (OT)
- Lack of tactile and haptic feedback of structures during surgery
- Comparatively longer operative time
- Longer time for docking and undocking of system and instruments

USES IN ENT (EAR, NOSE, THROAT) SURGERIES

- **TORS**
    - Tonsillectomy
    - Lingual tonsillar excision
    - Partial glossectomy
    - Base of tongue resection
    - Oropharyngeal carcinoma (T1, T2)
    - Supraglottic cancer (T1, T2)
    - Cordectomy (T1 lesions)
    - Total laryngectomy
    - Biopsy
- Transaxillary thyroidectomy
- Neck dissections
- Parathyroidectomy
- Facelift and retroauricular approaches such as parotidectomy, submandibular gland excision
- **Others:** Robotic skull base surgery, robotic surgery in pediatric airway, cochlear implantation.

DA VINCI SURGICAL ROBOTIC SYSTEM

Developed by Intuitive Surgical Inc., Sunnyvale, CA **(Fig. 2)**.

Two parts of this system are:
1. Surgeon control
2. Patient side cart

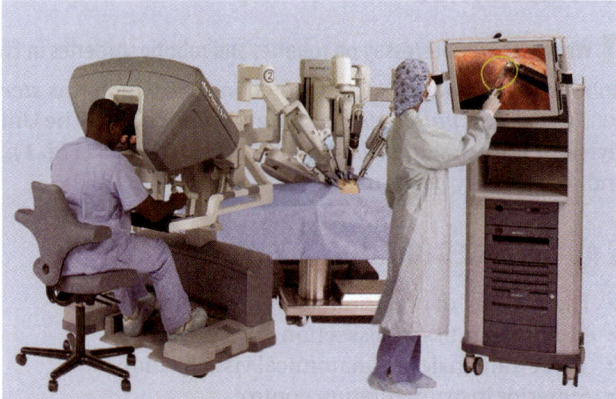

Fig. 2: The da Vinci surgical robotic system.

Surgeon Control

- Two control handles
- Virtual three-dimensional vision projection system
- Primary surgeon is in control of instruments
- Hand movements are perceived by sensors and relayed to robotic arms and instrument tips.

Patient Side Cart

- Around 3–4 arms
- Consists of video capture and EndoWrist technology
- Manages the instrument tray required for surgery
- Fourth arm holds the telescope for surgical field visualization.

Chapter 73

Chemotherapy in ENT

■ INTRODUCTION

Q. Briefly discuss the role of chemotherapy in various ENT disorders.

❖ Chemotherapy is one of the important modalities of treatment of malignancies including metastatic cancers. It is administered alone or in combination (like radiotherapy). Squamous cell carcinomas are the most common type of the head and neck malignancies.
❖ Many drugs are found to be effective against these cancer cells. Drugs like methotrexate, cisplatin, bleomycin and 5-fluorouracil are some of the commonly used chemotherapeutic agents.
❖ For non-squamous variety like adenoid cystic carcinoma, drugs like adriamycin has been used while dacarbazine has been used for melanomas. Lymphomas like Hodgkin and non-Hodgkin lymphoma are multi focal and are also treated by chemotherapy.

■ PRINCIPLES OF CHEMOTHERAPY

❖ Cancer is defined as the uncontrolled growth of cells coupled with malignant behavior—invasion and metastasis. It arises through a complex interaction between genetic and environmental factors, causing genetic mutations in oncogenes and tumor suppressor genes.
❖ Chemotherapy aims to exploit the resulting differences in biological and proliferative characteristics between normal and cancer cells where most cytotoxic drugs preferentially affect dividing cells in tumors.

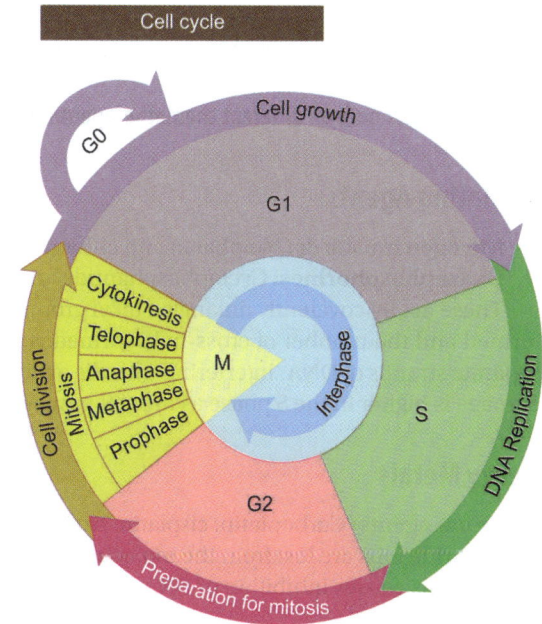

Cell Cycle

The cell cycle is divided into a number of phases which are:
1. **G1:** The growth phase in which the cell increases in size and prepares to copy DNA
2. **S (Synthesis):** Doubling of the chromosomal material takes place
3. **G2:** A further growth is seen before cell division
4. **M (Mitosis):** Where the chromosomes separate and cell divides.
   At the end of a cycle the daughter cells can either continue through the cycle, leave and enter the resting phase (G0) or become terminally differentiated. Most anticancer agents do not cause cell death during G0.

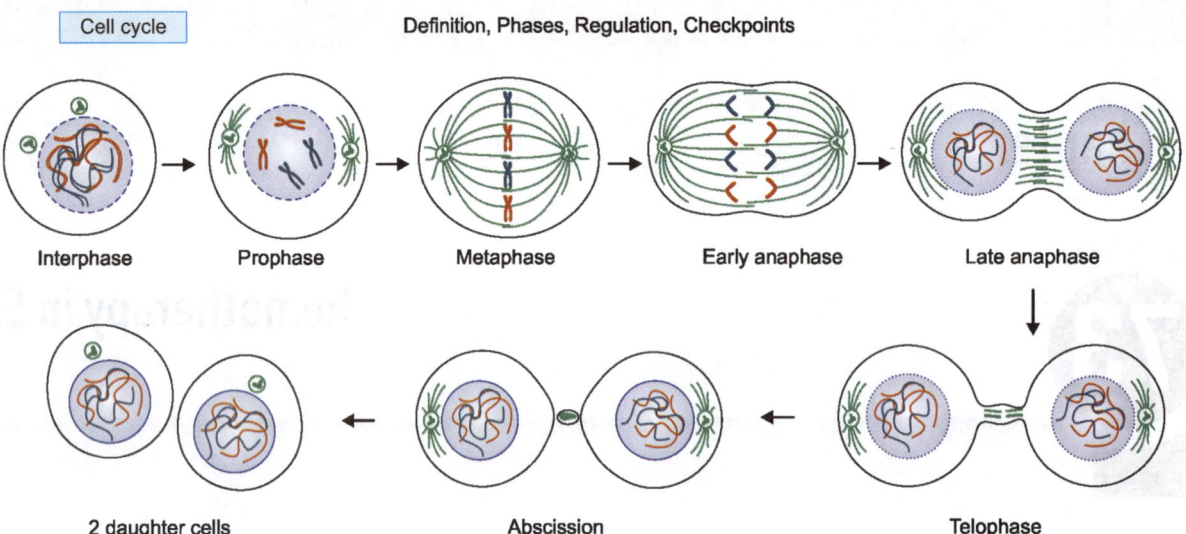

■ CLASSIFICATION OF CHEMOTHERAPEUTIC AGENTS

Cytotoxic chemotherapy agents are classified as phase-specific or non-phase-specific depending on the effect on the cell cycle.

Phase-specific Chemotherapy

These drugs (e.g. methotrexate, vinca alkaloids) kill proliferating cells only during a specific phase of the cell cycle. Antimetabolites such as methotrexate act on cells in the S phase whereas vinca alkaloids act more on M-phase.

Cell-cycle-specific Chemotherapy

Most chemotherapy agents are cell cycle specific that is they act predominantly on cells that are actively dividing. Some drugs have an equal effect on tumor and normal cells whether they are in the proliferating or resting phase (e.g. alkylating agents, platinum derivatives).

■ CLASSIFICATION AS PER THE MECHANISM OF ACTION

Q. Write a short note on different chemotherapeutic agents based on their mechanism of action.

Alkylating Agents

- **Nitrogen mustards:** Melphalan and chlorambucil
- **Oxazaphosphorines:** Cyclophosphamide and ifosfamide
  These act by covalently linking an alkyl group (R-CH2) in nucleic acids or proteins. The site at which the cross-links are formed and the number of cross-links formed is drug-specific. They can thus form bridges between a single strand or two separate strands of DNA, interfering with the action of the enzymes involved in DNA replication. This triggers apoptosis. The damage is higher in the S phase as the cell has less time to recover.

Heavy Metals

Platinum agents: Carboplatin, cisplatin, oxaliplatin.
  Chloride ions are lost from the molecule after it diffuses into a cell, forming cross links with the DNA, mostly to guanine groups. This causes inhibition of DNA, RNA and protein synthesis.

Antimetabolites

Antimetabolites are structural similar to vitamins, nucleosides or amino acids and compete with the natural substrate for the active site on an essential enzyme or receptor. Some are incorporated directly into DNA or RNA.

Most are phase specific, acting during the S phase of the cell cycle. They are usually given continuously. There are three main classes—folic acid antagonists, pyrimidine analogues and purine analogues.
- **Folic acid antagonists:** Methotrexate competitively inhibits dihydrofolate reductase.
- **Pyrimidine analogues:** Flourouracil (inhibits the synthesis of nucleic acids); Cytarabine (inhibits enzymes involved in DNA synthesis that is DNA polymerase); Gemcitabine (becoming incorporated into DNA).
- **Purine analogues:** 6 mercaptopurine (6MP) and thioguanine are derivatives of adenine and guanine respectively. A sulphur group replaces the keto group on carbon-6 in these compounds.

Cytotoxic Antibiotics

Antitumor antibiotics are produced from bacterial and fungal cultures (often *Streptomyces species*).
- **Anthracyclines**: Doxorubicin, daunorubicin, epirubicin (these intercalate with DNA and affect the topoisomerase II enzyme by stabilizing it).
- **Actinomycin D** intercalates between guanine and cytosine base pairs.
- **Bleomycin** consists of a mixture of glycopeptides that cause DNA fragmentation.
- **Mitomycin C** inhibits DNA synthesis by cross-linking DNA, acting like an alkylating agent.

Spindle Poisons

- **Vinca alkaloids:** Vincristine and vinblastine. These are mitotic spindle poisons. They bind to tubulin part of microtubules and prevent further assembly of the spindle during metaphase therefore inhibiting mitosis.
- Other agents are **vindesine and vinorelbine**.
- **Taxoids:** Paclitaxel (Taxol) and docetaxel (Taxotere) promote assembly of microtubules and inhibits their disassembly.

Topoisomerase Inhibitors

Topoisomerases are responsible for altering the 3D structure of DNA by a cleaving/unwinding/rejoining reaction. It also causes the manipulation of other cellular pathways within tumor cells.

These drugs are phase-specific and prevent cells from entering mitosis from G2. There are two broad classes:
- **Topoisomerase I inhibitors:** Irinotecan and topetcan which bind to the enzyme-DNA complex, stabilizing it and preventing DNA replication.
- **Topoisomerase II inhibitors:** Etoposide which stabilizes the complex between topoisomerase II and DNA that causes strand breaks and ultimately inhibits DNA replication.

TYPES OF CHEMOTHERAPY

Q. Write a short note on types of chemotherapy.

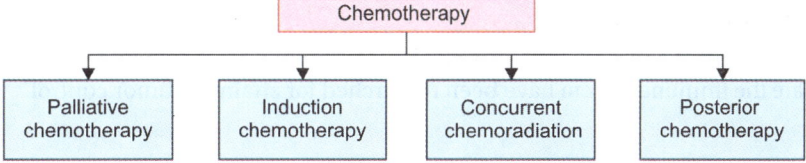

Palliative Chemotherapy

Here, cytotoxic drugs are administered for treatment of advanced, recurrent or metastatic disease in order to help relieving the symptoms.

Induction Chemotherapy

When chemotherapeutic drugs are given before surgery or radiation, it is called induction or anterior chemotherapy. This reduces tumor burden and micrometastases that is highly possible during surgery.

Concurrent Chemoradiation

When used along with radiotherapy, it has been found to be beneficial against cancer cells. It acts as a radiosensitizer by inhibiting cell repopulation and growth, killing hypoxic and microscopic cancer cells outside the tumor field as well as improving reperfusion to the cancer cells. This sensitizes radioresistant cells to radiotherapy.

Posterior Chemotherapy

When used after surgery or radiation in order to cure micrometastases and distant metastases.

■ SINGLE DRUG AND MULTIDRUG THERAPY

Methotrexate, cisplatin, bleomycin and 5-fluorouracil are commonly used as single agents in various dosage forms. Combination of drugs is also used so as to improve overall response rate and duration of response.

■ PREPARATION OF THE PATIENT BEFORE CHEMOTHERAPY

A candidate for cancer chemotherapy should undergo:
- Detailed history of presenting illness
- Significant past history and treatment history including surgeries underwent
- Complete clinical examination
- Proper staging of the disease (clinical and radiological staging)
- All routine hematological tests
- Urine routine examination
- Biochemistry
- Necessary radiological investigations which includes X-ray chest (bleomycin causes interstitial pulmonary fibrosis), CT scan/MRI where indicated, ultrasound of liver/spleen.
- Pulmonary function tests (for bleomycin)
- ECG (for adriamycin)
- Audiogram (cisplatin causes high frequency hearing loss)
- Nutritional status

■ TOXICITY OF ANTICANCER DRUGS

- These drugs act on rapidly dividing cells and can therefore affect normal cells as those of hair follicles, gastrointestinal mucosa and bone marrow causing alopecia, stomatitis, nausea, vomiting, diarrhea, anemia, leukopenia and thrombocytopenia.
- Some drugs have selective action on kidney (methotrexate, cisplatin), nerves (vincristine and cisplatin), heart (adriamycin) and bladder (cyclophosphamide).

■ NOVEL THERAPIES FOR THE FUTURE

Q. Write a short note on future of chemotherapy.

The management of advanced head and neck cancer is always challenging. More targeted mechanisms of action or agents that are able to manipulate the immune system have been researched for attaining tumor control.

Targeted Therapy

Targeted therapy aims to specifically act on a well-defined target or biologic pathway that, when inactivated, causes regression or destruction of the malignant process. This involves use of monoclonal antibodies or targeted small molecules.

Monoclonal antibodies can be:
- **Murine**—mouse antibodies
- **Chimeric**—part mouse and part human antibodies
- **Humanized**—engineered to be mostly human
- **Human**—fully human antibodies.

These induce apoptosis, block receptors needed for cell proliferation and function, form antibodies against cancer cell antigens thus amplifying an immune response to the tumor cell. They can also cause antibody dependent cellular cytotoxicity or complement-mediated cellular cytotoxicity.

Monoclonal antibodies against epidermal growth factor receptor (EGFR)—Chimeric IgG antibody **Cetuximab.**

Monoclonal antibodies against vascular endothelial growth factor receptor (VEGFR)—**Bevacizumab** (Avastin) is a humanized murine monoclonal antibody.

SOME IMPORTANT CHEMOTHERAPEUTICAL DRUGS USED IN HEAD AND NECK CANCERS

Q. Discuss briefly different drugs used in head and neck cancers.

Methotrexate

For squamous cell cancer, acute leukemia lymphomas given at 40 mg/m^2 IV weekly, high dose can be given with leucovorin rescue.

Side effects anticipated are:
- Maculopapular rash.
- Renal and hepatic toxicity

5-Fluorouracil (5-FU)

All Squamous cell cancers and some non-squamous tumors of breast and GI tract given at 10-15 mg/kg IV daily. Not more than 1 g is to be administered for 4-5 days.

Cyclophosphamide

Squamous cancers, lymphomas, leukaemia, neuroblastoma, multiple myeloma at 60-120 mg/m^2. Avoid barbiturates during therapy.

Dacarbazine

Melanoma, sarcomas. Dosage given is 250 mg/m^2 × 5 days every 3 weeks. It can cause severe nausea and vomiting, Myelosuppression flu-like symptoms (fever, malaise, myalgia), alopecia.

Bleomycin

Squamous cell cancer, lymphoma. Dosage is 10–20 mg/m^2 once or twice weekly. It causes pneumonitis (dry cough and rales) and pulmonary fibrosis. Hence, weekly chest X-ray is mandated. It can also cause fever and chills in first 24 hours of administration. Anaphylactic reactions, alopecia, erythema, hyperpigmentation, stomatitis is also seen.

Adriamycin (Doxorubicin)

Lymphoma, sarcomas, esthesioneuroblastomas, salivary gland cancer, pediatric malignancy. Dosage is 60–90 mg/m^2 IV every 3 weeks. Cardiomyopathy is seen if overdose happens. Other side effects are alopecia, stomatitis, nausea, vomiting, diarrhea, neutropenia, thrombocytopenia, urine may be red for initial few days.

Actinomycin-D

Rhabdomyosarcoma, given at 0.5 mg/m^2 IV × 5 days. It causes myelosuppression, nausea and vomiting, mucositis, diarrhea, alopecia, maculopapular rash.

Vincristine (Oncovin)

Lymphoma, squamous cell cancer, rhabdomyosarcoma. Dosage is at 1.5 mg/m^2 IV once or twice monthly. It is neurotoxic (sensory and motor neuropathy), constipation and alopecia.

Cisplatin

Squamous cell cancer at 80–120 mg/m^2 IV infusion every 3 weeks. It causes GIT (nausea, vomiting), renal toxicity, anemia, neutropenia, thrombocytopenia, peripheral neuropathy, ototoxicity (4–8 kHz).

Paclitaxel

Squamous cell cancer of head and neck at 135–350 mg/m^2 as 3 hour infusion every 3 weeks. It can cause neutropenia and infection, peripheral neuritis.

Chapter 74

Radiotherapy in ENT

■ INTRODUCTION TO RADIOTHERAPY

Q. Briefly discuss the role of radiotherapy in ENT.

- Radiotherapy is an important therapeutic modality in the treatment of early and advanced head and neck cancers. It causes direct damage to DNA by cascades of ionizations causing cell cycle arrest and death.
- Thus, cell replication of cancer cells is prevented. It induces apoptosis of cancer cells. The damage caused may be sublethal, potentially lethal or irreparable. Rapidly dividing cells like cancer cells have greater effect to radiotherapy than slowly dividing cells.
- 'Acute-reacting tissues' like bone marrow, skin, mucosa show effects of radiation within days. While connective tissue, bone manifest the effect later and hence are 'late-reacting tissues'. Squamous head and neck cancers behave as acute-reacting tissues.

■ FRACTIONATION

Treatment of head and neck cancers requires course of radiotherapy which conventionally takes several weeks consisting of numerous fractions. A fraction is the individual dose of radiation given in a single session of radiotherapy which constant throughout a course of radiotherapy. **Fractions are given once a day, five days per week typically for 4 to 6 weeks.**

Advantage of fractionation is that it maximizes damage to the cancer cell while damage to normal tissues is minimal. Subsequent fractions cause lethal damage to late reacting tissues and therefore effective cell damage to cancer cells. **Hyperfractionation** is similar to fractionation but the daily radiation dose is administered in 2 to 3 sessions in a day.

■ USES OF RADIOTHERAPY

- Independently for early cancers like glottic cancer (organ function preservation).
- As an adjuvant to surgery, administered before or after surgery in case of advanced cancers.
- As combination with chemotherapy.
- As a palliative management, in advanced stages to control local symptoms of pain, bleeding, obstruction to airway and esophagus where total control of disease is unlikely.
- As treatment of certain benign vascular lesions like angiofibroma or glomus tumor.
- Prevention of excessive scar formation in keloids.
- Gamma knife or cyberknife in management of acoustic neuroma.

■ IONIZING RADIATIONS

This radiation causes ionization of medium through which it passes. In tissue it can cause formation of highly reactive molecules which have oxidizing and reducing damaging effects on cells.

- **Photon beams**: The most common forms of radiation includes both X-rays and gamma rays. X-rays are formed when high energy electrons bombard a metallic target. Gamma rays are emitted by radioactive sources like cobalt 60.
- **Electron beams:** Second most common forms of radiation whose main characteristic is rapid dose build up and sharp dose fall off with very little scatter. The radiation dose to the target area is higher as compared to the adjoining vital structures. They are produced by linear accelerator, betatron and microtron.
- **Particle radiation like neutrons, protons:** Neutron radiations are used in malignant salivary gland tumors.

MODES OF RADIOTHERAPY

Q. Write a short note/essay on modes of radiotherapy.

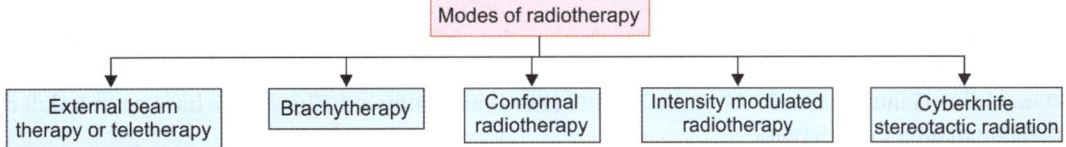

External Beam Therapy or Teletherapy

- Use of photons or electron beams
- It is directed to the target area through the skin.

Brachytherapy

- It uses radioactive materials close to the target area.
- It delivers high dose to the target area.
- Hence there is continuous radiation in low doses rather than intermittent which is effective against slow dividing and hypoxic cells.

Brachytherapy can be used for full dose of radiation or along with external beam radiation. Brachytherapy is delivered in three ways.

1. **Interstitial**: Radioactive material is implanted into the tumor.
2. **Intracavitary**: The radiation source is placed into the cavity like nasopharynx or maxillary antrum.
3. **Surface moulds**: Radioactive source is directly placed on the surface of tumor with the help of a mould.

Types of radioactive materials	
Permanent ones (short half-life)	
Gold seeds 198	Half-life 2.7 days
Iodine seeds 125	Half-life 60 days
Pallidium 103	Half-life 17 days
Temporary ones (long half-life and warrants removal)	
Radium 226 (needles)	Half-life 16–20 years
Cesium 137 (tubes and needles)	Half-life 30 years
Iridium 192 (wires and seeds)	Half-life 74 days

Conformal Radiotherapy (Three-Dimensional Radiotherapy)

Conformal radiotherapy conforms to the size and shape of the tumor. Radiation delivered maximum to the target area and minimal to the surrounding normal tissue and to critical areas. This is aided with the help of CT/MRI which give clear idea of the tumor size and depth. It has been used in the nasopharyngeal carcinoma.

Intensity Modulated Radiotherapy (IMRT)

It is a type of conformal radiotherapy. The primary tumor, lymphatic drainage and critical structures are identified. This is followed by radiation exposure by computer-controlled beams taking in account the depth, intensity and duration in a programmed manner. It has the greatest benefit of delivering a high radiation dose to tumor with least reactions to surrounding tissues. It is seen to be beneficial in the treatment of cancer of the nasopharynx, larynx and paranasal sinuses.

Cyberknife Stereotactic Radiation

Seen to be beneficial for recurrent head and neck cancers where no further radiation is possible due to acute and late complications. It is delivered by 6-million volts (MV) linear accelerator on a robotic arm with image guidance. Accurate radiation is given to the target area with sparing of surrounding normal tissues.

SOURCES OF RADIATION

Higher the energy of radiation then deeper is the penetration of radiation.

The various machines used for radiation are:

- **Kilovoltage machines**: Produce X-rays of 50–400 kV. They are the earliest machines used and can be divided into superficial 5-150 kV or orthovoltage 200-400 kV X-ray machines.
- **Cobalt 60 machine**: Gamma rays of 1.17 and 1.33 MeV (fixed) are produced. The source has its natural decay time and needs replacement after every 5 years.
- **Linear accelerator, betatron or microtron:** They are megavoltage machines which can produce photon or electron beams.
  - **Dual energy linear accelerators** can produce low-energy megavoltage X-rays (4–6 MV), high-energy megavoltage (15–25 MV) and also electron beams.
  - **Megavoltage therapy** has the advantages of:
    - Sparing the skin
    - Deep penetration of photon beam
    - Isodose distribution
      Electron beams are effective for superficial cancers and spares deeper tissues.
- **Radioactive material:** Radium 226 was used earlier in the form of needles. Now safer radionuclides like cesium 137 (pellets), iridium 192 (wire), gold 198 and iodine 125 (seeds or grain) are available.

UNITS OF RADIATION

Rad (radiation absorbed dose) and an international unit—Gray is the unit of radiation One Gray (Gy) is equivalent to one joule of energy deposited per kilogram of material.

One Gy equals 100 rads or 100 cGy.

MODES OF TUMOR TREATMENT WITH RADIATION

Radiation Alone

- It is delivered by teletherapy, brachytherapy or by combination of both.
- Dose will depend on extent of the tumor, the lymphatic field and tolerance of surrounding normal tissue.
- Usual dose delivered is:
  - 6000–6500 cGy for small tumors.
  - 6500–7000 cGy for large tumors.
  - 7000–7500 cGy for massive tumors.
- Initial dose covers tumor and its lymphatic bed safter which radiation portals are reduced to cover the tumor area as the target field shrinks with subsequent radiation cycles.

Radiation and Surgery

Preoperative Radiation

Preoperative dose is usually 4500 cGy delivered in 4–5 weeks.

Advantages:

- Reduction in tumor size
- Better response due adequate vascularity and oxygenation of tumor as compared to scarred field postsurgery.
- Blockage of lymphatics take place, hence tumor dissemination would be less during surgery.
- Eliminate microscopic islands of tumor cells away from tumor mass.
- Treatment portals are smaller.
- Sufficient to eradicate nearly 90% of micrometastases.

Disadvantages:

- It reduces the vitality of tissues
- Interferes with healing process
- Increases the chances of flap necrosis, fistula formation and carotid blow-out.
- Limitation for postoperative radiation in case of positive surgical margins.

Postoperative Radiation

Advantages:
- More effective as the bulk of tumor is excised surgically.
- Extension of tumor is well defined after surgery.
- Better postoperative healing.
- Higher dose of radiation can be given.
- Less chances of flap necrosis, wound dehiscence and infection as surgery.

Disadvantages:
- Fibrosis leads to diminished blood supply to the tissues. Hence, hypoxic cancer cells do not respond well.
- Surgical complications lead to delayed initiation of postoperative radiation. Poor results if delay exceeds 6 weeks.
- Tumor cells can get disseminated during surgery and hence greater chances of distant metastases.

Indications:
- Margins are positive or too close.
- There is involvement of bone or cartilage.
- Lymph nodes show extracapsular invasion.
- There is involvement of multiple nodes with size over 3 cm.
- Presence of perineural invasion.

Radiation and Chemotherapy

Chemotherapy has been combined with radiation as:
- Creating a synergistic effect against cancer cells
- Eliminate micrometastasis.
- Combination of modalities has resulted in better results.

Types:
- **Induction chemotherapy** (given before radiation)
- **Concurrent chemotherapy** (given simultaneously)

Radiotherapy for Palliation

- Advanced cancers with distant metastases
- Poor general condition of the patient

PLANNING RADIOTHERAPY

Radiotherapy can be given alone or in combination with surgery.

Decision making depends on:
- Whether radiation is for curative or palliative purposes. Palliative treatment can control local symptoms of pain or pressure symptoms.
- Tumor size.
- Nodal metastases.
- Histology and nature of tumor that is the grade of differentiation and if the tumor is rapidly or slowly proliferating.
- Ulcerative and infiltrative tumors respond poorly. While lymphoid tissue tumors respond quickly. Anaplastic tumors and those of embryonal origin respond well but recur early.
- General condition of the patient.

COMPLICATIONS OF RADIOTHERAPY

Q. Write short note on complications of radiotherapy.

Complications depend on the site, total dose delivered and the daily fraction of radiation used.

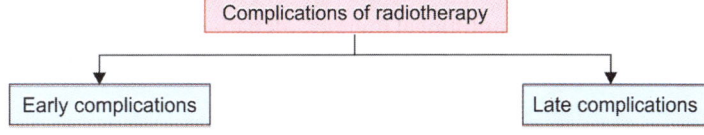

Early complications	Late complications
❖ Radiation sickness (loss of appetite, vomiting associated with nausea)	❖ Hematopoietic suppression
❖ Mucositis	❖ Permanent xerostomia
❖ Xerostomia	❖ Skin changes (atrophy of skin, subcutaneous fibrosis)
❖ Skin reactions (erythema, desquamation of skin)	❖ Decaying of teeth (secondary to xerostomia)
❖ Laryngeal edema	❖ Osteoradionecrosis (mandible more than maxilla)
❖ Candida infections	❖ Cartilage necrosis
❖ Acute transverse myelitis (rare)	❖ Trismus (fibrosis of TM joint and muscles)
	❖ Transverse myelitis (Lhermitte syndrome)
	❖ Radiation retinopathy and cataract
	❖ Endocrinal deficit (thyroid, pituitary)
	❖ Serous otitis media, sensorineural hearing loss and vestibular dysfunction
	❖ Radiation-induced malignancy (thyroid cancer, osteosarcoma of orbit)
	❖ Brain injury (Somnolence syndrome and brain necrosis)

■ CARE OF PATIENT DURING RADIOTHERAPY

Nutrition

Rich in protein, vitamins and iron is important. Nasogastric tube feeding may be necessary.

Care of Teeth

Dental evaluation and treatment of dental caries is important prior to radiation sessions.

Care of Skin

Skin reactions are common with orthovoltage or electron beam therapy to skin but the modern megavoltage therapy has a skin-sparing effect.
- ❖ Keep the area dry and avoid washing with soap and water.
- ❖ Avoid exposure to sunlight.
- ❖ Do not use adhesive plaster for dressings.
- ❖ Cover the area with soft cloth for free aeration of the skin.
- ❖ Avoid abrasive dressing.
- ❖ For moist desquamation use an antibiotic ointment.
- ❖ Topical steroid creams can be used to relieve itching and pain.

Care of Oral Cavity

For mucositis and xerostomia as they can interfere with feeding.
- ❖ Patient should avoid alcohol, tobacco, spicy food, irritating mouth washes.
- ❖ Milk of magnesia can be applied to the area of mucositis to give protective coating. It also neutralizes the acid pH and prevents caries of teeth.
- ❖ Pain and discomfort of mucositis can be relieved by use of lignocaine/xylocaine.
- ❖ Acute radiation mucositis usually persists 8–12 weeks after radiation.

Care Against Infection

Patients receiving radiotherapy are generally debilitated. They can get Candida infection of the oral cavity and pharynx. It can be treated by topical alone or with systemic antifungal therapy. All patients should ensure that they maintain good oral hygiene at all times.

PART 3

Miscellaneous Topics

Outline

75. Instruments in ENT
76. Radiology in ENT (X-rays)
77. CT Scan and MRI
78. Anesthesia in ENT
79. Pure Tone Audiogram and Impedance Audiometry

Chapter 75

Instruments in ENT

EN2.2: Demonstrate the correct use of head lamp, tongue depressor.
EN2.7: Identify and describe the use of common instruments used in ENT surgery.

◼ GENERAL ENT INSTRUMENTS

Headlight (Fig. 1) (scan QR code)

- It has inbuilt fiberoptic light.
- Used for outpatient ENT diagnostic procedure and ENT surgical procedures in OT.

Head Mirror (Fig. 2)

- It has adjustable head band to which concave mirror with central aperture is attached
- **Mirror:** Focal length- 23.6 cm
  - Diameter—2.9 cm
  - Central circular aperture—3.2 cm
- Used with Bull's Lamp. The light is reflected on the head mirror to the area to be examined.
- Binocular vision is retained and through the central aperture of mirror the right eye pupil coincides and clear visualization under illuminated light is possible
- Used for routine ear, nose, throat examination in outpatient department
- Both the handa are free so OPD procedures like IDL, anterior and posterior rhinoscopy, ear syringing, antral puncture can be done

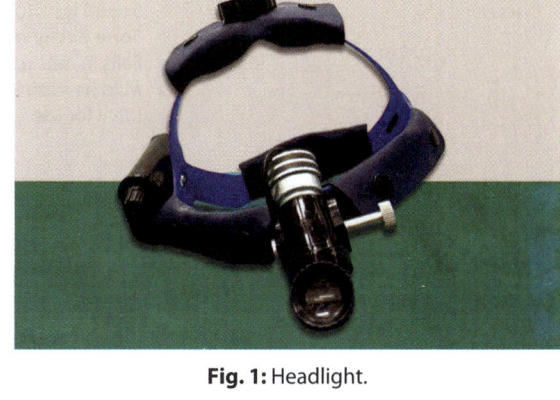

Fig. 1: Headlight.

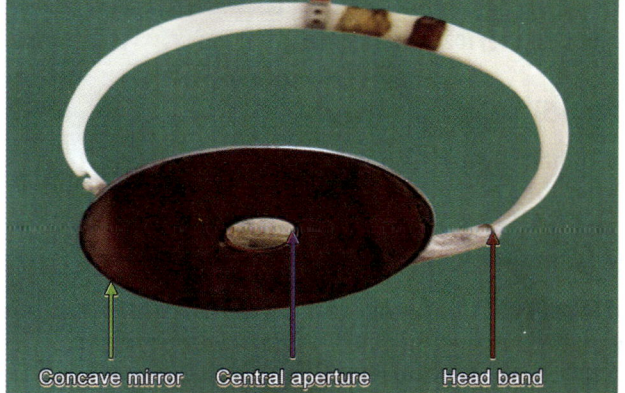

Fig. 2: Head mirror.

EAR INSTRUMENTS

Otoscope (Fig. 3)

It has inbuilt light bulb and good illumination.
- Magnified 2X view of tympanic membrane obtained
- Portable
- Different size speculum can be attached to the otoscope as per the size of external auditory canal in various age groups
- Used for ear (tympanic membrane, external auditory canal) examination in outpatient department
- Used to perform Siegelization test with Siegel's speculum

Tuning Fork

- Made up of stainless steel and has parts as prongs, shoulder, base, stem, foot plate
- It is stuck at the junction of upper 1/3rd and lower 2/3 rd of the prongs against hard surface
- It is used for checking hearing gloss and degree of hearing loss by doing Rinne's test, Weber's test, ABC test
- It comes in three frequencies 256, 512 and 1024 Hz

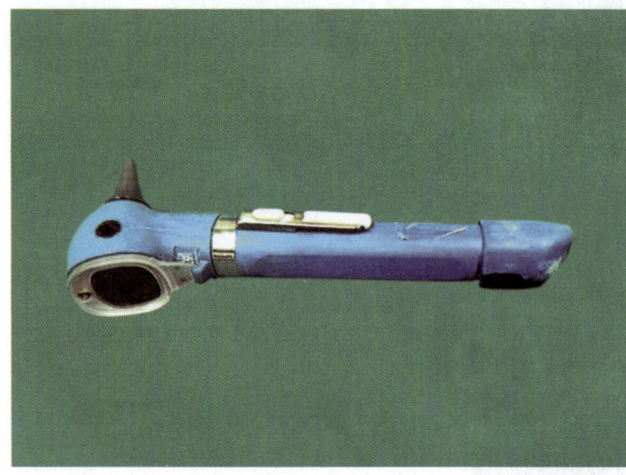

Fig. 3: Otoscope.

256 Hz tuning fork	512 tuning fork	1024 tuning fork
❖ Produces more overtrones ❖ Enhance perceptions by vibration sense	❖ **Overtones are minimal** ❖ Sound is more auditory than vibratory ❖ Sound lasts longer ❖ **Tone decay minimal** ❖ Falls in mid speech frequency ❖ Mild hearing loss can be detected ❖ Ideal for use	❖ Tone decay is very fast ❖ Detect degree of hearing loss

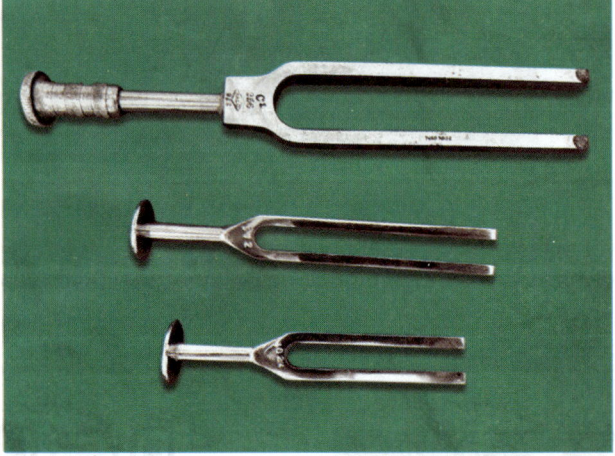

Fig. 4: Gardiner Brown tuning fork (256, 512, 1024 Hz).

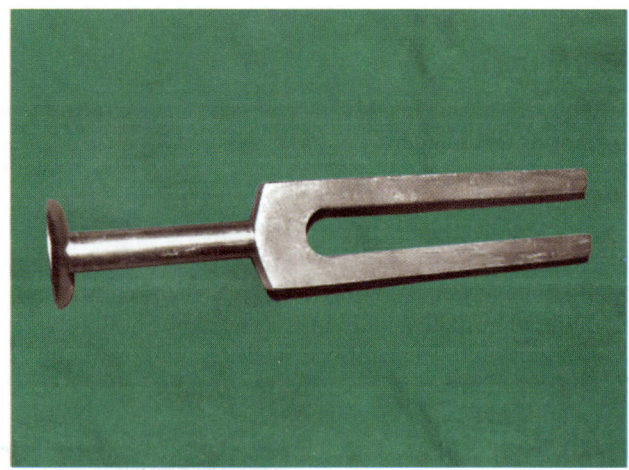

Fig. 5: Hartmann's tuning fork.

Types of Tuning Forks (Figs. 4 and 5)

- **Gardiner tuning fork:** Lighter, thinner, longer, slender.
- **Hartmann's tuning fork:** Heavier, thicker, shorter.

Simpson Aural Syringe (Fig. 6) (scan QR code)

- Made up of stainless steel and has got metallic syringe with a well fitting piston and nozzle
- It is used for wax removal and nonhygroscopic foreign body removal by syringing
- Sterile water at body temperature is used for syringing
- Syringing can lead to complications like vertigo, otitis externa, trauma, otomycosis, vasovagal attack

Complications of syringing	Vertigo	Due to stimulation of labyrinth
	Trauma	To external auditory canal and eardrum, followed by bleeding leading to otitis externa
	Otitis externa	Occurs due to trauma or unsterilized water
	Otomycosis	Occurs due to persistent dampness in external auditory canal
	Exacerbation of otitis media	Occurs if syringing done in ruptured tympanic membrane
	Vasovagal attack	

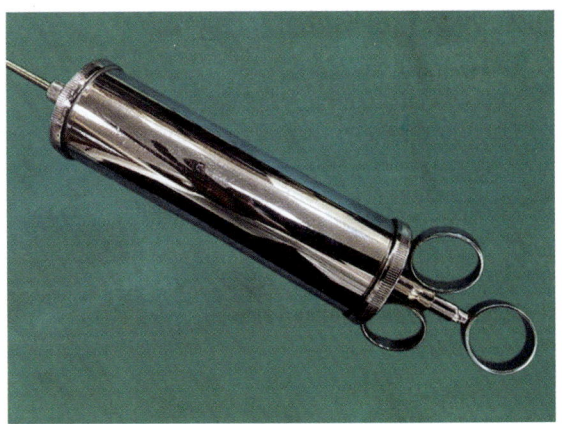

Fig. 6: Simpson's aural syringe.

Toynbee's Aural Speculum (scan QR code)

- It is made up of stainles steel and also comes in black carbon coated form. It can also be present with groove
- The carbon coated and the one with groove or slit is used for surgical procedures and the stainless steel one without groove is used for diagnostic purposed in outpatient department as well as in operation theater
- Used for Diagnostic and surgical procedures in ear, it is put in **rotatory or screwing motion in External cartilage only upto cartilaginous portion of EAC** after pulling pinna upward and backward. This prevents pain as bony meatus very sensitive it is not touched

Diagnostic uses	Therapeutic uses
Examination of external canal and removal of wax, foreign body, Otomycosis	Myringotomy
Examination of tympanic for diagnosing chronic otitis media, adhesive otitis media, retraction pocket, acute otitis media, granular myringitis	Myringotomy with grommet insertion, endaural , endomeatal tympanic neurectomy
	Aural polypectomy, removal of granulations
	Foreign body removal
	Endaural, endomeatal tympanoplasty
	Endaural, endomeatal stapedotomy

Different kinds of aural speculums (Figs. 7 to 10):

- Toynbee's aural speculum **(Figs. 7 and 8)**
- Farrier's aural speculum **(Fig. 9)**
- Politzer's aural speculum **(Fig. 10)**
- Health speculum
- Gruber speculum
- Zollner speculum
- Shea's aural speculum
- Rosen's aural speculum

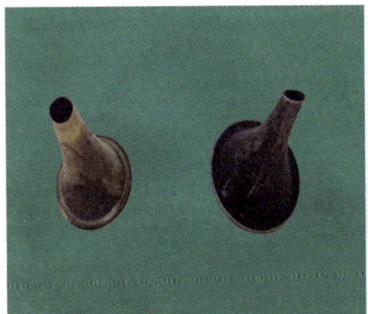

Fig. 7: Toynbee's aural speculum black carbon coated.

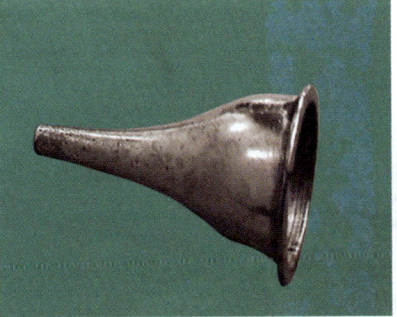

Fig. 8: Toynbee's aural speculum.

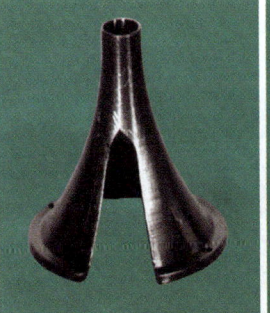

Fig. 9: Rosen's aural speculum (with slit).

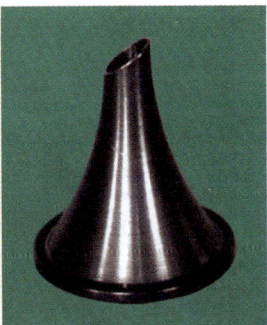

Fig. 10: Shea's aural speculum.

Eustachian Tube Catheter (Fig. 11)

- It is made up of stainless steel
- Sterilized by boiling, autoclaving
- Used for therapeutic purposes and diagnostic purposes.
  - Diagnostic uses:
    - To check Eustachian tube patency
  - Therapeutic uses:
    - To remove the nasal foreign bodies

Eustachian Tube Patency Tests
- Valsalva test
- Toynbee's test
- Politzer test
- Catheterization of eustachian tube
- Tympanometry
- Radiological test with radiopaque dye
- Sonotubometry
- Saccharin/methylene blue test
- Siegelization

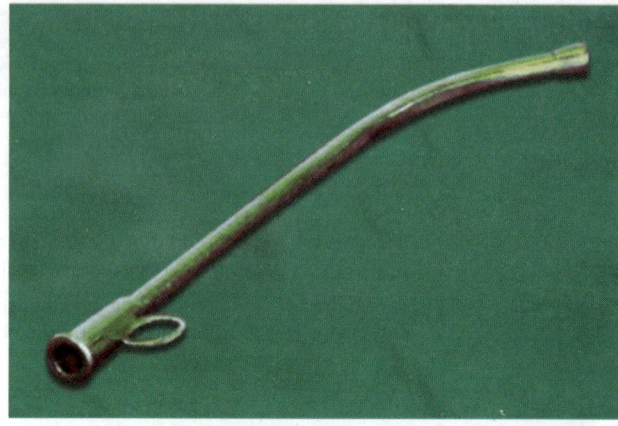

Fig. 11: Eustachian tube catheter.

Endaural Speculum (Fig. 12)

- Made up of stainless steel
- Sterilized by boiling and autoclaving
- Used for taking Lempert's endaural incision in ear surgeries like:
  - Tympanoplasty
  - Myringoplasty
  - Stepedotomy
  - Atticotomy

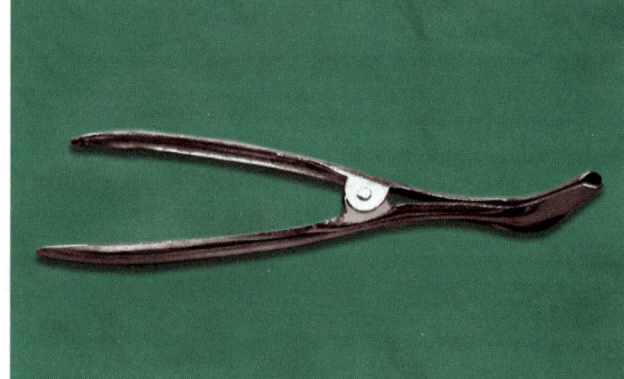

Fig. 12: Endaural speculum.

Jobson Horne Probe with Ring Curette (Fig. 13)

- Made up of stainless steel
- Has curette at one end and ring at the other end
- Its Curette is used for wax removal, foreign body removal and granulations removal from external auditory canal
- Its probe is used for probing polyp in external auditory canal, the probe with cotton swab is also used for aural toileting for cleaning the aural discharge and to apply medications in external auditory canal

Farabeuf's Periosteal Elevator (Fig. 14)

- Made up of stainless steel and has got broad end and thumb rest
- Used to elevate soft tissue and periosteum over
- Mastoid bone in tympanoplasty, mastoidectomy surgery
- Over canine fossa and antrum in Caldwell-Luc surgery
- Over maxilla in maxillectomy surgery
- Over nasal bone in external ethmoidectomy

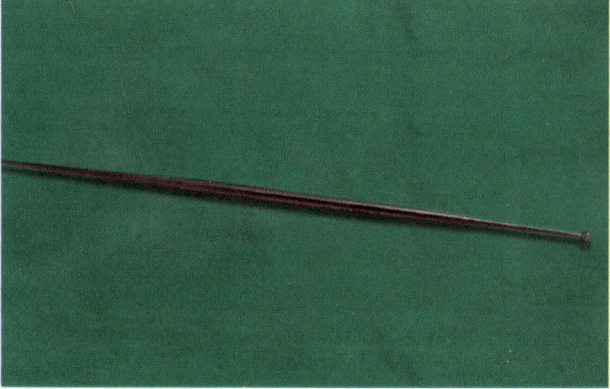

Fig. 13: Jobson Horne probe with ring curette.

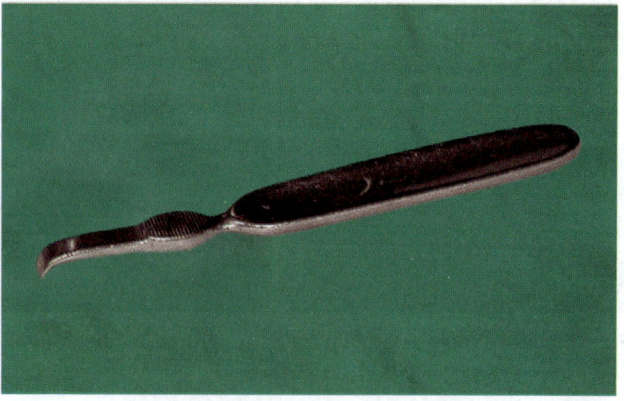

Fig. 14: Farabeuf's periosteal elevator.

Mollison's Self-retaining Hemostatic Mastoid Retractor (Fig. 15)

- Made up of stainless steel and autoclaved by boiling and autoclaving
- It opens on closing and has got Rachet Lock
- It is self-retaining and achieves hemostasis due to pressure exerted by teeth of retractor on the tissue
- It is used to remove temporalis fascia graft and retract tissues after taking incision in ear surgeries like tympanoplasty, mastoidectomy, facial nerve decompression, cochlear implant surgery
- Also used for surgeries like laryngofissure, external ethmoidectomy, optic nerve decompression, burr hole surgery

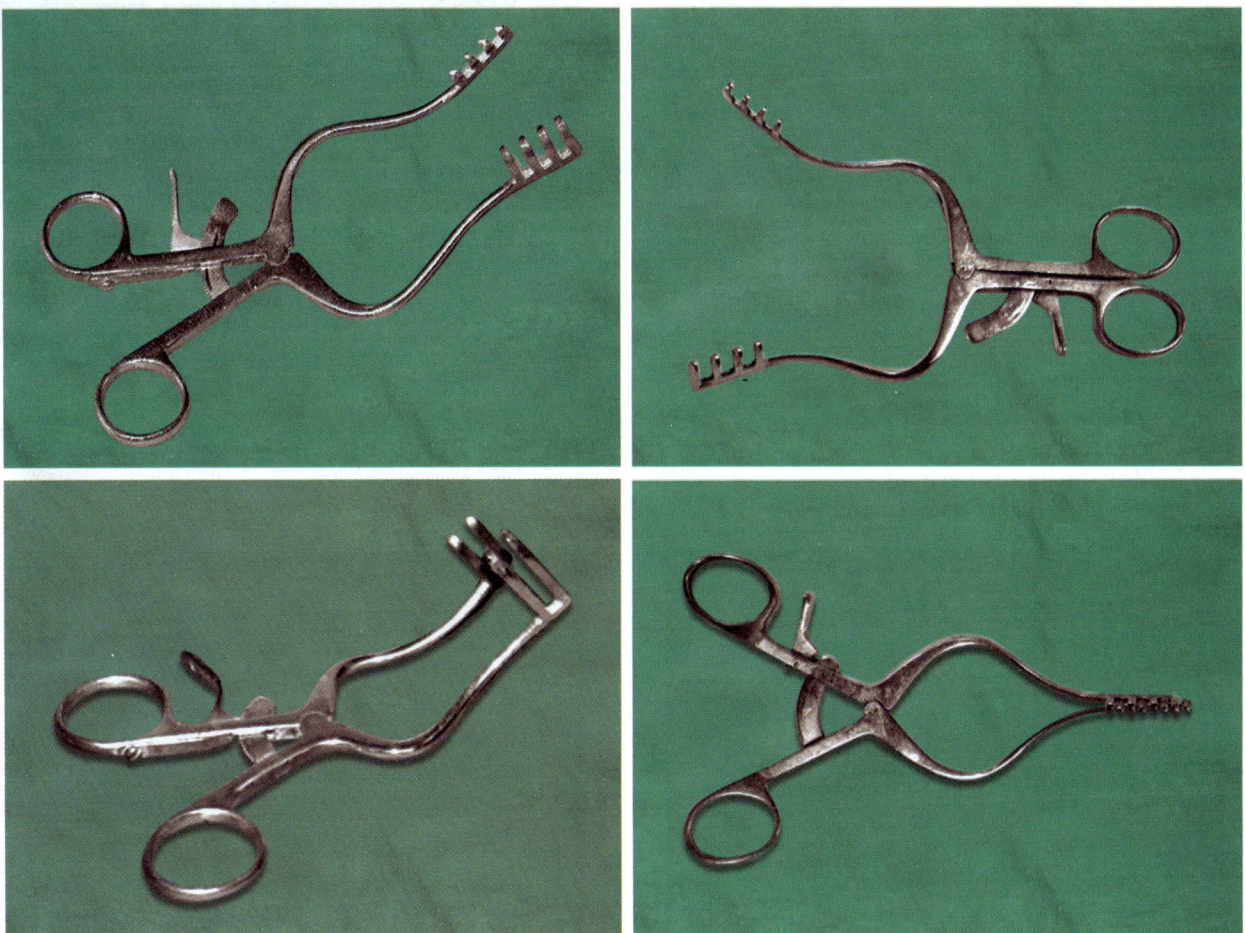

Fig.15: Mollison's self-retaining hemostatic mastoid retractor (2,3,4 teeth).

■ MICROEAR SURGERY INSTRUMENTS

Crocodile Forceps (Figs. 16 and 17)

- Made up of stainless steel
- Sterilized by boiling and autoclaving
- Used for microscopic ear surgeries
  - Tympanoplasty
  - Myringoplasty
- Stapedotomy/stapedectomy
- Atticotomy
- Mastoidectomy
- Myringotomy with grommet insertion

Crocodile forceps used in various microear surgeries
- To hold temporalis fascia graft
- To hold and insert grommet and ossiculoplasty prosthesis
- To remove ossicles
- To put adrenaline soaked cotton for achieving hemostasis

PART 3: Miscellaneous Topics

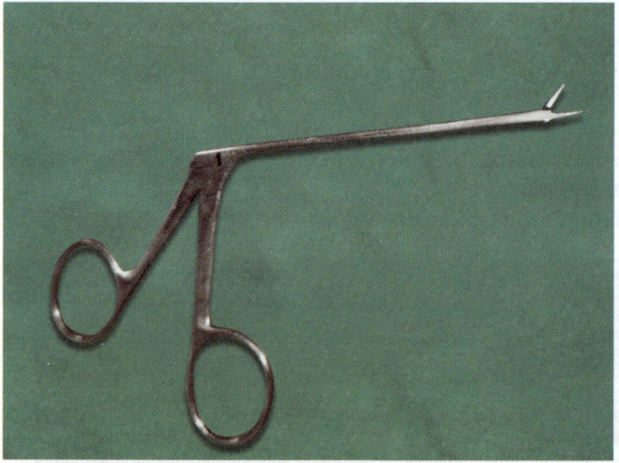

Fig. 16: Crocodile forceps.

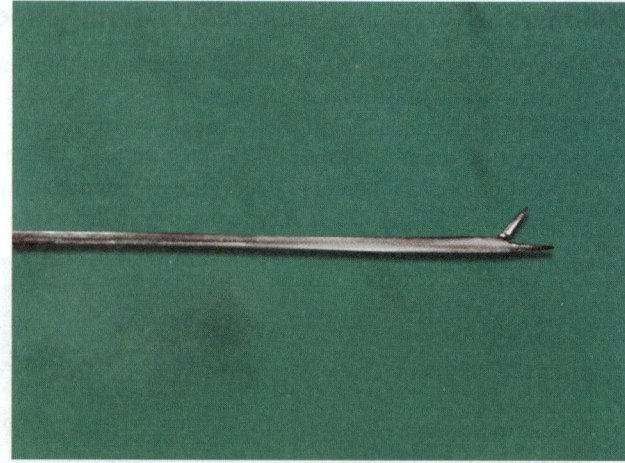

Fig. 17: Crocodile forceps with straight serrated tip.

Microsurgical Baluchi Scissors (Figs. 18 and 19)

- ❖ Made up of stainless steel
- ❖ Sterilized by boiling and autoclaving
- ❖ Used for microscopic ear surgeries like
  - ➢ Aural polypectomy
  - ➢ Chorda tympanic neurectomy
  - ➢ Stapedectomy (to cut stadial tendon)

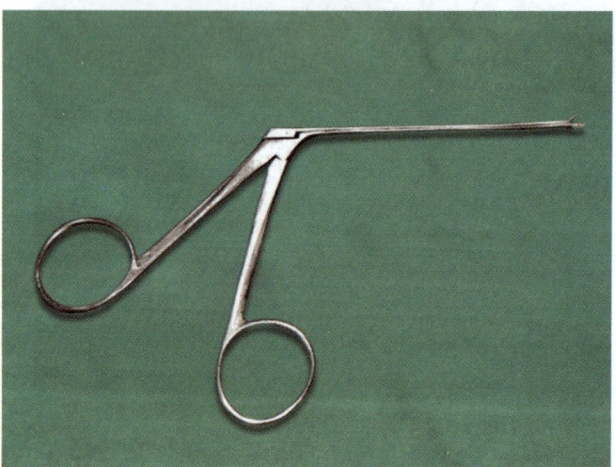

Fig. 18: Microear Baluchi scissors.

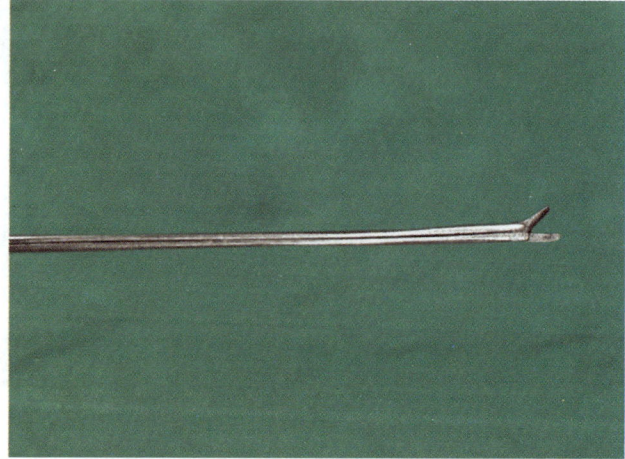

Fig. 19: Microear Baluchi scissors showing the sharp tip.

Straight Pick (Fig. 20)

Made up of stainless steel
- ❖ Sterilized by boiling and autoclaving
- ❖ Used for microscopic ear surgeries like:
  - ➢ Tympanoplasty
  - ➢ Myringoplasty
  - ➢ Stapedotomy/stapedectomy
  - ➢ Atticotomy
  - ➢ Mastoidectomy
  - ➢ Myringotomy with Grommet insertion

Pick- straight, angled (45°, 90°, 120°)

Straight pick is used to:
- ♦ To elevate tympanomeatal flap
- ♦ To separate chorda tympani nerve
- ♦ To remove cholestetoma matrix to check ossicular mobility and adjust ossicles in ossiculoplasty
- ♦ To separate incudostapedial joint and break the crura in stapedotomy surgery
- ♦ To tuck the temporalis fascia graft in tympanoplasty, mastoidectomy- to adjust grommet, teflon piston and cartilage

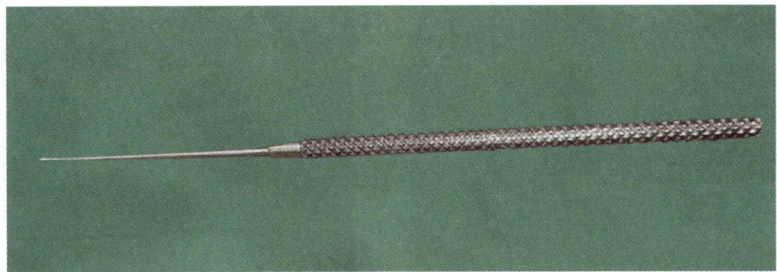

Fig. 20: Straight pick.

Sickle Knife (Figs. 21 and 22)

- ❖ Made up of stainless steel
- ❖ Sterilized by boiling and autoclaving
- ❖ Used for microscopic ear surgeries like
    - ➢ Tympanoplasty
    - ➢ Myringoplasty
    - ➢ Stepedotomy
    - ➢ Atticotomy
    - ➢ Mastoidectomy
    - ➢ Myringotomy with grommet insertion

Sickle knife is used in microear surgeries
- To elevate tympanomeatal flap in tympanoplsty and mastoidectomy
- To freshen the edges of perforation
- Ttuck the graft in tympanoplasty and mastoidectomy
- To maneuver ossicles in ossiculoplasty
- To remove granulations and cholesteatoma matrix
- To take incision in myringotomy
- To cut stapedius tendon
- To cut sac in endolymphatic sac decompression
- To cut facial nerve sheath in facial nerve decompression surgery

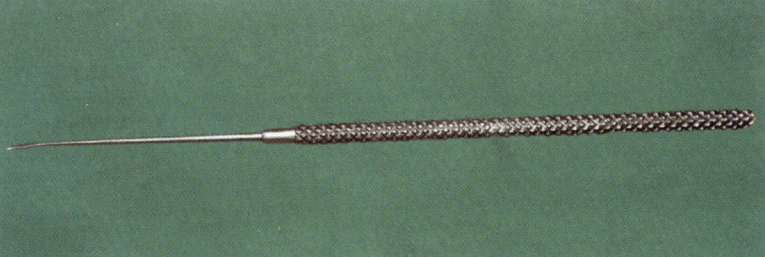

Fig. 21: Sickle knife.

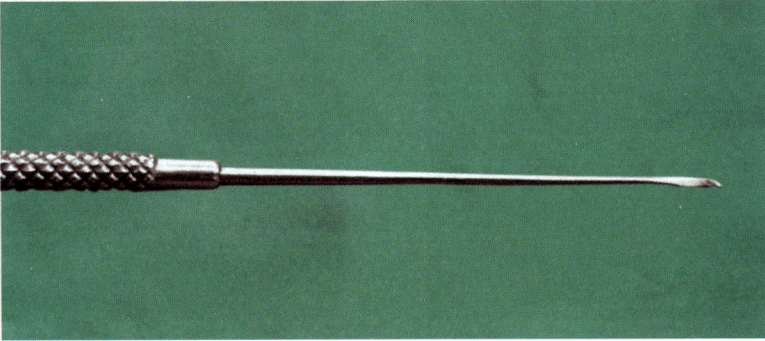

Fig. 22: Sickle knife showing the tip.

Rosen's Circular Knife (Figs. 23 and 24)

- ❖ Made up of stainless steel
- ❖ Sterilized by boiling and autoclaving
- ❖ Used for microscopic ear surgeries like:
    - ➢ Tympanoplasty
    - ➢ Myringoplasty
    - ➢ Stepedotomy
    - ➢ Atticotomy
    - ➢ Mastoidectomy

Rosen's knife is used in microear surgeries
- To elevate tympanomeatal flap in myringoplasty, tympanoplasty, mastoidectomy, stapedotomy
- To freshen the undersurface of perforation in myringoplasty, tympanoplasty, mastoidectomy
- To remove granulations and hidden cholesteatoma from sinus tymani

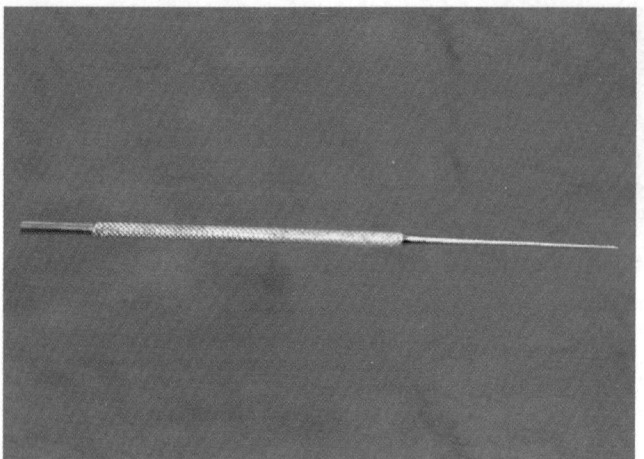

Fig. 23: Rosen's circular knife.

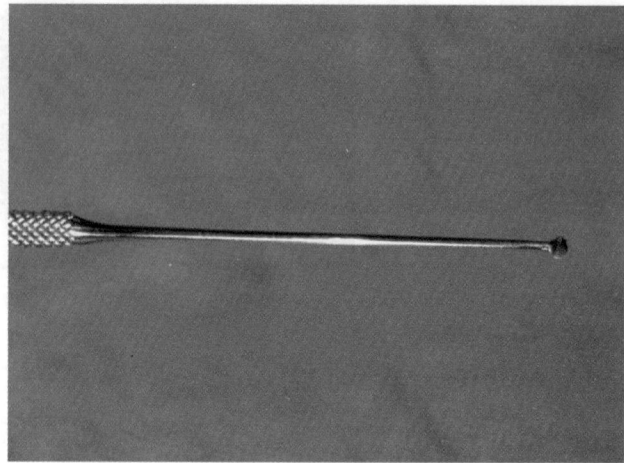

Fig. 24: Rosen's circular knife with angled circular tip.

Plester's Side Knife/Flag Knife (Figs. 25 and 26)

Made up of stainless steel
- ❖ Sterilized by boiling and autoclaving
- ❖ Used for microscopic ear surgeries like:
  - ▹ Tympanoplasty
  - ▹ Myringoplasty
  - ▹ Stepedotomy
  - ▹ Atticotomy
  - ▹ Mastoidectomy

> **Plester's knife/knife/side knife/flag knife is used in microear surgeries**
> - To take 12 o'clock and 6 o'clock incision in postaural, endaural and endomeatal tympanoplasty
> - To remove granulations from middle ear and mastoid antrum
> - To elevate chorda tympani nerve
> - To remove cholesteatoma matrix
> - To put bone dust to seal labyrinthine fistula

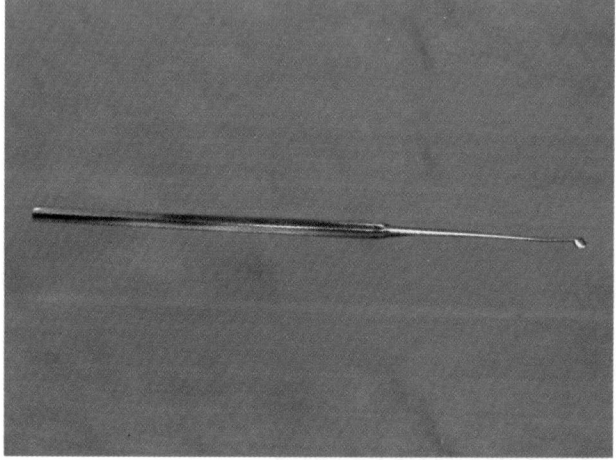

Fig. 25: Plester's side knife/Flag knife.

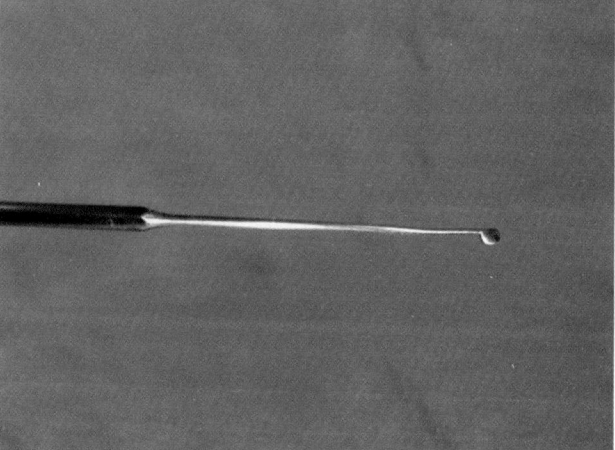

Fig. 26: Plester's side knife/ Flag knife showing circular tip at side of handle.

Mallet (With Chisel or Gouze) (Figs. 27 and 28)

- ❖ Also called as hammer.
- ❖ It is used to hammer bone for its removal in various surgeries like:
  - ▹ Mastoidectomy
  - ▹ Rhinoplasty (for osteotomies)
  - ▹ Septoplasty (for spur removal and maxillary crest removal along with gouze or chisel)
  - ▹ Caldwell-Luc operation (for creating window in canine fossa)
  - ▹ Mandibulectomy (osteotomy)
  - ▹ Maxillectomy (osteotomy using chisel)

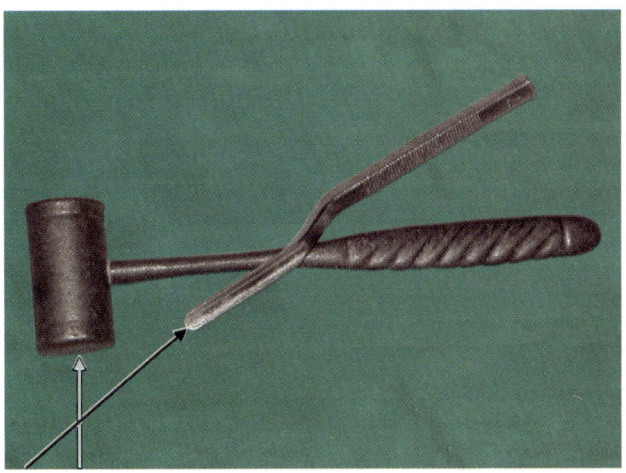

Fig. 27: Gouge with hammer.

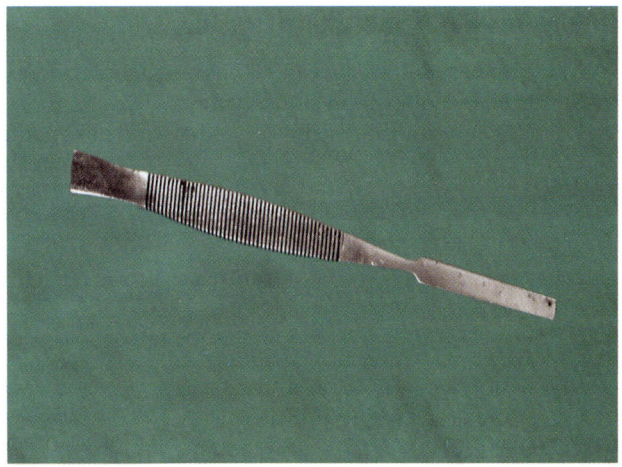

Fig. 28: Chisel.

Differences between Chisel, Gouze and Osteotome

	Chisel	Gouze	Osteotome
Tip	Sharp	Comparatively blunt	Sharp
Edge	Straight	No bevel	Double bevel
Shape	Straight without groove	Straight or bayonet with groove	Straight without groove

NOSE INSTRUEMENTS

St. Clair Thompson's Posterior Rhinoscopy Mirror (Fig. 29)

- ❖ It has **bayonet** shaped handle made up of stainless steel and mirror (0 to 5 size) without magnification
- ❖ Used for posterior rhinoscopy procedure
- ❖ Structures seen:
  - ➢ Posterior border of septum
  - ➢ Posterior margin of soft palate
  - ➢ Uvula
  - ➢ Fossa of Rosenmuller
  - ➢ Torus tubarius
  - ➢ Roof of nasopharynx
  - ➢ Posterior wall of nasopharynx
  - ➢ Tubal tonsils

Procedure (scan QR code):

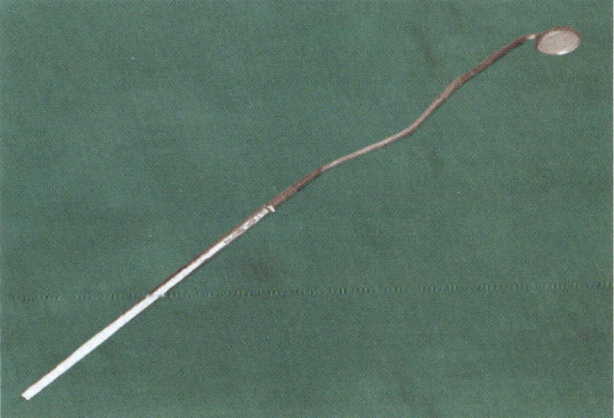

Fig. 29: St. Clair Thompson posterior rhinoscopy mirror.

Thudicum's Nasal Speculum (Fig. 30)

- Made up of stainless steel and it has one handle and two blades
- Sterilized by boiling and autoclaving
- Used for anterior rhinoscopy procedure and has got diagnostic and therapeutic uses

Diagnostic	Therapeutic
For anterior rhinoscopy to see	Removal of nasal foreign bodies
❖ Nasal septum, middle and inferior turbinates, floor of nose	Antral puncture
➤ Little's area	Nasal packing
➤ Pus in middle meatus	Nasal surgeries septoplasty, SMR, polypectomy
❖ Septal perforation and deviation, nasal spur	Application of medications
❖ Nasal mass, rhinolith, Foreign bodies	

Procedure (scan QR code):

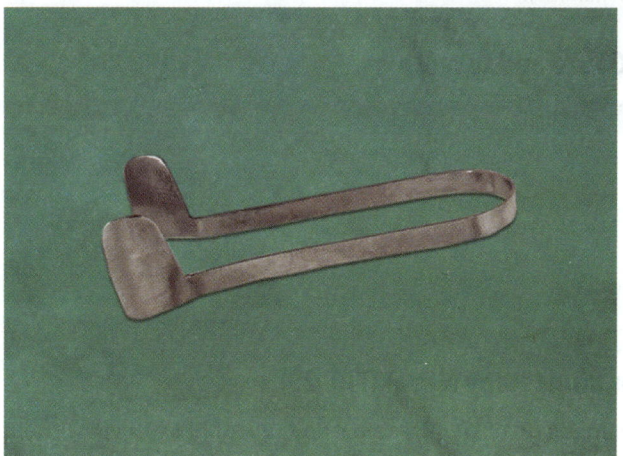

Fig. 30: Thudicum nasal speculum.

St. Clair Thompson Nasal Speculum (Fig. 31)

- Similar instruments like Thudicum's nasal speculum with long blades is called St. Clair Thompson's nasal speculum used for nasal surgeries.
- It has to be used only under general anesthesia.

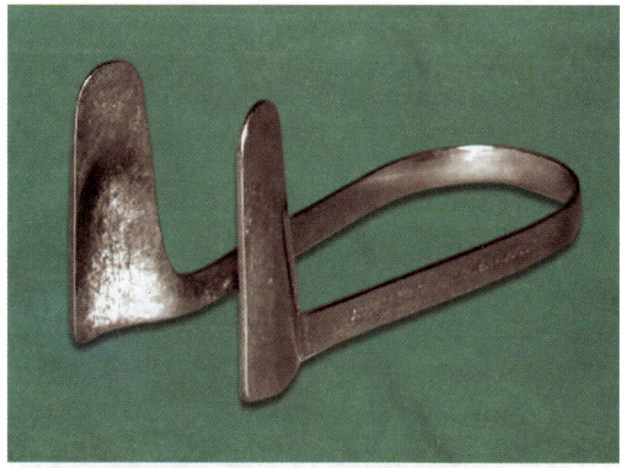

Fig. 31: St. Clair Thompson nasal speculum.

Hartmann's Dressing Forceps (Fig. 32)

❖ Made up of stainless steel and it is bayonet shaped and the tip is diamond or olive shaped with a groove in the center.
❖ Sterilized by boiling and autoclaving
❖ Used for:
  ➢ Removal of nasal pack
  ➢ Removal of nasal foreign bodies, bone chip, cartilage in nasal surgeries
  ➢ Introduction of cotton pledgets in nose for local anaesthesia

Tilley's Nasal Packing Forceps (Fig. 33)

❖ Made up of stainless steel and it is angled instrument and has got straight smooth tip with serrations at the end
❖ Used foe anterior nasal packing using ribbon gauze or net cell after nasal surgeries and in epistaxis to achieve hemostasis
❖ Anterior nasal packing is done parallel to floor of nose

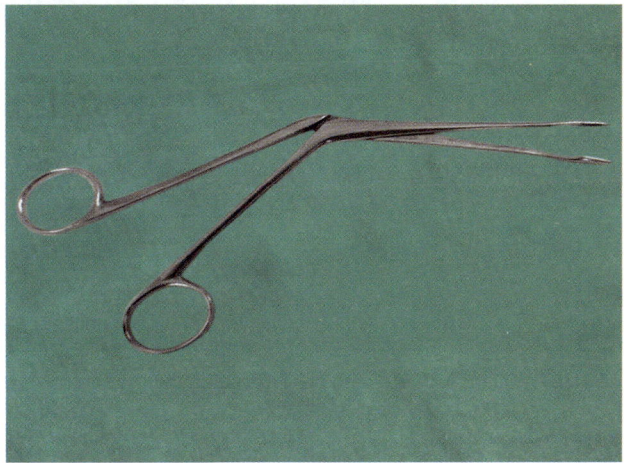

Fig. 32: Hartmann's dressing forceps.

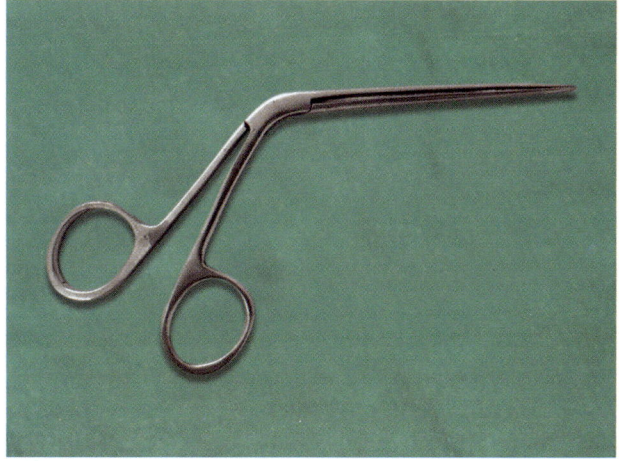

Fig. 33: Tilley's packing forceps.

Freer's Mucoperichondrial Elevator (Fig. 34)

❖ Made up of stainlesteel
❖ Sterilized by boiling and autoclaving
❖ Uses:
  ➢ To elevate mucoperichondrial flap in septoplasty, SMR surgeries
  ➢ To remove maxillary crestin in septoplasty, SMR surgeries
  ➢ To break inferior turbinate in antrostomy surgery
  ➢ To dislocate bony and cartilaginous junction in septoplasty, SMR surgeries
  ➢ To harvest cartilage in rhinoplasty surgery

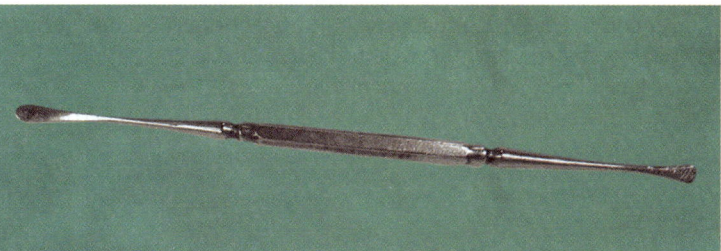

Fig. 34: Freer's mucoperichondrial elevator.

Lempert's Elevator (Fig. 35)

❖ Made up of stainless steel and has got one concave tip and one end with sharp end
❖ Sterilized by boiling and auto claving
❖ **Uses:**
  ➢ To elevate mucoperichondrial flap in septoplasty, SMR surgeries
  ➢ To remove maxillary crest in in septoplasty, SMR surgeries
  ➢ To break inferior turbinate in antrostomy surgery

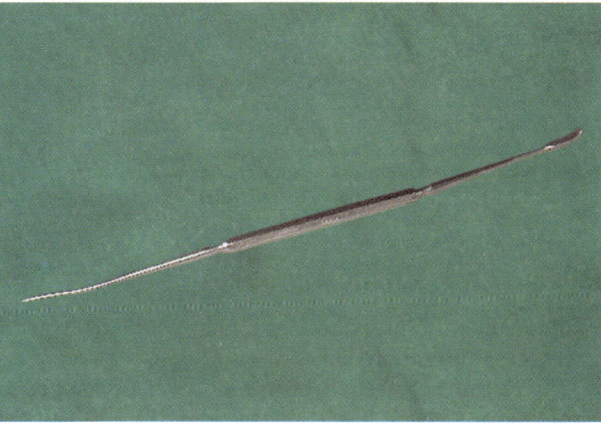

Fig. 35: Lempert's elevator.

- To dislocate bony and cartilaginous junction in septoplasty, SMR surgeries
- To harvest cartilage in rhinoplasty surgery
- To elevate periosteum in DCR surgery and tympanoplasty, mastoidectomy surgery

Killian's Self-retaining Nasal Speculum (Figs. 36 and 37)

- Made up of stainless steel and it opens when closed. It is self-retaining (screw) and blades can be adjusted which allows deeper structure visualization and surgeons both hands are free for instrumentation
- Sterilized by boiling and autoclaving
- Used for nasal surgeries like taking nasal mass biopsies, septoplast, SMR, rhinoplasty, anterior nasal packing

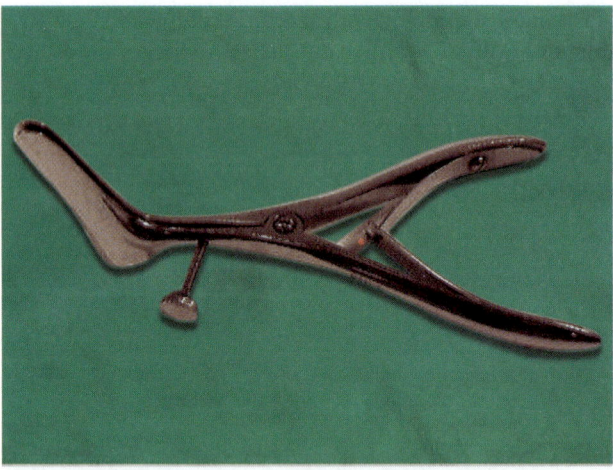

Fig. 36: Killians self-retaining nasal speculum (self-retaining with screw).

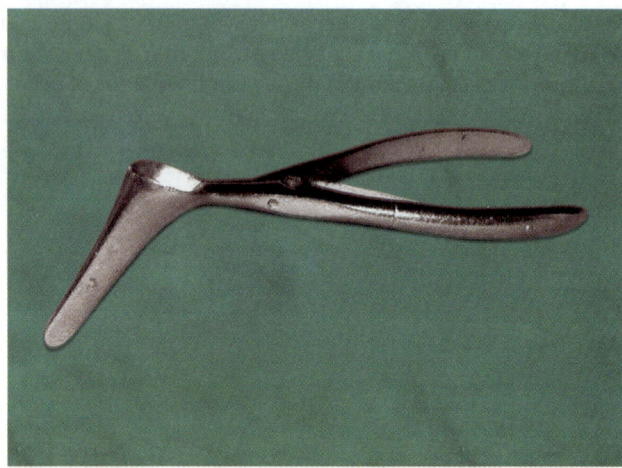

Fig. 37: Killians self-retaining nasal speculum (without screw).

Killian's Mucoperichondrial/Periosteal Elevator (Fig. 38)

- Made up of stainless steel. It is Bayonet shaped and has one flat side and other convex side, Flat side faces towards septum and convex towards mucoperichondrium or periosteum. It has thumb rest which faces upwards. Hence there are two separate instruments for right and left nostril
- Sterilized by boiling and autoclaving
- Used to elevate mucoperichondrial flap in septoplasty, SMR surgeries

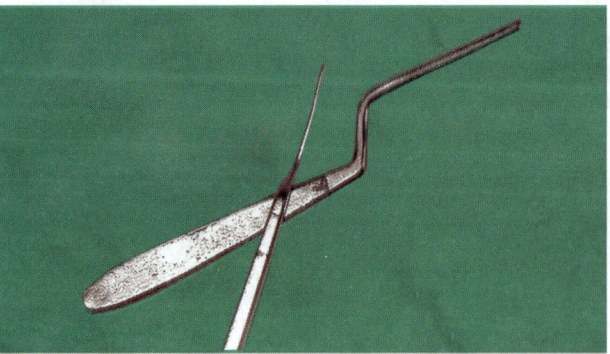
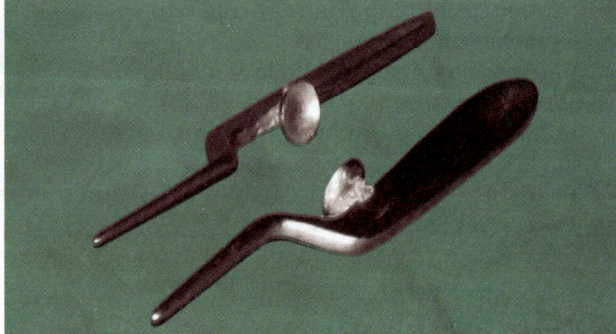

Fig. 38: Killian's elevator (right and left sided).

Ballenger Swivel Knife (Fig. 39)

- Made up of stainless steel and it has got blade which rotates at 360^0. It is called swivel knife as the cutting edge of knife revolves around two bars.
- This instrument needs to be introduced backward, downward and forwards after dislocation of bony cartilaginous junction of septum
- Sterilized by boiling and autoclaving
- Used for surgeries like septoplasty, smr, rhinoplasty and tympanoplasty to remove cartilage

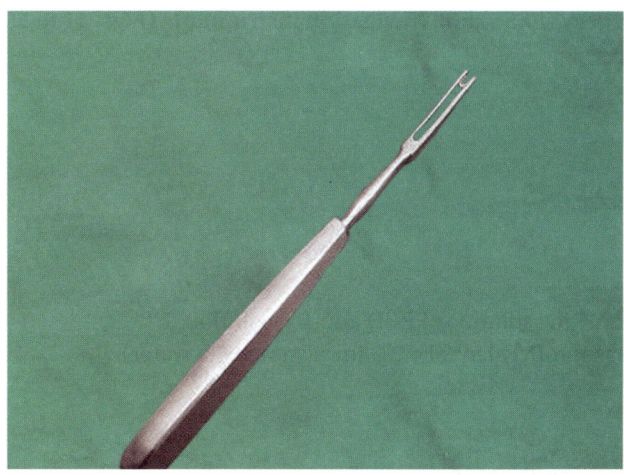

Fig. 39: Ballenger swivel knife.

Nasal Endoscope (Fig. 40)

0 degree endoscope: Green color
30 degree endoscope: Red color
45 degree endoscope: Black color
70 degree endoscope: Yellow color

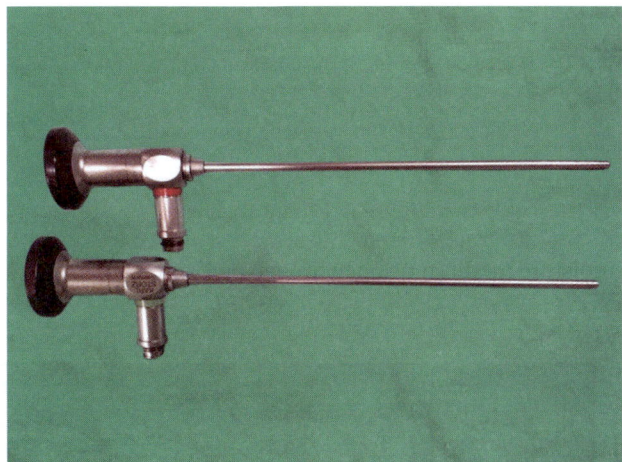
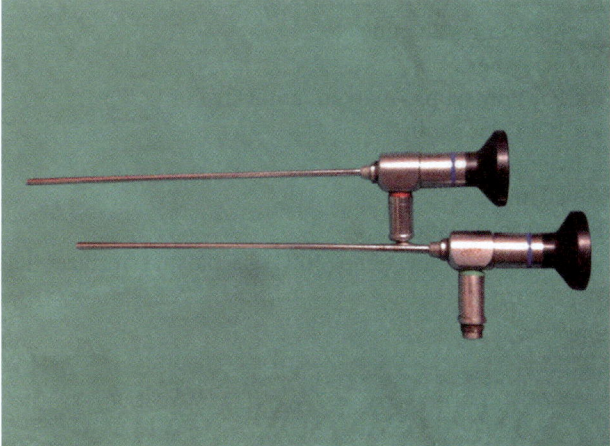
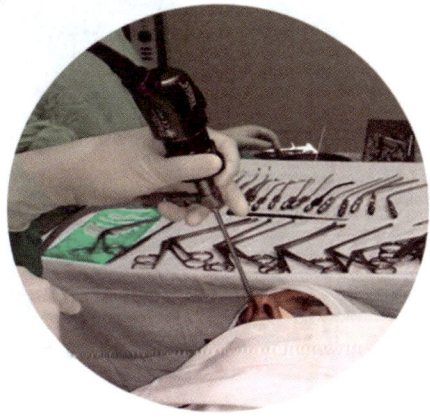

Fig. 40: Nasal endoscopes: 0°, 30°, 45°, 70°.

PART 3: Miscellaneous Topics

Functional endoscopic sinus surgery (FESS) and Navigation instruments (Figs. 41 to 55)

Sizes

- Adult size—4 mm
- Pediatric size—2.7 mm

Scopes—defogger

- Warm water
- Savlon
- Defogger anti-fog kit/ Dr Fog anti-fog solution/ FRED anti-fog solution
  - Market preparation (<15% isopropyl alcohol + 2% surfactant+ 85% water)

Scope—care

- Fragile. Handle with care
- Hold it by its eyepiece or body, never the tube
- Do not bend the tube
- Avoid contact between other instruments or surfaces
- If possible, store it individually
  Don't drop it

Scopes—sterilization

- Cidex
  - Activated glutaraldehyde
  - Contact period—12 min at 20°C
  - Max time—30 min
- Autoclaving
  - For only scopes marked "autoclave"
  - 134°C for 5 min
- Ethylene oxide
  - 60 min
- Plasma sterilization
  - STERRAD—low temp (50°C) gas plasma sterilizer in low moisture medium using hydrogen peroxide

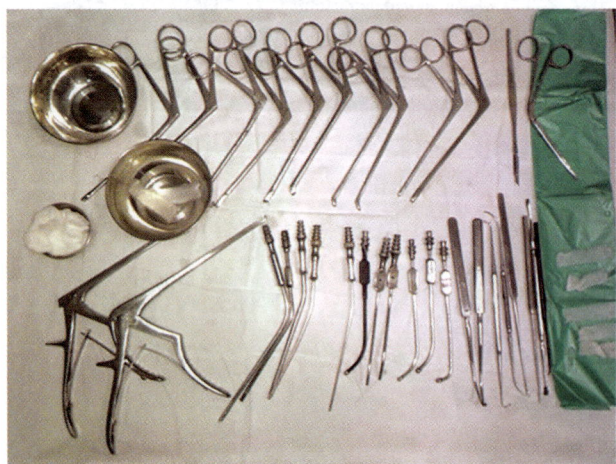

Fig. 41: Functional endoscopic sinus surgery (FESS) instruments.

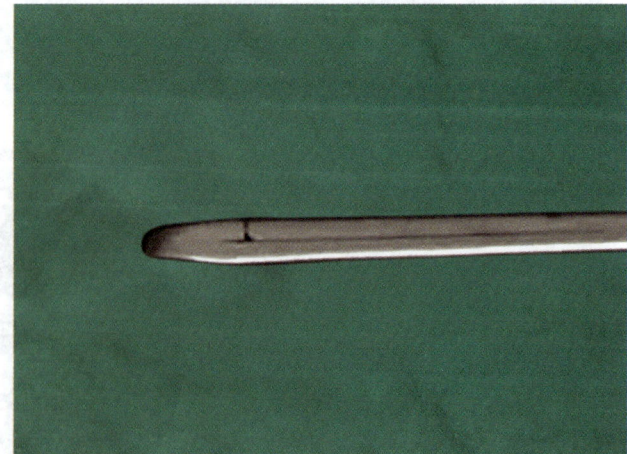

Fig. 42: Weil-Blakesley straight cupped forceps.

CHAPTER 75: Instruments in ENT

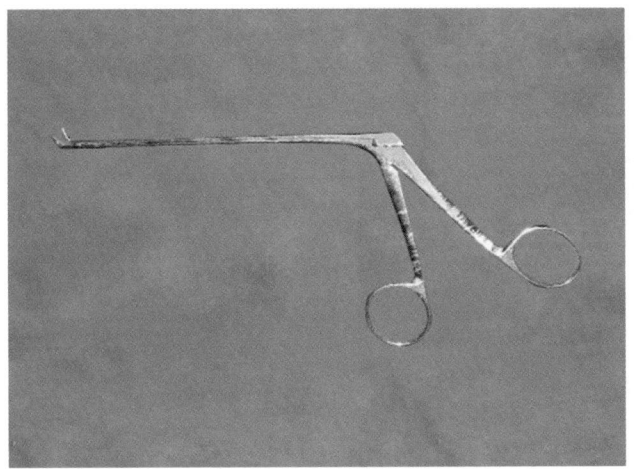

Fig. 43: Blakesley weil straight and upturned cupped forceps.

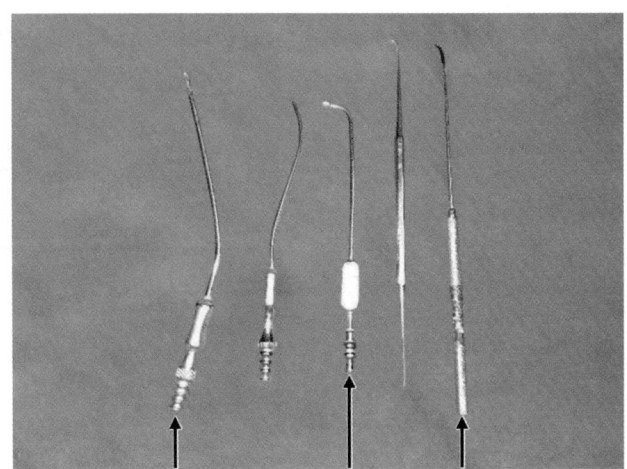

Fig. 44: Nasal suction tips, ballpoint, sickle knife.

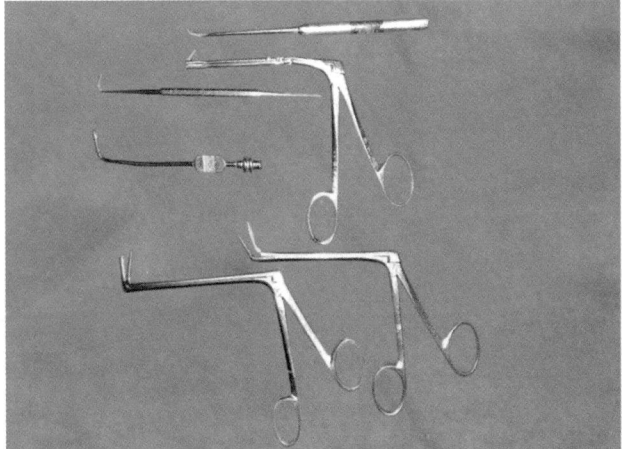

Fig. 45: Maxillary sinus FESS instruments.

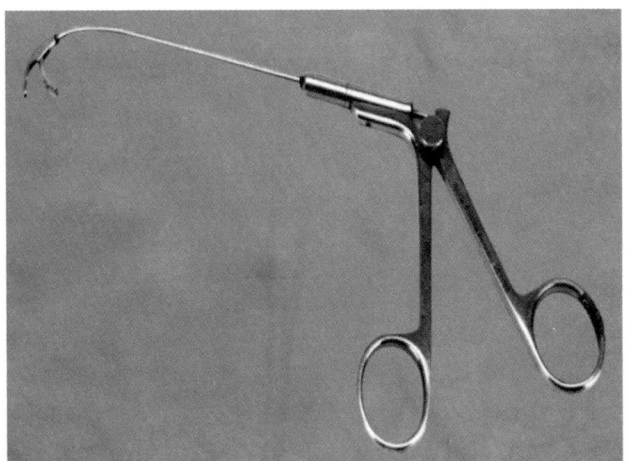

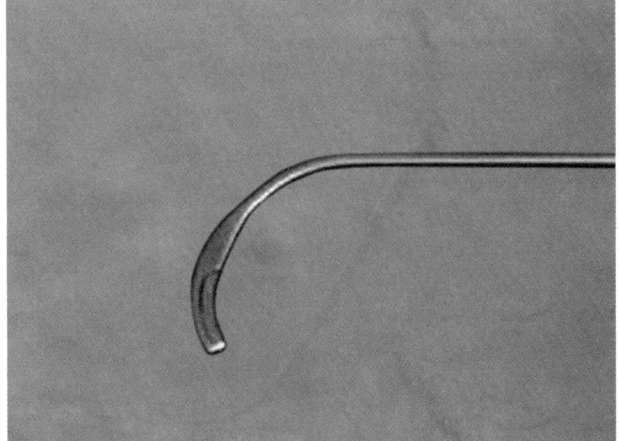

Fig. 46: Heuwieser antral grasping forcep (maxillary sinus FESS forceps).

PART 3: Miscellaneous Topics

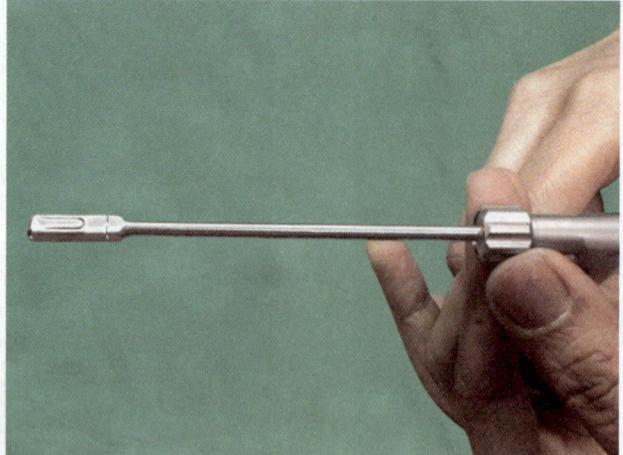

Fig. 47: Antrum punch rotating backbiter (maxillary sinus forceps).

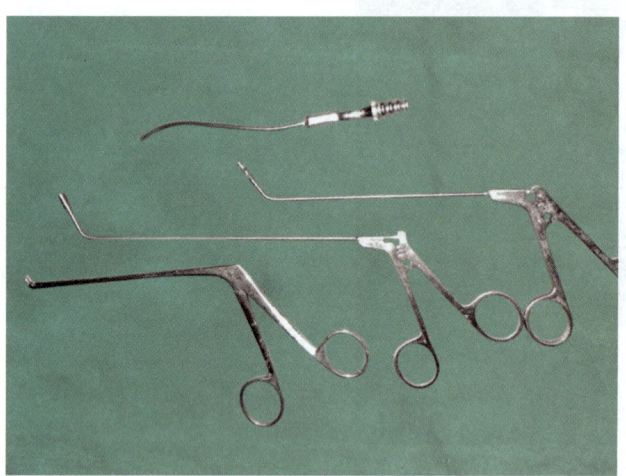

Fig. 48: Frontal sinus FESS instruments.

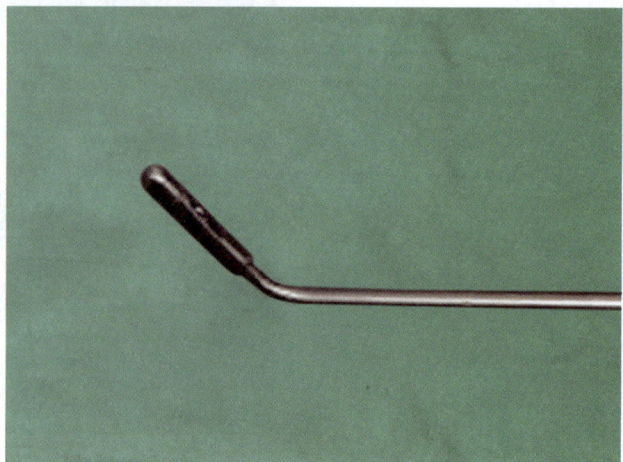

Fig. 49: Kuhn-Bolger frontal recess giraffe forceps.

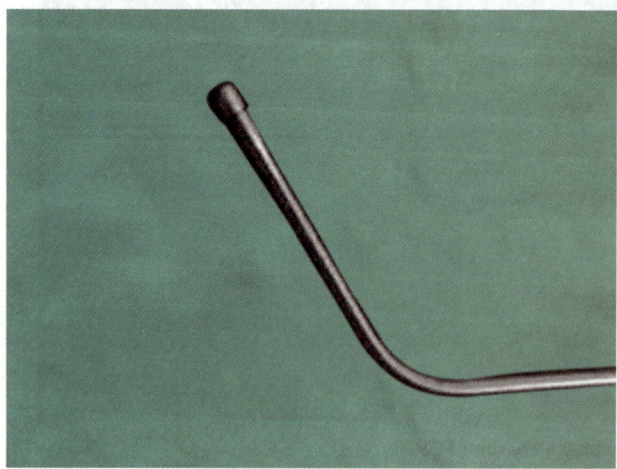

Fig. 50: Stammberger upturned mushroom punch for frontal sinus surgery.

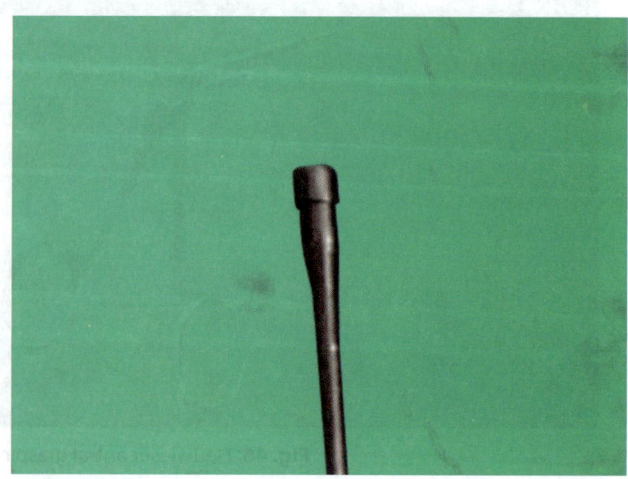

Fig. 51: Stammberger straight mushroom punch for frontal sinus surgery.

CHAPTER 75: Instruments in ENT

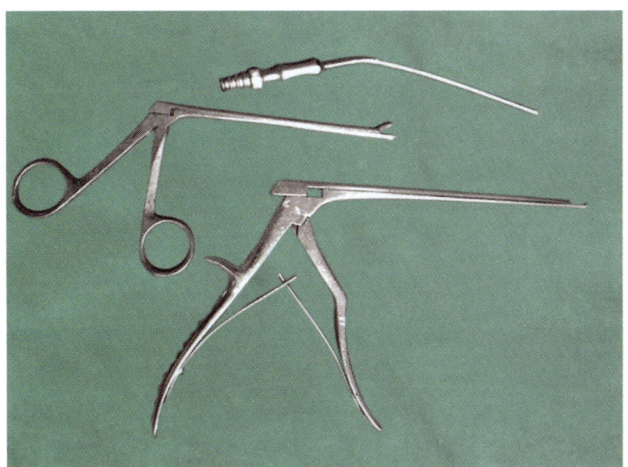

Fig. 52: Sphenoid sinus FESS instruments.

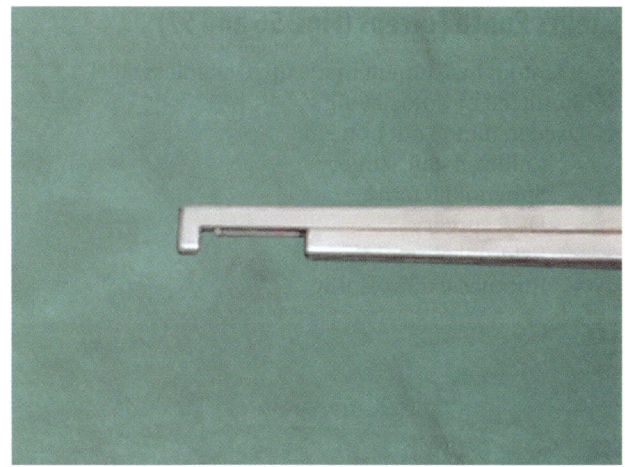

Fig. 53: Kerrison punch.

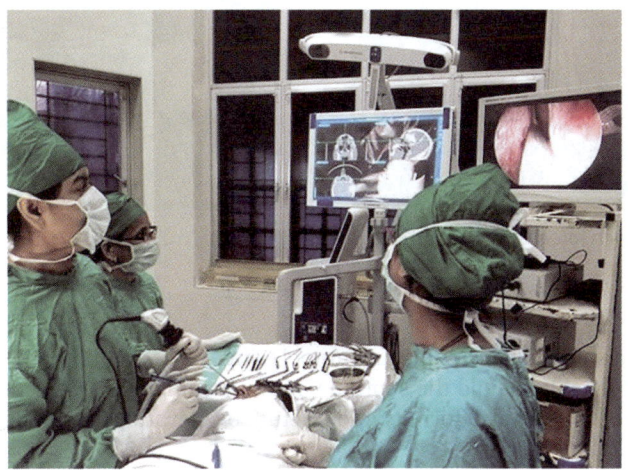

Fig. 54: FESS surgery using navigation system.

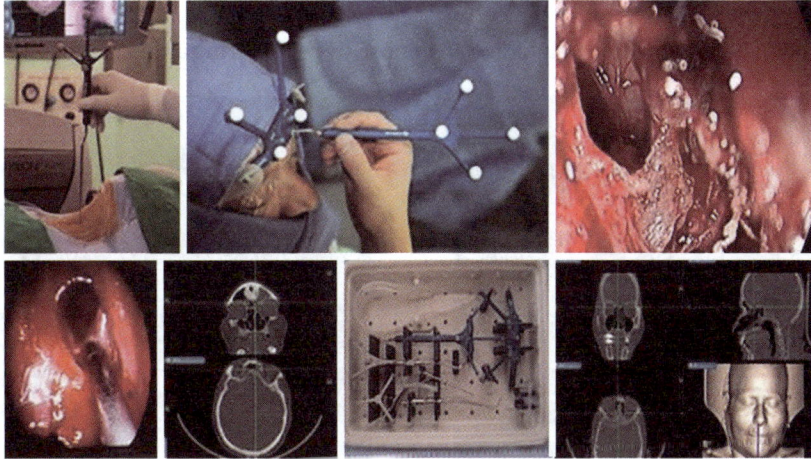

Fig. 55: Navigation system and instruments.

Citelli's Punch Forceps (Figs. 56 and 57)

- It is stout instrument made up of stainless steel
- Sterilized by autoclaving
- Used to punch out bone in:
  - Caldwell–Luc surgery
  - Sphenoidectomy
  - DCR surgery
  - External ethmoidectomy
  - Intranasal antrostomy

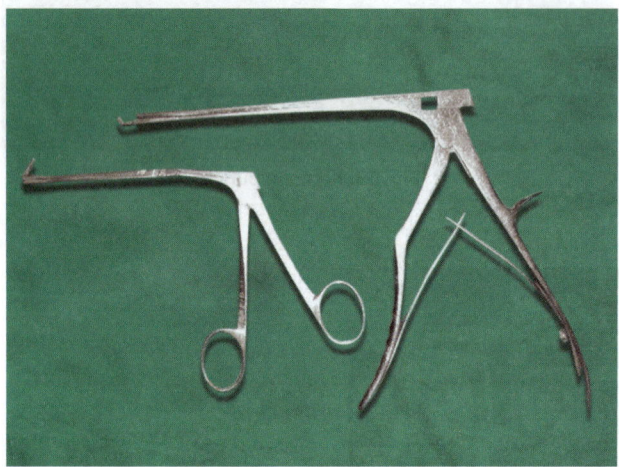

Fig. 56: Citelli's punch forceps.

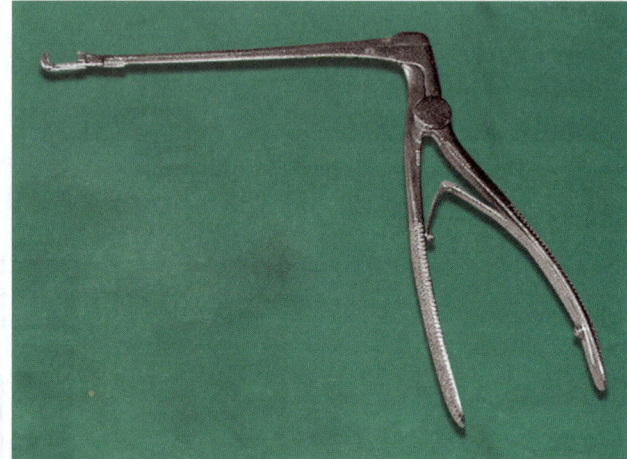

Fig. 57: Citelli's sphenoid punch.

Asch's Forceps (Fig. 58)

- Made up of stainless steel and sterilized by boiling and autoclaving.
- It has got a gap in between to enable to hold the septum without traumatizing the septum. Hence, it is used in fracture nasal bone reduction to reduce the septal deformity and fracture by elevating and straightening the septum.

Walsham's Forceps (Fig. 59)

- Made up of Stainless steeland sterilized by boiling and autoclaving.
- There is no gap in the blades of this forceps. Its tip is covered by rubber tubing to prevent trauma to skin over lateral wall of nose.
- It is used in fracture nasal bone reduction of lateral wall of nose by refracturing and disimpacting nasal bones.

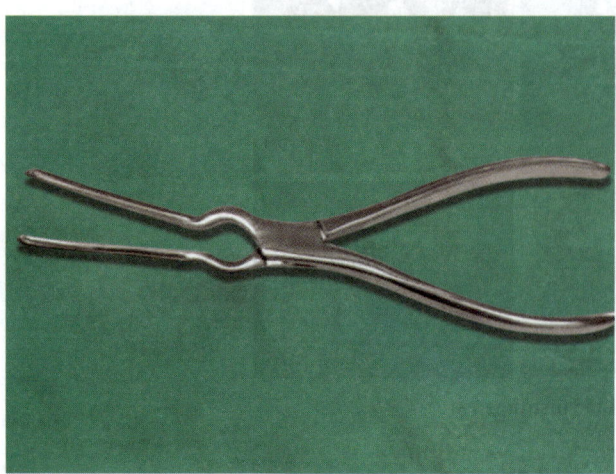

Fig. 58: Asch's forceps.

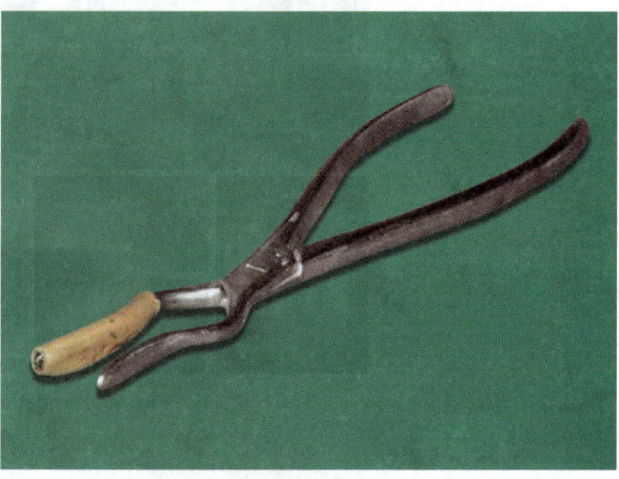

Fig. 59: Walsham's forceps.

Differences Between Walsham's forceps and Asch's Forceps

	Walshams forceps	*Asch's forceps*
Blades	Straight	Slightly angled
Covering of blades	Covered with rubber tubing to prevent trauma skin over lateral nose	Not covered
Gap in between blades	No gap	Gap to prevent trauma to septum
Fracture reduction	Used to refracture and disimpact fractured nasal bones	Used to elevate and straighten septum

Higginson's Rubber Syringe (Fig. 60)

❖ It is made up of rubber and has got rubber bulb and two tubings on either side. One end of tube has nozzle and it fits into Tilley Lichtwitz trocar and cannula. Other end of tubing has got **unidirectional valves** which allows inflow of fluid into the syringe.
❖ The capacity of this syringe is 3 oz (90 mL)
❖ It is used for:
  ➢ Antral wash after antral puncture and after antrostomy
  ➢ Nasal douching in atrophic rhinitis

Tilly Lichtwitz Antral Trocar and Cannula (Fig. 61)

❖ It is made up of stainless steel.
❖ Sterilized by boiling and autoclaving.
❖ It is used for antral puncture in maxillary sinus antrum. Antrostomy is made in the genue of inferior. Turbinate in the inferior meatus which is the thinnest bone there.
* **Direction:** While introducing trocar and cannula the direction should be between medial canthus of eye and tragus of ear. This prevents false passage and trauma to eyeball.

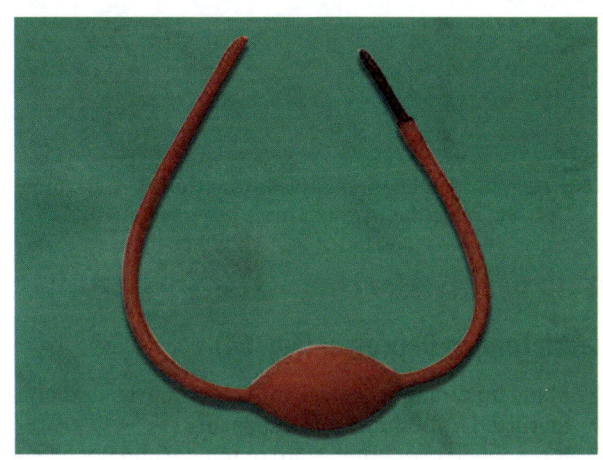

Fig. 60: Higginson's syringe.

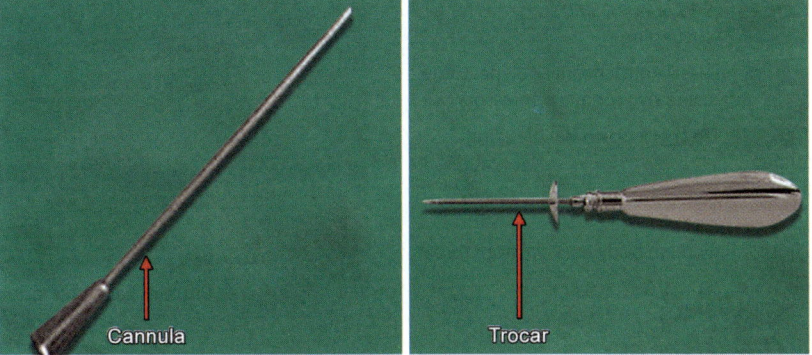

Fig. 61: Lichtwitz antral cannula and trocar.

Microdebrider Wand (Fig. 62)

Used for adenoidectomy, angiofibroma, nasal polyp/mass surgeries

Coblator Wand (Fig. 63)

Used for tonsillectomy, oral lesions/mass surgeries, adenoidectomy, uvulopalatopharyngoplasty surgery, angiofibroma surgery, laryngeal mass/polyp/cyst surgeries

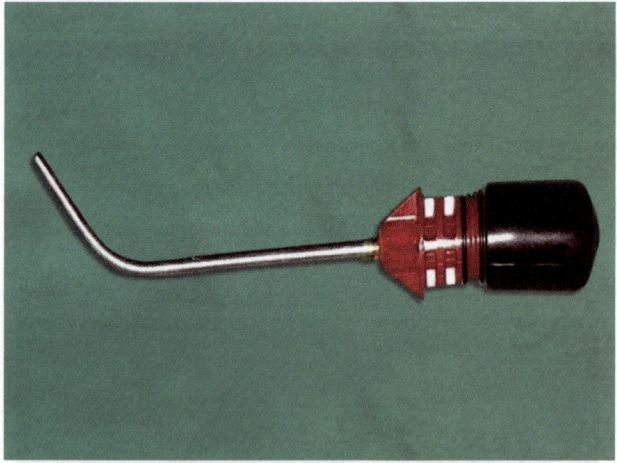

Fig. 62: Microdebrider angled blade (used for adenoidectomy and angiofibroma, nasal mass/polyp surgeries).

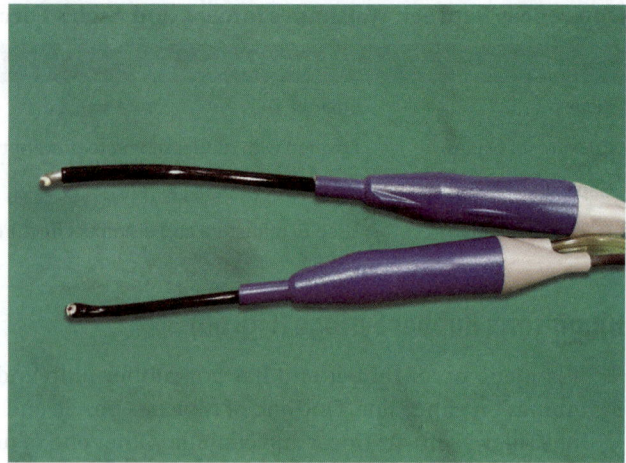

Fig. 63: Coablator wands (used for tonsil and oral mass lesions surgeries).

THROAT INSTRUMENTS

Lack's Tongue Depressor (Fig. 64)

- Made up of stainless steel and it has one flat and one curved end.
- Sterilized by boiling and autoclaving
- It is applied over outer 2/3rd of tongue and not over posterior 1/3rd to prevent gag reflex
- Uses are diagnostic and therapeutic

Diagnostic	Therapeutic
Examination of oral cavity, oropharynx, nasopharynx (two tongue depressors used)	• Oral and oropharyngeal lesion and tumors • Biopsy
To retract lip and cheek	Tonsillectomy surgery
To test gag reflex	Septoplasty, SMR surgeries for oral suctioning
In posterior rhinoscopy examination	Nasal antrochoanal polypectomy using two tongue depressors
To test nasal air blast/cold spatula test/Fogging over tongue depressor to check excelled air from both nostrils	To check postnasal bleeding
To squeeze cheesy material from tonsils	Foreign body removal from throat

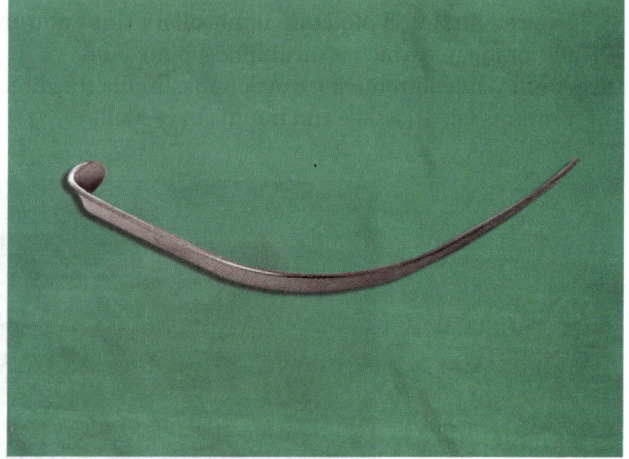

Fig. 64: Lack's tongue depressor.

Indirect Laryngoscopy Mirror (Fig. 65)

- It has straight handle made up of stainless steel mirror without magnification
- Used to see laryngeal inlet **structures**
- Base tongue
- Vallecula
- Median and lateral glossoepiglottic folds
- Aryepiglottic folds
- Arytenoids, true and false vocal cords In same plane
- Pyriform fossa

Procedure (scan QR code)

Structures not seen:
- Postcricoid region

- ❖ Anterior commissure
- ❖ Apex of pyriform fossa
- ❖ Laryngeal surface of epiglottis
- ❖ Ventricles

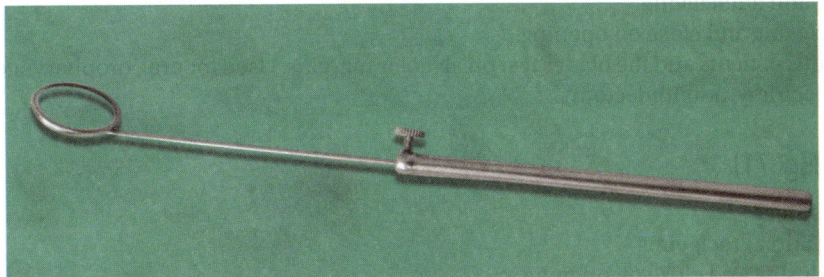

Fig. 65: Indirect laryngoscopy mirror.

Boyle Devis Mouth Gag with Tongue Depressor (Figs. 66 to 69)

- ❖ It is self-retaining mouth gag used with Draffin's bipods. Has inbuilt tongue depressor.
- ❖ It has Boyle' Blade and Davis gag.
- ❖ Used for various oral, oropharyngeal, nasopharyngeal surgeries like tonsillectomy, adenoidectomy, cleft palate, submucous cleft repair.
- ❖ No need of assistant as it is self-retaining.

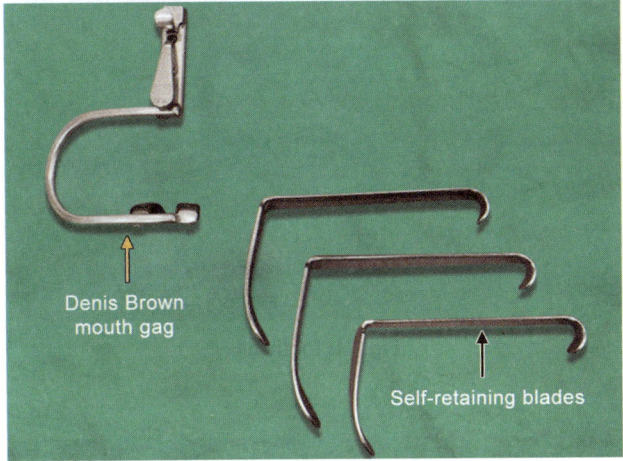

Fig. 66: Denis Brown mouth gag and self-retaining blades.

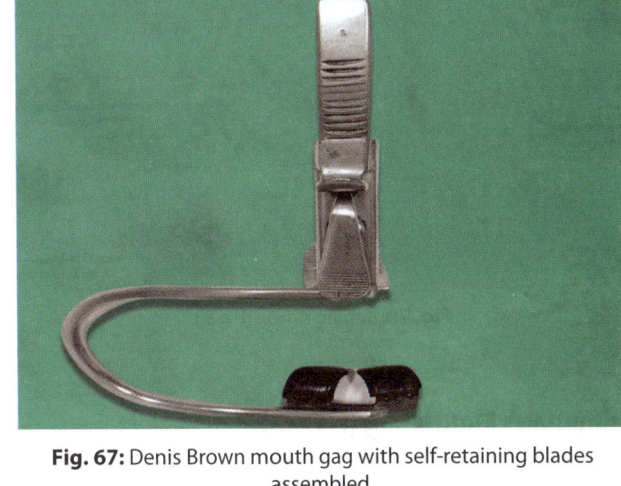

Fig. 67: Denis Brown mouth gag with self-retaining blades assembled.

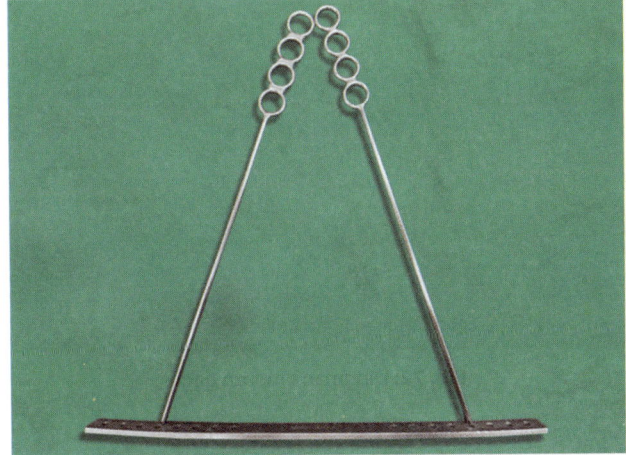

Fig. 68: Draffin's bipod, Maguaran plate assembled.

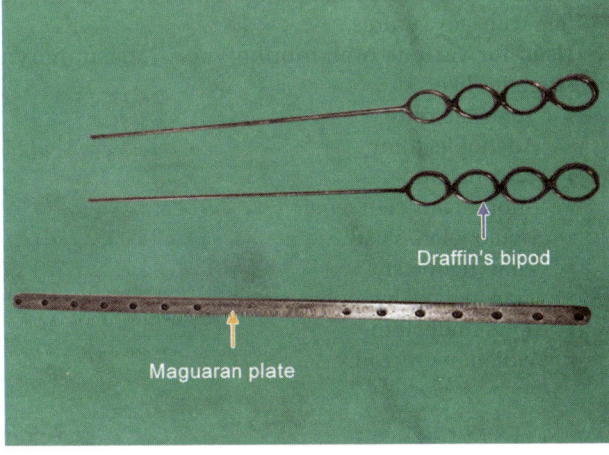

Fig. 69: Maguaran plate and Draffin's bipod.

Jening's Mouth Gag (Fig. 70)

- It is self-retaining mouth gag
- Made up of stainless steel.
- Sterilized by boiling and autoclaving.
- Its blades open on closing and close on opening.
- It is used in edentulous patients and the blades rest on alveolar margins. Used for oral, oropharyngeal and nasopharyngeal surgeries like tonsillectomy, adenoidectomy.

Doyen's Mouth Gag (Fig. 71)

- Made up of stainless steel.
- Sterilized by boiling and autoclaving.
- Its blades open on closing and close on opening
- Its tip are curved and covered with rubber tubing to prevent trauma to gums. It remains open by Rachet.
- The rubber tip ends are applied against first molar or second premolar teeth as these teeth have double root and they are strong, so less chances of intraoperative tooth fall.
- Used for operative procedures of oral cavity, oropharynx, nasopharynx, tongue tie release, tonsillectomy, oral lesion biopsies, improving movement of temporomandibular joint in trismus.

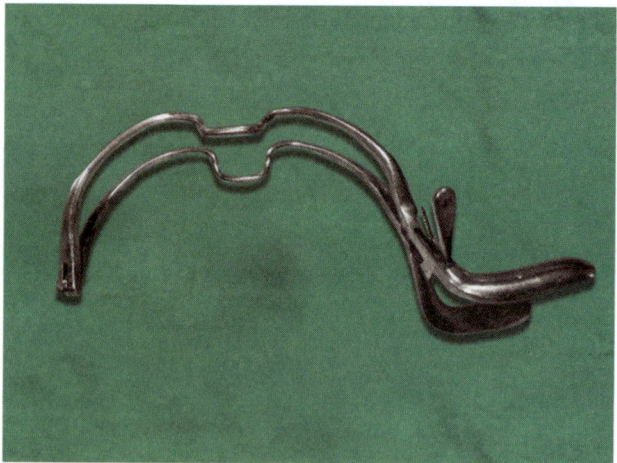

Fig. 70: Jening's mouth gag.

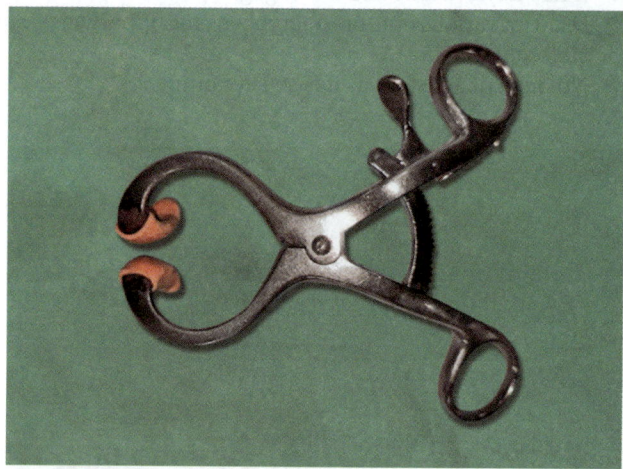

Fig. 71: Tooth fall.

Dingman's Mouth Gag (Fig. 72)

- It is self-retaining mouth gag. It has got tongue depressor, cheek retractor and wire spring which help to fix the palatal flap with stay sutures.
- Used for various oral, oropharyngeal, nasopharyngeal surgeries like:
  - Tonsillectomy
  - Adenoidectomy
  - Cleft palate
  - Submucous cleft repair
  - Uvulopalatoplasty
  - Pharyngoplasty
  - Transpalatal hypophysectomy
  - Sphenoidectomy
  - Vidian neurectomy

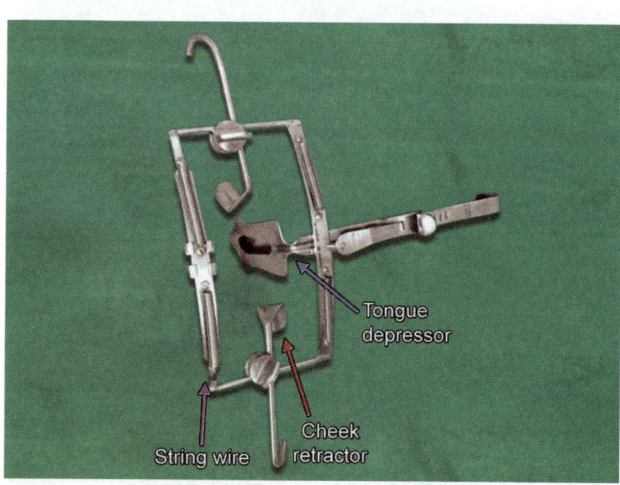

Fig. 72: Dingman's mouth gag.

Yankauer Suction Tube (Fig. 73)

- It has long suction cannula, large handle and rubber coated covered tip which makes it atraumatic.
- Multiple opening at the tip prevents blockage while suctioning due to its long handle and curved shaped the operating field is not obstructed.
- It is used for oral (tonsillectomy, adenoidectomy), oropharyngeal, palatal, nasal surgeries.

Mollison's Tonsillar Artery Forceps (Fig. 74)

- Made up of stainless steel.
- Sterilized by boiling and autoclaving.
- Used for controlling bleeding tonsil by cross clamping and tying a knot with sutures.

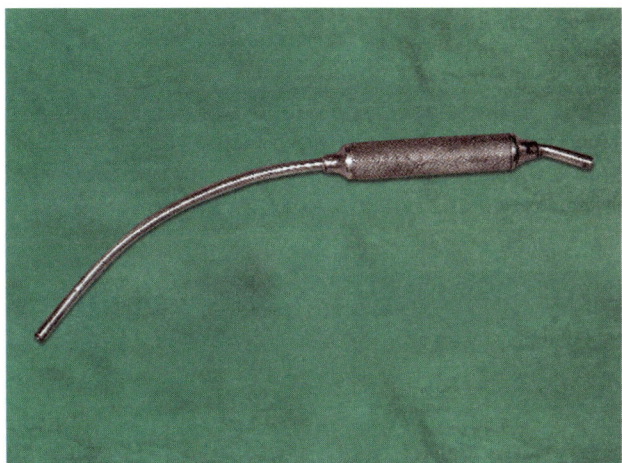

Fig. 73: Yankauer suction tube.

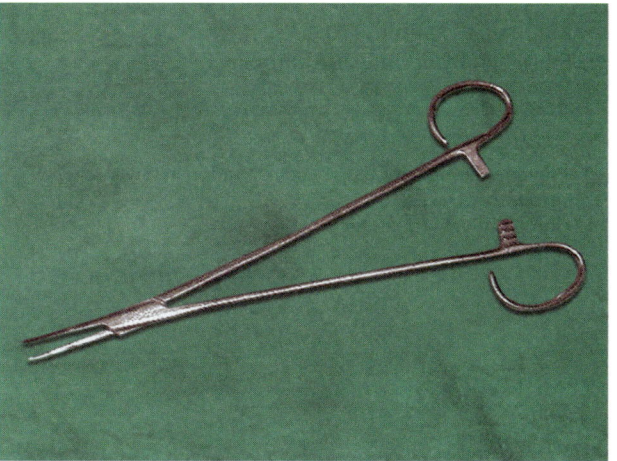

Fig. 74: Mollison's tonsillar artery forceps.

Eve's Tonsillar Snare (Fig. 75)

- Made up of stainless steel
- Sterilized by boiling and autoclaving
- It has a wire loop which is 3 inches long and thickness of 28 gauge.
- It is used for tonsillectomy surgery to remove tonsil by snaring. It **catches, crushes and cuts the tonsillar pedicle at lower pole.** Crushing releases thromboplastin which causes vasoconstriction, platelet aggregation and helps in hemostasis.

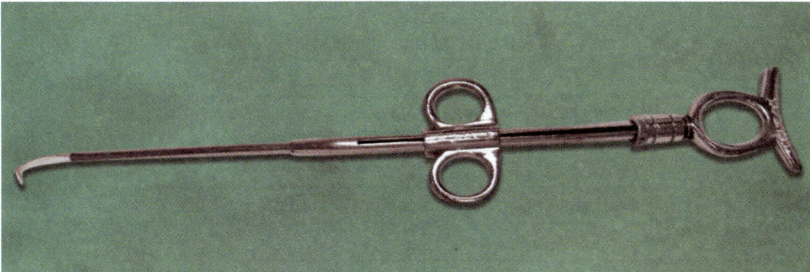

Fig. 75: Eve's tonsillar snare.

Mollison's Tonsillar Dissector with Anterior Pillar Retractor (Fig. 76)

- Made up of stainless steel
- Sterilized by boiling and autoclaving
- Used for tonsillectomy surgery. Dissector is used to separate capsule from tonsillar bed. Retractor helps to retract the anterior tonsillar pillars to look for bleeding points and tonsillar tags or retained gauze pieces in tonsillar fossa after removal of tonsil.

PART 3: Miscellaneous Topics

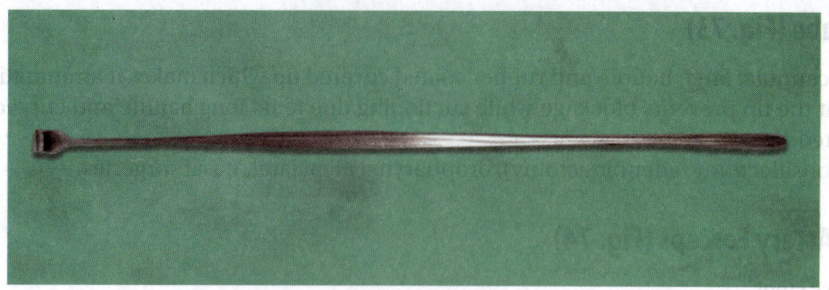

Fig. 76: Mollison's tonsillar dissector with anterior pillar retractor.

St. Clair Thomson Adenoid Curette (Fig. 77)

❖ Made up of stainless steel.
❖ Sterilized by boiling and autoclaving.

St. Clair Thomson adenoid curette with cage	St. Clair Thomson adenoid curette without cage
❖ Used for adenoidectomy	❖ Used for tubal tonsil removal around Eustachian tube
❖ Prevents slippage of tissue and aspiration in lower respiratory tract ❖ Comparatively traumatic	❖ Used for removal of remnants of adenoid tissue ❖ Relatively atraumatic

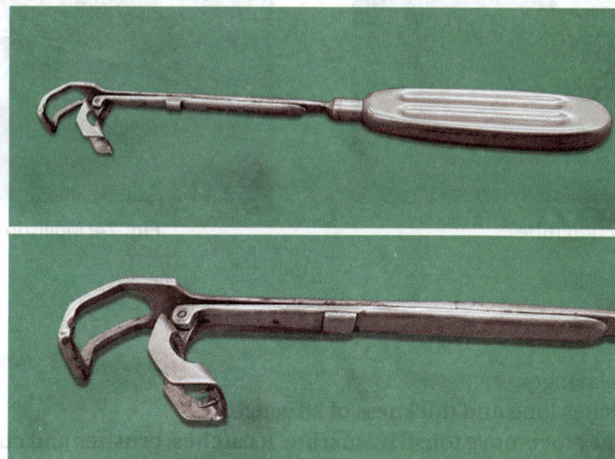

Fig. 77: St. Clair Thomson adenoid curette with guard.

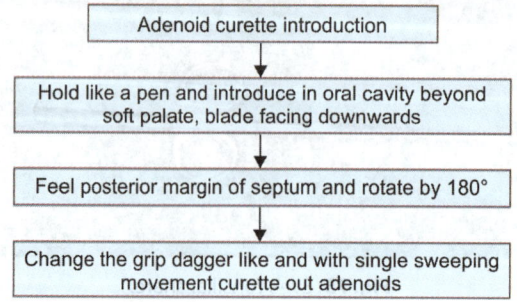

Denis Browne Tonsil Holding Forceps (Figs. 78 and 79)

❖ Made up of stainless steel. **Upper fenestrated jaw fits over lower larger jaw**.
❖ Sterilized by boiling and autoclaving.
❖ Used for holding tonsils during tonsillectomy surgery.

CHAPTER 75: Instruments in ENT

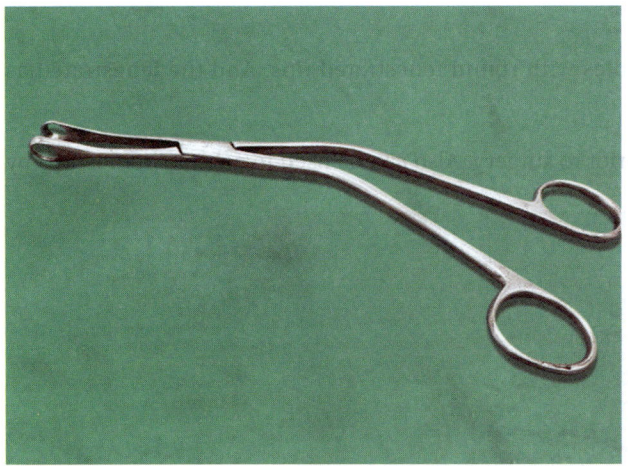

Fig. 78: Denis Browne tonsil holding forceps.

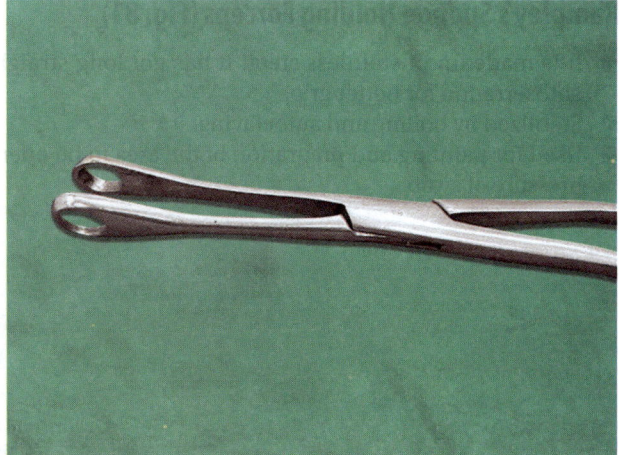

Fig. 79: Upper fenestrated jaw fits over lower larger Jaw of Denis Browne tonsil holding forceps.

Luc's Forceps (Fig. 80)

- Made up of stainless steel.
- Sterilized by boiling and autoclaving.
- It has a screw joint and two fenestrated sharp ended blades. They secure grip on tissue held and the tissue bulges through the fenestra and this prevents crushing of tissue.
- Used for punch biopsy of oral, nasal, nasopharyngeal lesions/tumors
- Used for surgeries like septoplasty, SMR (removal of cartilage, bone), removal of adenoid tags
- Two Luc's forceps are used for antrochonal polypectomy.

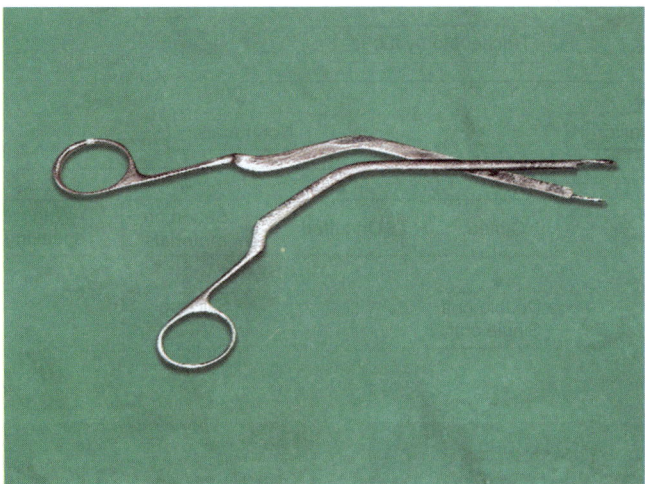

Fig. 80: Luc's forceps.

Differences between Luc's forceps and Denis Browne tonsil holding forceps

	Luc's forceps	Denis Browne tonsil holding forceps
1	Screw Joint	Box joint
2.	Same size tips of jaws	Upper fenestrated jaw fits over lower larger Jaw
3.	Sharp tips of Jaw	Comparatively blunt tips of fenestrated jaws
4.	Good for taking biopsy as two fenestrated sharp ended blades secure grip on tissue held and the tissue bulges through the fenestra and this prevents crushing of tissue	Not good for biopsy

PART 3: Miscellaneous Topics

Rampley's Sponge Holding Forceps (Fig. 81)

- It is made up of stainless steel. It has got long straight handles with round fenestrated tips. And the fenestrate has gotbserration for better grip.
- Sterilized by boiling and autoclaving.
- Used for painting and prepration of the area to be operated prior to surgery. Also can be used to achieve hemostasis by pressure of swab.

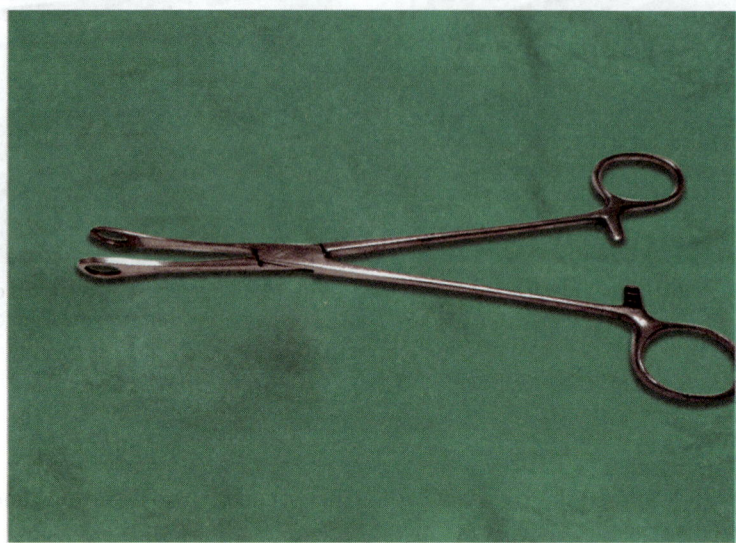

Fig. 81: Sponge holding forceps.

Tracheostomy Tubes (Figs. 82 to 85)

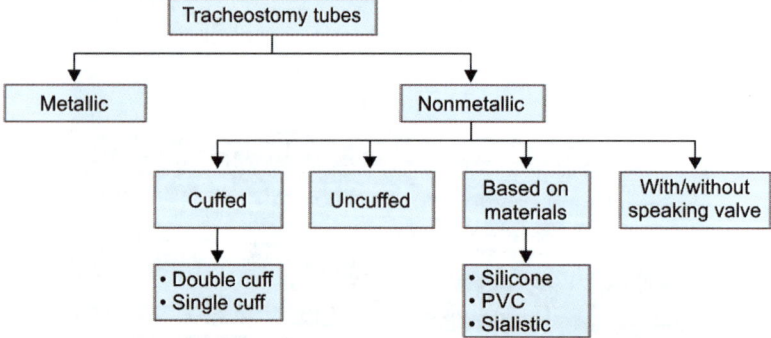

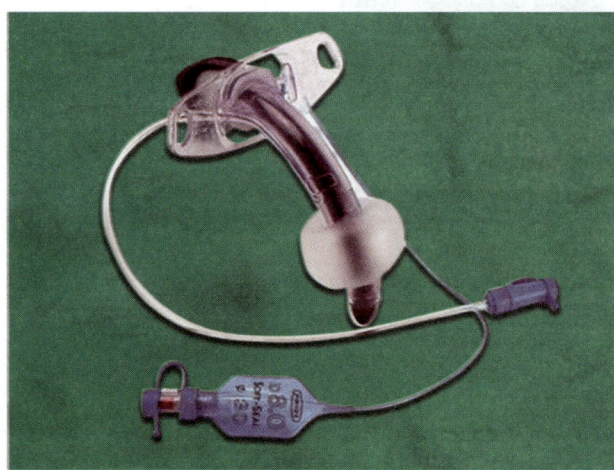

Fig. 82: Portex tracheostomy tube (cuffed).

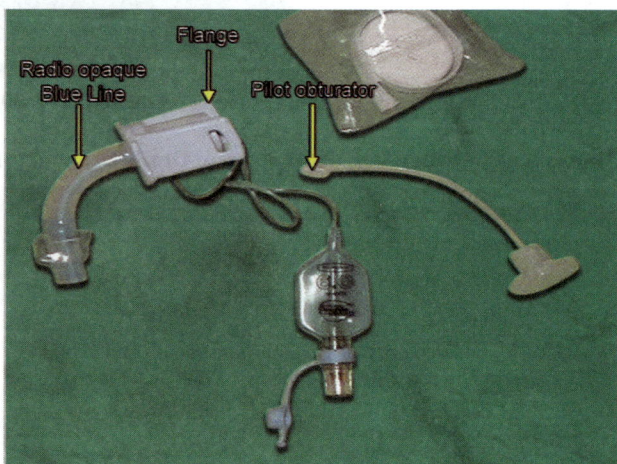

Fig. 83: Portex blue line tracheostomy disposable tube.

CHAPTER 75: Instruments in ENT

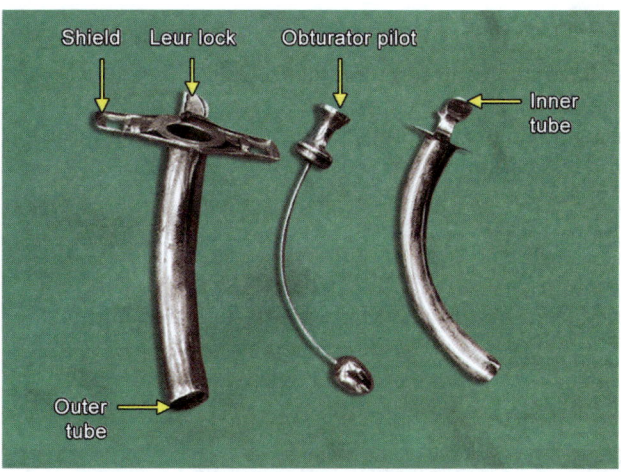

Fig. 84: Jackson's metallic tracheostomy tube.

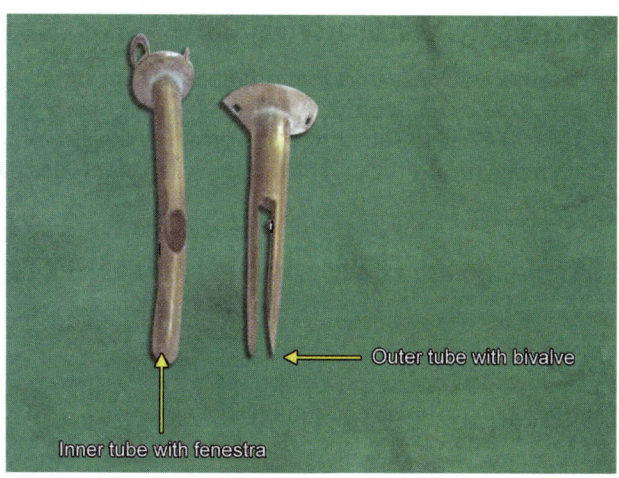

Fig. 85: Fuller's bivalve metallic tube.

Differences Between Metalic and Portex (Nonmetalic) Tubes

Metallic tracheostomy tube	Nonmetallic cuffed/uncuffed tracheostomy tube
Made up of metal German silver/stainless steel	Synthetic
Parts: Outer tube, inner tube, pilot obturator, shield, Leur lock	Parts: Portex tube, pilot, flange, cuff
Does not have cuff (nonself-retaining)	Comes in both cuffed (self-retaining) and noncuffed form
Used for permanent tracheostomy	Used for temporary tracheostomy tube
Can be reused after cleaning, boiling	Disposable hence cannot be reused
Cannot be used for patients on ventilator who requires intermittent positive pressure (IPPV) ventilation	Can be used for patients on ventilator who requires intermittent positive pressure (IPPV) ventilation as it has cuff which snuggly fits the tube
Does not have radio opaque blue line	Have blue radio opaque line which confirms the midline position of tube in trachea after tracheostomy
Two tubes (outer and inner)	Single tube
	❖ Used for patients on radiotherapy patients having aspiration ❖ For general anaesthesia

Double Hook Retractor (Fig. 86)

❖ It is metallic blunt instrument with two hooks.
❖ Sterilized by boiling and autoclaving.
❖ Used in tracheostomy procedure to retract pretracheal layers or strap muscles.
❖ Used to retract skin, subcutaneous tissue, strap muscles on both sides of incision. Also to retract parotid tissue during parotidectomy surgery.
❖ **Cricoid single hook (Fig. 87)** is used to retract the thyroid gland in tracheostomy and to retract cricoid in laryngeal airway surgeries.

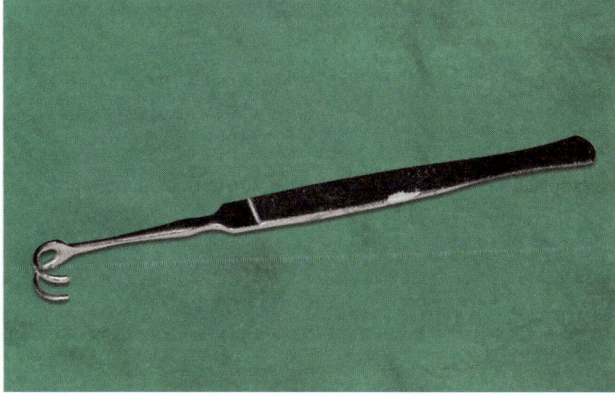

Fig. 86: Cricoid hook (double).

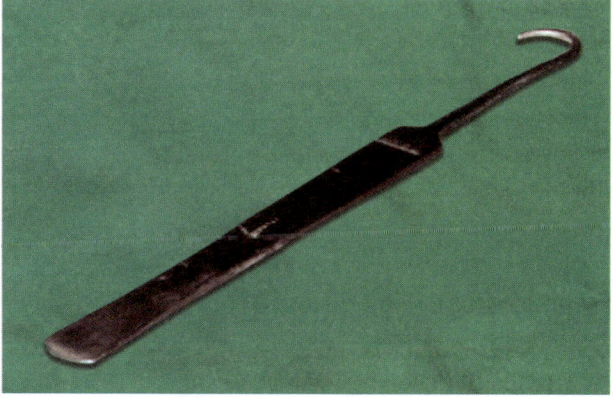

Fig. 87: Cricoid hook (single).

Trousseu's Tracheal Dilator (Fig. 88)

❖ It is made up of stainless steel. It opens when closed. It does not have catch and serrations at tip.
❖ Sterilized by boiling and autoclaving
❖ Used to dilate the opening made on anterior wall of trachea during tracheostomy procedure. This allows easier insertion of tracheostomy tube. There are less chances of false passage and less complications.

St. Claire Thomson Quinsy Draining Forceps (Fig. 89)

❖ Made up of stainless steel and it has a guard at some distance from tip to prevent deeper penetration and further complications.
❖ Sterilized by boiling and autoclaving
❖ Used to drain quinsy or peritonsillar abscess.

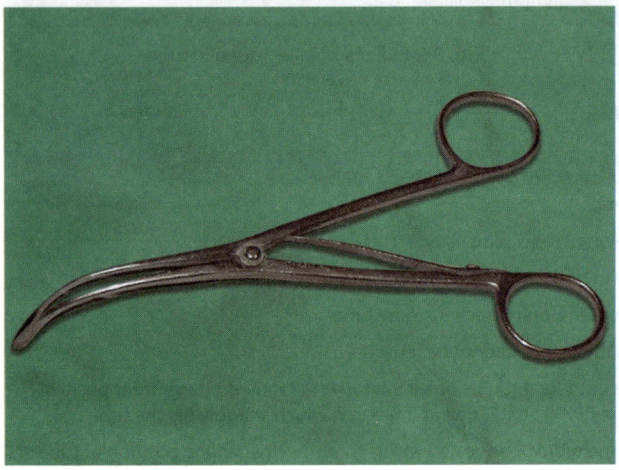

Fig. 88: Trosseau's tracheal dilator.

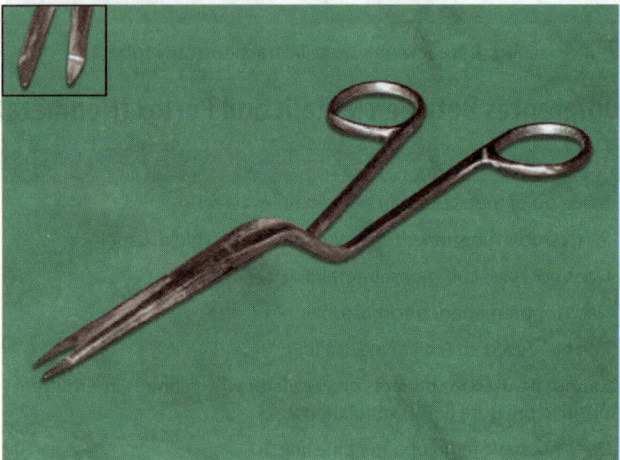

Fig. 89: St. Claire Thomson quinsy draining forceps.

■ VARIOUS SCOPES IN ENT

❖ Bronchoscopes
❖ Esophagoscope
❖ Cricopharyngoscope
❖ Microlaryngoscope
❖ Direct laryngoscope

There are two patterns of endoscopes:
1. Negus
2. Jackson

TABLE 2: Showing Differences between Jackson and Negus pattern of endoscopes.		
	Jackson	*Negus*
Illumination	Distal	Proximal
Lumen	Single	Double
Tip	Tapering	Broad
Advantage	Instrumentation better	Diagnostic procedure better
Disadvantage	Secretions cover the illumination frequently	Secretions cover the illumination less frequently but due to poor illumination instrumentation is comparatively difficult

Esophagoscope (Figs. 90 and 91)

❖ Made up of stainless steel.
❖ **Sterilization:** Boiling and autoclaving
❖ Used for diagnostic (biopsy) and theraputic esophagoscopy (foreign body removal)

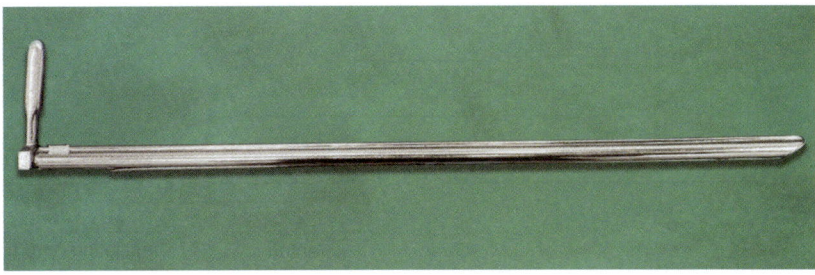

Fig. 90: Esophagoscope.

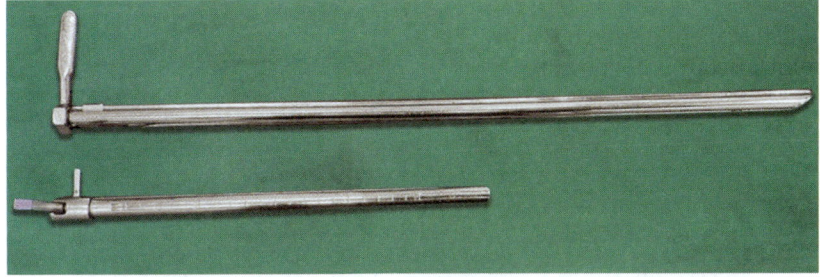

Fig. 91: Esophagoscope and cricopharyngoscope showing shorter cricopharyngeus.

Cricopharyngoscope (Figs. 91 and 92)

- Made up stainless steel and shorter than esophagoscope in length
- **Sterilization:** Boiling and autoclaving
- Used for diagnostic (biopsy) and therapeutic cricopharyngoscopy (foreign body removal from cricopharynx which is narrowest sphincter of esophagus).

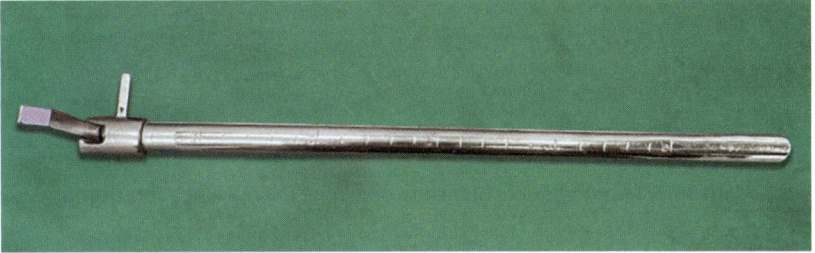

Fig. 92: Cricopharyngoscope.

Telescope with Forceps (Fig. 93)

- Better illuminationand with optical forceps
- Foreign bodies can be removed easily.
- Can be seen on screen monitor hence documentation and teaching possible using this instrument
- Documentation photography, videography is possible.

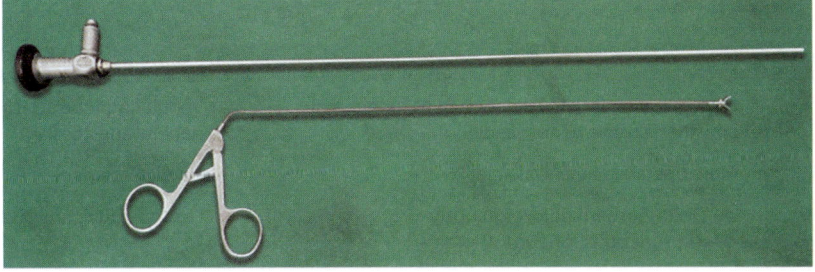

Fig. 93: Telescope and telescope forceps.

Bronchoscope

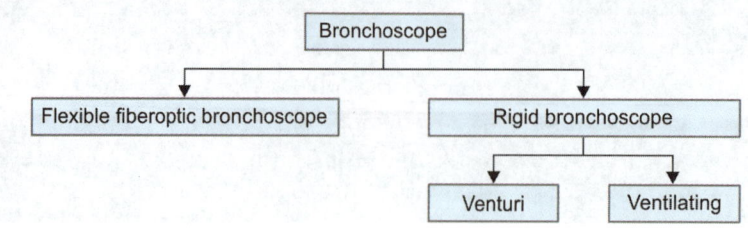

Flexible Fiberoptic Bronchoscope (Fig. 94)

- Used for diagnostic and therapeutic bronchoscopy.
- Useful where rigid bronchoscopy is not possible.

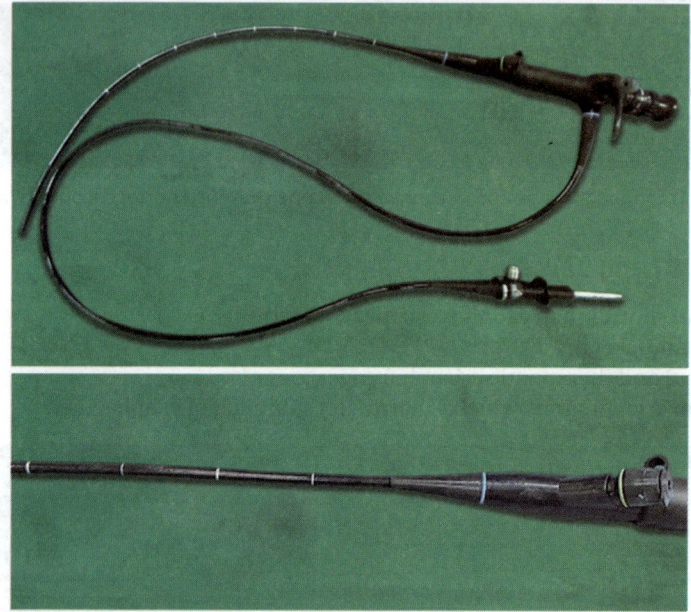

Fig. 94: Fiberoptic flexible bronchoscope (note the markings at the tip).

Rigid Bronchoscope (Figs. 95 to 98)

- Used for diagnostic and theraputic bronchoscopy.

Types: Venturi and ventilating bronchoscopes
Age and size:
- Neonate: 2.2–3 mm
- 1–2 years: 3.5–4 mm
- 3–9 years: 4.5–5 mm
- 9–14 years: 6 mm

TABLE 1: Differences between venturi and ventilating rigid bronchoscopy.

	Venturi Bronchoscope	Ventilating bronchoscopes
Anesthesia	High pressure air/jet ventilation used for general anesthesia using 16 no. needle	Ventilating tube attached to bronchoscope for general anesthesia
Advantage	More operative time available	No displacement of Foreign body/ rupture bulla
Disadvantage	• Dislodgement of foreign body • Rupture bulla, pneumothorax	Less operative time available

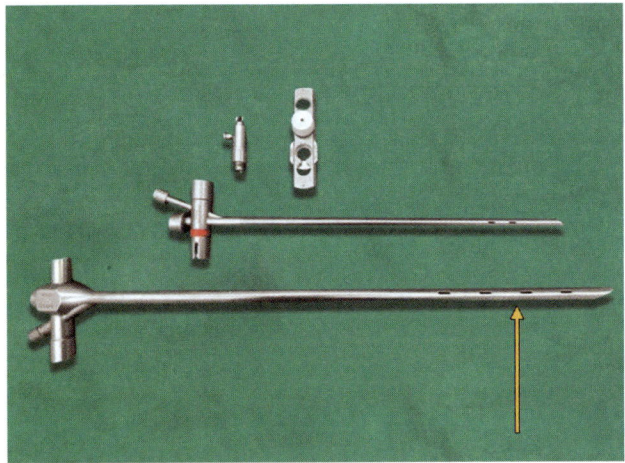

Fig. 95: Rigid bronchoscope with prism and glass eyepiece (note vents over distal end of scope).

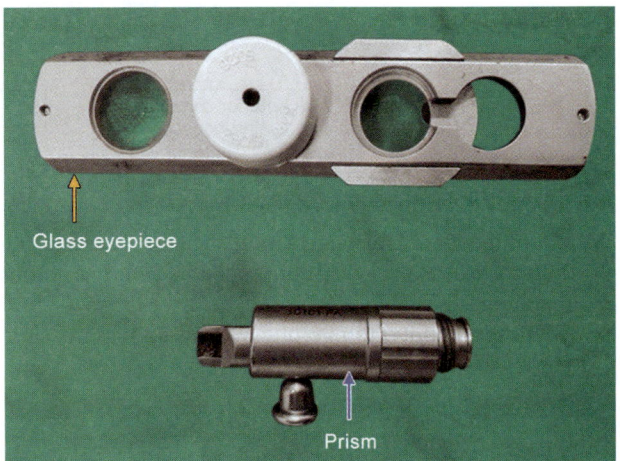

Fig. 96: Glass eyepiece and prism.

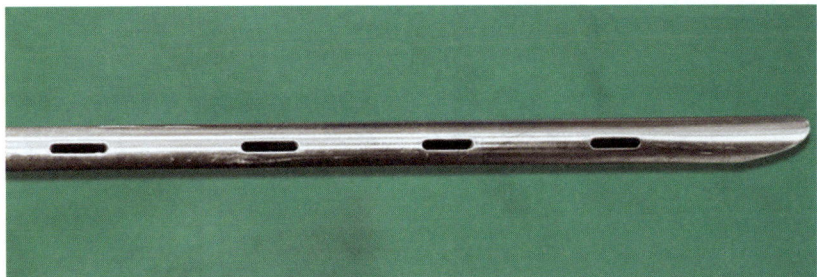

Fig. 97: Tip of bronchosope showing vents over distal end of scope for ventilation of other lung to prevent collapse of lung when bronchoscope is introduced in one main bronchus.

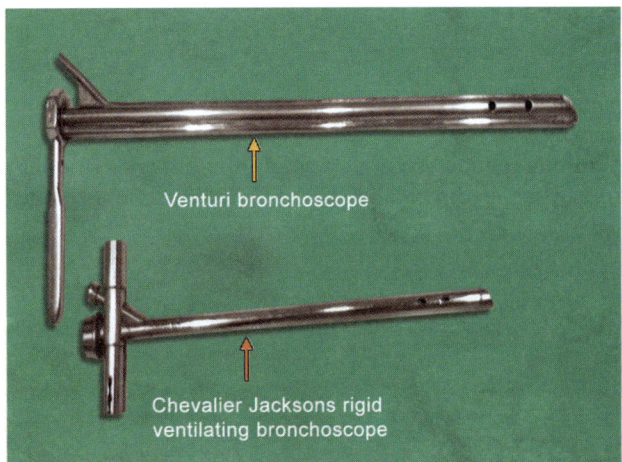

Fig. 98: Chevalier Jacksons rigid ventilating bronchoscope and venturi bronchoscope.

Kleinsasser's Microlaryngoscope with Chest Piece (Figs. 99 and 100)

- Made up of stainless steel.
- Has proximal wider and distal narrow aperture, flat lower surface on lower teeth of patient allows even distribution of force
- It is self-retaining. It is fixed with **chest piece (Riecker's chest holder).**
- It is used with **operating microscope with 400 mm lens**
- Used for diagnostic (biopsy) and therapeutic scopy of laryngeal pathologies.

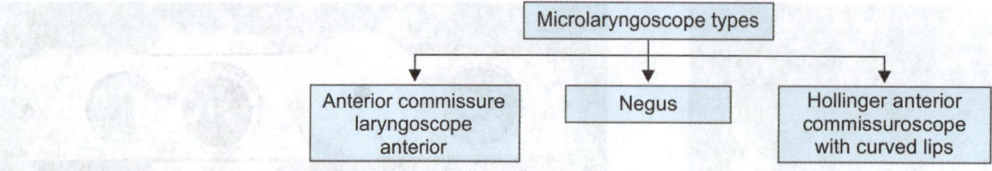

Advantages over direct laryngoscopy:

- Magnified view of laryngeal inlet structures seen as it is used with microscope
- Both true and false vocal cords seen in different planes
- Teaching is possible.
- Documentation, photography, videography is possible.

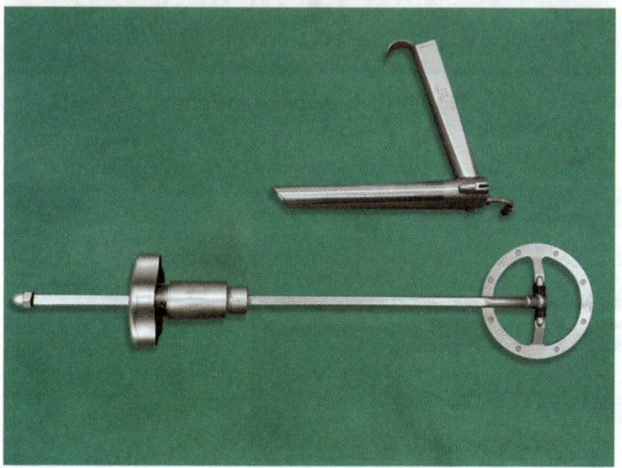

Fig. 99: Kleinsasser's microlaryngoscope with chest piece.

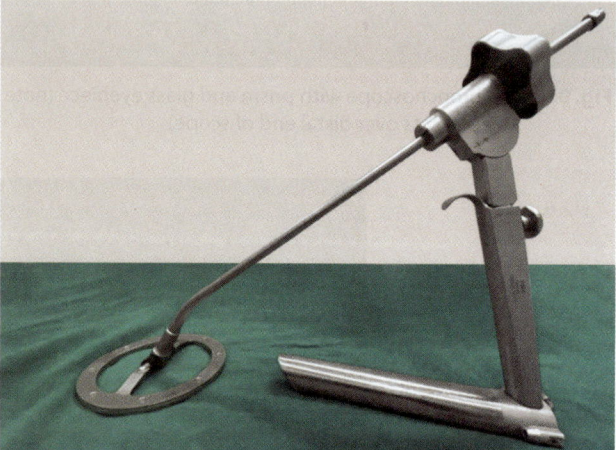

Fig. 100: Showing assembly of microlaryngoscope with chest piece.

Direct Laryngoscope (Fig. 101)

- It is U-shaped. Made up of German silver.
- Sterilized by boiling and autoclaving.
- Used for diagnostic (biopsy) and therapeutic scopy of laryngeal pathologies (benign lesions from vocal cords), while bronchoscopy to introduce bronchoscope (direct laryngoscope with detachable blade used).

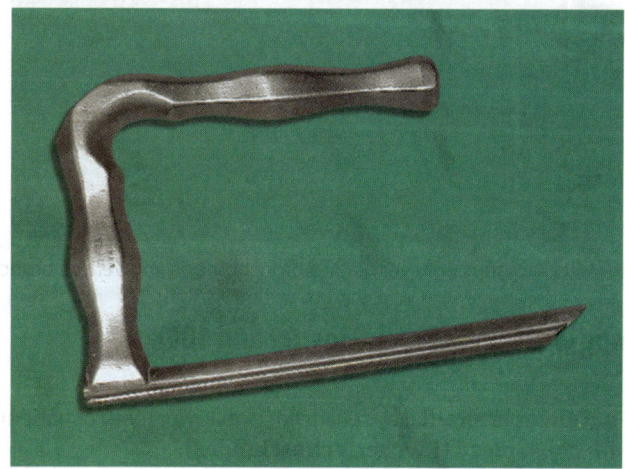

Fig. 101: Chevalier Jackson direct laryngoscope.

Chapter 76

Radiology in ENT (X-rays)

EN2.6: Choose correctly and interpret radiological, microbiological and histological investigations relevant to the ENT disorders.

■ X-RAY OF PARANASAL SINUSES

Q. What are the different views of X-ray of paranasal sinuses (PNS)?

- ❖ **Water's view** (occipitomental view)
  - ➢ Chin and tip of nose touches film
  - ➢ Mouth open—to see sphenoid sinus and nasopharynx
- ❖ **Caldwell's view** (occipitofrontal view)
  - ➢ Forehead and tip of nose touches the film
  - ➢ X-ray beams take angle of 20 with orbitomeatal line
  - ➢ Maxillary antrum not well demonstrated as they overlap with petrous bone
- ❖ **Lateral view:** Sphenoid sinus is well visualized

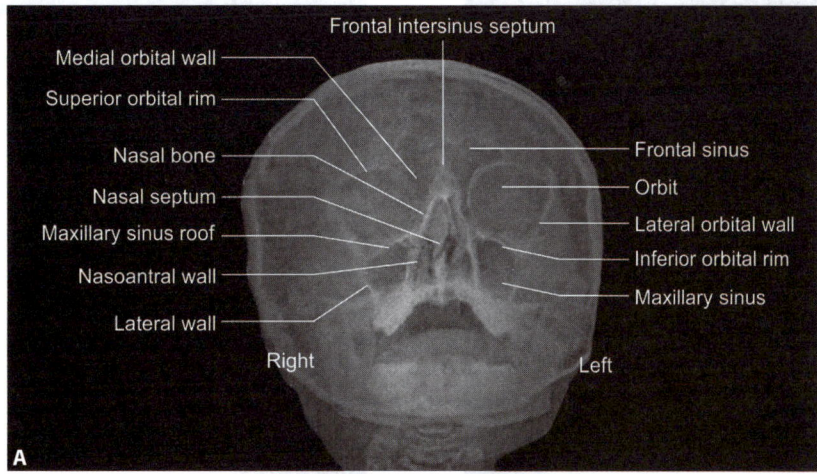

Fig.1A

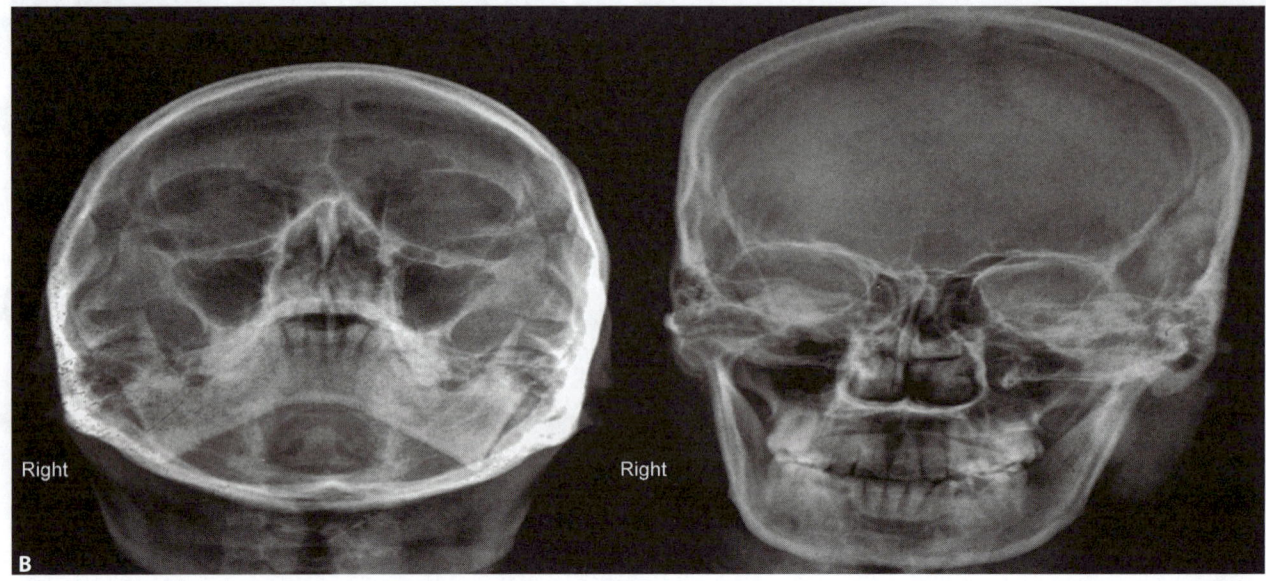

Fig.1B

Figs. 1A and B: (A) X-ray of paranasal sinus (PNS) Water's view and (B) Caldwell's view—normal X-rays.

Q. What are the differential diagnosis of unilateral maxillary sinus haziness?

- Maxillary sinusitis
- Antrochoanal (AC) polyp
- **Maxillary sinus cyst:** Retention cyst, dental cyst
- Post-traumatic hematoma in maxillary sinus
- **Neoplasm:** Inverted papilloma, carcinoma, etc.

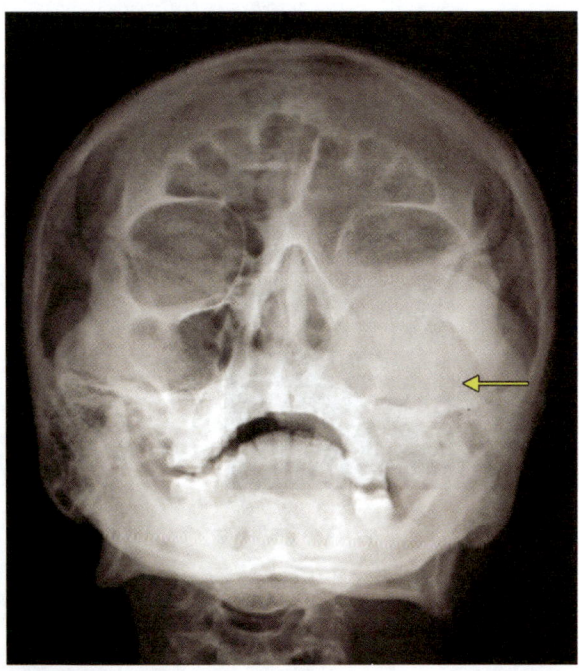

Fig. 2: X-ray of PNS Water's view showing soft tissue in one maxillary sinus.

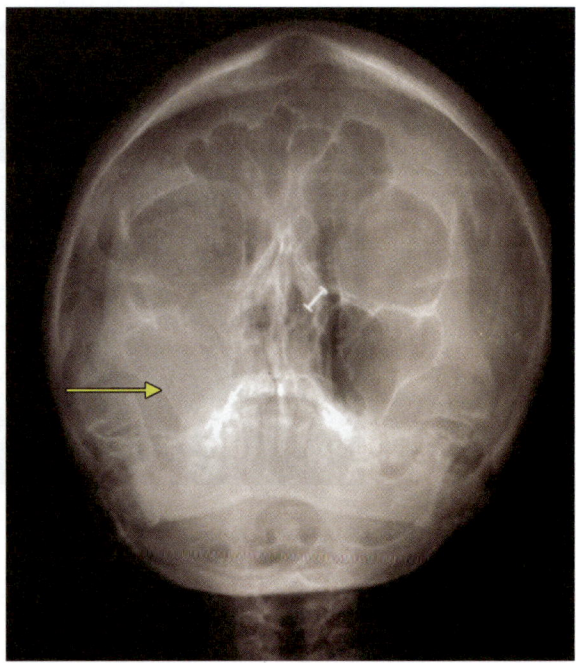

Fig. 3: X-ray of PNS Water's view showing complete haziness in one maxillary sinus.

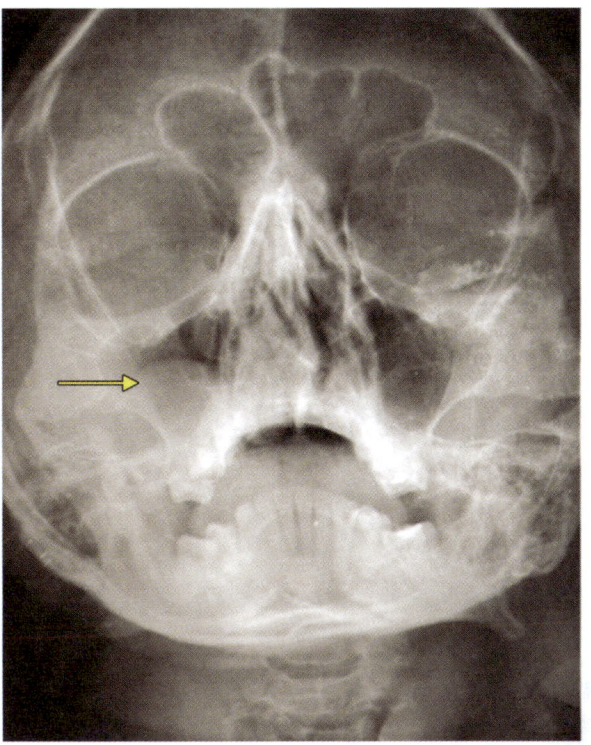

Fig. 4: X-ray of nose and PNS Water's view showing soft tissue in one maxillary sinus and nasal cavity (antrochoanal polyp).

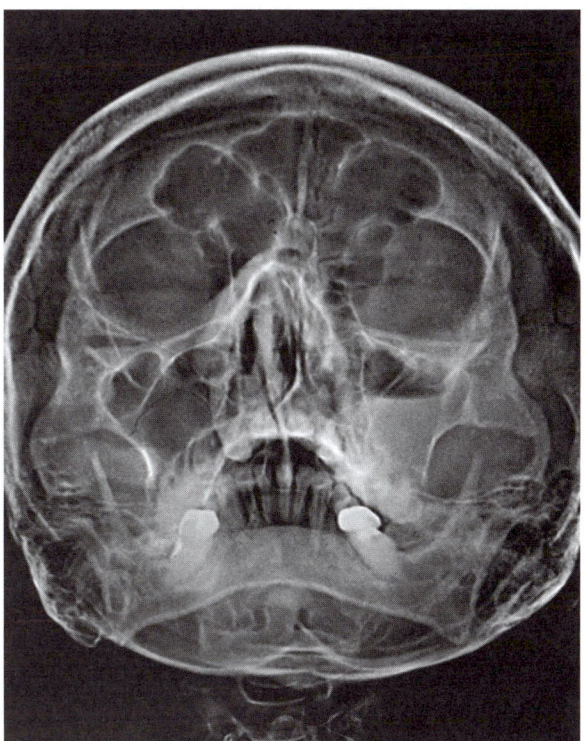

Fig. 5: X-ray of PNS Water's view showing **air-fluid level** in one maxillary sinus suggestive of maxillary sinusitis.

Q. What are the causes of unilateral nasal obstructions?
- Deviated nasal septum (DNS)
- Unilateral chonal atresia
- Foreign body
- Hypertrophied turbinate
- AC polyp
- Rhinosporidiosis
- Inverted papilloma
- Synechia

Q. What are the causes of nasal obstructions in children?
- Foreign body
- Adenoids
- Rhinitis
- Choanal atresia
- Nasal diphtheria

X-RAY OF NASOPHARYNX

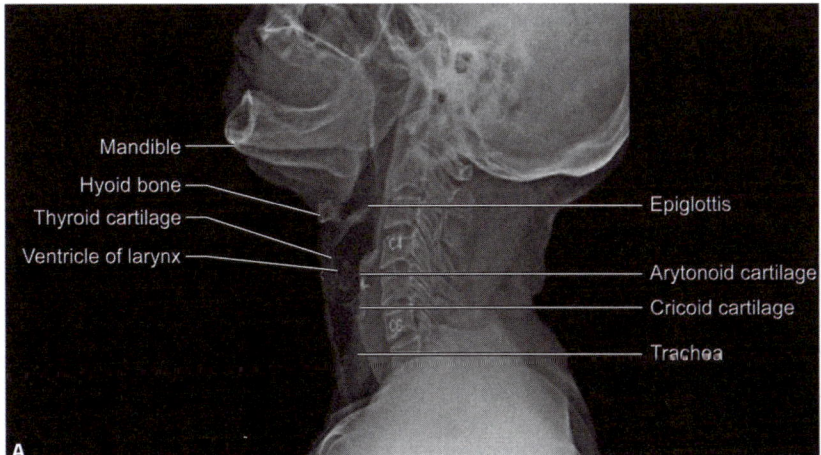
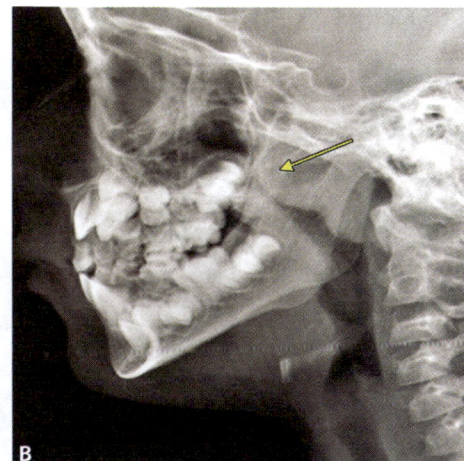

Figs. 6A and B: X-ray of nasopharynx. Lateral view showing soft tissue in nasopharynx.

PART 3: Miscellaneous Topics

Q. What are the features of adenoids?
- Sunken eyes
- Narrow piched nostril
- Open mouth
- High-arched palate
- Crowded teeth
- Loss of nasolabial fold
- Dull mask-like face
- Rhinorrhea
- Everted upper lip
- Protruding teeth
- Drooling of saliva

Aural manifestation in adenoids
- Otalgia
- Secretory otitis media
- Acute otitis media
- Atelectasis
- Endotracheal (ET) block
- Chronic otitis media

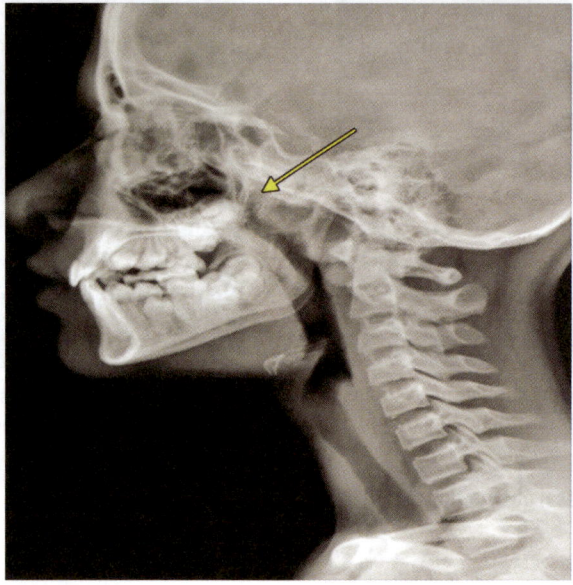

Q. What are the other methods to detect adenoids?
- Posterior rhinoscopy
- Digital palpation
- Examination under general anesthesia (GA)

Q. What is differential diagnosis of adenoids?
- Thornwaldt's cyst
- High-arched palate

■ USE WRITTEN REPORT IN CASE OF MANAGEMENT OF THIS PARANASAL SINUS PATHOLOGY

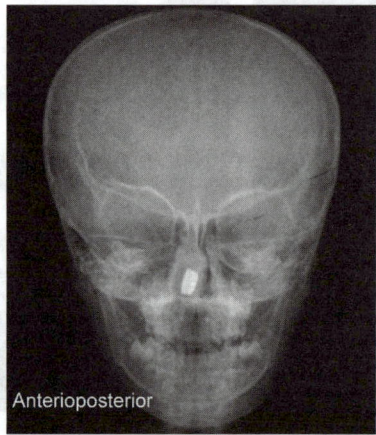
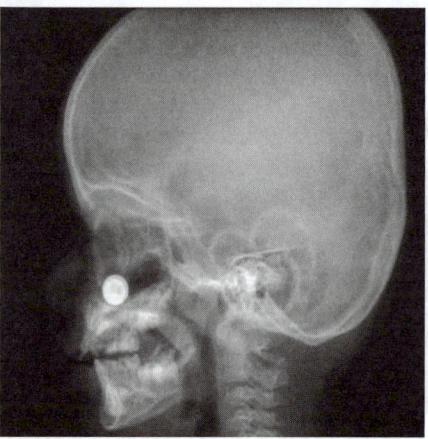

Fig. 7: X-ray of nose: Anteroposterior (AP) and lateral view showing metallic foreign body (battery cell).

CHAPTER 76: Radiology in ENT (X-rays)

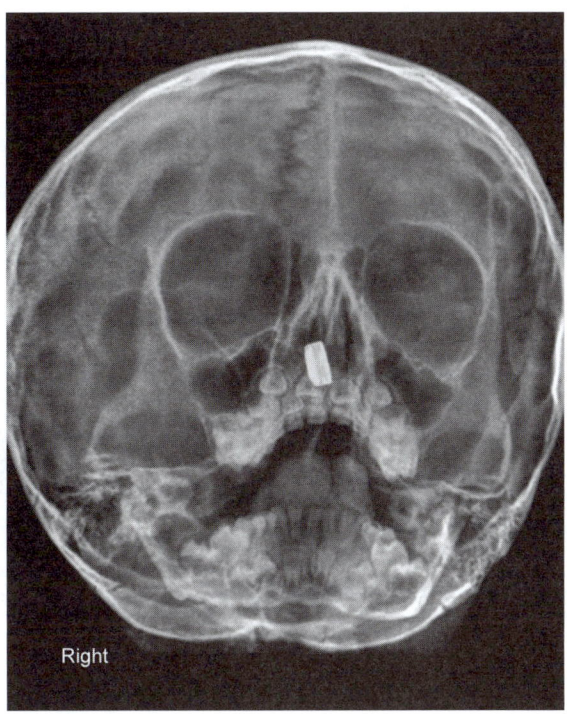

Fig. 8: X-ray of nose: Anteroposterior (AP) view showing metallic foreign body (battery cell).

Q. **Identify the foreign body.**

- **Management:** Manual or endoscopic removal of foreign body
- **Possible complications:**
  - Bleeding from nose (epistaxis)
  - Septal perforation due to chemical release from battery cell

■ INTERPRET THE X-RAY OF MASTOID

- **Type of pneumatization:** Cellular (well pneumatized), acellular (sclerotic), diploic
- Position of: Dural plate, sinus plate
- Presence of bone destruction
- Presence of mastoid cavity
- Presence of choleasteatoma
  When reading an X-ray of mastoid, never forget to comment on the following points:

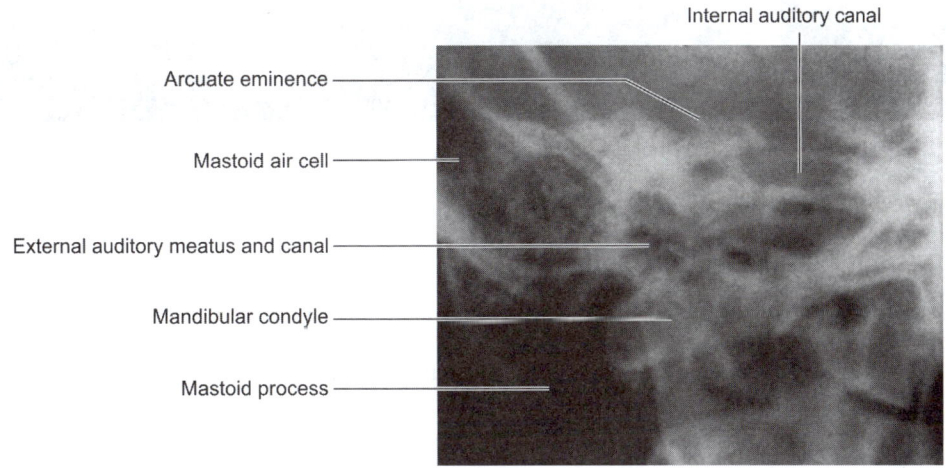

Q. Interpret the following mastoid pathologies:

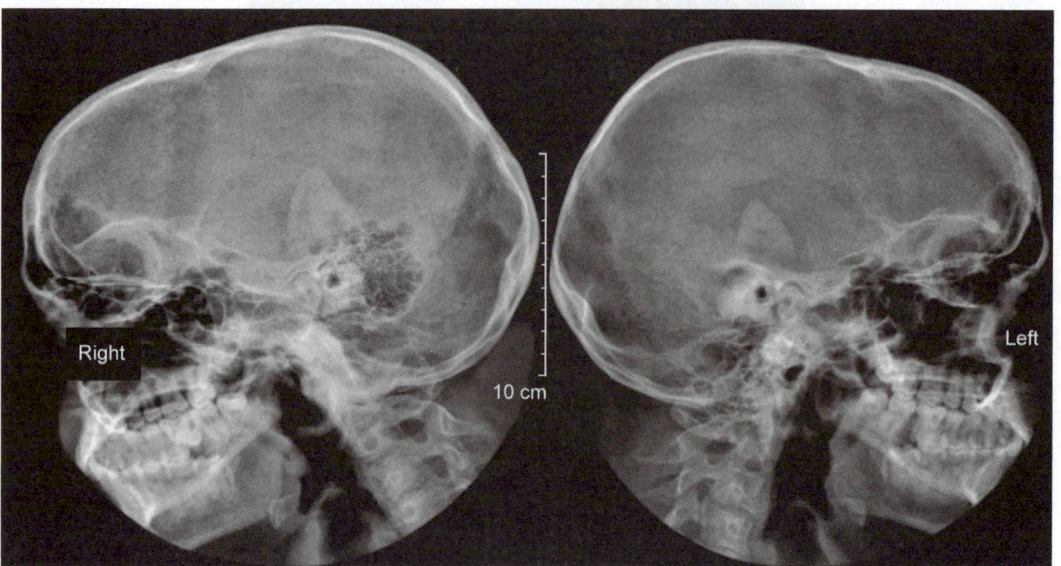

- Right mastoid is pneumatic.
- Left mastoid is sclerotic.

Q. What are the types of mastoid?

- Pneumatic, diploic, and sclerotic

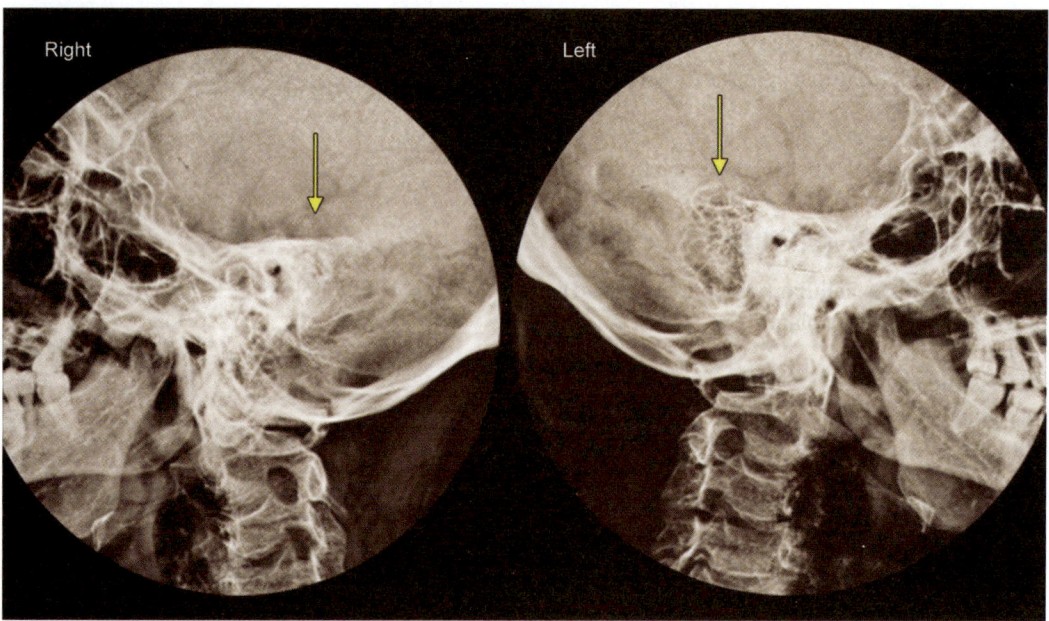

Fig. 9: X-ray of mastoid: Shuller's view showing right sclerotic and left pneumatic mastoid.

Q. What are different views?

Schuller's or Rugnstrom View (30° Lateral Oblique)

- Similar to Law's view but cephalocaudal beam makes an angle of 30° instead of 15°
- **Structures seen:**
    - External auditory canal (EAC) superimposed on internal auditory canal (IAC)

- Mastoid air cells
- Tegmen
- Lateral sinus plate
- Condyle of mandible
- Sinodural angle
- Attico-antral region

❖ **Structures seen:**
- External auditory canal (EAC) superimposed on internal auditory canal (IAC)
- Mastoid air cells
- Tegmen
- Lateral sinus plate
- Temporomandibular joint

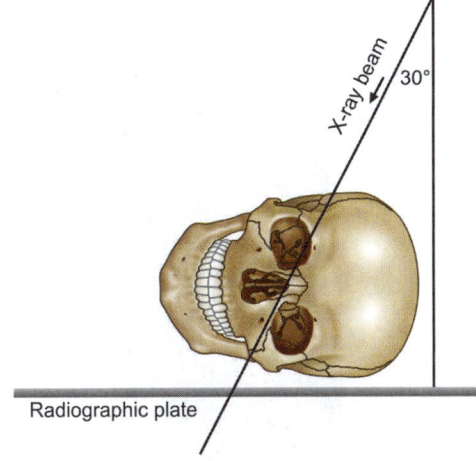

Law's View (15° Lateral Oblique)

❖ Sagittal plane of the skull is parallel to the film and X-ray beam is projected 15° cephalocaudal.
❖ It is the standard view of mastoids.

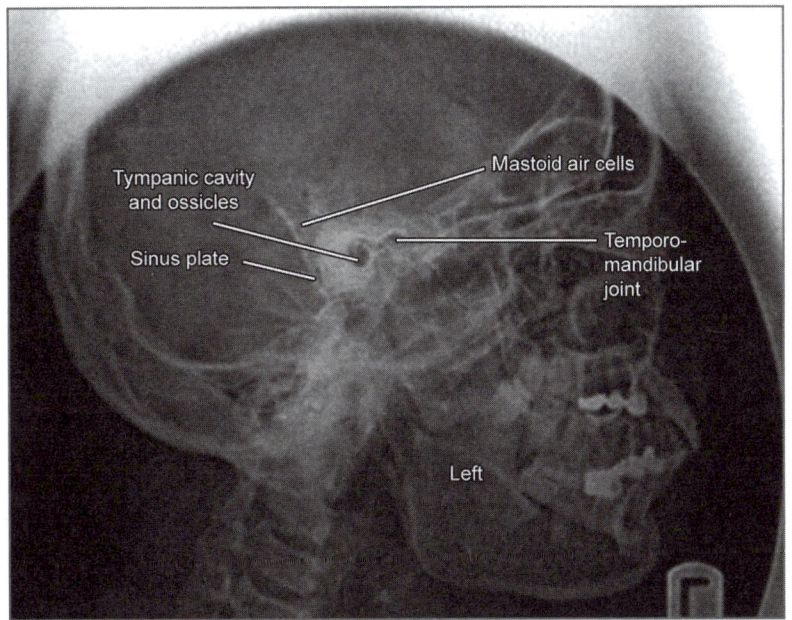

Towne's View

- **Towne's view** (30° fronto-occipital axial): **Anteroposterior** view at 30° tilt from above and in front
- It shows:
  - IAC of both sides
  - Petrous apex
  - Cochlea
  - Semicircular canals
  - Middle ear
  - Both external canal

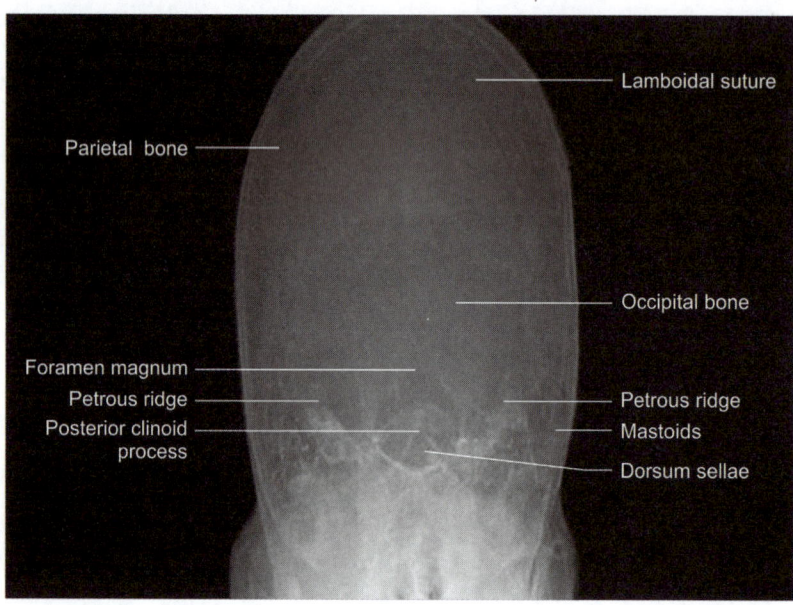

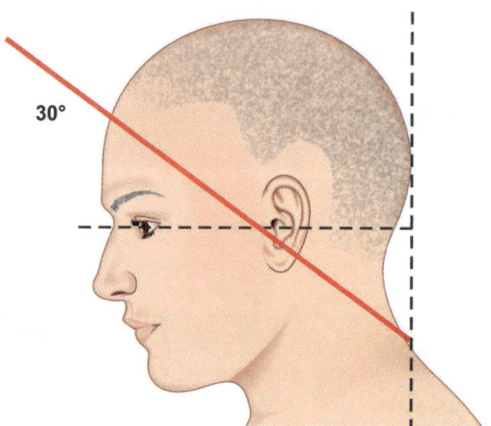

- **Submentovertical view (full axial):** Chin raised and neck hyperextended until orbitomeatal line is parallel to the film and the beam is projected at right angles to the film from submental area.

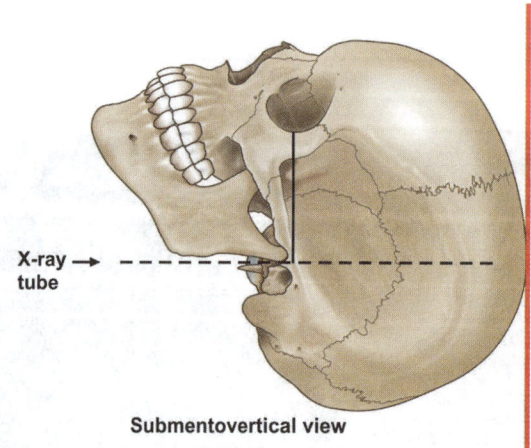

Transorbital View (Anteroposterior or Posterior Anterior)

AP or PA view with orbitomeatal line perpendicular to the film and the X-ray beam also perpendicular to the film.
- This is an anteroposterior view of skull
- Orbitomeatal line is at right angles to the film
- X-ray beam passes through the orbit
- **Structures seen:** IAC, cochlea, labyrinth and both petrous pyramids projected through the orbits
- **Clinical applications:** Acoustic neuroma and petrous pyramid

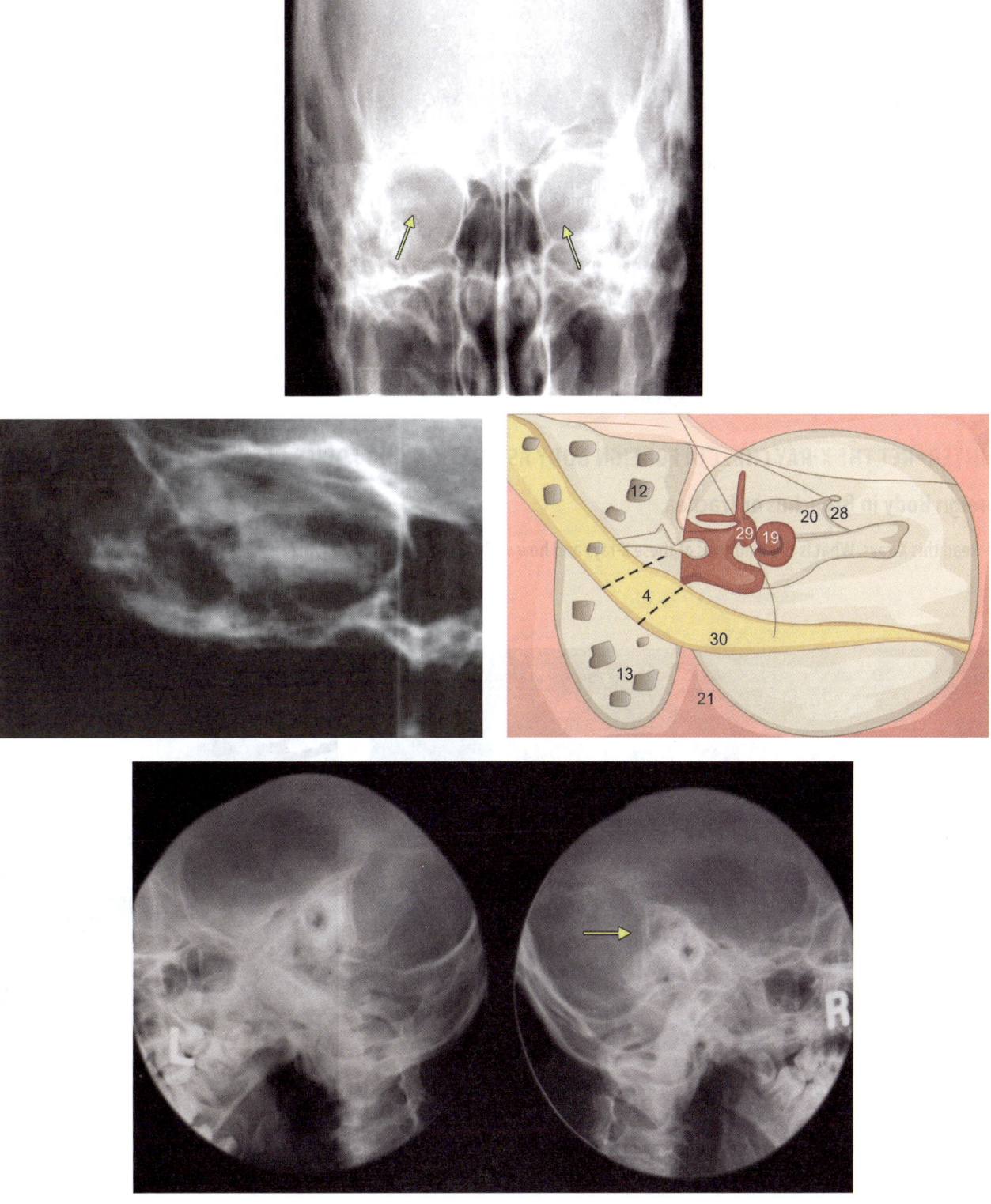

Fig. 10: X-ray of mastoid: Shuller's view showing radiolucent cavity in right mastoid.

Stenver's View (Axio-Anterior Oblique Posterior)

Facing the film and head slightly flexed and rotated to 45° to the opposite of side under examination and X-ray beam is angulated 14° caudal.

It shows:
- IAC
- Cochlea
- Semicircular canal
- Mastoid process
- Petrous apex

Q. Read this X-ray and give the diagnosis.

Q. What are the causes of radiolucent cavity within mastoid?
- Cholesteatoma
- Operated mastoidectomy
- Large antral cell
- Malignancy
- Eosinophic granuloma
- Tuberculosis
- Multiple myloma
- Metastasis from kidney, bronchus, and breast

INTERPRET THE X-RAY CHEST IN FOREIGN BODY ASPIRATION AND LOWER RESPIRATORY TRACT INFECTION

Foreign Body in Bronchus or Trachea

Q. Read this X-rays. What is the diagnosis of these X-rays and how will you manage this patient?

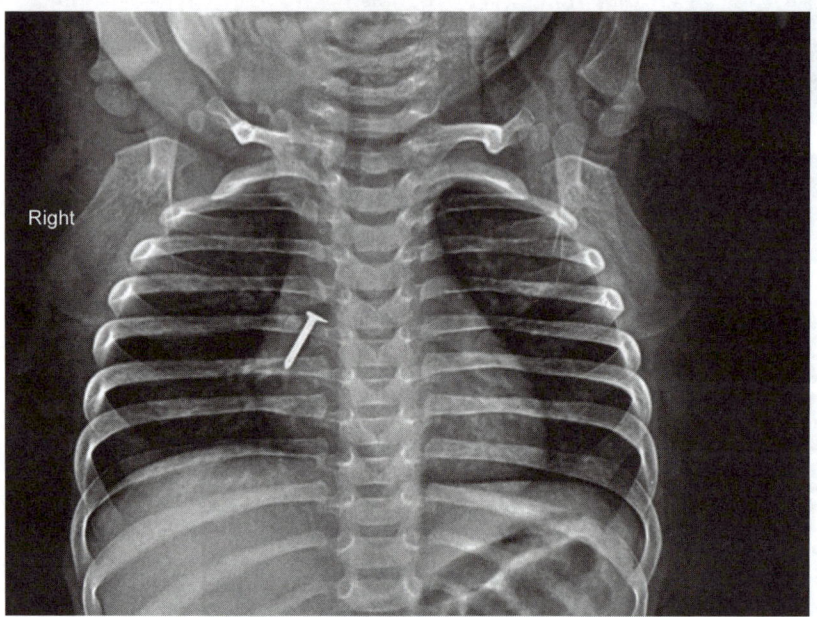

Fig. 11: X-ray of chest: PA view showing metallic foreign body (nail) in right main bronchus.

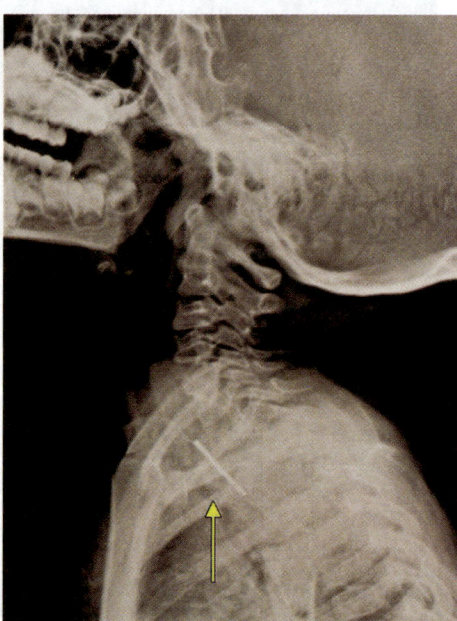

Fig. 12: X-ray of chest and neck: Lateral view showing metallic foreign body (nail) in bronchus.

CHAPTER 76: Radiology in ENT (X-rays)

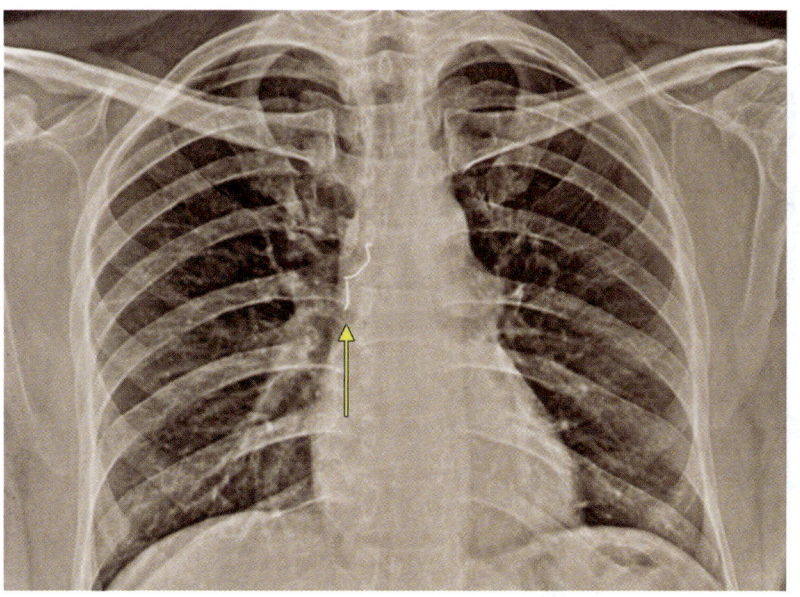

Fig. 13: X-ray of chest: PA view showing metallic foreign body (wire) in right main bronchus.

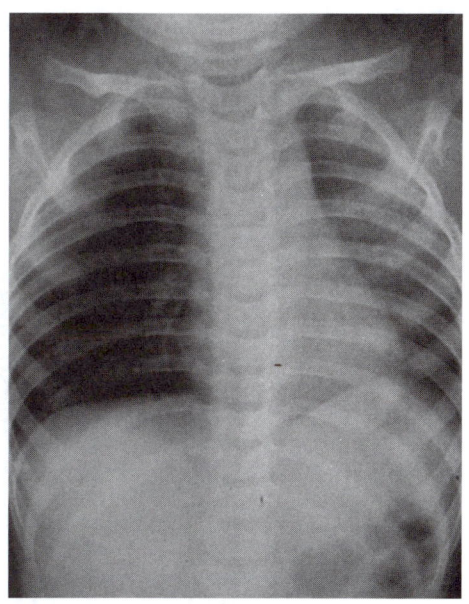

Fig. 14: X-ray of chest showing unilateral lung collapse.

Q. What is a diagnosis of these X-rays and how will you manage this patient?

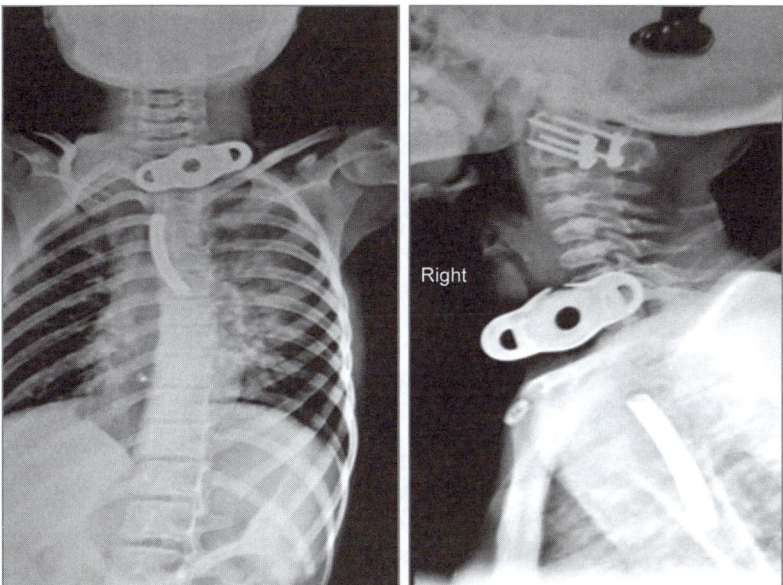

Fig. 15: X-ray of neck: AP and lateral view showing metallic foreign body (broken metallic tracheostomy tube).

Treatment: Removal of foreign body using bronchoscope and forceps

X-RAY OF NECK: LATERAL VIEW

Interpret X-ray of the Neck

- Foreign body
- Foreign body aspiration
- Parapharyngeal
- Retropharyngeal abscess

PART 3: Miscellaneous Topics

Q. What is the diagnosis of these X-rays and how will you manage this patient?

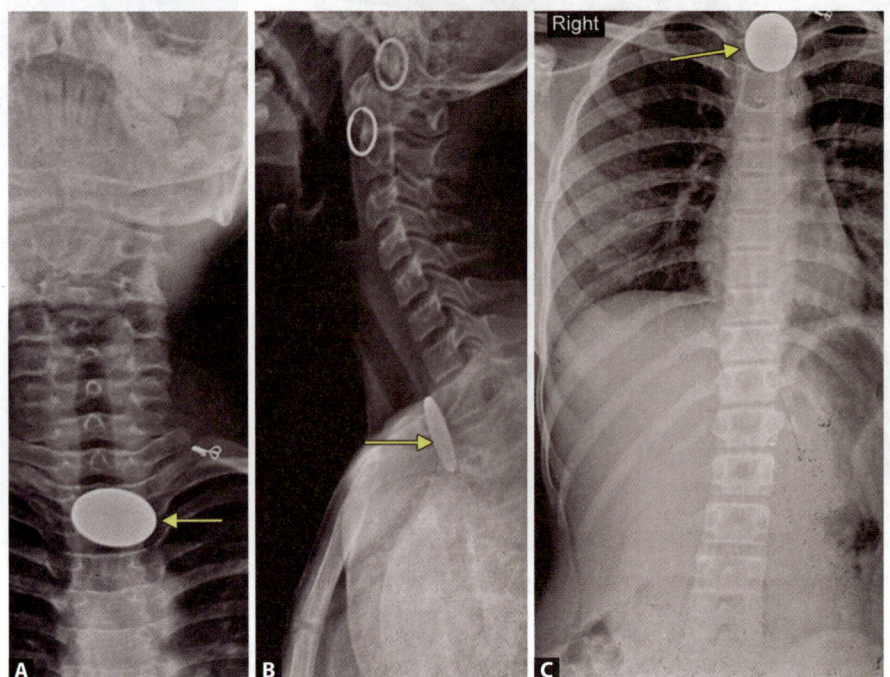

Figs. 16A to C: X-ray of neck: AP, lateral view, and (B and C) X-ray of chest: PA view showing metallic foreign body (coin) in esophagus (at the level of cricopharynx, which is the narrowest constriction of esophagus).

❖ **Management:** Removal of foreign body by esophagoscopy/cricopharyngoscopy surgery using forceps

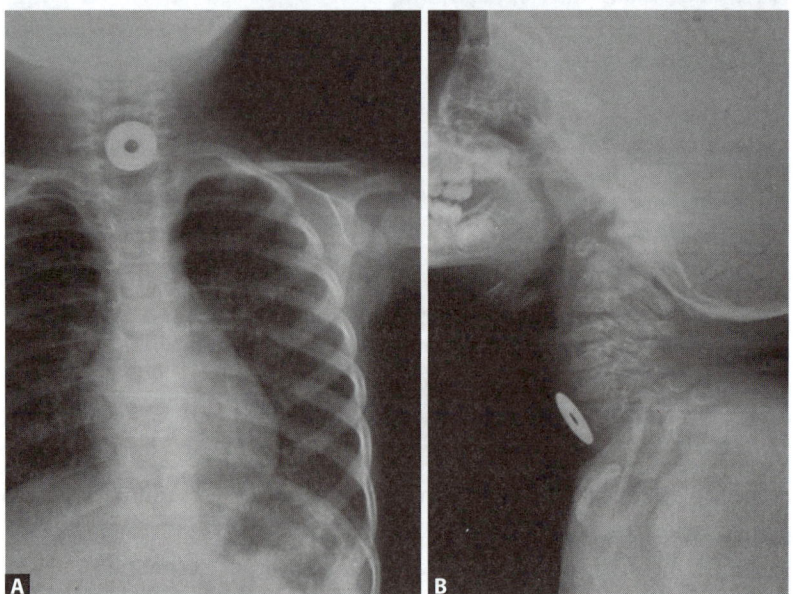

Figs. 17A and B: X-ray of neck AP, lateral view, and (B) X-ray of chest: PA view showing metallic foreign body (whistle) in esophagus (at the level of cricopharynx, which is the narrowest constriction of esophagus).

CHAPTER 76: Radiology in ENT (X-rays)

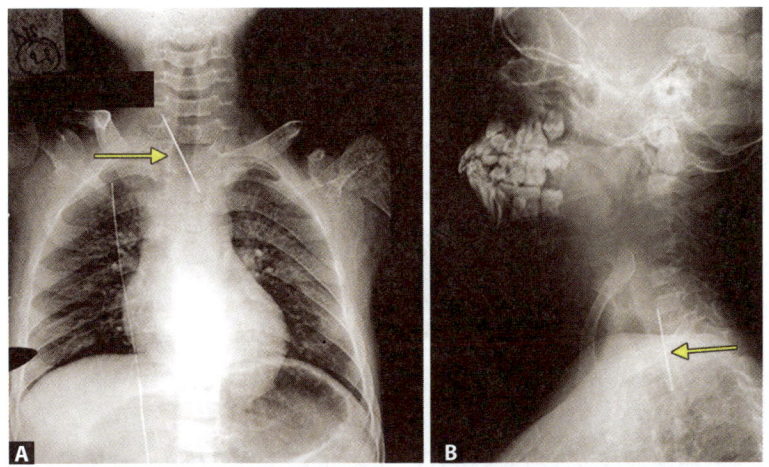

Figs. 18A and B: X-ray of neck AP, lateral view, and (B) X-ray of chest: PA view showing metallic foreign body in esophagus (at the level of cricopharynx, which is the narrowest constriction of esophagus)—needle.

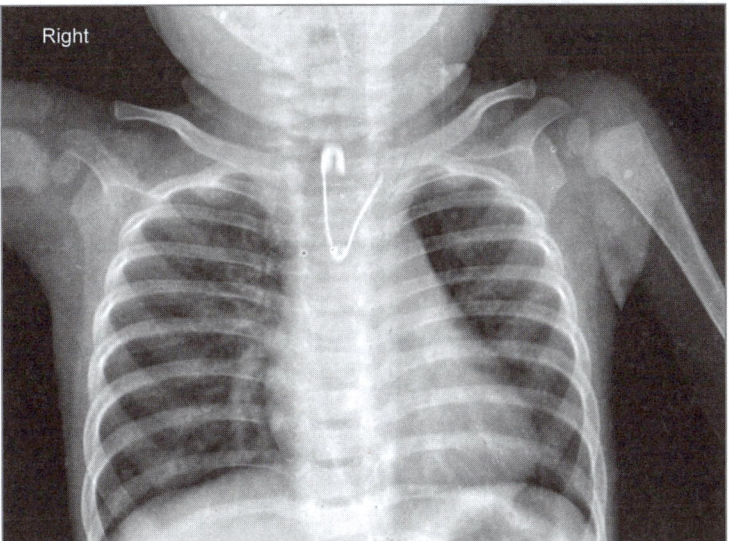

Fig. 19: X-ray of neck and chest: PA view showing metallic foreign body in esophagus (at the level of cricopharynx, which is the narrowest constriction of esophagus)—open safety pin in favorable lie.

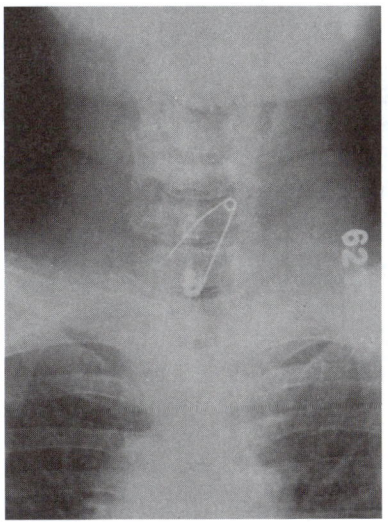

Fig. 20: X-ray of neck and chest: PA view showing metallic foreign body in esophagus (at the level of cricopharynx, which is the narrowest constriction of esophagus)—open safety pin in unfavorable lie.

PART 3: Miscellaneous Topics

Q. How will you remove safety pin in unfavorable lie?

RETROPHARYNGEAL ABSCESS

Q. Read this X-rays. What is the diagnosis?

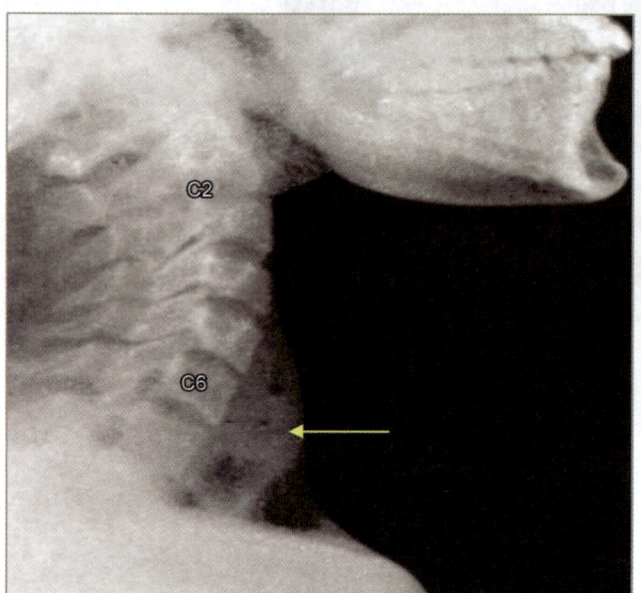
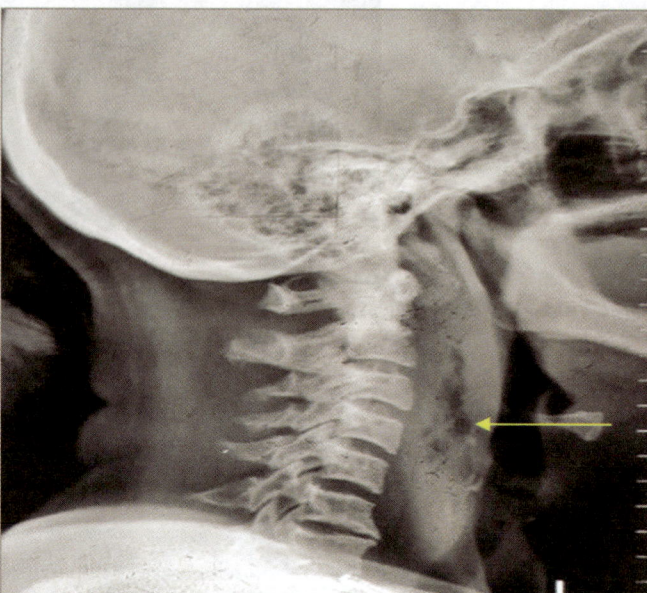

Fig. 21: X-ray of neck: Lateral view showing retropharyngeal abscess with air bubbles in abscess soft tissue.

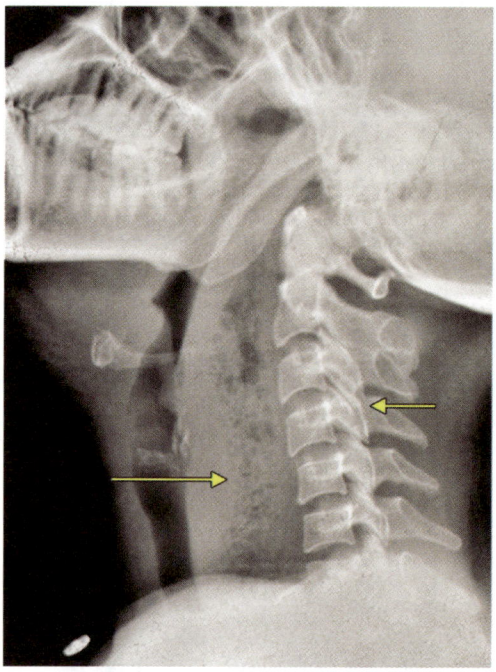

Fig. 22: X-ray of neck: Lateral view showing retropharyngeal abscess with air bubbles in abscess soft tissue and straightening of cervical spine.

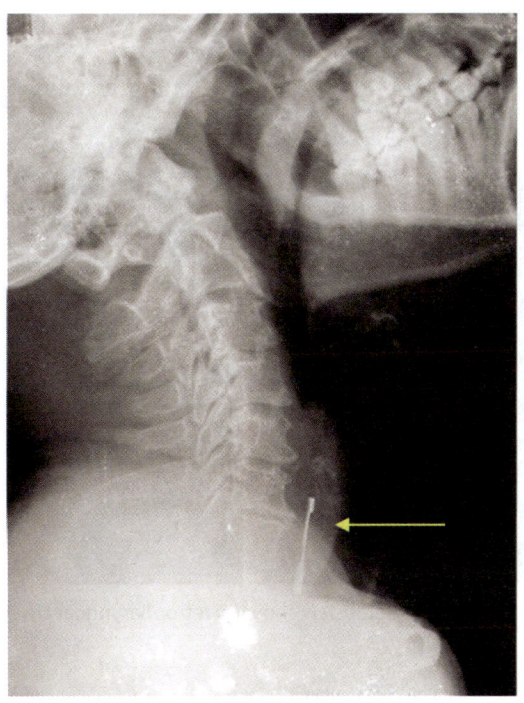

Fig. 23: Diagnosis: X-ray of neck—lateral view showing retropharyngeal abscess with foreign body safety pin.

Q. What are the cases of retropharyngeal abscess?

- Most common cause in children—tuberculosis (TB)
  - Can be missed due to calcified cartilage
  - Also look for impending retropharyngeal abscess formation

Change of management protocol:

- **Most common cause in adults:** Penetrating foreign bodies such as chicken bone, fish bone, etc.
- **Management of retropharyngeal abscess:** Acute/chronic

Q. What is Lincoln Highway? Enumerate its importance.

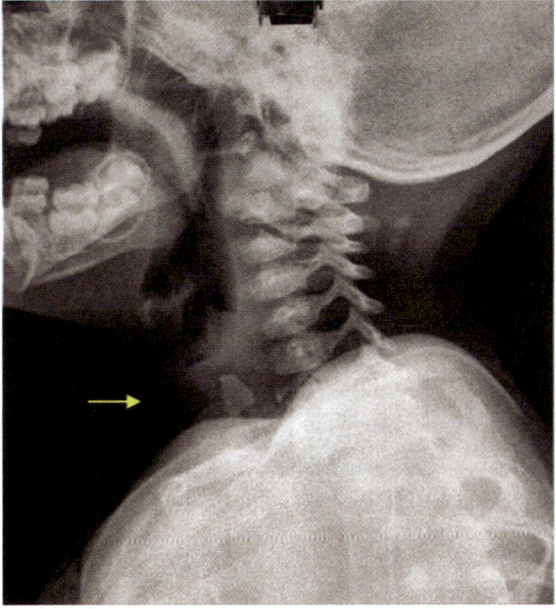

Fig. 24: X-ray of neck: Lateral view showing retropharyngeal abscess with chicken bone.

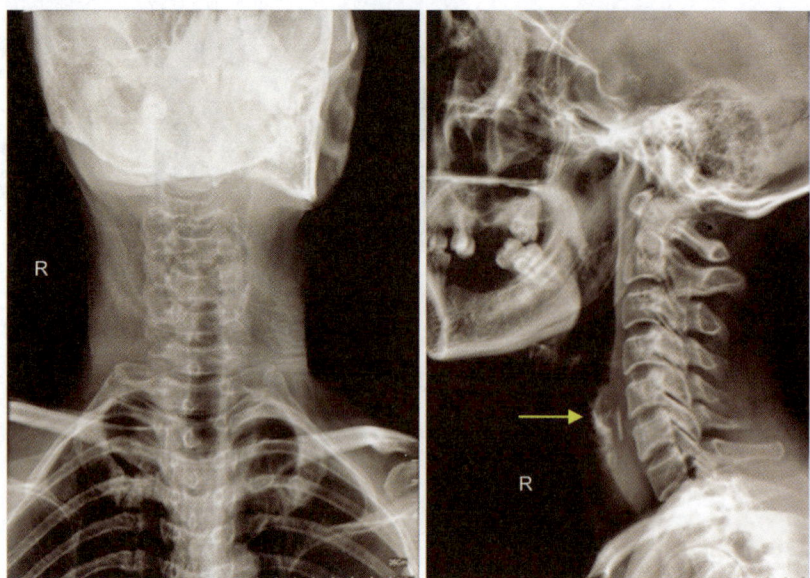

Fig. 25: X-ray of neck: AP and lateral view showing retropharyngeal abscess with fish bone.

X-ray nasal bone:
- Types of nasal bone fracture
- Classification of Lee Forte's facial fracture
- Management of patient with nasal bone fracture
- Septal hematoma and septal abscess

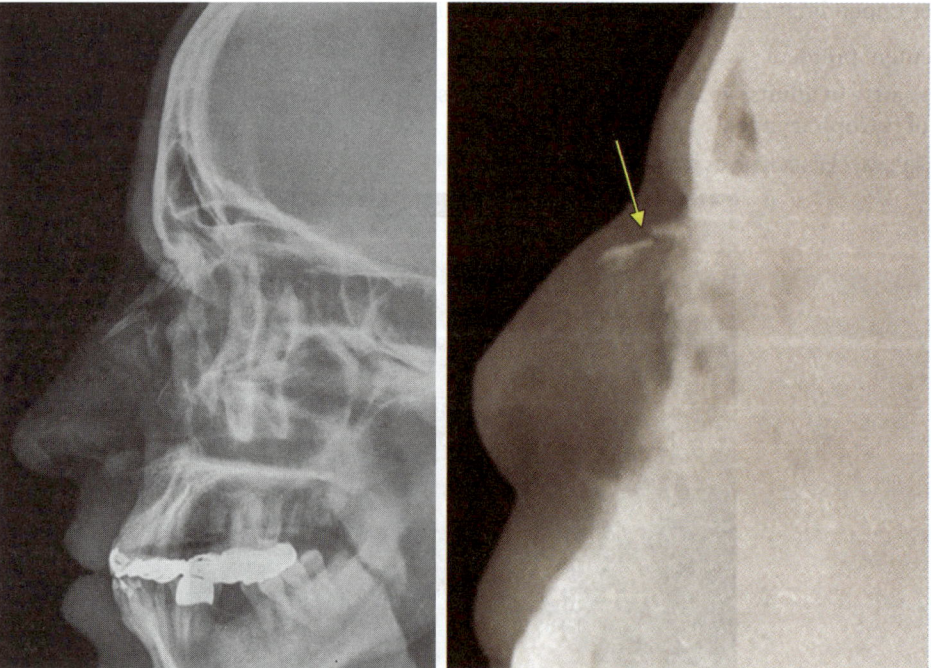

Fig. 26: X-ray of nasal bone—lateral view showing displaced fracture of nasal bone.

CHAPTER 76: Radiology in ENT (X-rays)

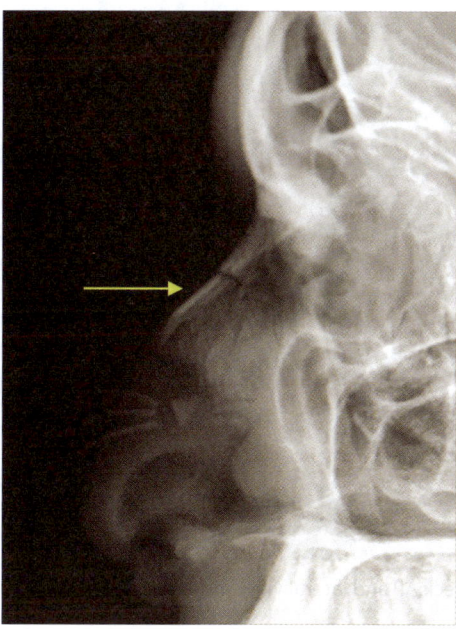

Fig. 27: X-ray of nasal bone—lateral view showing undisplaced fracture of nasal bone.

Esophagoscopy

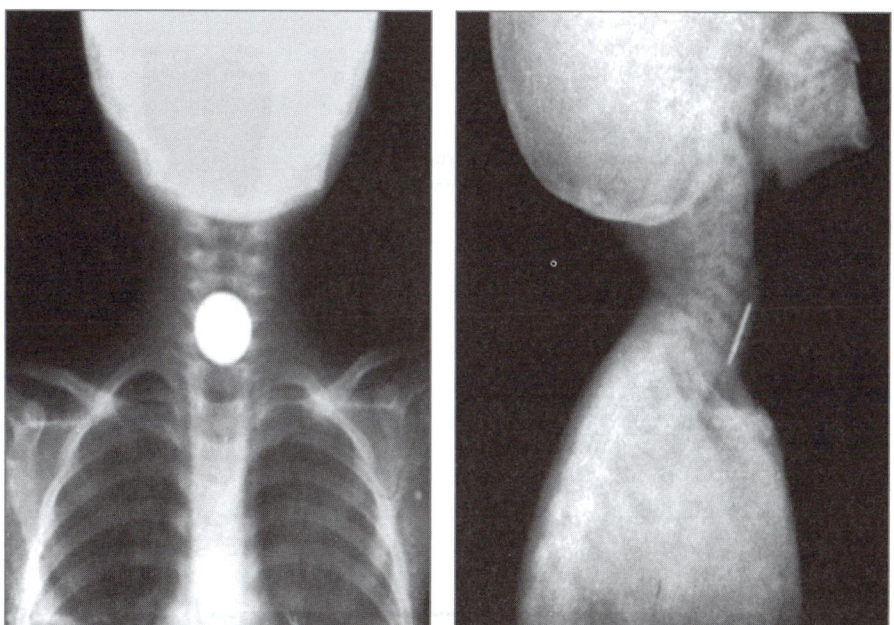

Fig. 28: X-ray of neck: AP and lateral view showing battery cell.

Q. Identify the type of foreign body—coin/pebble/battery.

Q. Where it is located? Esophagus/trachea

Q. What is significance of battery cell foreign body in esophagus? How to manage?

PART 3: Miscellaneous Topics

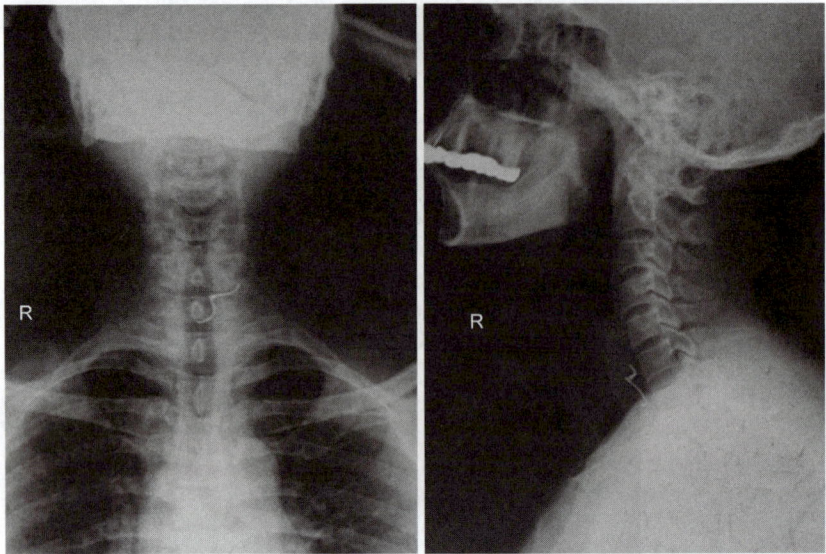

Fig. 29: X-ray of neck: AP and lateral view showing foreign body (wire) in esophagus.

- History
- Management
- Possible complications

Q. What are the common sites of obstructions in esophagus?

Q. What are the constrictions in esophagus?

Natural constrictions

Site	Vertebral level	Distance from central incisor
Cricopharynx	C 6	15 cm
Aortic arch	T 4	25 cm
Left main bronchus	T 5	28 cm
Esophageal hiatus	T 10	40 cm

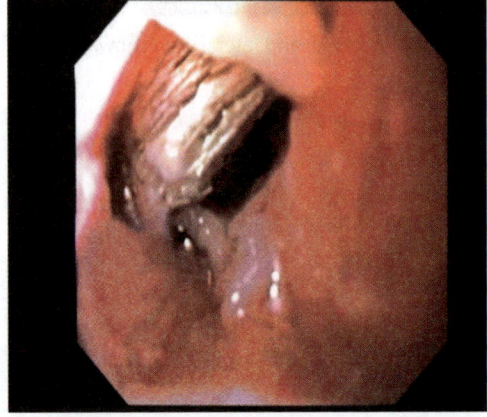

Fig. 30: Flexible esophagoscopy.

Chapter 77: CT Scan and MRI

EN2.6: Choose correctly and interpret radiological, microbiological and histological investigations relevant to the ENT disorders.

CT SCAN / MRI OF EAR

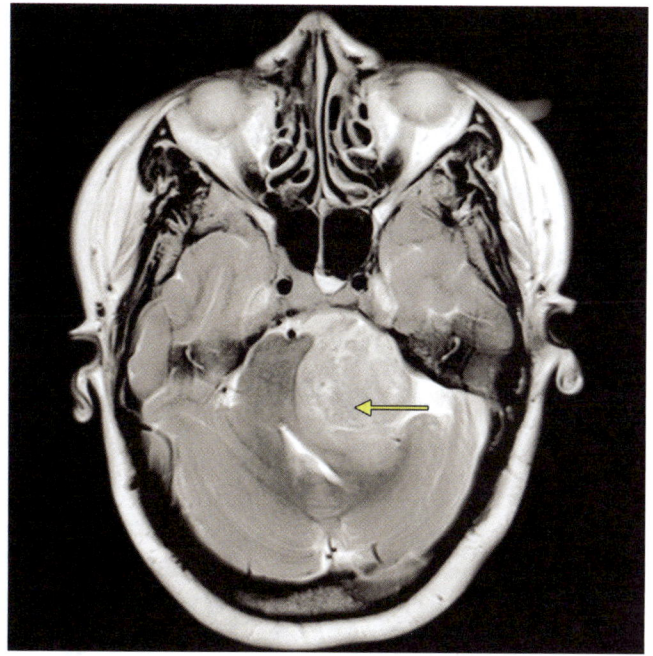

Fig.1: MRI showing acoustic neuroma.

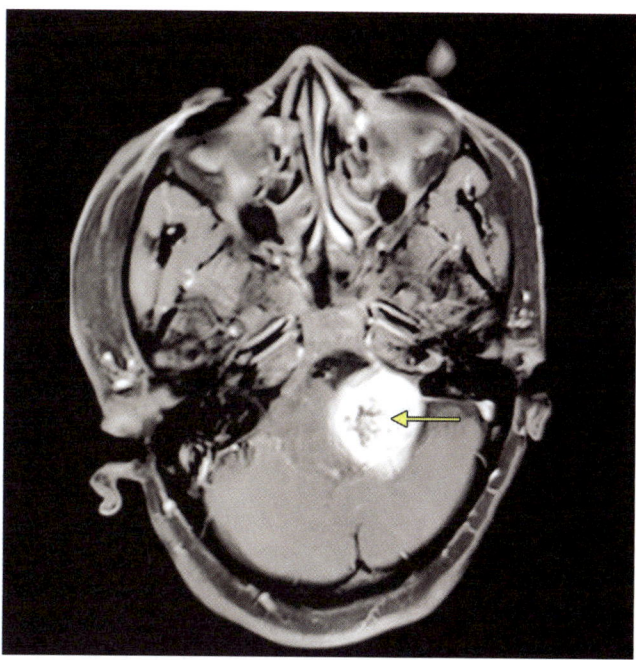

Fig. 2: MRI contrast showing acoustic neuroma.

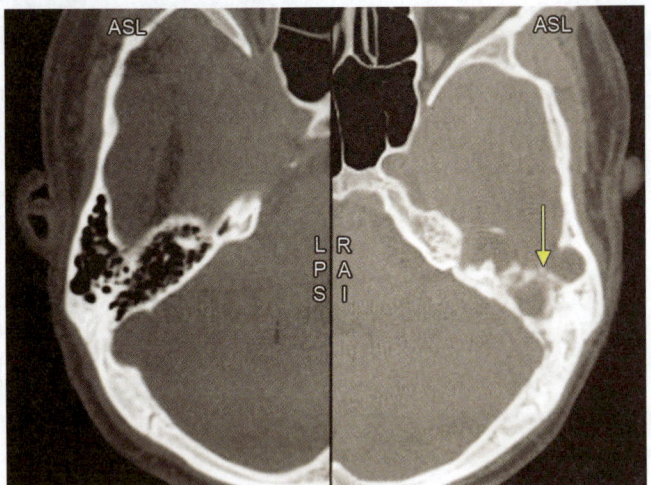

Fig. 3: High resolution computed tomography (HRCT) temporal bone with brain showing petrous apex erosion with sclerosis of mastoid and dural plate erosion (Gradenigo's syndrome).

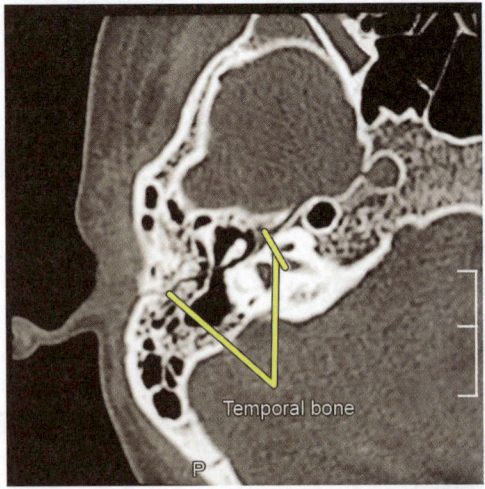

Fig. 4: High resolution computed tomography (HRCT) temporal bone showing longitudinal fracture of temporal bone (axial cut).

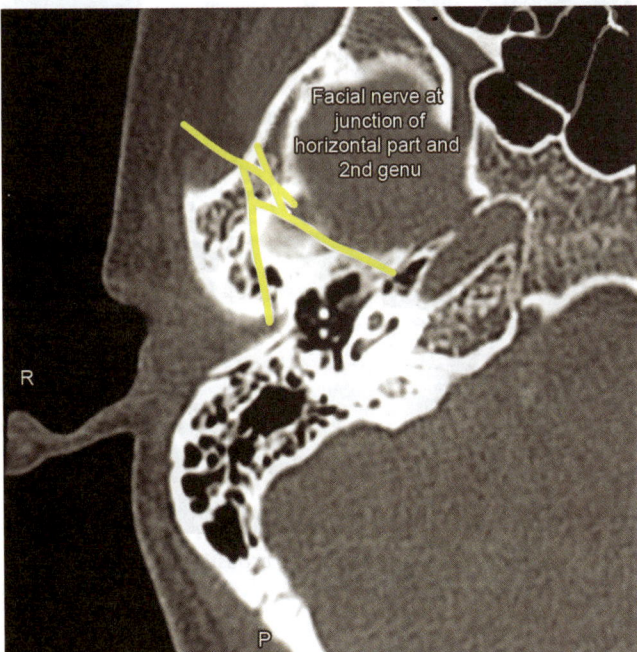

Fig. 5: High resolution computed tomography (HRCT) temporal bone showing fracture of temporal bone going through second genu of facial nerve.

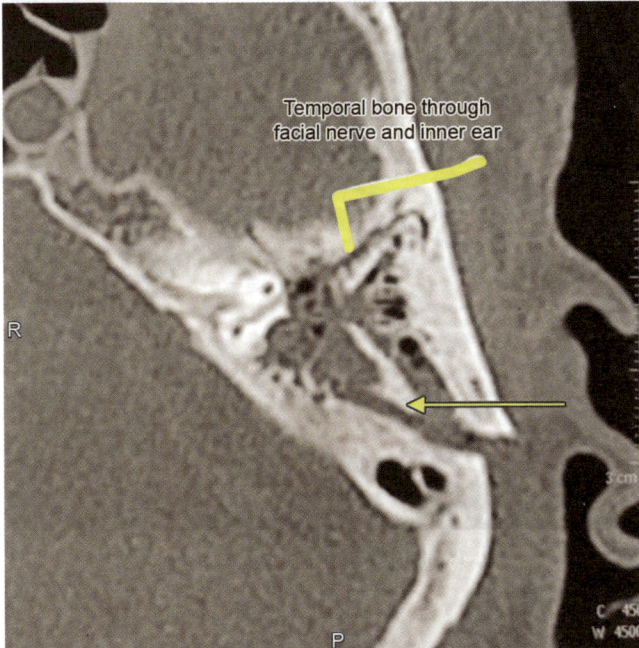

Fig. 6: High resolution computed tomography (HRCT) temporal bone showing extensive mixed fracture going through inner ear and facial nerve.

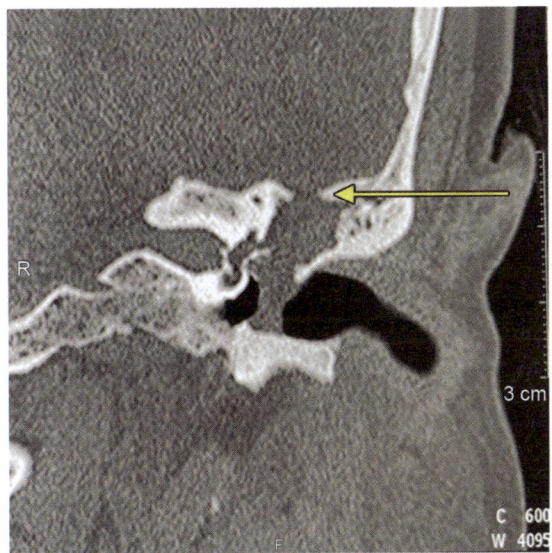

Fig. 7: High resolution computed tomography (HRCT) temporal bone showing soft tissue in middle ear, mastoid cavity with erosion of dural plate.

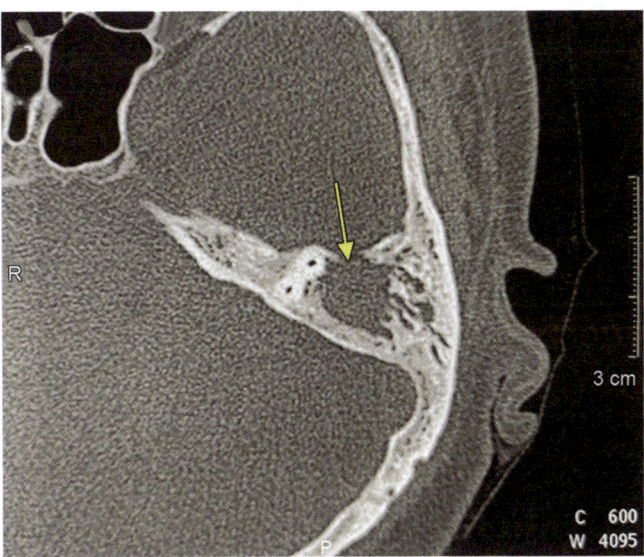

Fig. 8: High resolution computed tomography (HRCT) temporal bone showing erosion of dural plate.

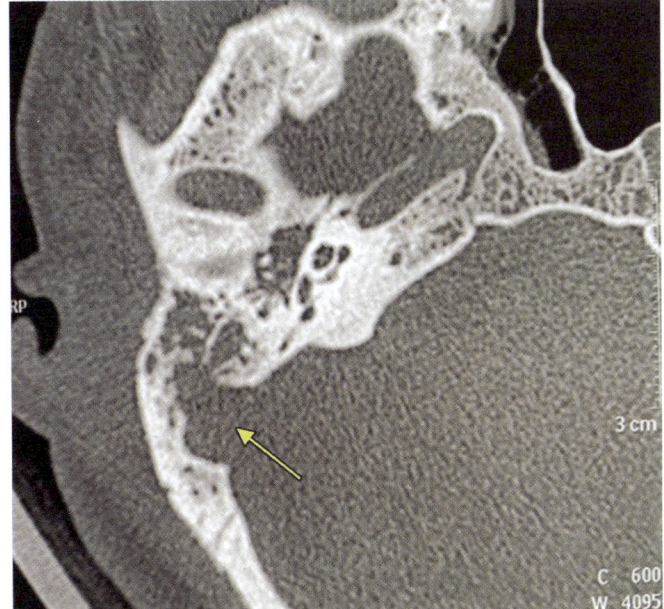

Fig. 9: High resolution computed tomography (HRCT) temporal bone showing soft tissue, sclerosis of mastoid with erosion of sinus plate.

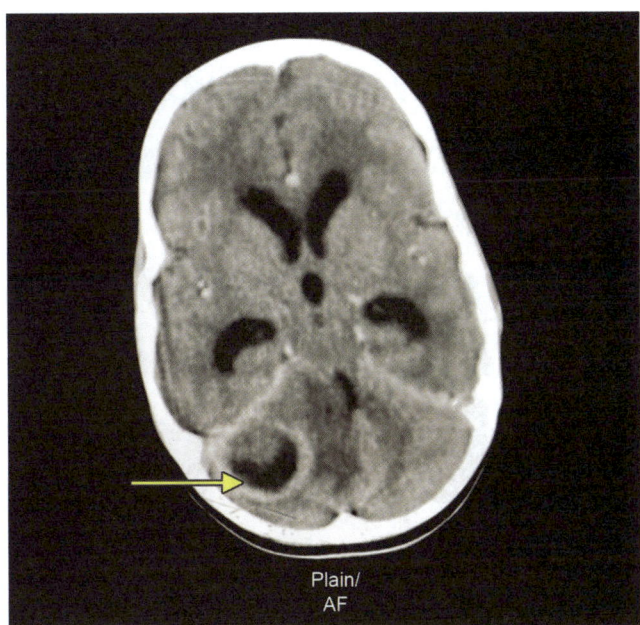

Fig. 10: CT scan showing cerebellar abscess.

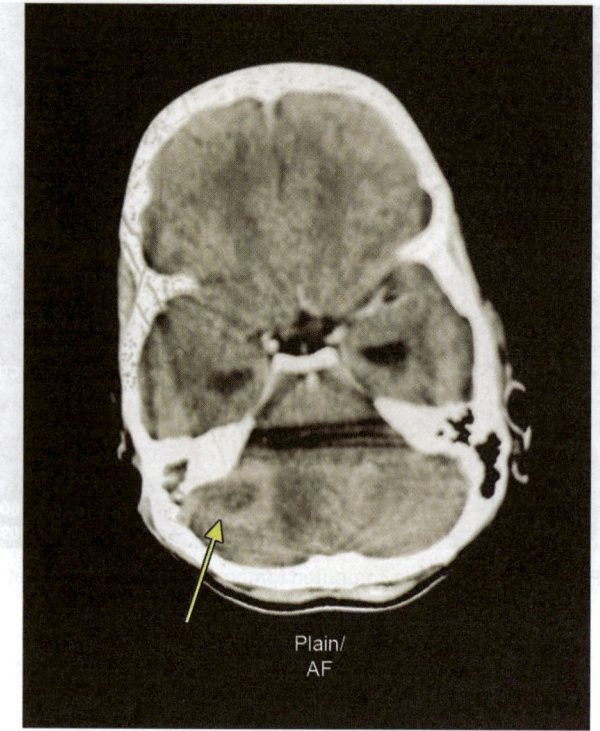

Fig. 11: CT scan showing sclerosis of mastoid with erosion of sinus plate and cerebellar abscess.

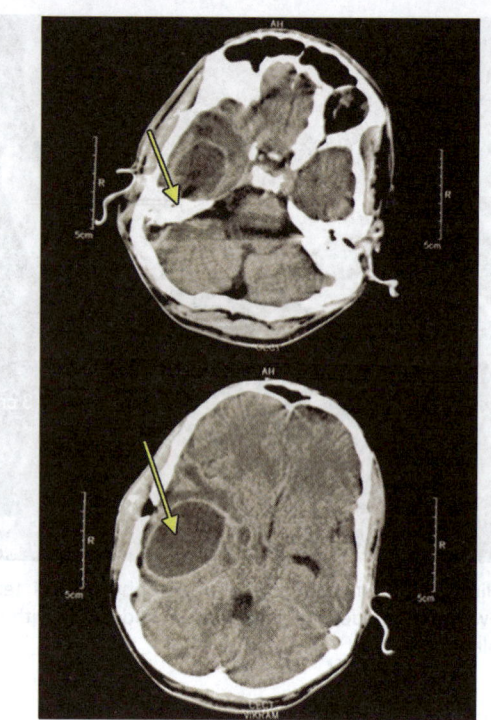

Fig. 12: CT scan showing scerotic mastoid with temporal lobe abscess with ring enhancement.

CT SCAN/MRI OF NOSE AND PARANASAL SINUSES

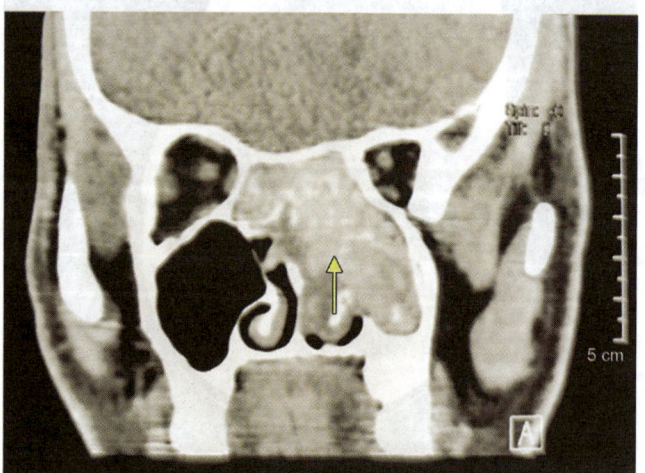

Fig. 13: CT scan showing contrast-enhancing mass in nose and shenoid sinus (angiofibroma), salt and pepper appearance.

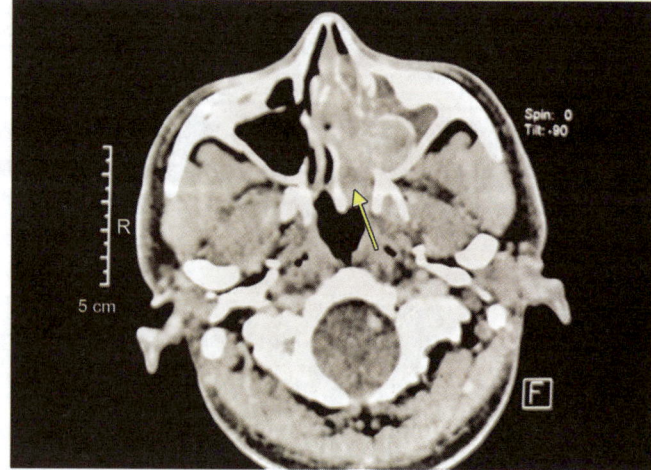

Fig. 14: CT paranasal sinus (PNS) showing angifibroma with widening of sphenopalatine foramina.

CHAPTER 77: CT Scan and MRI

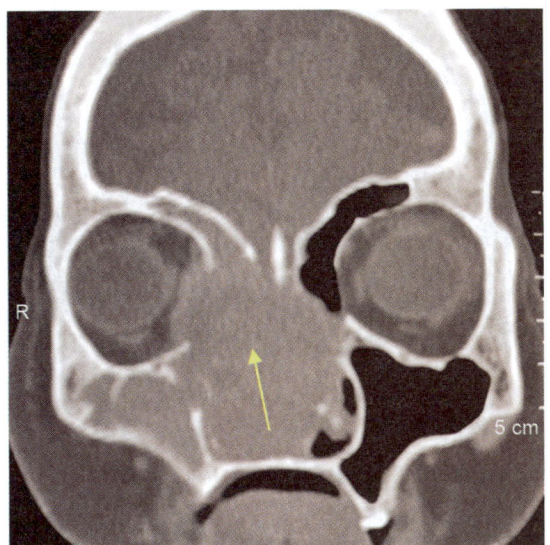

Fig. 15: CT scan of nose and paranasal sinus (PNS) showing nasal mass erroding nasal septum, maxillary sinus, and lamina papyracea suggestive of carcinoma maxilla.

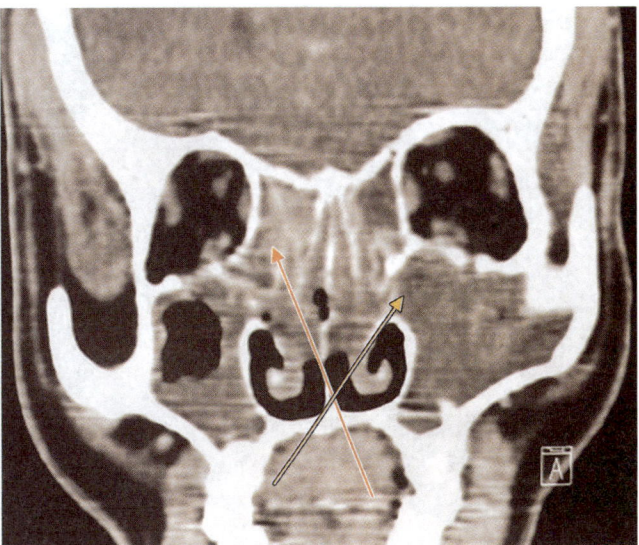

Fig. 16: CT nose and paranasal sinus (PNS) showing maxillary and ethmoid sinusitis.

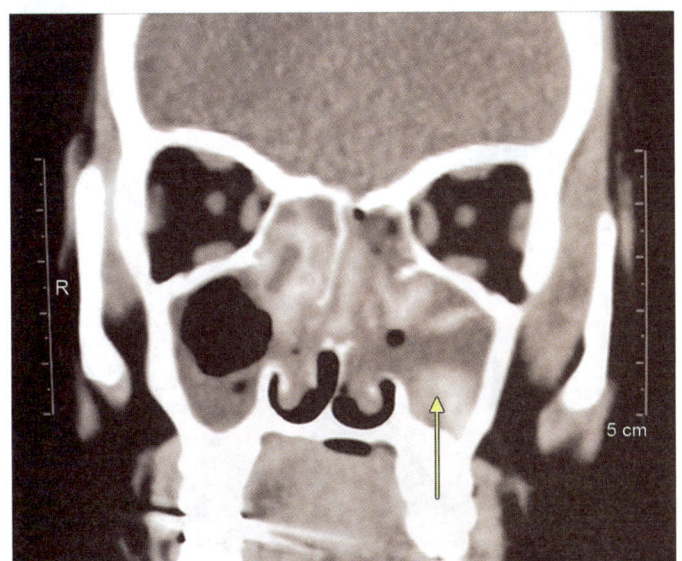

Fig. 17: CT paranasal sinus (PNS) showing fungal concretions in maxillary and ethmoid sinuses suggestive of allergic fungal sinusitis (AFS).

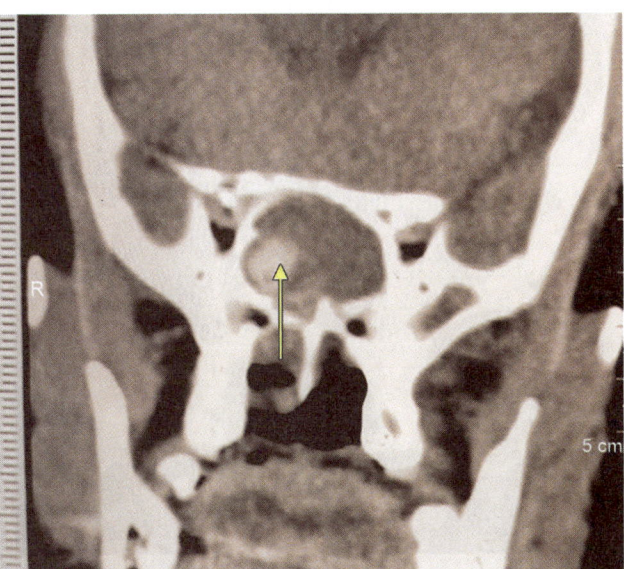

Fig. 18: CT paranasal sinus (PNS) showing fungal concretions of allergic fungal sinusitis (AFS) in sphenoid sinus.

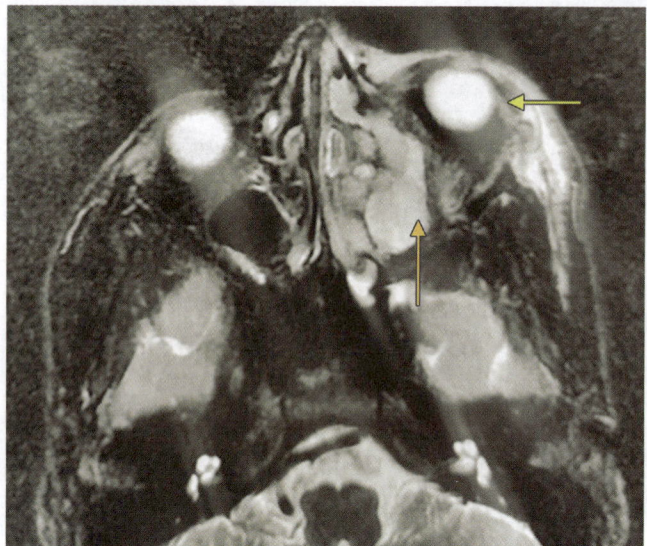

Fig. 19: MRI paranasal sinus (PNS) and nose showing ethmoid and sphenoid sinusitis with orbital proptosis.

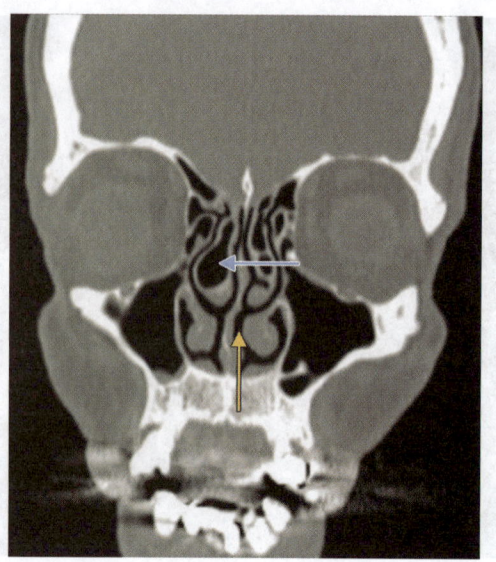

Fig. 20: CT nose and paranasal sinus (PNS) showing "S"-shaped deviated nasal septum (DNS) with concha bullosa of right middle turbinate.

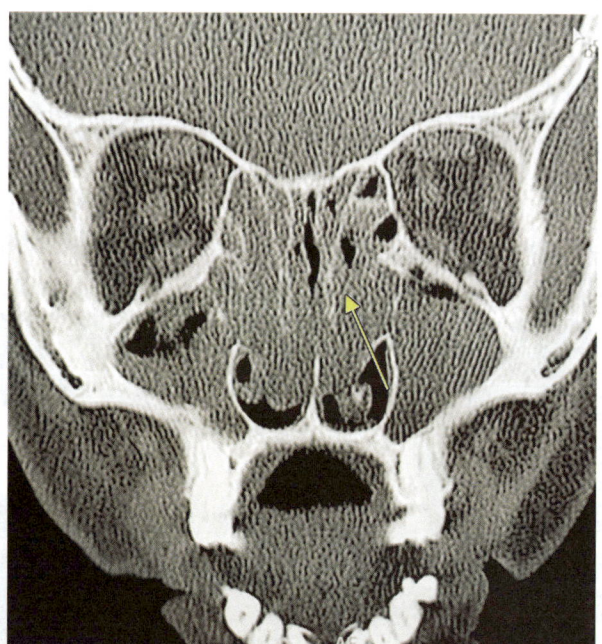

Fig. 21: CT paranasal sinus (PNS) showing nasal polyps in maxillary and ethmoid sinus.

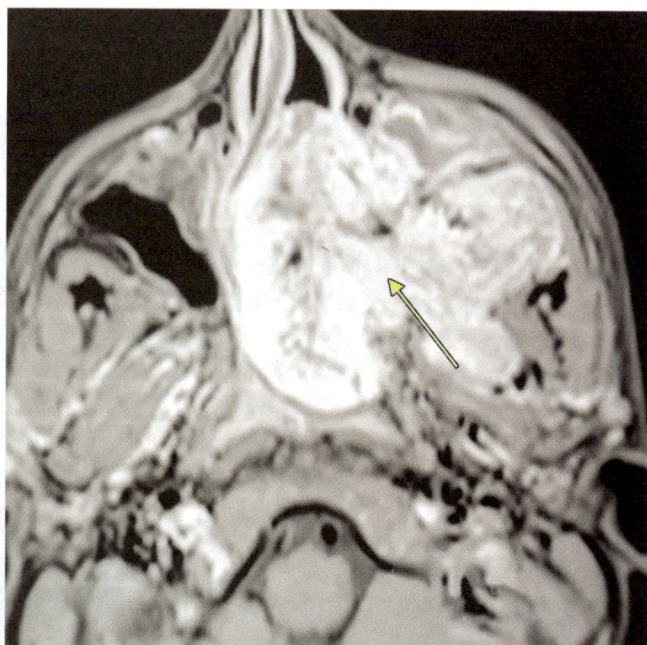

Fig. 22: MRI nose and paranasal sinus (PNS) showing contrast-enhanced mass-extensive angiofibroma extending into infratemporal fossa.

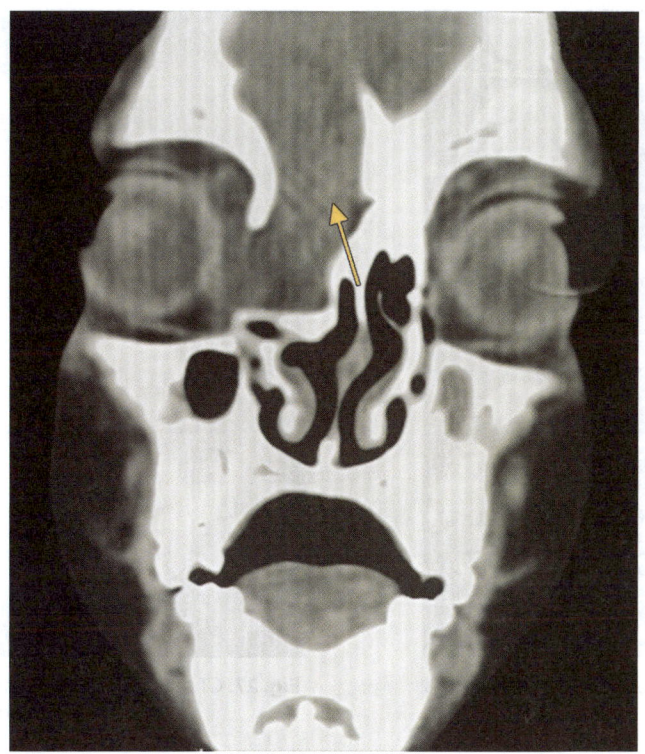

Fig. 23: CT paranasal sinus (PNS) showing defect in the roof of nose suggestive of meningoencephalocele.

CT SCAN/MRI OF NECK

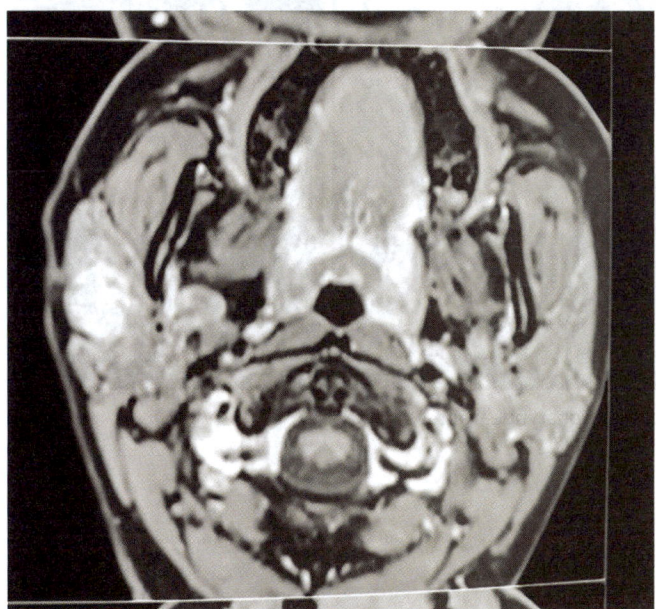

Fig. 24: MRI neck showing mass in right parotid gland suggestive of pleomorphic adenoma.

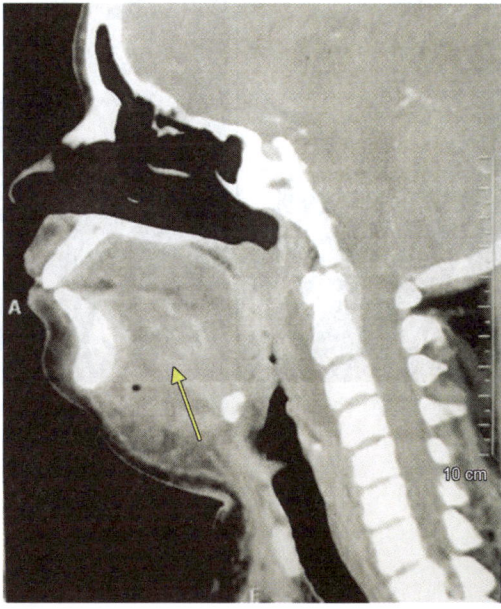

Fig. 25: CT scan of neck lateral view showing Ludwig's angina.

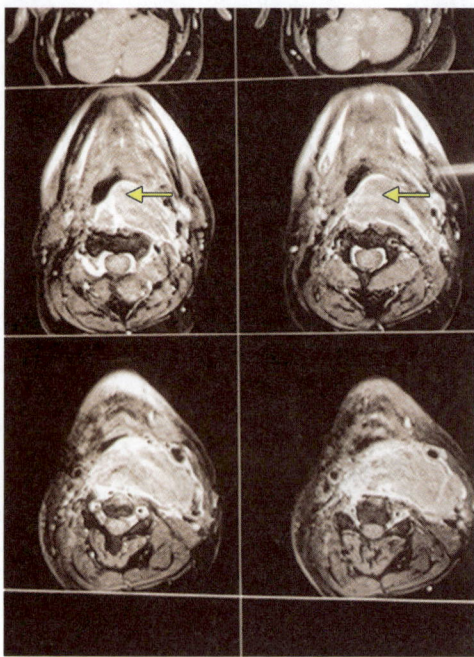

Fig. 26: MRI neck showing parapharyngeal abscess.

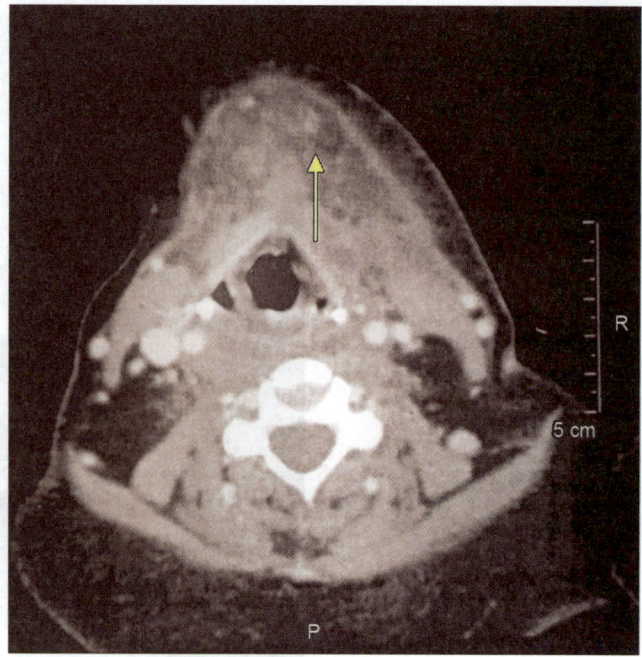

Fig. 27: CT scan of neck showing abscess in submandibular space, Ludwig's angina.

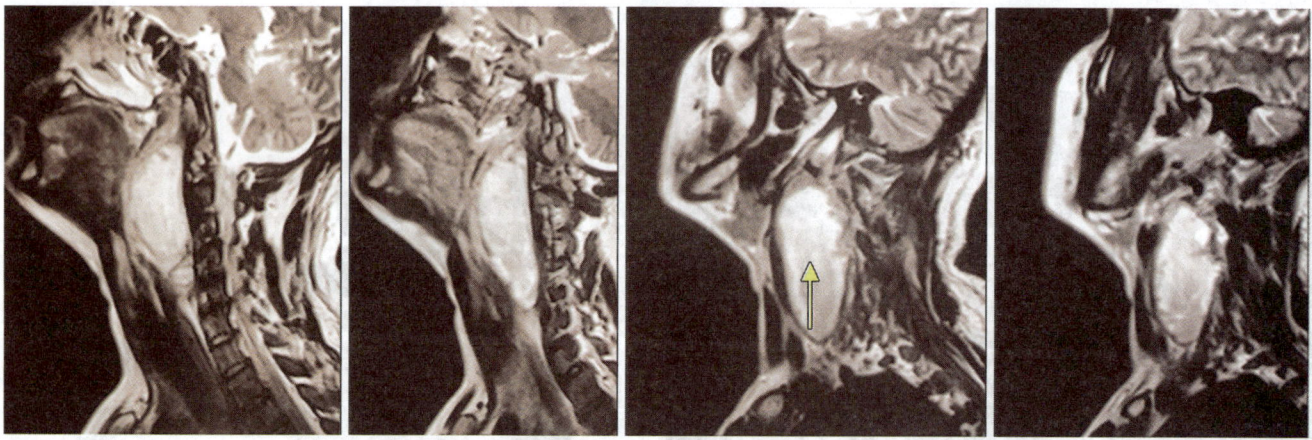

Fig. 28: CT scan of neck showing retropharyngeal abscess.

Chapter 78

Anesthesia in ENT

EN2.11: Demonstrate the correct technique to instilling topical medications into the ear, nose and throat in a simulated environment.

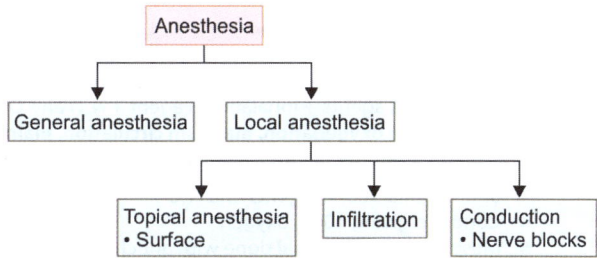

GENERAL PRINCIPLES

Q. Write a short note on general principles of use of anesthesia in ENT surgeries.

To secure airway, to achieve deep level of anesthesia for rapid recovery.
- Preoperative assessment
- Investigations
- Consent
- Preoperative fasting
- Monitoring
- Premedication

1. Preoperative assessment	<ul><li>General, systemic examination</li><li>History of drug allergy, medication, previous anesthesia</li><li>Airway assessment, nasal passage, dentition, mouth opening, neck mobility</li></ul>
2. Investigations	<ul><li>Blood investigations: Hb, CBC, LFT, RFT, HIV, HbsAg, HpCV, HIV, BT, CT, prothrombin time, platelet count</li><li>X-ray chest, ECG</li></ul>
3. Consent	<ul><li>Written/informed/valid consent</li></ul>
4. Preoperative fasting	<ul><li>For solid: Not less than 6 hours</li><li>For liquid: Not less than 4 hours</li></ul>
5. Monitoring	<ul><li>Blood pressure, pulse, ECG, pulse oximetry, CVP, end tidal CO_2</li></ul>
6. Premedication	<ul><li>Antisialogogues. Atropine, glycopyrolate</li><li>Antiemetics: Metoclopramide, ondanseteron</li><li>Anxiolytics/sedatives/tranquilizers: Midazolam, diazepam, promethazine</li><li>Opioids: Pentazocine, pethidine, tramadol, fentanyl</li></ul>

(BT: bleeding time; CBC: complete blood count; CT: clotting time; CVP: central venous pressure; ECG: electrocardiograph; HbsAg: hepatitis B surface antigen; LFT: liver function test; RFT: renal function test)

PART 3: Miscellaneous Topics

■ GENERAL ANESTHESIA

Q. Write a short note on general anesthesia.

- ❖ Preoxygenation
- ❖ Induction
- ❖ Maintenance
- ❖ Reversal and extubation
- ❖ Postoperative pain relief

A. Preoxygenation	100% oxygen given with mask for 3–5 minutes

B. Induction	❖ **Intravenous (fast):** Intravenous agent + muscle relaxant
	➢ Intravenous agents
	  » Pentothal: 5–7 mg/kg
	  » Propofol: 1–2 mg/Kg
	  » Ketamine: 1–2 mg/kg
	➢ **Muscle relaxant:**
	  » Scoline: 1–2 mg/kg
	  » Pancuronium: 0.08 mg/kg
	  » Vecuronium: 0.08 mg/kg
	  » Atracurium: 0.5 mg/kg
	❖ **Inhalational (slow)**
	➢ $O_2 + N_2$ + inhalation agent
	➢ Inhalational agents: Halothane/isoflurane/sevoflurane

C. Maintenance	Any one of the following used ❖ Intravenous agents + N_2O and O_2 ± muscle relaxant ❖ Inhalational agents + N_2O and O_2 ± muscle relaxant ❖ Intravenous agents + inhalational agent + N_2O and O_2 ± muscle relaxant **Keep adequate oxygenation, maintain circulation, maintenance of normothermia, IV fluids (5% dextrose/Ringer lactate/DNS), replacement for actual blood loss/urine output**
D. Reversal and extubation	❖ Shutoff inhalational agents and N_2O ❖ Continue giving 100% oxygen ❖ Muscle relaxant reversal done with anticholinesterase like neostigmine/prostigmin ❖ With return of airway reflexes remove throat pack, deflate endotracheal tube ❖ With the return of consciousness, protective airway reflexes and muscle power extubate the patient ❖ Keep patient nil by mouth
E. Postoperative pain relief	**Any suitable analgesics** Diclofenac sodium: 2–3 mg/kg IM or Tramadol: 1–2 mg/kg IM/IV **Prior to extubation**

■ LOCAL ANESTHESIA

Q. Briefly describe various local anesthesia used in ENT.

Topical anesthesia	4% Xylocaine/10% Xylocaine spray/2% viscous lignocaine, 0.5, 1.0, 1.5% lignocaine	
Infiltration anesthesia	2% lignocaine with/without adrenaline	
Conduction (nerve blocks) anesthesia	2% lignocaine with/without adrenaline	❖ **Superior laryngeal nerve block** ➢ On either side of greater cornu of hyoid bone local infiltration is given ❖ **Translaryngeal block** ➢ Anesthetize trachea below vocal cords and puncture cricothyroid membrane and infiltrate 3–5 mL of local anesthetic drug ❖ **Glossopharyngeal nerve block** ➢ Inject 5 mL of anesthetic solution at base of posterior tonsillar pillar to anesthetize posterior 1/3rd of tongue, pharynx and superior surface of epiglottis

CHAPTER 78: Anesthesia in ENT

Local Anesthetic Agents/Drugs

Q. Discuss various local anesthetic agents/drugs for ENT surgeries.

Drugs	Uses	Dosage	Effects
❖ 4% and 10% lignocaine sprays are used for surface anesthesia ❖ Lignocaine/xylocaine ➤ 2% lignocaine with/without adrenaline: Available as 0.5, 1.0, 1.5, 2, 4, and 10% solution with/without adrenaline (1:50,000, 1:1,00,000, 1:200,000) used for infiltration anesthesia 4% and 10% lignocaine sprays are used for surface anesthesia **(Figs. 1A and B)**	**Maintenance in ENT surgical procedures lasting for more than 20 minutes**	**Maximum safe dose** ❖ **With adrenaline** (1: 200,000) 5 µg/kg, 1 mL of adrenaline in 200 mL solution, 7 mg/kg ❖ **Without adrenaline** 4 mg/kg ❖ Topical ❖ Infiltration ❖ Transtracheal ❖ Superior laryngeal nerve block	**Duration** 45 minutes to 1 hour 1 to 1.5 hours ❖ It has antiarrhythmic effect ❖ It attenuates the pressor response (tachycardia and hypotension) to intubation
❖ Bupivacaine/marcaine ➤ Amino amide local anesthetic: It is available as 0.25% and 0.5% solution with/without adrenaline (1: 2,00,000)		**Maximum safe dose** ❖ **With adrenaline** 3 mg/kg, improves quality of analgesia ❖ **Without adrenaline** 2 mg/kg	If the dose exceeds the maximum safe dose level, it can cause refractory cardiac arrest and death
❖ Adrenaline ➤ Inotropic agent it activates both alpha and beta adrenergic receptors 1 mg/mL	Used with local anesthetic to reduce their absorption thereby lessening the potential systemic toxicity	**Maximum safe dose** 0.5–1.0 mg/100 mL (1:1,00,000–1:2,00,000) **The dose should not exceed 10 mL of 1:1,00,000 over a 10 minutes period**	❖ Increased myocardial activity ❖ Increases blood pressure, heart rate Dilatation of skeletal muscle vasculature ❖ Decreases renal blood flow, urinary output ❖ Ventricular arrhythmias ❖ Angina

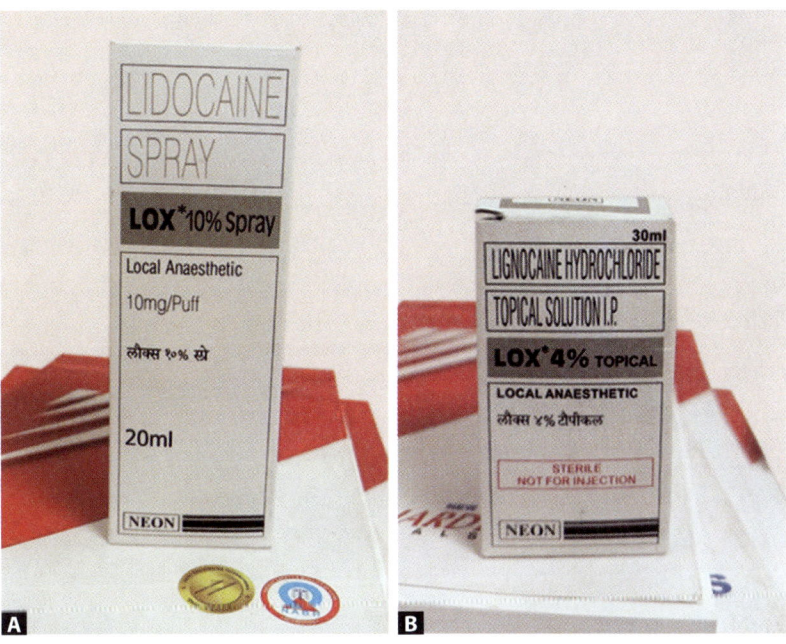

Figs. 1A and B: (A) 10% lignocaine solution; (B) 4% lignocaine solution.

ANESTHESIA INSTRUMENTS

Q. Enumerate anesthetic instruments.

- Mask
- Airway (oral, nasopharyngeal)
- Laryngeal mask airway (LMA)
- Endotracheal tubes
- Laryngoscope
- Magill's forceps
- Anesthesia machine **(Fig. 2)**
- Breathing system (circuit)
- Resuscitation bag
- Oxygen cylinder
- Oxygen flow meter
- Oxygen mask
- Nasal catheter/prongs
- Monitors: Blood pressure monitor, cardioscope, pulse oximeter, capnometer, respiratory gas monitor

Note: Hypotensive anesthesia required for ENT surgeries

- Parotidectomy
- Functional endoscopic sinus surgery (FESS)

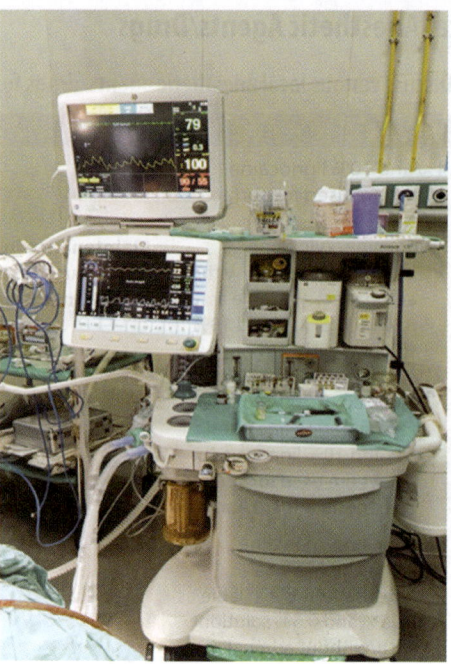

Fig. 2: Anesthesia machine.

Chapter 79

Pure Tone Audiogram and Impedance Audiometry

EN2.4: Demonstrate the correct technique to perform and interpret pure tone audiogram and impedance audiogram.

■ PURE TONE AUDIOGRAM

Q. What is pure tone audiometry? Describe briefly how you perform it.

Introduction

Pure tone audiogram (PTA) is the most basic assessment of hearing sensitivity.

Pure tone means a tone with single nominal frequency. Basically in pure tone audiometry we detect the persons hearing threshold at different frequencies from 250 Hz to 8000 Hz and intensities from 0 to 120 dBnHL. During air conduction (AC) testing hearing sensitivity is assessed at octave intervals from 250 Hz to 8000 Hz and during bone conduction (BC) testing hearing sensitivity is assessed at octave intervals from 250 to 4,000 Hz. Threshold is referred as the lowest intensity at which the person can detect the presence of pure tone stimulus at least 50% of the times.

Method

Case History

Case history is an important parameter of PTA. It should cover following points:
- ❖ Hearing loss
- ❖ Otorrhea
- ❖ Otalgia
- ❖ Tinnitus
- ❖ Vertigo
- ❖ Noise exposure

Method (scan QR code)
- ❖ During PTA testing, patient should be seated in such a way that he/she cannot see the audiometer and the audiologist.
- ❖ Ask the patient to remove earrings, glasses, all the things which cause discomfort to them during the testing. During the AC testing, place the headphones appropriately on patients' ears, i.e., the red headphone should be placed on the patient's right ear and the blue headphone should be placed on the patient's left ear. During the placement of AC headphones make sure that the diaphragm of the headphones should be placed in front of the opening of external auditory canal (EAC).
- ❖ During the BC testing vibrator should be placed on the mastoid grooves/process of the patients.
- ❖ Give proper, clear instructions to the patient, i.e., they have to raise their hand whenever the stimulus to be heard to them and immediately after that they need to take their hand down as soon as the stimulus will be off. Very importantly they need to provide attention to the softest sound also.

Technique

PTA can be carried out by using **ascending method or descending method**.

PTA testing needs to always start with the patient's better ear. During case history procedure, audiologist can make some guess about persons hearing, based on that starting level of audiometry test can be decided. After the initial response decrease the intensity by 10–15 dB steps until no response obtained. After the inaudibility reached increase the intensity of signal in 5 dB steps until the patient responds. Similarly the procedure should be carried out in 5 dB up, 10 dB down till threshold is obtained.

Interpretation

Interpretation of PTA based on the degree and type of hearing loss.

Pure tone average (PTA) is calculated for each ear. It basically involves average of 500, 1000, 2000 Hz AC thresholds, which help to summarize the degree of hearing loss.

Degree of hearing loss	Hearing loss range (dBHL)
Normal	-10 to 25
Mild	26–40
Moderate	41–55
Moderately severe	56–70
Severe	71–90
Profound	91+

Symbols (Fig. 1)

Symbols for interpreting AC and BC threshold on audiogram:

Legends	Right ear	Left ear
Air	O	X
Air masked	Δ	□
Bone	<	>
Bone masked	[	]
No response	↓	↓

Hearing loss: Type of hearing loss depends on which part of your hearing is damaged.

There are three basic types of hearing loss:
1. Conductive hearing loss
2. Sensorineural hearing loss
3. Mixed hearing loss

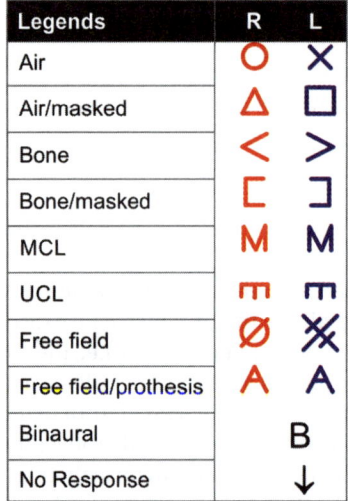

Fig. 1: Various symbols used for audiogram.
(MCL: most comfortable loudness level; UCL: uncomfortable loudness level)

CHAPTER 79: Pure Tone Audiogram and Impedance Audiometry

■ IMPEDANCE AUDIOMETRY

Q. Write a short note on impedance audiometry. Briefly describe its procedure and interpretation.

Introduction

- ❖ Impedance audiometry is an objective assessment method of the function of the middle ear.
- ❖ Impedance audiometry is also termed as tympanometry.
- ❖ Impedance audiometry provides information about:
  - ▷ Middle ear pathologies
  - ▷ Middle ear muscle contractions due to the acoustic reflex
- ❖ Tympanometry involves measuring the acoustic admittance of the ear with various amounts of pressure in the ear canal. (Gelfund)
- ❖ For tympanometry, we use 226 Hz (or 220 Hz) probe tone because 226 Hz tone is sensitive to changes in stiffness reactance, comprising a major part of the normal ears impedance.
- ❖ In tympanometry, we measure three basic parameters, i.e., (1) ear canal volume, (2) static compliance, (3) middle ear pressure.
  - ▷ *Ear canal volume:* Normal ear canal volumes vary as a function of age. Typically for children ear canal volume ranges from 0.5–1.5 cc; while for adults ear canal volume ranges from 0.5–2.0 cc
  - ▷ *Static compliance:* Normal range for static compliance is 0.3–1.5 cc
  - ▷ Middle ear pressure: Middle ear pressure ranges from +50 to -200 daPa
- ❖ All this information obtained in tympanometry testing plotted on tympanogram.
- ❖ On tympanogram, X-axis represents pressure in daPa, Y-axis represents static compliance in mmhos.

Tympanometry Procedure (scan QR code)

- ❖ **Give proper instructions to the patient:** Do not swallow, cough, yawn, or raise hand during testing.
- ❖ The first step in tympanometry involves proper insertion of probe tip so that it makes hermetic seal with the EAC.
- ❖ Observe the graphical representation of the tympanogram on the screen and interpret the tympanogram.

Tympanometry Interpretation (Fig. 2)

Type of tympanogram	EAV value (cc)	Static compliance value (cc)	Middle ear pressure value (daPa)	Interpretation
A type	0.5–1.5	0.3–1.3	± 100	Normal middle ear functioning
As type	0.5–1.5	Below 0.2	± 100	Otosclerosis
Ad type	0.5–1.5	Beyond 1.5	± 100	Hypermobile TM or ossicular chain discontinuity
B type	0.5–1.5	Below 0.2	Flat	Middle ear effusion
B type	More than 1.5	Below 0.2	Flat	TM perforation or patent grommet
B type	Below 0.5	Below 0.2	Flat	Probe is blocked or wax in the EAC
C type	0.5–1.5	0.3–1.3	Low pressure (more than -100)	Eustachian tube dysfunction

(EAC: external auditory canal; EAV: external auditory volume; TM: tympanic membrane)

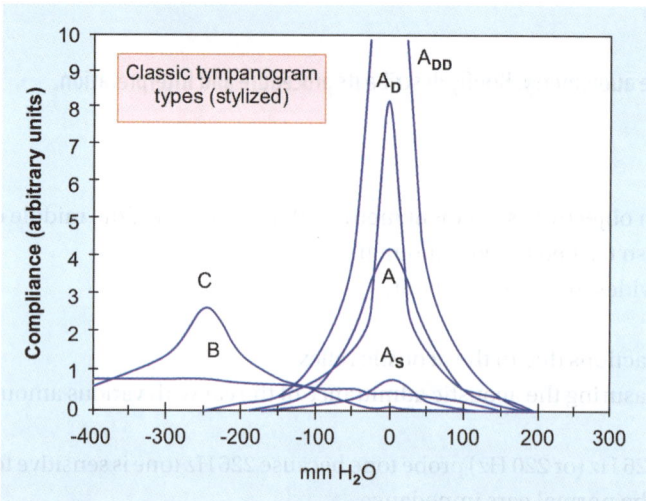

Fig. 2: Various impedance audiometry curves—A_D, A_S, B, C, and C type on tympanogram. (X-axis shows compliance and Y-axis shows middle ear pressure).

AUDIOGRAMS AND INTERPRETATION

Q. Read the pure tone audiogram (PTA) showing in the Figures 3 to 9, give the diagnosis, and enumerate the causes.

Normal Hearing (Fig. 3)

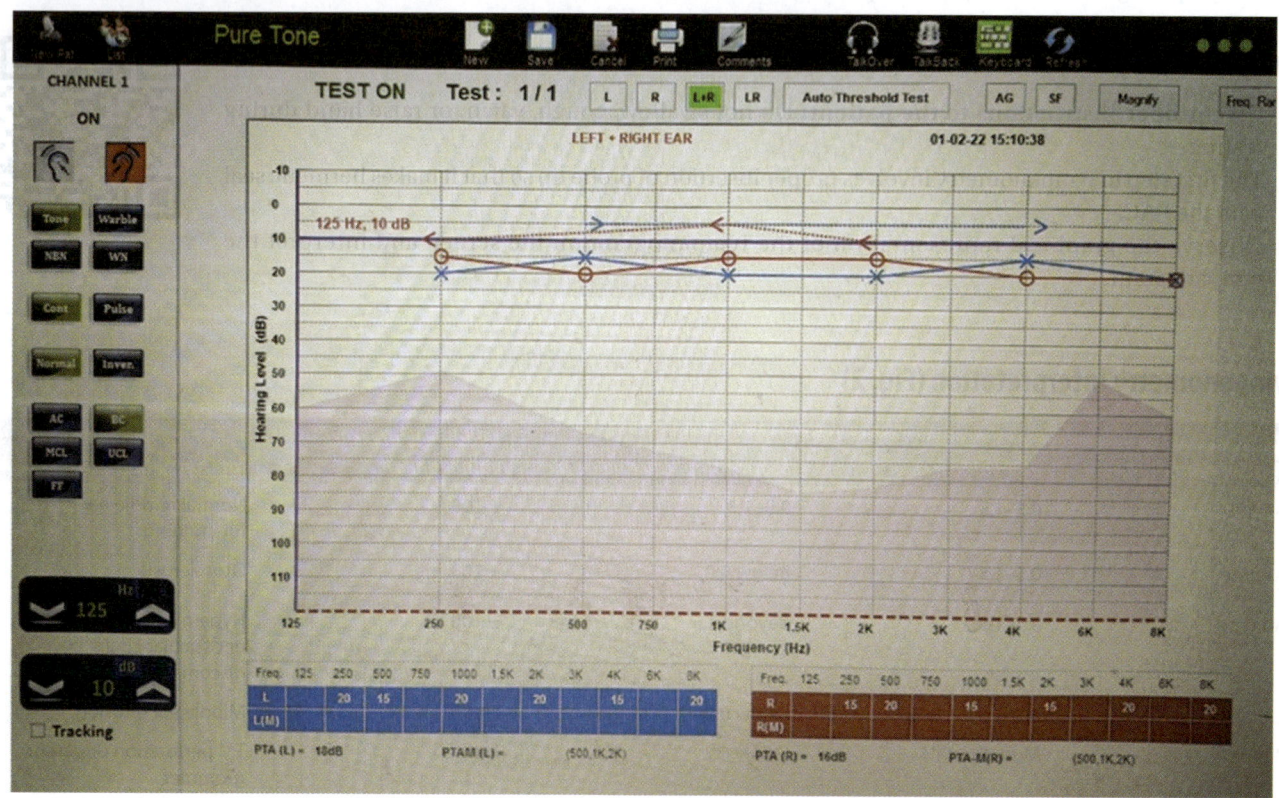

Fig. 3: PTA: Showing normal hearing (X-axis—hearing loss in decibels and Y-axis—frequencies in hertz).

Noise-induced Hearing Loss (Fig. 4)

- Sensorineural hearing loss with notch at 4 KHz
- **Causes:** Blast injuries, Prolonged exposure to loud sound

CHAPTER 79: Pure Tone Audiogram and Impedance Audiometry

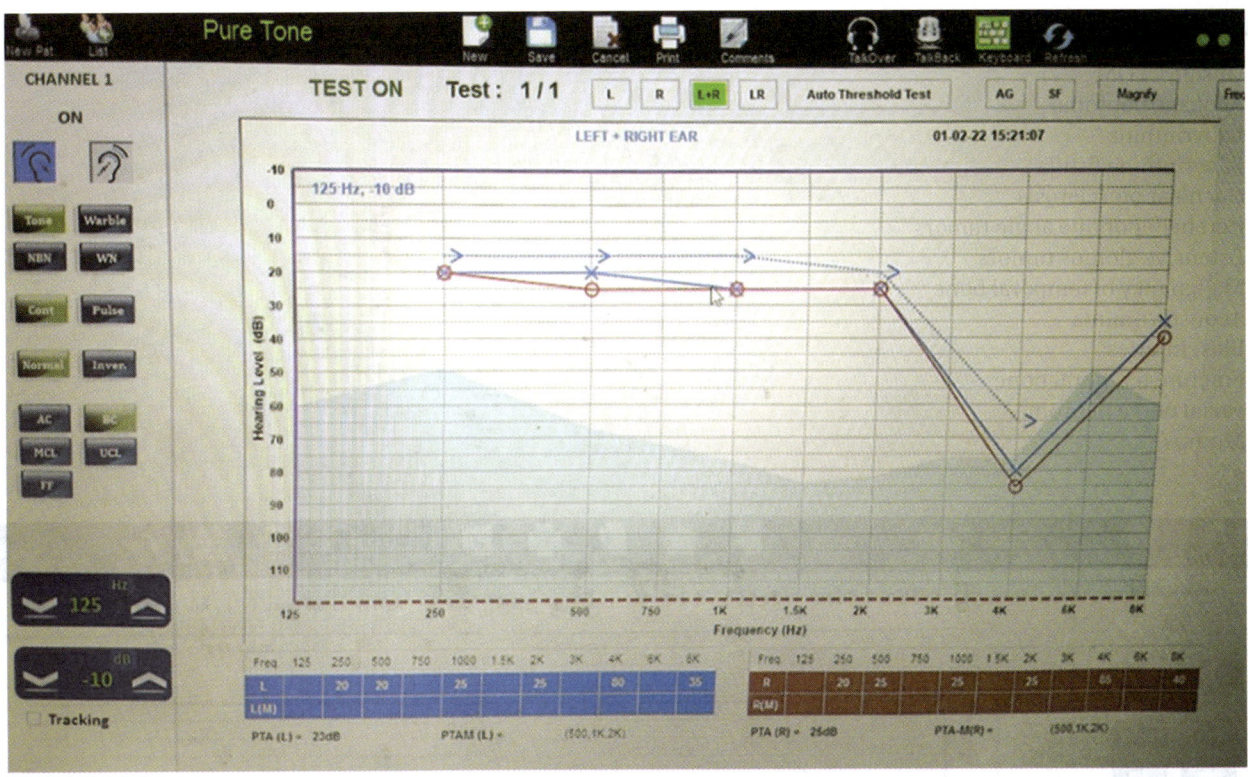

Fig. 4: PTA: Showing bilateral noise-induced hearing loss (4 kHz notch).

Causes of Unilateral/Bilateral Mixed Hearing Loss (Fig. 5)
- Unsafe chronic suppurative otitis media (CSOM)
- Labyrinthitis
- Glomus tumors

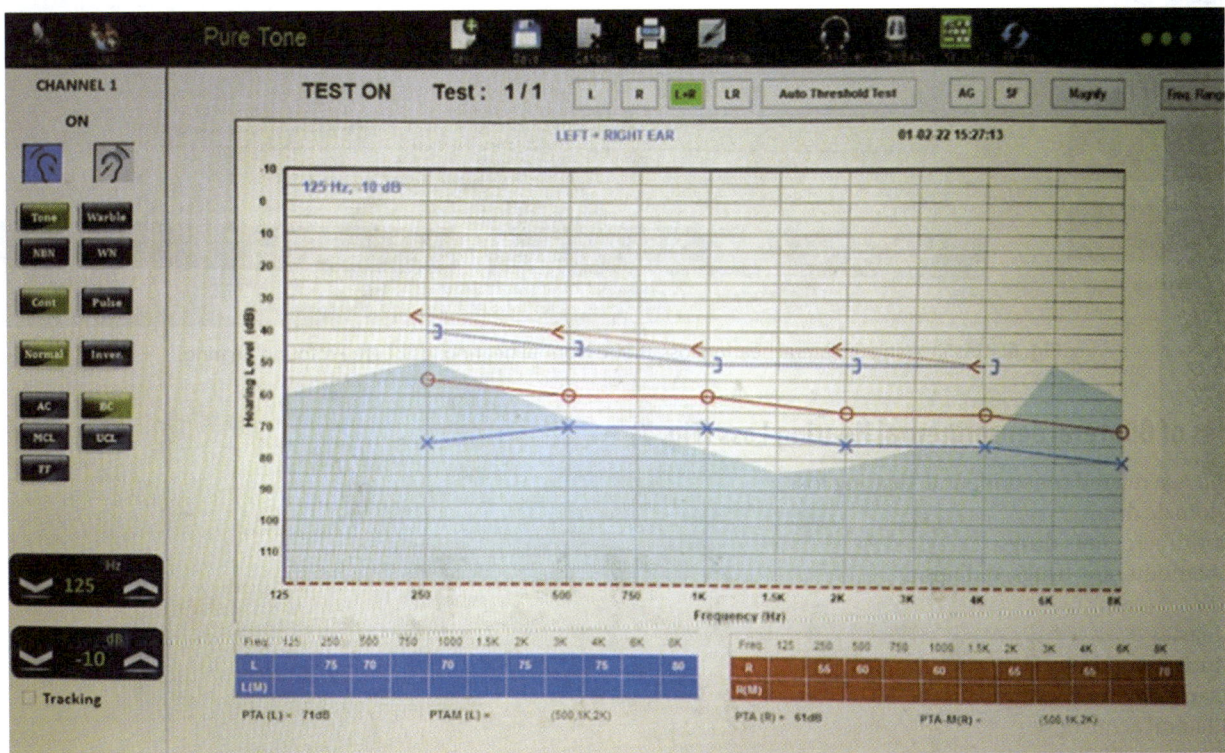

Fig. 5: PTA: Showing severe mixed hearing loss. Right: Moderately severe mixed hearing loss; Left: Severe mixed hearing loss.

Causes of Unilateral Profound Hearing Loss (Fig. 6)

- Unsafe CSOM
- Acoustic neuroma
- Labyrinthitis
- Labyrinthine fistula
- Cochlear otosclerosis
- Cerebellopontine angle tumors
- Extensive glomus tumors,
- Malignancy of temporal bone
- Acoustic trauma
- Blast injuries
- Fracture temporal bone
- Facial nerve neuroma
- Mumps

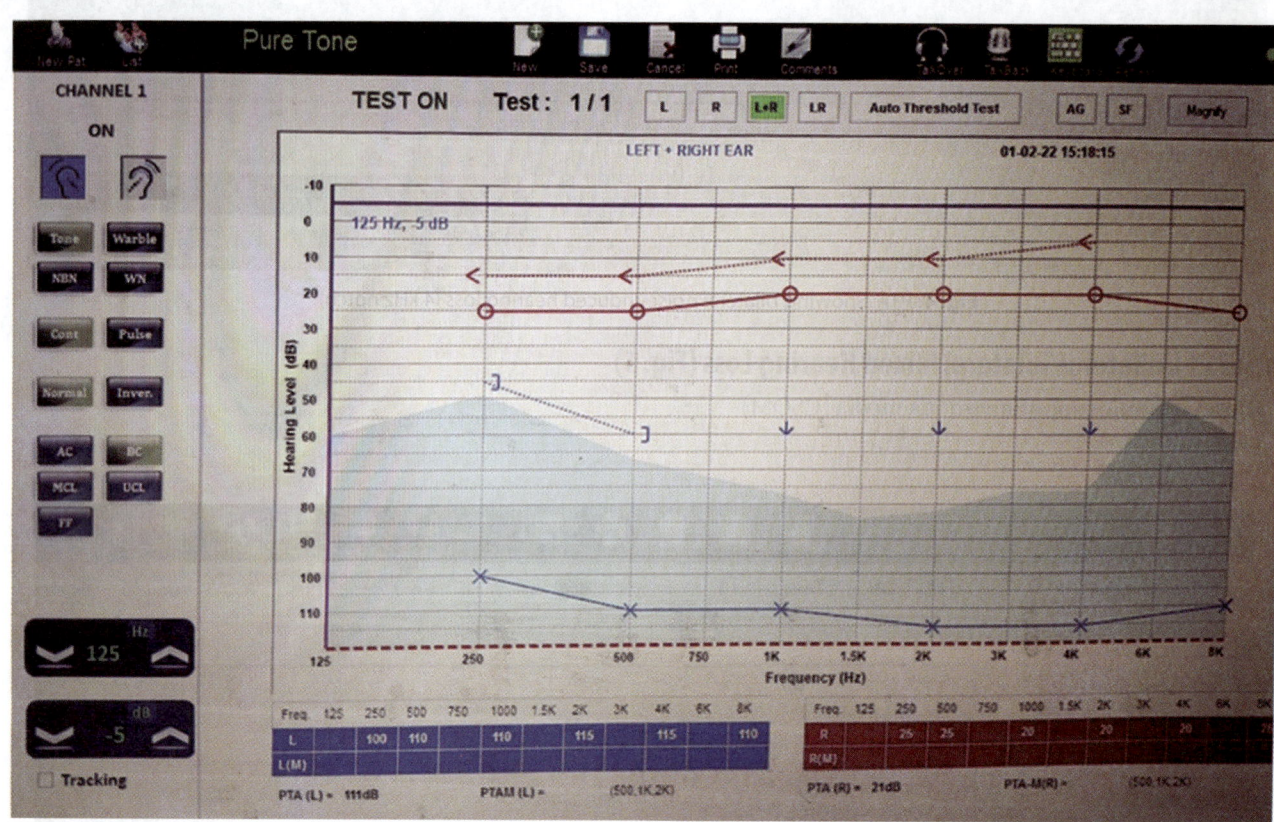

Fig. 6: PTA: Showing unilateral hearing loss. Right: Normal hearing loss; Left: Profound hearing.

Causes of Bilateral Sensorineural Hearing Loss (Fig. 7)

- Old age related sensorineural hearing loss
- Ototoxic drugs
- Antituberculous drugs
- Chemotherapy drugs, radiation
- HIV
- Measles
- Mumps
- Exanthematous fever
- Bilateral acoustic
- Neuroma, diabetes

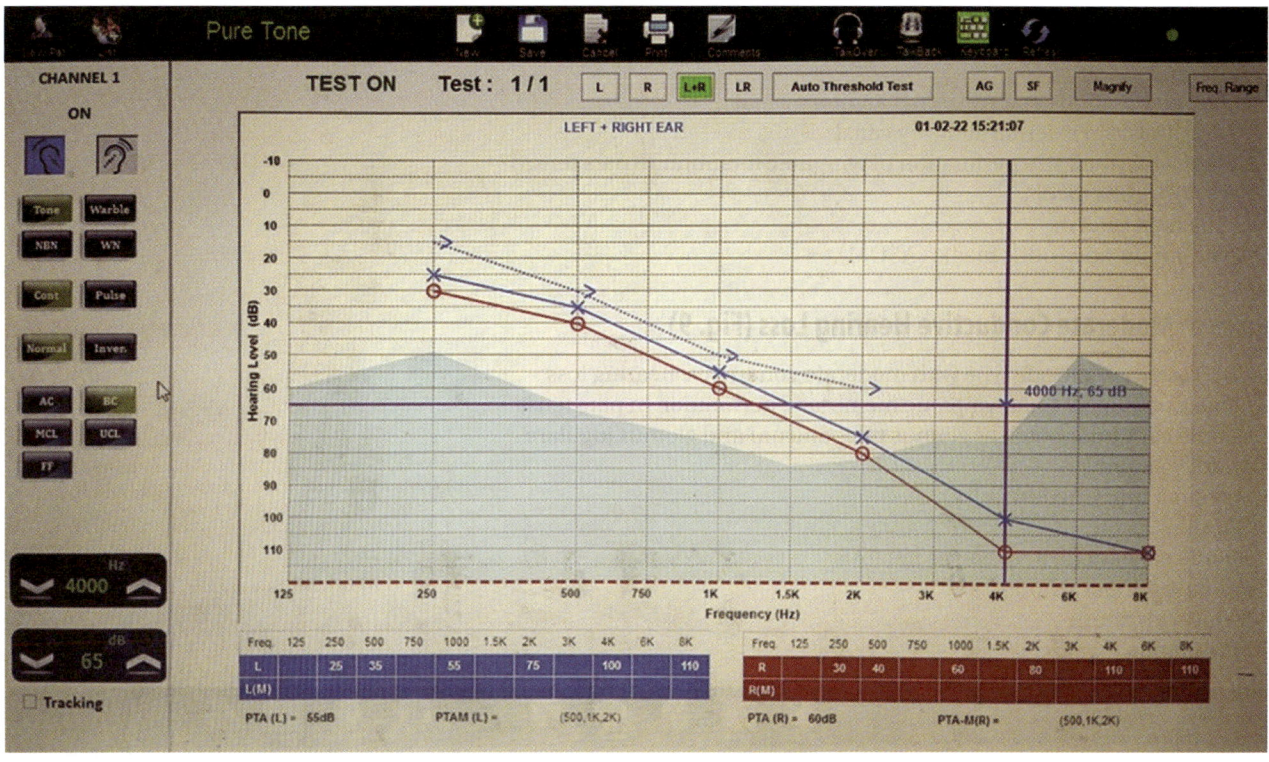

Fig. 7: PTA: Showing bilateral mild to profound sloping sensorineural hearing loss (presbycusis).

Causes of Bilateral Mild Conductive Hearing Loss (Fig. 8)
❖ Otosclerosis
❖ Tympanosclerosis

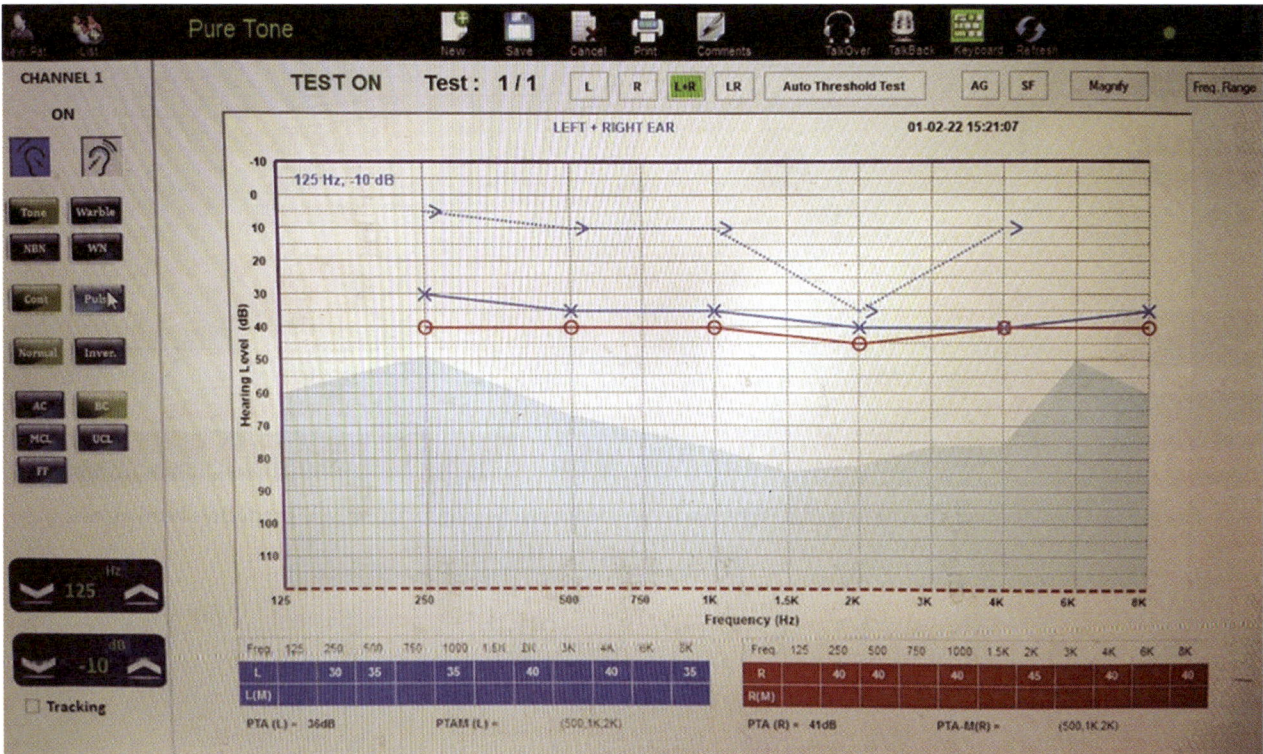

Fig. 8: PTA: Showing bilateral mild conductive hearing loss (2 kHz Carhart notch).

Causes of Mild Conductive Hearing Loss

- Wax, otomycosis
- Polyp, granulations in the external auditory canal
- Partial atresia of external auditory canal
- CSOM with small size perforation of tympanic membrane (pars tensa)
- Secretory otitis media
- Eustachian catarrh
- Acute suppurative otitis media (ASOM)

Causes of Moderate Conductive Hearing Loss (Fig. 9)

- CSOM safe and unsafe type with moderate conductive hearing loss
- Large, subtotal, or total tympanic membrane perforation in pars tensa
- Middle ear tumors such as glomus tympanicum and glomus jugulare
- Middle ear polyp
- Secretory otitis media
- Glue ear
- Middle ear ossicular erosion or necrosis
- Fracture temporal bone
- Hemotympanum
- Barotrauma

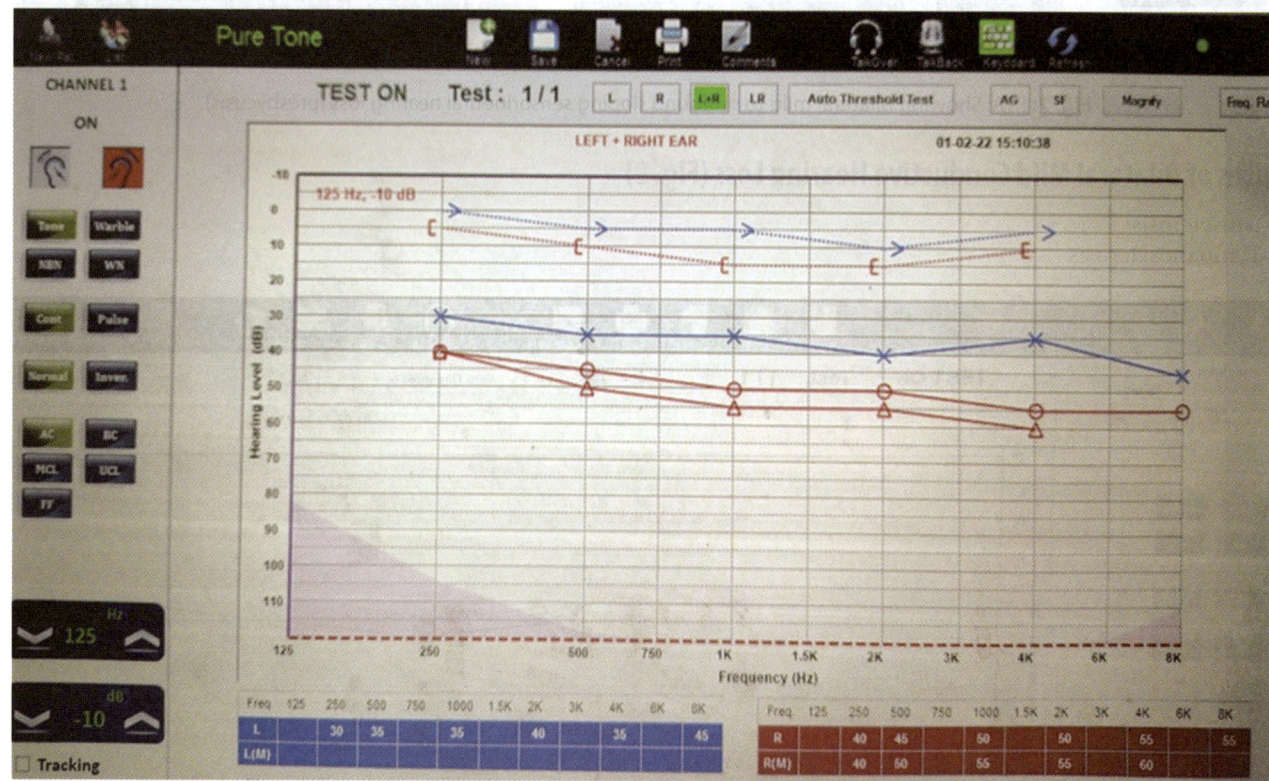

Fig. 9: PTA: Showing conductive hearing loss. Right: Moderate conductive hearing loss; Left: Mild conductive hearing loss.

PART 4

Questions

Outline

80. Objective Structured Clinical/Practical Examination (OSCE)
81. Operative Specimens in ENT
82. Mock Questions Papers
83. Multiple Choice Questions (MCQs)
84. Long Cases and Short Cases in ENT

Chapter 80

Objective Structured Clinical/Practical Examination (OSCE)

■ STATION 1

Q. Perform the ear examination of this patient and write your findings.
(Do not take any history).

■ STATION 2

Q. A. Identify the instrument and what are its parts?
B. Mention its use.
C. Mention the components of Waldeyer's internal ring.

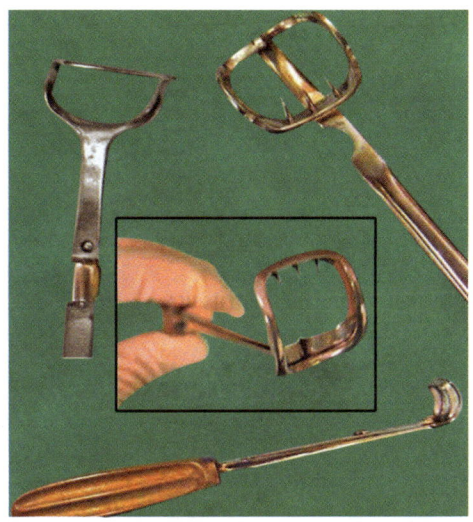

■ STATION 3

Q. A. Describe the lesion.
B. What is probable diagnosis?
C. Name the organisms causing it.

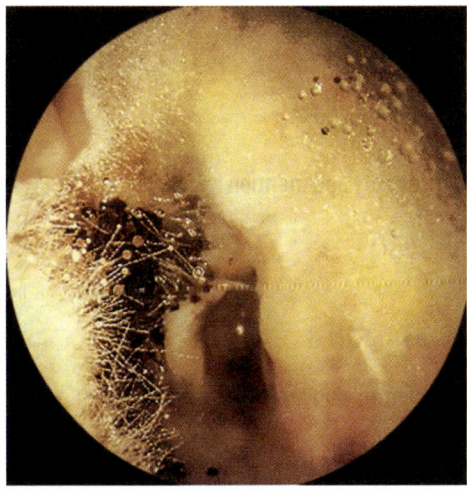

STATION 4

Q. A. What clinical signs help with diagnosis?
   B. Name the surgery done.

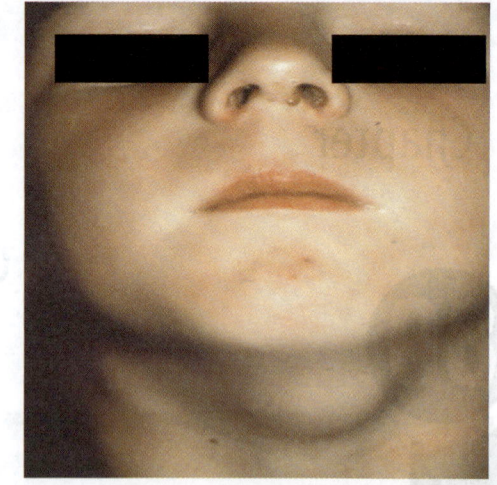

STATION 5

Q. Identify and mention its use.

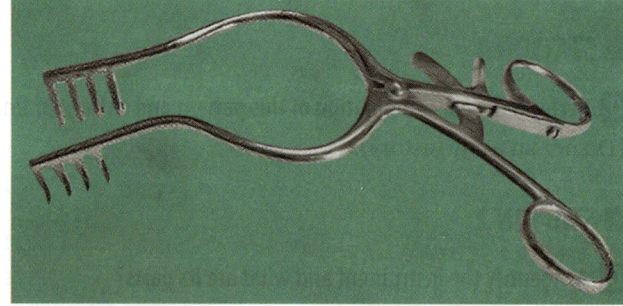

STATION 6

Q. Identify and mention its use.

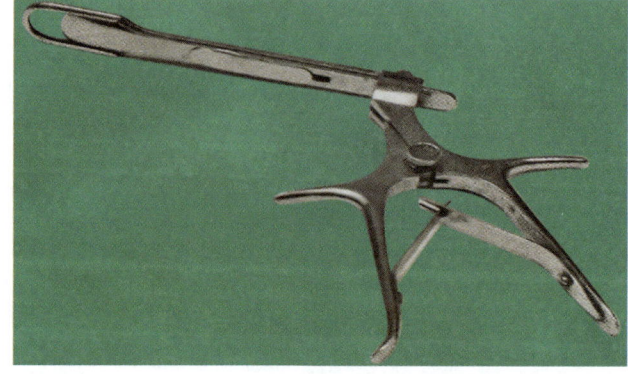

STATION 7

Q. Identify and mention its use.

STATION 8

Q. Identify and mention its use.

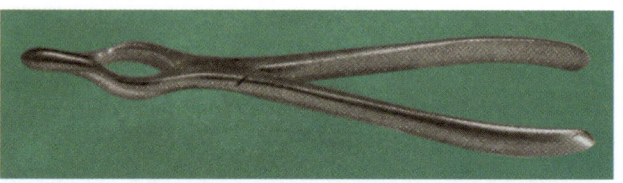

STATION 9

Q. Identify and mention its use.

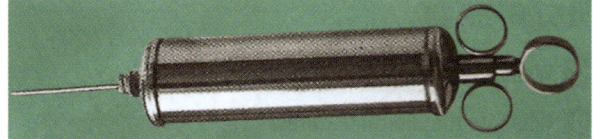

STATION 10

Q. Identify the view.
   A. Give its importance.
   B. Mention other important views.
   C. Mention types of mastoid.
   D. Enumerate differential diagnosis of radiolucency in mastoid.

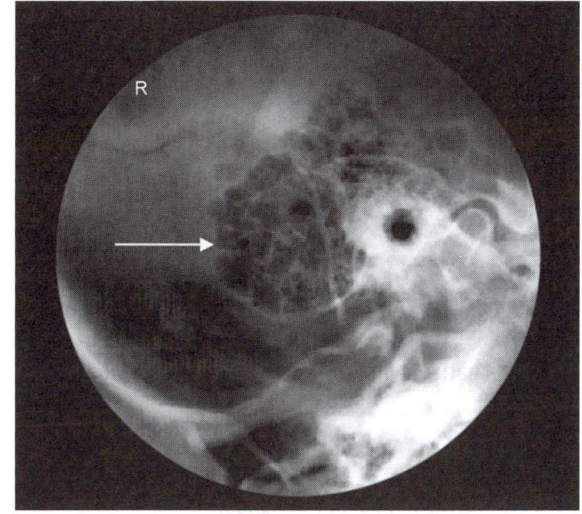

STATION 11

Q. Identify the specimen.

Q. What are the gross findings?

Q. What may be the probable diagnosis?

Q. What is the extent of the lesion?

Q. What is the TNM staging?

Q. What are the methods used for rehabilitation after such procedure?

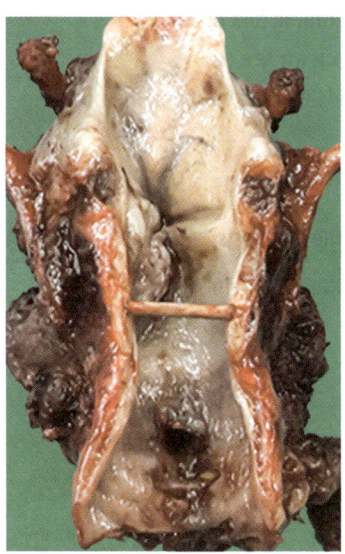

STATION 12

Q. Identify the pathology.

Q. Enumerate few etiological factors.

Q. Mention its clinical features.

Q. What are management options?

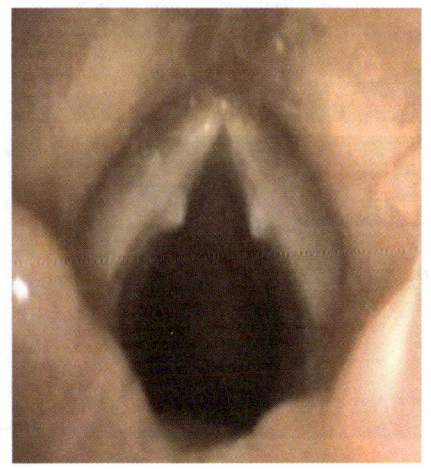

PART 4: Questions

STATION 13

Q. What is your diagnosis?

Q. What are the clinical features?

Q. What is the treatment?

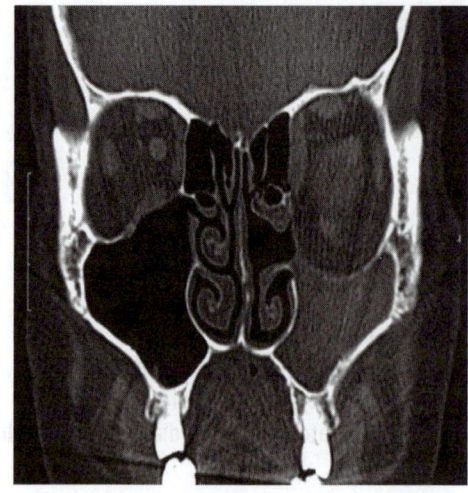

STATION 14

Q. I am a patient with nasal polyposis. Counsel me about the management.

STATION 15

Q. Examine the left ear of this patient.

Q. Perform tuning fork tests.
  ❖ Do not clean the ear

Q. Draw and label left tympanic membrane.

STATION 16

Q. What is the diagnosis?

Q. What is the management?

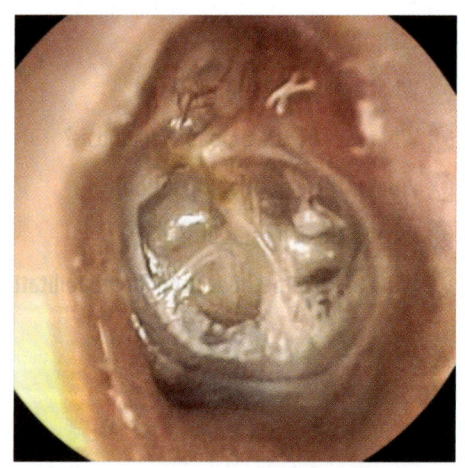

STATION 17

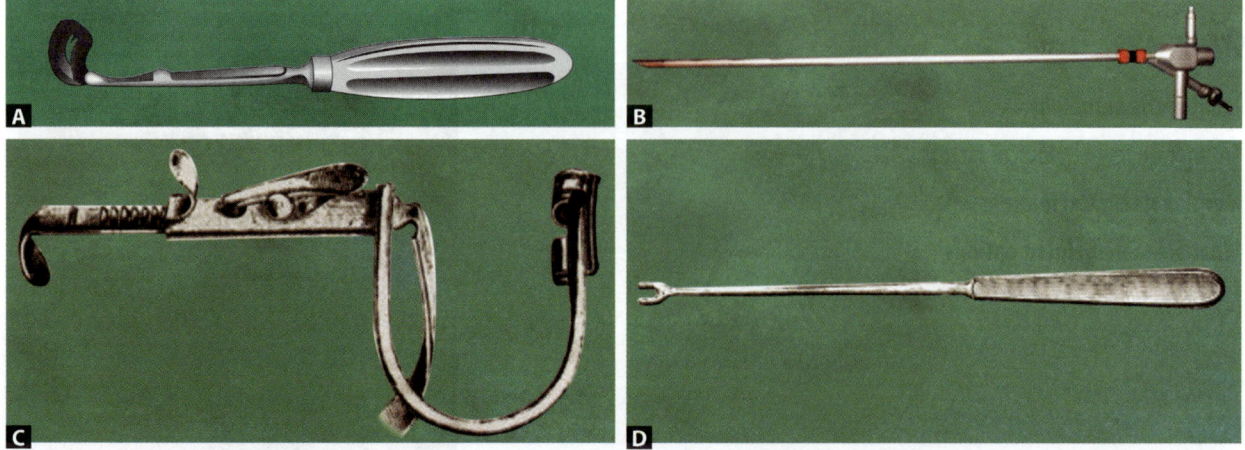

CHAPTER 80: Objective Structured Clinical/Practical Examination (OSCE)

Q. Identify instruments by function.
  A. Adenoid curette for adenoidectomy
  B. Boyle-Davies mouth gag for tonsillectomy
  C. Rigid bronchoscope
  D. Negus knot pusher for tonsillectomy

■ STATION 18

Q. What is a diagnosis?

Q. What are the commonest organism?

Q. What is the management of this case?

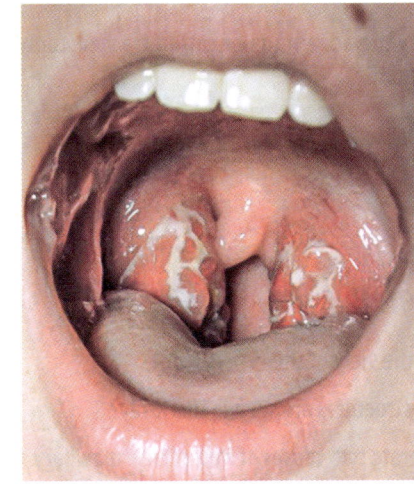

■ STATION 19

Q. What is a diagnosis?

Q. What is a management?

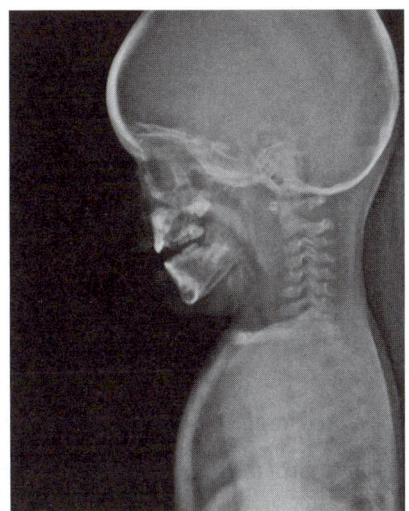

■ STATION 20

Q. Identify the procedure.

Q. Draw the diagram of the normal structures seen on this procedure.

Q. What are the indications of this procedure?

Q. Name of the instrument used in this procedure and its peculiarity.

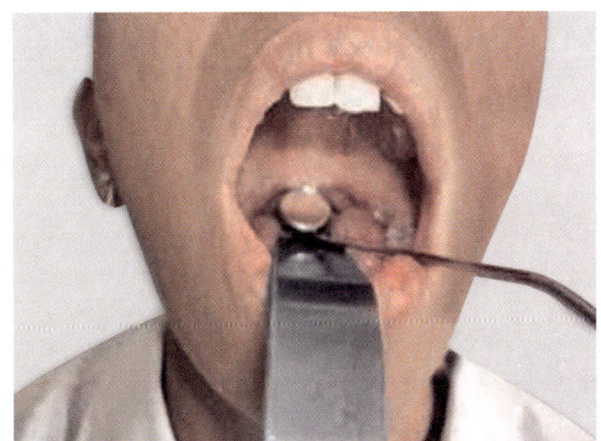

PART 4: Questions

STATION 21

Q. Write full name of this instrument.

Q. Describe the parts of this instrument.

Q. What are the advantages of this instrument?

Q. What is the advantage of cuffed tracheostomy tube over uncuffed tube?

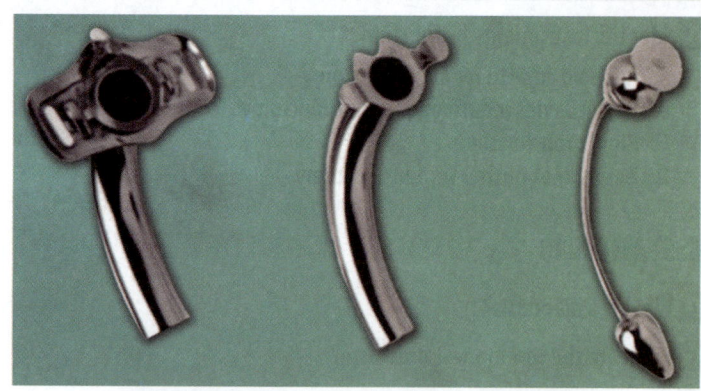

STATION 22

Q. Name the view of this X-rays.

Q. Which structures are seen in this X-ray?

Q. Enumerate two causes of hyperdense maxillary sinus.

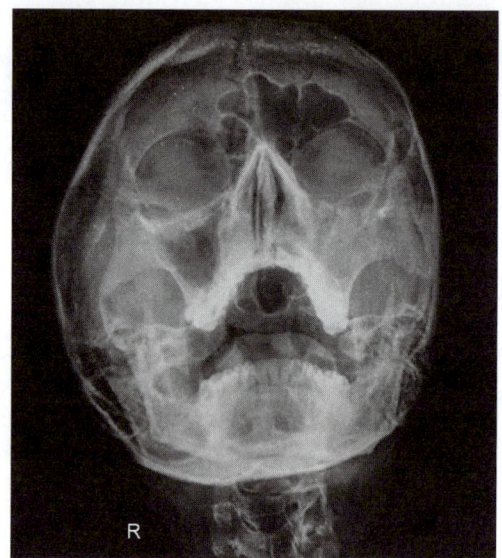

STATION 23

Q. Name the procedure and the instrument used in this procedure.

Q. Draw the diagram of the structures seen in this procedure.

Q. How to defog this instrument used in this procedure?

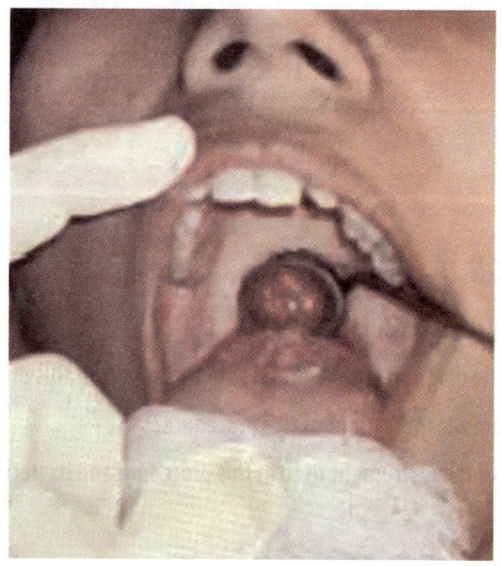

■ STATION 24

Q. What is diagnosis based on following audiometry chart?

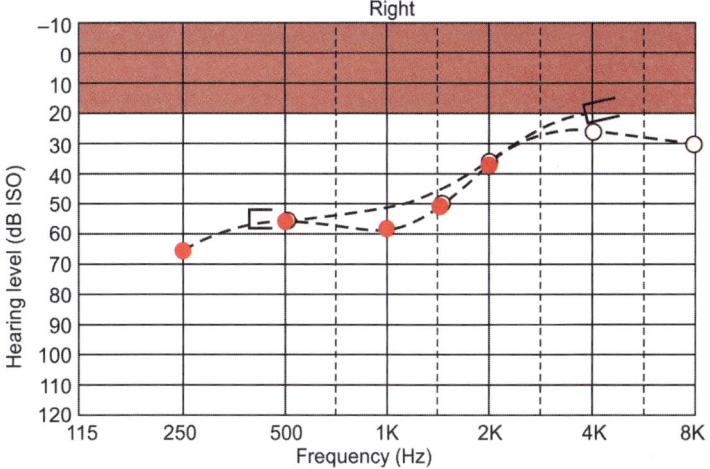

(pure tone audiogram showing sensorineural hearing loss)

■ STATION 25

Q. Name the investigation and view shown.

Q. What is the diagnosis?

Q. What is the management of this case?

Q. What possible symptoms can this patient present with?

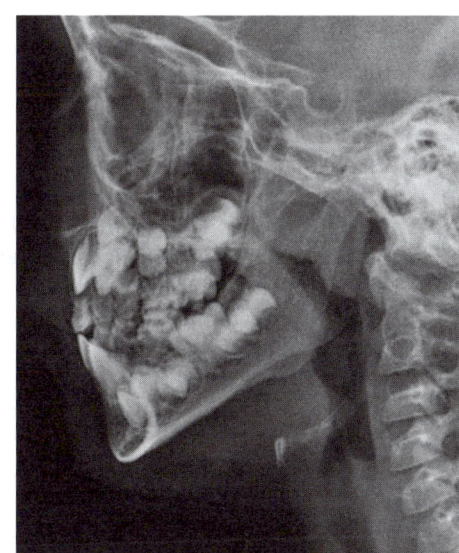

■ STATION 26

Q. Name the procedure.

Q. What is the diagnosis?

Q. What is the management?

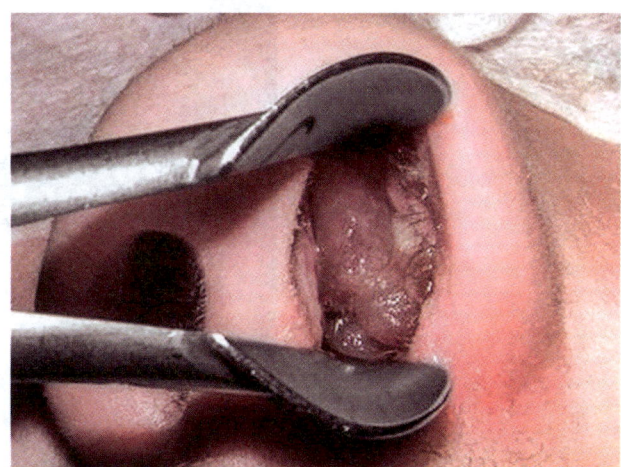

Chapter 81

Operative Specimens in ENT

- ❖ **Parameters under which a resected surgical specimen should be studied:**
  - ➢ Identification of the specimen
  - ➢ Specific findings in the specimen
  - ➢ Extent of the resection
  - ➢ Indications for the surgical resection
  - ➢ Preoperative work-up required for the procedure
  - ➢ Operative procedure and variants if any
  - ➢ Reconstructive options if any
  - ➢ Postoperative management
  - ➢ Complications of the procedure
- ❖ **Following specimens are discussed here:**
  - ➢ Partial and total maxillectomy
  - ➢ Total laryngectomy
  - ➢ Total thyroidectomy
  - ➢ Hemiglossectomy
  - ➢ Antrochoanal polyp (AC polyp)
  - ➢ Juvenile angiofibroma (JA)
  - ➢ Superficial parotidectomy
  - ➢ Submandibular gland with calculus (sialolith)

  (Relevant and most commonly asked questions in the examination pertaining to the specimen are given. Readers are advised to go through the relevant chapters to look for the answers.)

■ SPECIMEN 1.1: PARTIAL MAXILLECTOMY

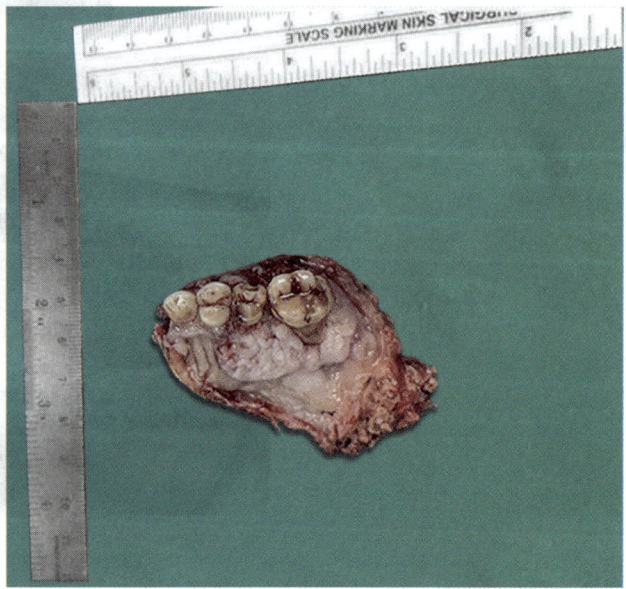

CHAPTER 81: Operative Specimens in ENT

Q. Identify and describe the specimen.

This is an operated specimen of partial maxillectomy seen from inferior aspect and showing the inner surface of the alveolar process of the maxilla, teeth, and the maxillary sinus. An ulceroproliferative cauliflower-like growth is seen extending from the alveolar process to the interior of the maxillary sinus highly suggestive of maxillary sinus carcinoma. There is a clear demarcation seen between the growth and the normal maxillary sinus mucosa.

Q. What is the most common microscopic finding (histopathology) for carcinoma of the maxilla?

Squamous cell carcinoma is the most common. Second most common is the adenoid cystic carcinoma.

Questions for Viva Voce

- What are the indications of partial maxillectomy?
- Name the different types of maxillectomies.
- Name the incision used for maxillectomy by open approach.
- What are the complications of the maxillectomy?
- What are the modalities of treatment available for treating maxillary sinus carcinoma?
- What are the reconstruction options available for maxillectomy surgery postoperatively?

■ SPECIMEN 1.2: TOTAL MAXILLECTOMY—OUTER SURFACE

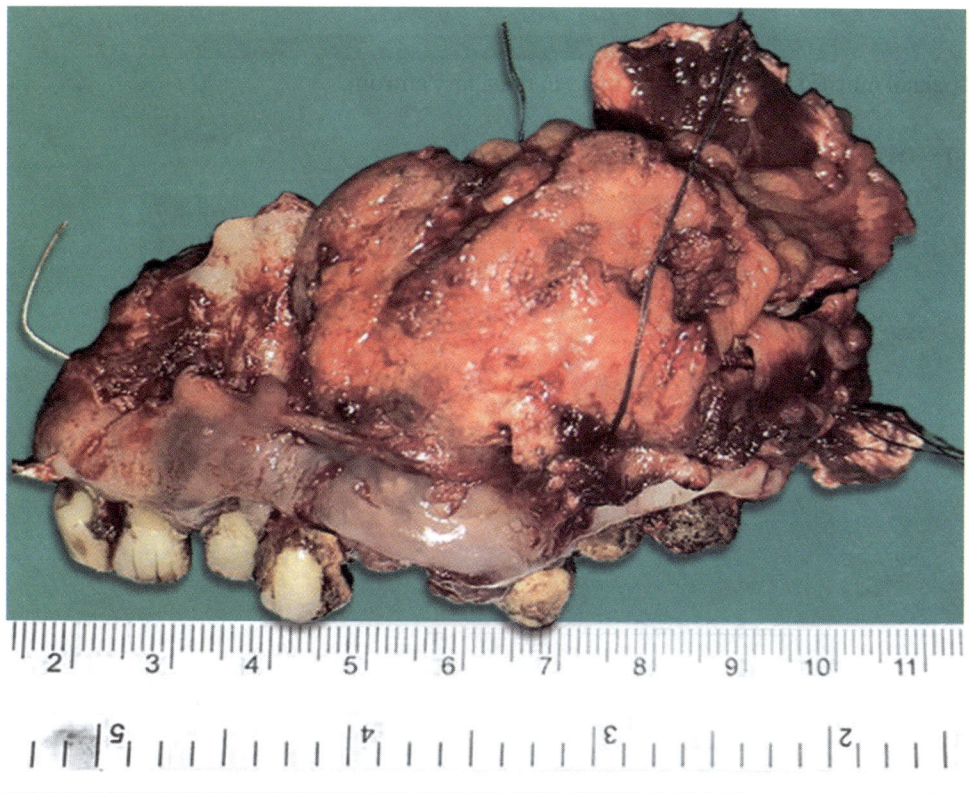

This is an operated specimen of the total maxillectomy of left side seen from lateral aspect. The white thread shows anterior border of the maxilla while the black thread shows the posterior border. A well-circumscribed cauliflower-like proliferative growth is seen occupying the whole of the interior of the maxillary sinus and extending to the adjacent sites such as alveolar process of maxilla evidenced by its edematous, indurated greyish white appearance. There is no clear demarcation between the normal mucosa and the tumor. So, this specimen is highly suggestive of the carcinoma of the maxilla.

■ SPECIMEN 1.3: TOTAL MAXILLECTOMY—INNER SURFACE (SEEN FROM MEDIAL ASPECT)

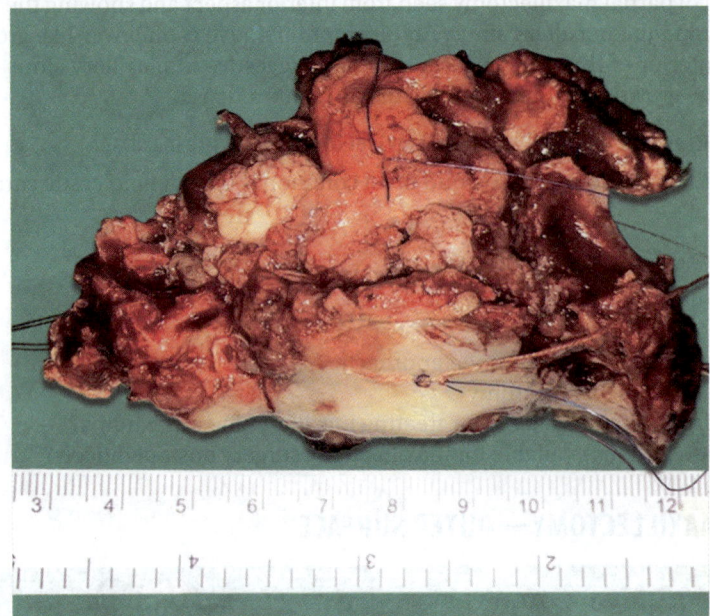

Showing normal palatal mucosa, loose teeth and mass in maxillary antrum.

■ SPECIMEN 2.1: TOTAL LARYNGECTOMY (POSTERIOR SURFACE)

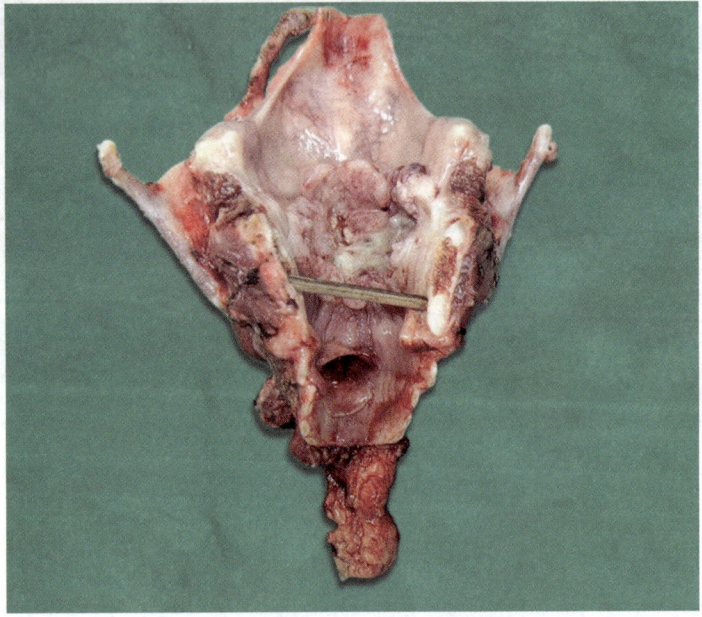

Q. Identify and describe the specimen.

This is an operated specimen of the total laryngectomy. Specimen has been split open to show the following structures:
- Epiglottis
- Arytenoid cartilage
- Aryepiglottic folds
- Thyroid cartilage
- Cricoid cartilage
- Subglottis

  A small wooden stick is placed to demarcate the lower level of glottis and upper level of the subglottis.

  An ulceroproliferative cauliflower-like growth with everted margins, circumferentially involving the glottis, i.e., true vocal cords, false vocal cords, ventricle, anterior commissure, and left vocal process of the arytenoid cartilage. It is involving supraglottis also. Growth seems to be extending approximately 5 mm above the level of the true vocal cords. Thus, the specimen is highly suggestive of glottis-supraglottis carcinoma.

Q. What is the most common microscopic finding (histopathology) for carcinoma of the larynx?

Squamous cell carcinoma is the most common finding.

Questions for Viva Voce

- What are the indications for total laryngectomy?
- What are the contraindications for total laryngectomy?
- What are the types of laryngectomies?
- What are the important points to consider while taking consent for the total laryngectomy procedure?
- What are the complications of the total laryngectomy?
- What is the most common site of the squamous cell carcinoma of the larynx?
- Give TNM classification for the glottis carcinoma.

■ SPECIMEN 2.2: TOTAL LARYNGECTOMY—GLOTTIS CARCINOMA

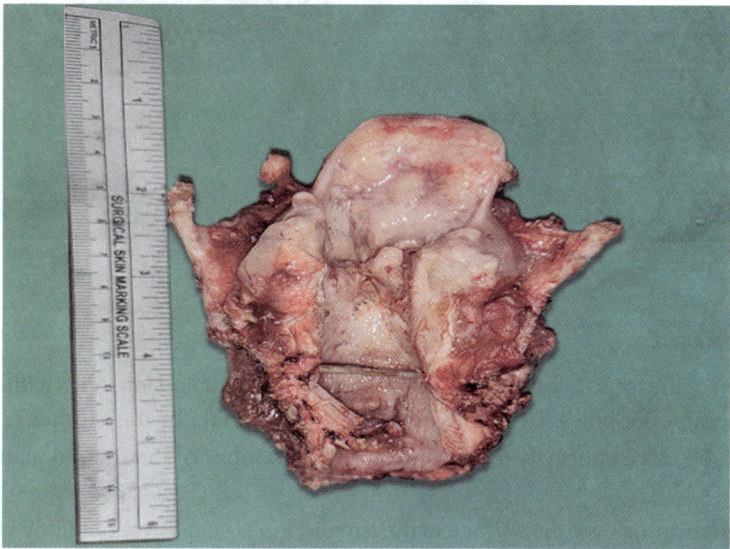

For explanation *see* Specimen 2.1.

■ SPECIMEN 2.3: TOTAL LARYNGECTOMY (ANTERIOR SURFACE)

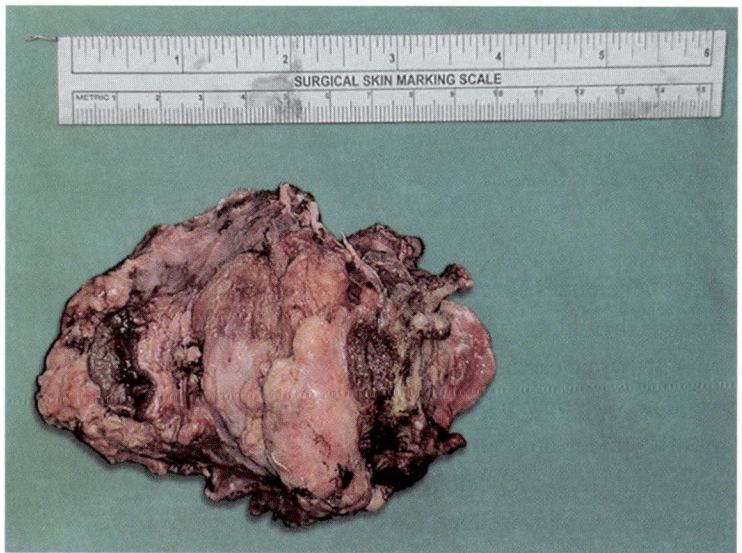

Anterior surface of larynx showing normal epiglottis, hyoid bone, thyroid cartilages without infiltration of tumor.

SPECIMEN 3: TOTAL THYROIDECTOMY (ANTERIOR ASPECT)

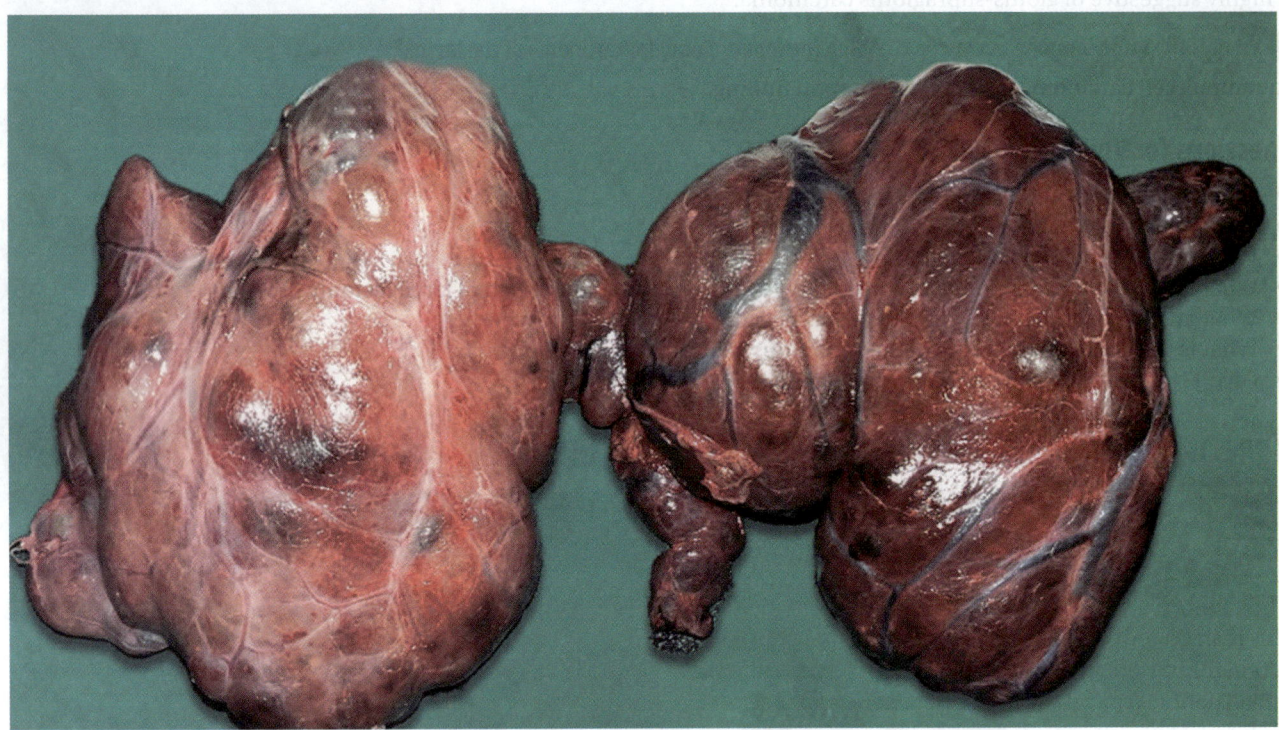

Q. Identify and describe the specimen.

This is an operated specimen of the total thyroidectomy identified by the right and left lobes with superior and inferior poles, showing tapering toward the superior poles. Two lobes are joined in the center by the isthmus is seen.

Lateral surface of each lobe has a concavity facing anteriorly. Both lobes of the thyroid gland are enlarged in size with multiple nodules seen.

Prominent veins are seen running over the surface of the thyroid lobes suggestive of highly vascular tissue of the thyroid gland. There are some areas of hemorrhage seen over the lobes.

So, the specimen is highly suggestive of multinodular goiter.

Q. What are the most common microscopic findings (histology) in cases of thyroid carcinomas?

- Papillary thyroid carcinoma (PTC)
- Follicular carcinoma
- Follicular variant of the papillary cancer
- Oncocytic carcinoma

Questions for Viva Voce

- Mention different types of thyroidectomies.
- What are the indications for total thyroidectomy?
- Mention most common types of thyroid carcinomas.
- Mention the blood supply and nerve supply of the thyroid gland.
- What are the complications of thyroidectomy surgery?
- What are the parameters one should monitor postoperatively in a case of thyroidectomy?
- Mention differential diagnosis for a thyroid swelling.

■ SPECIMEN 4: HEMIGLOSSECTOMY SPECIMEN (DORSAL SURFACE)

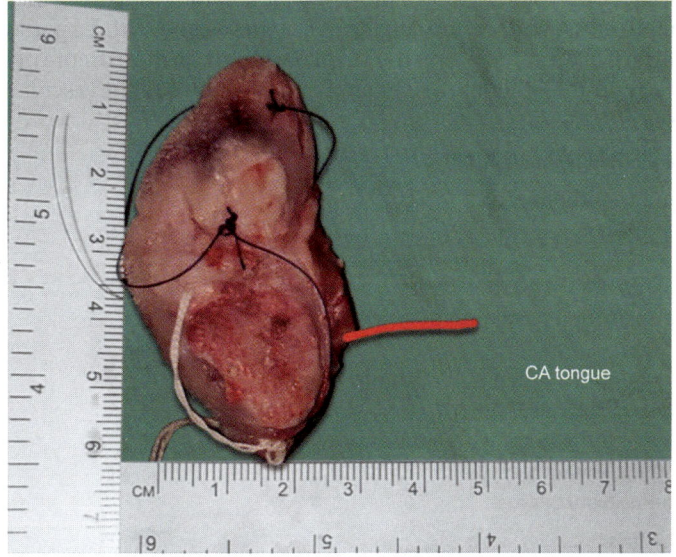

Q. Identify and describe the specimen.

This is an operated specimen of the hemiglossectomy identified by the papillae seen over the anterior two-third of the tongue and highly vascular pinkish white tissue seen. White thread denotes the posterior one-third of the tongue; while the black thread denotes the tip of the tongue. There is an ulcerative lesion involving posterior one-third aspect of the tongue along with the base of the tongue on the dorsal surface with well-demarcated thick margins. Area adjacent to the ulcer shows induration. So, this is highly suggestive of the carcinoma of the tongue.

Q. What is the most common microscopic finding (histology) in a case of carcinoma of the tongue?

Squamous cell carcinoma is the most common finding.

Questions for Viva Voce

- What are the different modalities of treatment for carcinoma of tongue?
- What are the indications of hemiglossectomy?
- Mention the blood supply and nerve supply of the tongue.
- What are the complications of hemiglossectomy?
- Give TNM classification of the carcinoma of tongue.
- Give the differential diagnosis for an ulcer over the tongue.
- How will you manage a case of hemiglossectomy postoperatively?

■ SPECIMEN 5: ANTROCHOANAL POLYP

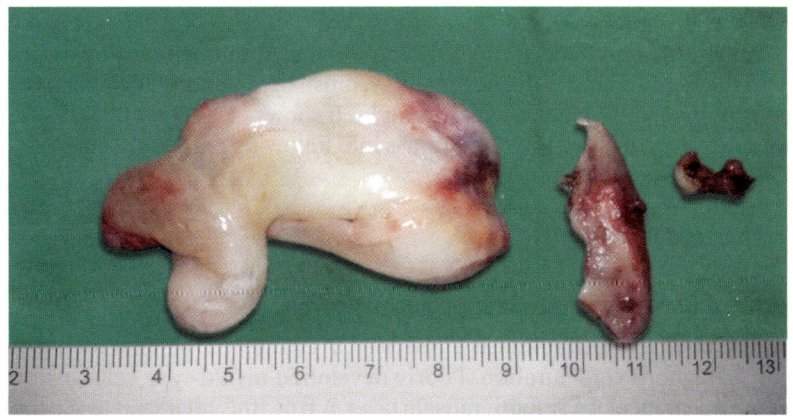

Q. Identify and describe the specimen.

This is an operated specimen of an AC polyp that shows a prolapsed edematous mucosa of the sinuses/nasal cavity with a pale grape-like appearance with smooth glossy surface and soft in consistency. It shows three parts as shown in the picture—antral part on the extreme left, choanal part in the middle, and the small nasal part on the extreme right. It shows two constrictions—one at the maxillary ostium area and the other at the choanal area. It shows slight vascularity at the periphery due to the long-standing nature of the disease.

Q. What is the microscopic picture (histology) of an AC polyp?

Pseudostratified ciliated columnar epithelium.

Questions for Viva Voce

- What is the differential diagnosis for a nasal polyp?
- Define nasal polyp.
- Mention four differences between AC polyp and ethmoid polyp.
- What are the treatment options for a nasal polyp?
- What are the clinical features of the patient with a nasal polyp?
- What is functional endoscopic sinus surgery (FESS)?
- Mention salient steps of the FESS surgery.

■ SPECIMEN 6: JUVENILE ANGIOFIBROMA

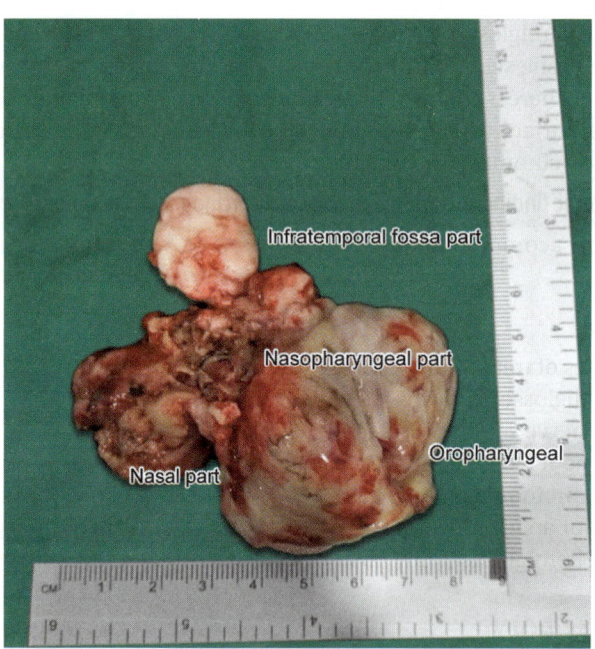

Q. Identify and describe the specimen.

It is an operated specimen showing a well-circumscribed, multilobulated, dumbbell-shaped mass showing whitish gray area in the center of the mass and the reddish area at the periphery. Whitish area denotes the fibrous core while the reddish area is indicative of the vascularity of the tumor; highly suggestive of JA. It shows three constrictions—one constriction anteriorly and two constrictions posteriorly thus dividing the tumor mass into following parts:

- Nasal part anteriorly
- Nasopharyngeal part posteriorly
- Infratemporal fossa part posterolaterally
- Oropharyngeal part inferiorly

Q. What is the microscopic picture (histology) of a juvenile angiofibroma?

It shows vascular and fibrous stromal tissue (fibroblasts embedded in collagen). The intervening vessels vary in size, ranging from slit-like to ectatic with a staghorn configuration. Poorly developed myoid-type cells surround the endothelial-lined vascular channels, giving the appearance of a smooth muscle layer. A true muscular coat or elastic lamina is totally absent.

Questions for Viva Voce

- What is the common age group affected by the JA?
- What are the clinical features of a patient with JA?
- What is the differential diagnosis of patient presenting with a nasal bleed and a nasal mass?
- What are the surgical techniques available for the excision of JA?
- What are the complications of the JA surgery?
- What is the most common blood supply of the JA?
- JA—is it a benign tumor or a malignant tumor?

SPECIMEN 7: SUPERFICIAL PAROTIDECTOMY

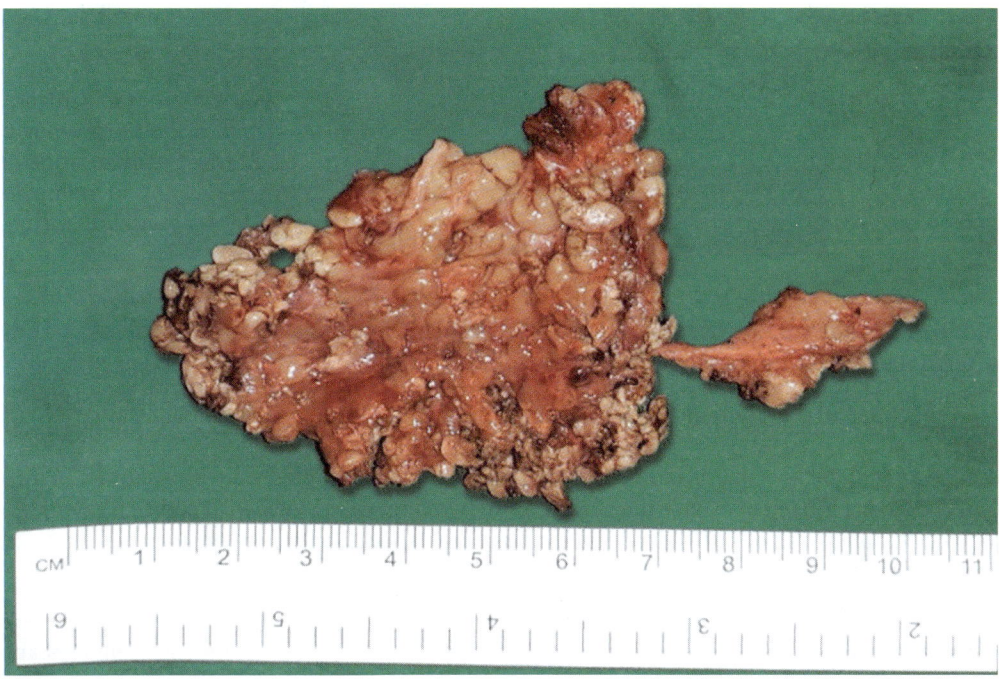

Q. Identify and describe the specimen.

This is a pear-shaped specimen of the salivary gland showing multiple lobulations of the parenchyma (small grayish white grape-like structures) separated by the connective tissue septa (myxoid stroma). Left hand side of the specimen shows the inferior pole of the gland while the middle part denoting the superior pole of the gland. On the extreme right of the specimen there is a parotid gland duct seen with the adjacent fibrofatty tissue.

Inferiorly, areas of cystic degeneration with hemorrhage and necrosis (mahogany-colored areas) are seen well separated from the normal gland parenchyma. So, this specimen is highly suggestive of pleomorphic adenoma of the parotid gland.

Q. Describe the microscopic picture (histology) of the pleomorphic adenoma of the parotid gland.

Tumor is circumscribed by a fibrous capsule demarcating it from the normal glandular serous acini. It consists of myoepithelial cells and small striated ducts within a chondromyxoid stroma. Serous acini surround the striated ducts. Cells can be spindled, epithelioid, plasmacytoid or have clear cytoplasm.

Questions for Viva Voce

- Mention benign and malignant tumors of the parotid gland.
- Name the incision used for superficial parotidectomy.
- Mention different types of parotidectomies.
- What are the landmarks used for identifying the facial nerve during parotidectomy?
- What are the complications of superficial parotidectomy?
- Name two important preoperative investigations for a parotid swelling.
- What is Frey's syndrome?

SPECIMEN 8: SUBMANDIBULAR GLAND WITH CALCULUS (SIALOLITH)

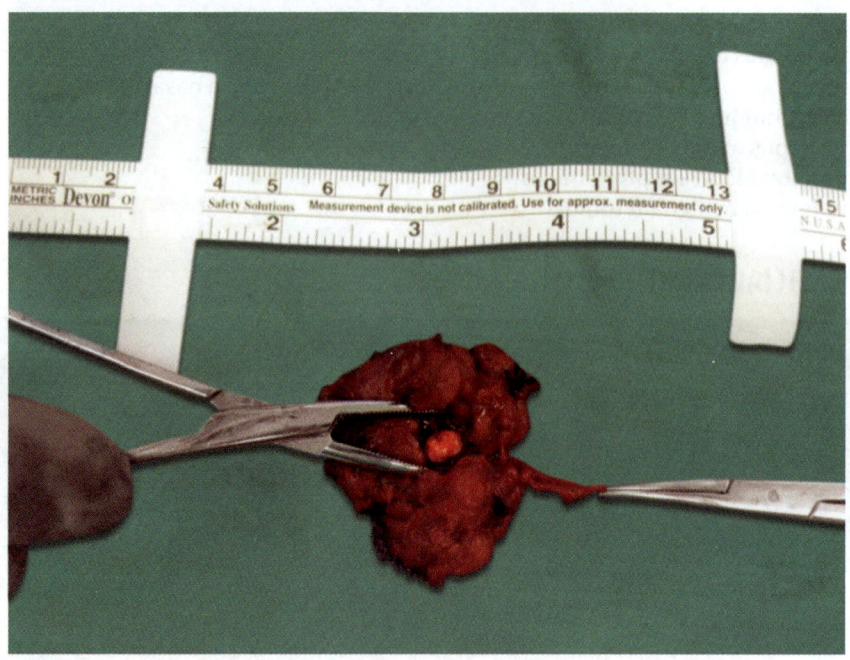

Q. Identify and describe the specimen.

This is an operated specimen of the submandibular salivary gland with its lobulated appearance and reddish white areas of the fibrous stroma.

On the right hand side of the specimen; submandibular gland duct is seen grasped with a curved hemostat. On the left hand side, a curved hemostat is used to expose the gland parenchyma revealing yellowish cod-like calculus.

Gland seems to be enlarged in size as a result of the calculus. Thus, specimen is highly suggestive of submandibular gland excision for the calculi (sialolithiasis) by open approach.

Q. What is the microscopic picture (histology) of a normal submandibular gland?

Both serous and mucous secreting cells are seen. Serous cells are arranged in acini while mucous cells are capped with serous demilune cells. Serous cells are generally spherical and show eosinophilic zymogen granules while mucous cells are tubular with pale staining cytoplasm and nuclei that are pushed against the basal cell membrane.

Questions for Viva Voce

- Mention the indications for submandibular gland excision.
- What are the different types of salivary gland calculi seen commonly?
- What is alternative surgical technique for submandibular gland stone extraction apart from open surgical technique?
- What are the boundaries and contents of the submandibular gland triangle?
- What are the complications of submandibular gland excision by open approach?
- What are the clinical features of a patient with salivary gland calculi?
- What are different types of salivary glands you know of?

Mock Question Papers

THEORY

Section A (20 Marks)

Multiple choice questions (Total 20 MCQs of one mark each) *(1 ×20 = 20)*

1. Stapes footplate covers:
   a. Round window
   b. Oval window
   c. Interior sinus tympani
   d. Pyramid
2. Ceruminous glands present in the ear are:
   a. Modified eccrine glands
   b. Modified apocrine
   c. Mucus gland
   d. Modified holocrine gland
3. All are true for Gradenigo's syndrome, *except*:
   a. It is associated with conductive hearing loss
   b. Caused by abscess in the petroux apex
   c. Involvement of CN V and VI
   d. Characterized by retro-orbital pain
4. Which among the following is an absolute indication for cortical mastoidectomy
   a. Acute coalescent mastoiditis
   b. SOM
   c. Severe ASOM
   d. CSOM safe type
5. The most common complication of CSOM is:
   a. Subperiosteal abscess
   b. Mastoiditis
   c. Brain abscess
   d. Meningitis
6. The palatine tonsil receives its arterial supply from all of following, *except*:
   a. Facial
   b. Ascending palatine
   c. Sphenopalatine
   d. Dorsal lingual
7. The most common cause of epistaxis in 4-year-old boy is:
   a. Chronic rhinitis
   b. Nasal polyp
   c. Foreign body
   d. Nose packing
8. A laryngocele arises from the:
   a. True vocal cord
   b. Subglottis
   c. Saccule of the ventricle
   d. Anterior commissure
9. Which one of the following statements truly represents Bell's paralysis?
   a. Hemiparesis and contralateral facial nerve paralysis
   b. Combined paralysis of the facial, trigeminal, and abducens nerves
   c. Idiopathic ipsilateral paralysis of the facial nerve
   d. Facial nerve paralysis with a dry eye
10. The etiology of anterior ethmoidal neuralgia is:
    a. Inferior turbinate pressing on the nasal septum
    b. Middle turbinate pressing on nasal septum
    c. Superior turbinate pressing on nasal septum
    d. Causing obstruction of sphenoid opening
11. Pars flaccid of TM is also called as:
    a. Reissner's membrane
    b. Sharpnell's membrane
    c. Basillar membrane
    d. Secondary TM

12. **The most common site of otosclerosis:**
    a. Round window
    b. Oval window
    c. Utricle
    d. Incus
13. **Tuberculous otitis media is characterized by all, *except*:**
    a. Pain
    b. Pale granulation
    c. Thin odorless fluid
    d. Multiple perforations
14. **In which of the following conditions is sialography contraindicated:**
    a. Ductal calculus
    b. Chronic parotitis
    c. Acute parotitis
    d. Recurrent Sialadenitis
15. **Trotter's triad includes all, *except*:**
    a. Seizures
    b. Mandibular neuralgia
    c. Deafness
    d. Palatal palsy
16. **Use of Seigel's speculum during examination of ear provides all, *except*:**
    a. Magnification
    b. Assessment of movement of TM
    c. Removal of foreign body
    d. Application of powdered antibiotic
17. **Recruitment phenomenon is seen in:**
    a. Otosclerosis
    b. Meniere's disease
    c. Acoustic schwannoma
    d. Otitis media with effusion
18. **All of the following open into middle meatus, *except*:**
    a. Anterior ethmoidal sinus
    b. Middle ethmoidal sinus
    c. Posterior ethmoidal sinus
    d. Maxillary sinus
19. **Epiglottitis in a 2-year-old child is to infection with:**
    a. Influenza virus
    b. *Staphylococcus aureus*
    c. *Haemophilus influenzae*
    d. Repsiratory synctial virus
20. **The most common and earliest manifestation of Ca glottis is**
    a. Hoarseness
    b. Hemoptysis
    c. Cervical lymphadenopathy
    d. Stridor

Section B (40 Marks)

Long answer questions (Any 2 out of 3) (Structured case based) *(2 × 10 = 20)*

Q1. What are the causes of epistaxis? How will you manage a patient with intractable epistaxis?

Q2. Enumerate the causes of conductive hearing loss with intact tympanic membrane. Describe the clinical features and management of safe chronic suppurative otitis media (CSOM).

Q3. What is stridor? Discuss the various causes and management of stridor.

Short answer questions (attempt all) [1 attitude, ethics and communication (AETCOM), 2 clinical reasoning question]
(4 × 5 = 20)

Q1. Foreign body in the nose

Q2. Gradenigo's syndrome

Q3. Rinne's test

Q4. Draw and label diagram of left tympanic membrane.

Section C (40 Marks)

Long answer question (Any 2 out of 3) (Structured case based) *(2 × 10 = 20)*

Q1. Draw a well-labeled diagram of nasal septum and its blood supply. Enumerate difference between septoplasty and submucosal resection (SMR). Enumerate the complications of SMR.

Q2. Describe in brief about the clinical features and management of chronic tonsillitis. Add a note on complications of tonsillectomy.

Q3. Discuss the etiopathogenesis, clinical features, management of Ca larynx in a 50 years male who is chronic tobacco chewer.

Short answer questions (Any 4 out of 5) (Minimum 2 clinical reasoning question) *(4 ×5 = 20)*

Q1. Serous otitis media
Q2. Surgical management of atrophic rhinitis
Q3. Management of fractured nasal bone
Q4. Enumerate instruments required for IDL and its procedure
Q5. Post-tracheostomy care

■ PRACTICAL EXAMINATION

Case	OSCE				Table viva		
❖ Long case ❖ Short case	OSCE 1 (Clinical skills)	OSCE 2 (Clinical skills)	OSCE 3 (Certifiable skills)	OSCE 4 (AETCOM skills)	❖ Surgical pathology ❖ Radiology	Instruments and surgical procedure	Journal and log book

(OSCE: Objective Structured Clinical and Practical Examination)

Multiple Choice Questions (MCQs)

EAR

1. **Tympanic membrane develops from:**
   a. Ectoderm
   b. Mesoderm
   c. Endoderm
   d. All the three germinal layers

2. **Stapes footplate covers:**
   a. Round window
   b. Oval window
   c. Sinus tympani
   d. Pyramid

3. **Inner ear malformation in fetus can occur when mother during pregnancy is exposed to:**
   a. Radiation
   b. German measles
   c. Cytomegalovirus
   d. Thalidomide
   e. All of the above

4. **Which of the following is not a typical feature of Meniere's disease?**
   a. Sensorineural deafness
   b. Pulsatile tinnitus
   c. Vertigo
   d. Fluctuating deafness

5. **Treatment of choice for glue ear is:**
   a. Conservative
   b. Myringotomy with cold knife
   c. Myringotomy with ventilation tube insertion
   d. Myringotomy with diode laser

6. **The posterosuperior retraction pocket, if allowed to progress, will lead to:**
   a. Sensorineural hearing loss
   b. Secondary cholesteatoma
   c. Tympanosclerosis
   d. Tertiary cholesteatoma

7. **Which is the investigation of choice in assessing hearing loss in neonates?**
   a. Impedance audiometry
   b. Brain stem evoked response audiometry (BERA)
   c. Free field audiometry
   d. Behavioral audiometry

8. **All are true for Gradenigo's syndrome, *except*:**
   a. It is associated with conductive hearing loss
   b. It is caused by an abscess in the petrous apex
   c. It leads to involvement of cranial nerves V and VI
   d. It is characterized by retro-orbital pain

9. **Otoacoustic emissions are produced by:**
   a. Inner hair cells
   b. Outer hair cells
   c. Basilar membrane
   d. Auditory nerve

10. **Speech frequencies include:**
    a. 125, 250, 500 Hz
    b. 250, 500, 1000 Hz
    c. 500, 1000, 2000, Hz
    d. 1000, 2000, 3000 Hz

11. **On Dix-Hallpike testing, nystagmus of central origin:**
    a. Can be easily fatigued on repeated testing
    b. Has a fixed direction
    c. Appears immediately as soon as head is in critical position without a latent period
    d. Lasts for a few seconds

12. **Phelps sign is seen in:**
    a. Glomus jugulare
    b. Vestibular schwannoma
    c. Meniere's disease
    d. Neurofibromatosis
13. **Brown's sign is seen in:**
    a. Glomus tumor
    b. Meniere's disease
    c. Acoustic neuroma
    d. Otosclerosis
14. **Extracranial complications of chronic suppurative otitis media (CSOM):**
    a. Epidural abscess
    b. Facial nerve palsy
    c. Labyrinthitis
    d. Sigmoid sinus thrombosis
15. **Picket fence graph of temperature is seen in:**
    a. Otitic hydrocephalus
    b. Lateral sinus thrombosis
    c. Extradural abscess
    d. Meningitis
16. **Aim of mastoid surgery in CSOM which should receive first priority is:**
    a. Making the ear dry
    b. Improvement in hearing
    c. Preservation of hearing
    d. Rendering the ear safe
17. **Otosclerosis is:**
    a. Autosomal dominant
    b. Autosomal recessive
    c. X-linked disease
    d. Mitochondrial disorder
18. **Most common site for initiation of stapedial otosclerosis is:**
    a. Fissula ante-fenestram
    b. Fissula post-fenestram
    c. Footplate of stapes
    d. Margins of stapes
19. **Schwartze's sign is:**
    a. Swelling over the mastoid
    b. Reddish hue seen in the hypotympanum behind an intact tympanic membrane
    c. Improved hearing in noisy surroundings
    d. Reddish hue seen over the promontory
20. **The triad of Van der Hoeve syndrome includes all, *except*:**
    a. Osteogenesis imperfecta
    b. Conductive hearing loss
    c. Blue sclera
    d. Preauricular sinuses
21. **Meniere's disease is characterized by:**
    a. Conductive hearing loss and tinnitus
    b. Vertigo, ear discharge, tinnitus, and headache
    c. Vertigo, tinnitus, hearing loss, and headache
    d. Vertigo, tinnitus, and hearing loss
22. **The most common cause of peripheral episodic vertigo is:**
    a. Meniere's disease
    b. Acoustic neuroma
    c. Benign paroxysmal positional vertigo
    d. Vascular occlusion of labyrinthine artery
23. **A cochlear implant has the following components, *except*:**
    a. Microphone
    b. Speech processor
    c. Electrode array
    d. Amplifier

Answer Key

1. d	2. b	3. e	4. b	5. c	6. b	7. b	8. a	9. b	10. c
11. c	12. a	13. a	14. b, c, d	15. b	16. d	17. a	18. a	19. d	20. d
21. d	22. c	23. d							

NOSE AND PARANASAL SINUSES

1. **A 20-year-old female from Uttar Pradesh presented with nasal obstruction and crusting of nose. Examination revealed an infiltrating lesion involving the nasal vestibule and upper lip with broadening of nasal dorsum. Likely diagnosis is:**
    a. Rhinosporidiosis
    b. Rhinoscleroma
    c. Fungal granuloma
    d. Nasal diphtheria
2. **A biopsy is taken from a granulomatous lesion of nose revealed Mikulicz's cells and eosinophilic structures in the cytoplasm of the plasma cells, the likely diagnosis is:**
    a. Mucormycosis
    b. Rhinosporidiosis
    c. Rhinoscleroma
    d. Nasal leprosy
3. **All of the following are associated with Kartagener syndrome (immotile cilia syndrome), *except*:**
    a. Bronchiectasis
    b. Sterility
    c. Chronic sinusitis
    d. Cleft palate
4. **Pott's puffy tumor is related to:**
    a. Infected cell in middle turbinate
    b. Tuberculous sinusitis
    c. Pyogenic infection of frontal sinus
    d. Cavernous sinus thrombosis

PART 4: Questions

5. Type of carcinoma of the sinonasal tract in wood workers is:
   a. Adenocarcinoma
   b. Adenoid cystic carcinoma
   c. Squamous cell carcinoma
   d. Olfactory neuroblastoma
6. In paranasal sinuses, osteoma commonly involves:
   a. Frontal sinus
   b. Maxillary sinus
   c. Ethmoid sinus
   d. Sphenoid sinus
7. Which of the following drug is linked with rhinitis medicamentosa?
   a. Intranasal steroid spray
   b. Ipratropium bromide
   c. Xylometazoline
   d. Cocaine
8. In Caldwell–Luc operation, entry into the maxillary sinus is made through:
   a. Transethmoid approach
   b. Canine fossa
   c. Maxillary alveolus
   d. Middle meatal antrostomy
9. Which of the following ganglion is associated with lacrimation?
   a. Otic
   b. Ciliary
   c. Sphenopalatine
   d. Gasserian
10. Complications following septal abscesses include all, *except*:
    a. Severe epistaxis
    b. Depression of nasal bridge
    c. Meningitis
    d. Cavernous sinus thrombophlebitis
11. Rhinophyma is associated with:
    a. Hypertrophy of sebaceous glands
    b. Hypertrophy of sweat glands
    c. Hyperplasia of endothelial cells
    d. Hyperplasia of epithelial cells
12. A 4-year-old child presents with bleeding from right side of nose. He also gets purulent discharge from the same side. The likely diagnosis is:
    a. Septal deviation with right maxillary sinusitis
    b. Unilateral channel atresia
    c. Antrochoanal polyp
    d. Foreign body
13. "Bleeding polyp" of the nose is another name for:
    a. Antrochoanal polyp
    b. Juvenile angiofibroma
    c. Hemangioma of nasal septum
    d. Rhinosporidiosis
14. The space between bulla ethmoidalis and uncinate process is called:
    a. Agger nasi
    b. Olfactory cleft
    c. Frontonasal duct
    d. Hiatus semilunaris
15. Arteries which take part in Kiesselbach's plexus include all, *except*:
    a. Anterior ethmoid
    b. Greater palatine
    c. Superior labial
    d. Inferior labial
16. Constituents of nasal septum include all, *except*:
    a. Vomer
    b. Perpendicular plate of palatine
    c. Quadrangular cartilage
    d. Maxillary crest
17. Opening of nasolacrimal duct is situated in:
    a. Superior meatus
    b. Middle meatus
    c. Ethmoid infundibulum
    d. Inferior meatus
18. Trismus accompanying peritonsillar abscess is due to spasm of which muscles?
    a. Masseter
    b. Pharyngeal constrictors
    c. Medial pterygoid
    d. Temporalis
19. Lymphoid tissue called Waldeyer's ring is situated in:
    a. Nasopharynx
    b. Oropharynx
    c. Both nasopharynx and oropharynx
    d. Base of tongue
20. Which of the following statement is not correct for ethmoidal polyp?
    a. Allergy is an etiological factor
    b. Occur in the first decade of life
    c. Are bilateral
    d. Are often associated with bronchial asthma
21. The most common site for CSF rhinorrhea:
    a. Sphenoid sinus
    b. Frontal sinus
    c. Petrous
    d. Cribriform plate
22. CSF rhinorrhea is diagnosed by:
    a. Beta 2 microglobulin
    b. Beta 2 transferrin
    c. Thyroglobulin
    d. Transthyretin
23. Nasopharyngeal chordoma originates from:
    a. Torus tubarius
    b. Rathke's pouch
    c. Notochord
    d. Pharyngeal bursa

CHAPTER 83: Multiple Choice Questions (MCQs)

24. Juvenile angiofibroma commonly arises from:
    a. Fossa of Rosenmuller
    b. Posterior border of nasal septum
    c. Sphenopalatine foramen
    d. Posterior wall of nasopharynx
25. Antral (Holman–Miller) sign is a feature of:
    a. Acoustic neuroma
    b. Glomus tumor
    c. Nasopharyngeal fibroma
    d. Coalescent mastoiditis
26. Thornwaldt's cyst is seen in:
    a. Larynx
    b. Nasopharynx
    c. Base of tongue
    d. Floor of mouth
27. Horner's syndrome consists of all of the following features, *except*:
    a. Ptosis
    b. Dilated pupil
    c. Anhidrosis
    d. Endophthalmos
28. Pharyngeal bursa is a site of origin for:
    a. Craniopharyngioma
    b. Chordoma
    c. Thornwaldt's cyst
    d. Rathke's pouch
29. A 6-year-old child presented with history of recurrent upper respiratory tract infections, mouth breathing, nasal obstruction, and hearing impairment. Management will be:
    a. Tonsillectomy
    b. Adenoidectomy with grommet insertion
    c. Myringotomy with grommet
    d. Myringotomy

Answer Key

1. b	2. c	3. d	4. c	5. a	6. a	7. c	8. b	9. c	10. a
11. a	12. d	13. c	14. d	15. d	16. b	17. d	18. c	19. c	20. b
21. d	22. b	23. c	24. c	25. c	26. b	27. b	28. c	29. b	

■ LARYNX

1. Which of the following lesions in the oral cavity has a malignant potential?
    a. Hypertrophic candidiasis
    b. Leukoderma
    c. Erythroplasia
    d. White sponge nevus
2. Taste buds are seen in all of the following papillae except:
    a. Circumvallate
    b. Fungiform
    c. Filiform
    d. Foliate
3. In which of the following locations (spaces), there is collection of pus in quinsy?
    a. Peritonsillar space
    b. Parapharyngeal space
    c. Retropharyngeal space
    d. Within tonsil
4. Type of voice in nasopharyngeal fibroma is:
    a. Rhinolalia aperta
    b. Rhinolalia clausa
    c. Hot-potato voice
    d. Staccato voice
5. Most common site for carcinoma of oral tongue is:
    a. Tip
    b. Dorsum
    c. Lateral border
    d. Ventral surface
6. All of the following statements about Zenker's diverticulum are correct, *except*:
    a. Arises from posterior part of hypopharynx
    b. Is a traction diverticulum
    c. Causes regurgitation of undigested food
    d. Treated by diverticulectomy and cricopharyngeal myotomy
7. Radiographic findings of achalasia cardia include all, *except*:
    a. Esophageal dilatation
    b. Rat-tail appearance
    c. Failure of lower esophageal sphincter to relax
    d. Diffuse esophageal spasm
8. A 50-year-old man had drinks followed by a heavy dinner. He had severe vomiting and chest pain and collapsed. X-ray of chest showed hydropneumothorax. The likely diagnosis is:
    a. Mallory–Weiss syndrome
    b. Boerhaave syndrome
    c. Ruptured duodenal ulcer
    d. Myocardial infarction
9. Characteristic features of submucous cleft palate include all, *except*:
    a. Bifid uvula
    b. Notch in posterior border of hard palate
    c. Deficient palatal muscles
    d. Common association with cleft lip

10. **Main blood supply to tonsil comes from:**
    a. Ascending pharyngeal artery
    b. Dorsal lingual branches of lingual artery
    c. Tonsillar branches of facial artery
    d. Descending palatine from maxillary

11. **Pulsatile swelling in tonsillar fossa can be due to:**
    a. Normal external carotid artery
    b. Carotid body tumor
    c. Aneurysm of internal carotid artery
    d. Peritonsillar abscess

12. **All of the following causes a gray-white membrane on the tonsils, *except*:**
    a. Infectious mononucleosis
    b. Ludwig's angina
    c. Streptococcal tonsillitis
    d. Diphtheria

13. **A 30-year-old male presented with trismus, fever, swelling pushing the tonsils medially and spreading laterally posterior to the middle of sternocleidomastoid. He gives a history of extraction of third molar few days back for dental caries. The diagnosis is:**
    a. Retropharyngeal abscess
    b. Ludwig's angina
    c. Submental abscess
    d. Parapharyngeal abscess

14. **A patient presented with a 3.5 cm size lymph node enlargement, which was hard and present in the submandibular region. Examination of the head and neck did not yield any lesion. Which of the following investigations should follow?**
    a. Chest X-ray
    b. Triple endoscopy
    c. Supravital oral mucosa staining
    d. Laryngoscopy

15. **Tonsil develops from:**
    a. First pouch
    b. Second pouch
    c. Second cleft
    d. First cleft

16. **Fordyce's spots in oral cavity arise from:**
    a. Mucous glands
    b. Sebaceous glands
    c. Taste buds
    d. Minor salivary glands

17. **Major amount of saliva, when salivary glands are not stimulated is contributed by:**
    a. Parotid glands
    b. Submandibular glands
    c. Sublingual glands
    d. Minor salivary glands

18. **What percentage of calculi in the submandibular gland is radiolucent?**
    a. 20%
    b. 30%
    c. 50%
    d. 80%

19. **Most common site of origin of pleomorphic adenoma:**
    a. Parotid gland
    b. Submandibular salivary gland
    c. Minor salivary glands of soft and hard palate
    d. Minor salivary glands of lip

20. **Most common malignant tumor of submandibular salivary gland is:**
    a. Mucoepidermoid carcinoma
    b. Squamous cell carcinoma
    c. Adenoid cystic carcinoma
    d. Adenocarcinoma

21. **Cricoid cartilage is a derivative of which branchial arch?**
    a. IIIrd arch
    b. IVth arch
    c. Vth arch
    d. Hypobranchial eminence

22. **Sensory nerve supply above the level of vocal cords is:**
    a. Glossopharyngeal
    b. Superior laryngeal
    c. Recurrent laryngeal
    d. Pharyngeal branch of vagus

23. **All of the following laryngeal muscles are adductors of vocal cord, *except*:**
    a. Lateral cricoarytenoid
    b. Posterior cricoarytenoid
    c. Thyroarytenoid
    d. Oblique arytenoid

24. **Paralysis of recurrent laryngeal nerve does not affect function of:**
    a. Thyroarytenoid
    b. Lateral cricoarytenoid
    c. Vocalis
    d. Cricothyroid

25. **Which of the following muscle is tensor of vocal cord?**
    a. Posterior cricoarytenoid
    b. Transverse arytenoid
    c. Lateral cricoarytenoid
    d. Cricothyroid

26. **Type of epithelium lining the vocal cords is:**
    a. Keratinizing stratified squamous
    b. Nonkeratinizing stratified squamous
    c. Pseudostratified ciliated columnar
    d. Cuboidal

27. **Laryngeal crepitus is seen in:**
    a. Normal persons
    b. Fractures of thyroid cartilage
    c. Postcricoid carcinoma
    d. Prevertebral abscess

CHAPTER 83: Multiple Choice Questions (MCQs)

28. Reinke's edema is responsible for:
    a. Vocal nodule
    b. Vocal polyp
    c. Diffuse polypoid degeneration of vocal cords
    d. Laryngeal cyst
29. Phonation in dysphonia plica ventricularis is produced by:
    a. Anterior thirds of vocal cords only
    b. False cords
    c. Cricopharyngeal segment
    d. Palatopharyngeal fold
30. The best way to diagnose laryngomalacia is:
    a. Symptoms and signs of disease only
    b. Soft tissue lateral view neck
    c. Direct laryngoscopy under general anesthesia
    d. Flexible fiberoptic laryngoscopy
31. Laryngeal web most commonly involves region of:
    a. Supraglottis
    b. Glottis
    c. Subglottis
    d. Both a and b
32. Acute epiglottitis in children is mostly caused by:
    a. Para influenza type I and II
    b. Respiratory syncytial virus
    c. *Streptococcus pneumoniae*
    d. *Haemophilus influenzae* type B
33. Virus responsible for juvenile papillomatosis of larynx is:
    a. Cytomegalovirus
    b. EBV
    c. Adenovirus
    d. Papovavirus
34. Laryngocele arises from:
    a. Vallecula
    b. Laryngeal saccule
    c. Laryngeal ventricle
    d. Aryepiglottic fold
35. Hoarseness is the earliest symptom of carcinoma of:
    a. Glottis
    b. Subglottis
    c. Supraglottis
    d. All of the above
36. In cancer of pyriform fossa, pain is referred to ipsilateral ear via:
    a. CN IX
    b. CN X
    c. CN XI
    d. CN XII
37. Type I thyroplasty is for:
    a. Vocal cord medialization
    b. Vocal cord lateralization
    c. Vocal cord shortening
    d. Vocal cord lengthening
38. All are true about external laryngocele, *except*:
    a. Produces a swelling in the neck on Valsalva
    b. Communicates with laryngeal ventricle
    c. Can be seen on CT
    d. Herniates through cricothyroid membrane
39. Steeple sign seen on posterosuperior view of neck in a child with stridor is indicative of:
    a. Acute epiglottitis
    b. Acute laryngotracheobronchitis
    c. Laryngeal papillomatosis
    d. Bilateral abductor paralysis

Answer Key

1. c	2. c	3. a	4. b	5. c	6. c	7. d	8. b	9. d	10. c
11. c	12. b	13. d	14. b	15. b	16. b	17. b	18. d	19. a	20. c
21. c	22. b	23. b	24. d	25. d	26. b	27. a	28. c	29. b	30. d
31. b	32. d	33. d	34. b	35. a	36. b	37. a	38. d	39. b	

Case Presentation

■ LONG CASE: EAR

My patient Mrs XYZ, 35-year-old, female, resident of Dadar, Mumbai, plumber by occupation, and Hindu by religion came with the chief complaints of:

KEY POINTS

- Demographic details include name, age, sex, address, occupation, and religion.
- Name gives identity.
- Certain diseases occur at particular age group, sex, and geographical region.
- Occupation is important for knowing occupational hazards. For example, noise-induced hearing loss for factory workers, allergic rhinitis in gardeners due to pollen, rhinosporidiosis in farmers.

KEY POINTS

- Chief complaints are to be mentioned in descending order of duration.
- Important to mention the side involved (right, left, or bilateral).

Chief Complaint

- ❖ Right ear discharge since 7 years
- ❖ Right ear reduced hearing since 4 years
- ❖ Left ear discharge since 2 years
- ❖ Left ear reduced hearing since 1 year

History of Present Illness (HOPI)

My patient was apparently asymptomatic when he complained of the following:

KEY POINTS

- Each symptom to be described as mentioned in under history. Ask for onset (sudden/insidious), duration, progression (rapid/gradual), periodicity (intermittent/continuous), frequency, severity, and aggravating/relieving factors for each symptom.
- History of presenting illness (HOPI) needs to be described as per patients' words.

- ❖ Right-sided otorrhea since 7 years which was sudden in onset, gradually progressive, initially ear discharge was present occasionally but now present every 3 months, intermittent in nature.
- ❖ The otorrhea was mucopurulent in nature, whitish in color, sticky in consistency, profuse in amount, nonfoul smelling, and nonblood stained.

- ❖ The otorrhea aggravates with upper respiratory tract infection (URTI) and relieves completely with medications. Last episode of ear discharge was present around 1 month back.
- ❖ The patients also complained of left-sided otorrhea since 2 years which was sudden in onset, gradually progressive, initially ear discharge was scanty and noticed while ear cleaning but now present associated with hearing loss, continuous in nature and does not resolve completely. The otorrhea was purulent in nature, yellowish in color, nonsticky in consistency, scanty in amount, foul smelling, and occasionally blood stained.
- ❖ The otorrhea has no aggravating factors and does not relieve completely with medications.

KEY POINTS

For ear discharge ask for:
- Nature: Mucoid [otitis media with effusion (OME)]/mucopurulent [mucosal chronic otitis media (COM)]/purulent (squamosal COM)
- Color
- Consistency: Watery [cerebrospinal fluid (CSF) otorrhea]/sticky (due to mucin production seen in mucosal COM)
- Amount: Scanty (discharge noticed while ear cleaning)/moderate (discharge fills ear canal)/profuse (discharge comes out of ear canal and fills concha)
- Foul smelling (seen in squamosal COM) or nonfoul smelling
- Blood stained or not
- Mucosal COM usually aggravates with URTI

The patient complained of:
- ❖ Right ear reduced hearing since 4 years which was gradual in onset and progression, initially was not able to hear whispers but now not able to hear normal conversations clearly. The hearing loss is continuous and has no aggravating or relieving factors.
- ❖ The patient also complained of left ear reduced hearing since 1 year which was gradual in onset and progression, initially was not able to hear whispers but now not able to hear loud conversations. The hearing loss is continuous, associated with ear discharge and has no relieving factors.

KEY POINTS

- Types of hearing loss—conductive, sensorineural, and mixed type
- Hearing loss can be constant or fluctuant.
- Fluctuant hearing loss is seen in Meniere's disease [sesorineural hearing loss (SNHL) at low frequency], Eustachian tube dysfunction, OME [conductive hearing loss (CHL)].
- Hearing loss can be sudden onset.
- Can be associated with poor speech discrimination and background noise (ototoxicity).
- Paracusis Willisii: Person with CHL hears better in noisy environment. Seen in otosclerosis.

- ❖ No history of otalgia (earache), aural fullness
- ❖ No history of postaural swelling, pain behind the ear, and neck swelling
- ❖ No history of giddiness and tinnitus
- ❖ No history of facial weakness or facial asymmetry
- ❖ No history of diplopia/double vision, retro-orbital pain/pain behind the eye
- ❖ No history of fever, vomiting, headache, and altered sensorium
- ❖ No history of visual disturbances, altered speech, seizures, and ataxia
- ❖ No history of trauma, exposure of loud noise, and frequent ear cleaning habits
- ❖ No history of use of ototoxic drugs.
- ❖ No history of nasal obstruction, recurrent rhinorrhea, excessive sneezing, facial heaviness, postnasal drip, and epistaxis
- ❖ No history of recurrent throat pain, dysphagia, odynophagia, dyspnea, cough, and change in voice

KEY POINTS

- First each symptom to be described as mentioned above.
- Negative history: To rule out associated symptoms with complications of COM.
- Ear pain (otalgia) is not feature of COM but associated with otitis externa or dural inflammation.
- Postaural swelling, pain behind the ear, neck swelling: Feature of postauricular abscess, Bezold abscess.
- Giddiness, tinnitus associated with vomiting: Feature of irritative labyrinthitis, labyrinthine fistula.
- Facial weakness or facial asymmetry: Feature of facial nerve palsy.
- Diplopia/double vision, retro-orbital pain/pain behind the eye associated with persistent ear discharge: Feature of petrositis/petrous apicitis
- Fever, vomiting, headache, altered sensorium, history of visual disturbances, altered speech, seizures, ataxia- To rule out intracranial complications of COM.

- No history of trauma, exposure of loud noise, frequent ear cleaning habits.
- No history of use of ototoxic drugs.

Past History

- No history of diabetes mellitus, hypertension, asthma, known allergies, tuberculosis, tuberculosis contact, or thyroid disorders.
- No history of previous otological or other major surgeries in the past.

KEY POINTS

- Diabetes and ENT: Malignant otitis externa, otomycosis, delayed wound healing
- Hypertension and ENT: Epistaxis, SNHL
- Tuberculosis and ENT: Tubercular otitis media, tubercular laryngitis, tubercular lymph node enlargement
- Asthma and ENT: Associated allergic rhinitis, allergic conjunctivitis, and allergic dermatitis

Personal History

- **Sleep:** Normal
- **Appetite:** Normal
- **Bowel and bladder habits**: Normal
- Vegetarian diet
- No history of any addictions
- **Menstrual history:** Last menstrual period (LMP) (mention date), regular in flow and duration.

Family History

No history of similar complaints in the family.

KEY POINT

Family history of congenital ear disease, otosclerosis is important.

Examination

General Physical Examination

- Patient is conscious, cooperative, well oriented to time, place, and person.
- **Built:** Thin
- **Nourishment:** Well nourished
- **Vitals:**
  - **Temperature**: Afebrile
  - **Pulse rate:** 79/min with good volume
  - **Respiratory rate:** 20/min, regular rhythm
  - **Blood pressure:** 120/80 mm Hg in sitting position/supine position
  - **Saturation/SpO$_2$:** 100% on room air
- No pallor, icterus, cyanosis, clubbing, lymphadenopathy, and edema.

Systemic Examination

- **Respiratory system:** Air entry bilaterally equal, no added sounds
- **Cardiovascular system:** S1 S2 heard, no murmurs
- **Central nervous system:** Conscious, well oriented to time, place, person
- **Cranial nerves:** Intact except VIII

CHAPTER 84: Case Presentation

- **Per abdominal examination:**
  - Soft, no tenderness/guarding/rigidity
  - Liver/spleen not palpable

ENT Local Examination

Ear Examination

Ear	Right	Left
Pinna	Normal in size, shape, and position	Normal in size, shape, and position
Preauricular region	Normal	Normal
Infra-auricular region	Normal	Normal
Postauricular region	Normal	Normal
External auditory canal	Normal	Normal
Tympanic membrane (TM)	Large central perforation involving all four quadrants of tympanic membrane, seen in pars tensa	❖ Perforation with cholesteatoma flakes in pars flaccid/epitympanum/attic ❖ Just above neck of malleus from 9 o'clock to 11 o'clock position. Pars tensa shows Grade I retraction and tympanosclerotic patch in posterosuperior quadrant
TM mobility	Cannot be assessed	TM mobile

Tuning Fork Tests

	Right	Left
Rinne's test 256 Hz	Negative (-)	Negative (-)
Rinne's test 512 Hz	Negative (-)	Negative (-)
Rinne's test 1024 Hz	Positive (+)	Negative (-)
Weber's test 512 Hz		Lateralizes to left ear →
Absolute bone conduction (ABC) test	Normal	Normal

- **Mastoid tenderness**: Not present bilaterally
- **Fistula test:** Negative bilaterally
- **Facial nerve**: Intact, no facial asymmetry
- **No spontaneous: Nystagmus**
- **Gaze test**: No nystagmus
- Otoneurological tests
- **Rhomberg's test**: No swaying, negative
- **Untenberger's test**: No swaying
- **Tandem walking**: Normal

Three point tenderness:
1. Mastoid tip
2. Root of zygoma, and
3. Cymba concha

- ❖ **Head impulse test**: No nystagmus
- ❖ **Cerebellar signs**: Coordination normal, No dysdiadochokinesia
- ❖ **Cranial nerves**: Intact except VIII
- ❖ **Dix Hallpike maneuver (scan QR code)**: No nystagmus or giddiness

Nose Examination

- ❖ **External nose:**
  - ➢ No external deformity or scars/sinuses/swelling over dorsum of nose
  - ➢ *Philtrum:* Normal
  - ➢ *Columella:* Normal
  - ➢ *Vestibule:* Normal on both sides
- ❖ **Anterior rhinoscopy (scan QR code):**
  - ➢ Mucosa of nose is normal on both sides
  - ➢ Mild "C" shaped deviated from nasal septum to right side with small spur present inferiorly
  - ➢ Left inferior turbinate hypertrophy present
  - ➢ No discharge seen along floor of nose on both sides

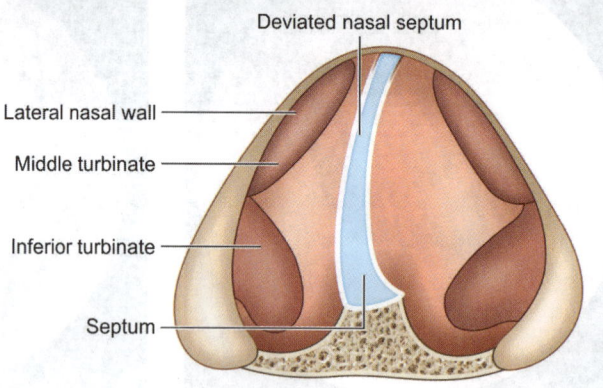

Fig. 1: Anterior rhinoscopy showing DNS.

- ❖ **Posterior rhinoscopy (scan QR code):**
  - ➢ *Posterior part of septum:* Normal
  - ➢ *Posterior part of middle and inferior turbinates:* Normal on both sides
  - ➢ *Nasopharynx (roof and posterior wall):* Normal
  - ➢ *Eustachian tube opening:* Normal
  - ➢ No discharge or secretions (postnasal drip) seen

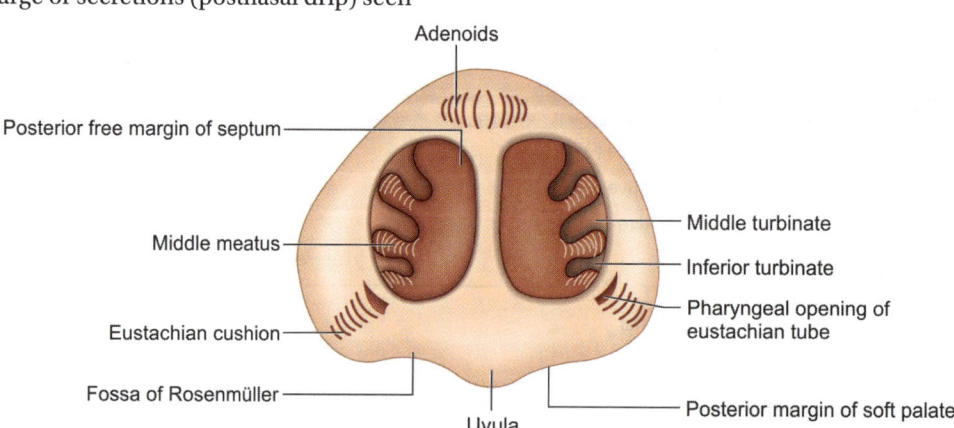

Fig. 2: Posterior rhinoscopy.

- ❖ **Paranasal sinuses (PNS):** No PNS tenderness
- ❖ **Tests for nasal patency:**
  - ➢ *Cold spatula test:* Adequate fogging on both sides **(scan QR code)**
  - ➢ *Cotton wool test:* Air blast adequate on both sides
  - ➢ *Cottle's test:* No improvement in nasal airway **(scan QR code)**
- ❖ **Tests for smell:** Intact

Oral Cavity and Throat

- **Lips**: Normal
- **Teeth and gingiva**: Normal
- **Tongue (anterior two-third)**: Normal; Tongue movements: Normal
- **Floor of mouth**: Normal, no bulge seen
- **Hard palate**: Normal
- **Buccal mucosa**: Mucosa normal
- **Retromolar trigone**: Normal
- **Uvula**: Normal, midline
- **Soft palate and hard palate**: Normal
- **Anterior pillars**: Normal
- **Tonsils (palatine)**: Not enlarged
- **Posterior pillars**: Normal
- **Base of tongue** (posterior one-third of tongue): Normal
- **Posterior pharyngeal wall (PPW) and oropharynx**: Clear, no postnasal drip
- **Indirect laryngoscopy** (IDL) **(scan QR code)**

Neck Examination

- No neck nodes or swelling palpable
- Laryngeal crepitus present **(scan QR code)**
- **Laryngeal framework:** Normal
- **Trachea:** Palpable in midline

Diagnosis (Provisional)

Right chronic otitis media (COM), mucosal, inactive with right moderate conductive hearing loss (CHL) with left chronic otitis media, squamosal, active with left severe CHL without any complications with "C" shaped deviated nasal septum (DNS) to right and spur.

KEY POINTS

- Complete diagnosis is to be mentioned.
- Management of the case includes investigations and treatment.
- Pure tone audiometry is to be done for hearing assessment.
- Ear toileting needs to be done if ear discharge is present and should be sent for culture and sensitivity.
- Examination under microscopy
- X-ray mastoid Schuller's view/high resolution computed tomography (HRCT) temporal bone [in chronic suppurative otitis media (CSOM) with complications]
- Treatment in this case would be medical management with left ear mastoidectomy followed by right ear tympanoplasty

■ SHORT CASE 1: THROAT (TONSILLITIS)

"My patient Mr. XYZ, 6–year-old, male child, resident of Sion, Mumbai, and Muslim by religion came with the **chief complaints of......**"

- Pain in the throat on and off since 5 years
- Difficulty in swallowing
- Complaint of fever since 3 days

History of Presenting Illness

- My patient was apparently asymptomatic when he complained of odynophagia (pain in the throat)
- Patient has more than three episodes of odynophagia since 5 years. Patient has pain while swallowing. Odynophagia is associated with fever and URTI.
- Patient also complaints of halitosis (bad breath)
- No history of dysphagia, dyspnea, hemoptysis, hematemesis, change in voice
- No history of swelling in the neck

PART 4: Questions

- No history of otalgia, fullness/blocking in the ear, decreased hearing
- No history of heaviness in the head, pain over PNS area, giddiness, headache
- No history of trauma
- No history of tuberculosis/any major illness

KEY POINTS

- Take history of etiology like URTI, trauma, foreign body.
- History of complications such as CSOM, acute suppurative otitis media (ASOM), suppurative otitis media (SOM), pharyngitis, sinusitis.

Local Examination of Throat and Neck

- **Temperature:** Afebrile
- **Pulse:** 80/minute
- **Blood pressure:** 110/70 mm Hg
- **Respiratory rate:** 24 breaths/minute

Neck Examination

- **Bilateral jugulodigastric lymph nodes are enlarged 2 × 2.5 cm in size, nontender, firm, and mobile**
- No neck swelling palpable
- Laryngeal crepitus present
- **Laryngeal framework:** Normal
- **Trachea:** Palpable in midline

Throat Examination

- **Lips**: Normal
- **Teeth and gingiva**: Normal
- **Tongue (anterior two-third)**: Normal; Tongue movements: Normal
- **Floor of mouth**: Normal, no bulge seen
- **Hard palate**: Normal
- **Buccal mucosa**: Mucosa normal
- **Retromolar trigone**: Normal
- **Uvula**: Normal, midline
- **Soft palate and hard palate**: Normal

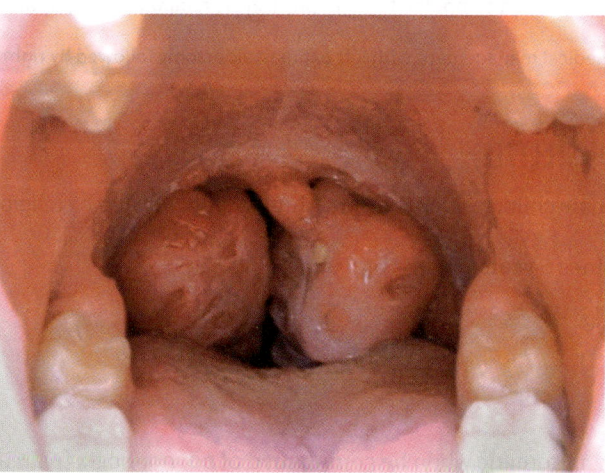

Fig. 3: Bilateral tonsillar hypertrophy.

- **Anterior pillars**: Congested
- **Tonsils (palatine)**: Bilateral palatine Grade 3 tonsillitis are enlarged reaching up to uvula and congested **(Fig. 3)**
- **Posterior pillars**: Not visualized due to tonsillar hypertrophy
- **Base of tongue (posterior one-third of tongue):** Normal
- **Posterior pharyngeal wall (PPW) and oropharynx:** Clear, no postnasal drip

KEY POINTS

- Management includes investigations and treatment.
- In this case, medical management first to reduce acute stage in terms of antibiotics/analgesics/anti-inflammatory drugs/antiseptic gargles to be given fist.
- Followed by tonsillectomy with or without adenoidectomy surgery.

Ear and Nose Examination

No abnormality detected

Provisional Diagnosis

Bilateral palatine acute on chronic nonfollicular palatine tonsillitis with bilateral jugulodigastric lymph node enlargement without any other complications.

■ SHORT CASE 2: THROAT

"My patient Mr. ABC, 14-year-old, male, resident of Wadala, Mumbai, student, and Hindu by religion came with the chief complaints of…"

"…….**Chief complaints** of recurrent throat pain since 3 years"

History of Presenting Illness

- My patient was apparently well when he complained of recurrent throat pain, which was sudden in onset, gradually progressive, intermittent in nature, initially present once every 6 months but now present around 4–5 episodes in a year. It is associated with fever and odynophagia during each episode. The throat pain aggravates with URTI and relieves with medications.
- Patient complaints of **fever** with each episode of throat pain, **low grade, intermittent, associated with chills and malaise, not associated with rigors, relieves with medications.** Patients also complaints of **odynophagia** with each episode, **both for solids and liquids, intermittent in nature, and relieves with medications.**

KEY POINTS

- Onset, duration, and progression of throat pain should always be elicited in history.
- Ask for number of episodes in a year.
- Does it affect daily routine activity and schooling in children?
- Associated symptoms with throat pain should be asked.

- No history of dysphagia
- No history of dyspnea
- No history of cough, change in voice, and vomiting
- No history of recurrent rhinorrhea, nasal obstruction, and excessive sneezing
- No history of facial heaviness, postnasal drip, and epistaxis
- No history of mouth breathing, snoring
- No history of headache, nasal pain, and nasal swelling
- No history of smell disturbances/altered or decreased smell/excessive lacrimation
- No history of trauma
- No history of ear pain, ear discharge
- No history of reduced hearing, aural fullness, tinnitus, and giddiness

Ask history related to adenoid hypertrophy also.

Local Examination

Oral Cavity and Throat

- **Lips:** Normal
- **Teeth and gingiva:** Normal

- ❖ **Tongue (anterior two-third):** Normal; Tongue movements: Normal
- ❖ **Floor of mouth:** Normal, no bulge seen
- ❖ **Hard palate:** Normal
- ❖ **Buccal mucosa:** Mucosa normal
- ❖ **Retromolar trigone:** Normal
- ❖ **Uvula:** Normal, midline
- ❖ **Soft palate:** Normal
- ❖ **Anterior pillars:** Flushed ++
- ❖ **Tonsils:** Grade 3 enlarged tonsils present **(Fig. 4)**
- ❖ Both tonsils are not congested.

> Look for cardinal signs of chronic tonsillitis

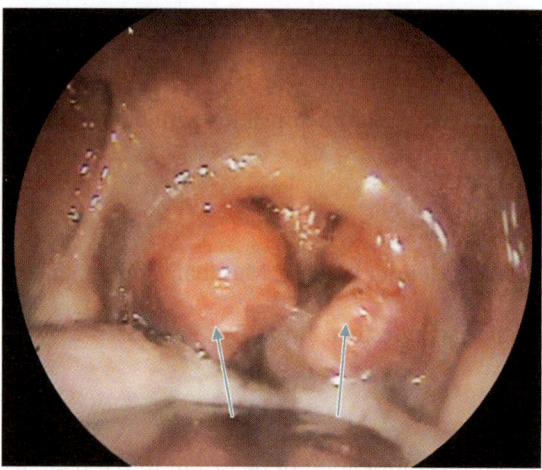

Fig. 4: Bilateral tonsillar hypertrophy.

- ❖ **Posterior pillars:** Not visible due to tonsillar enlargement
- ❖ **Base of tongue (posterior one-third of tongue):** Normal
- ❖ **PPW:** Clear, no postnasal drip
- ❖ **Indirect laryngoscopy (IDL):** Normal

Neck

- ❖ Jugulodigastric neck nodes are palpable on both sides
- ❖ No neck swelling palpable
- ❖ Laryngeal crepitus present
- ❖ **Laryngeal framework:** Normal
- ❖ **Trachea:** Palpable in midline

Nose

- ❖ **External nose examination:**
  - ▷ No external deformity or scars
  - ▷ *Philtrum:* Normal
  - ▷ *Columnella:* Normal
  - ▷ *Vestibule:* Normal on both sides
- ❖ **Anterior rhinoscopy:**
  - ▷ Mucosa of nose is normal on both sides
  - ▷ *Septum:* Midline
  - ▷ No turbinate hypertrophy present
  - ▷ No discharge seen along floor of nose on both sides
- ❖ **Posterior rhinoscopy:**
  - ▷ *Posterior part of septum:* Normal
  - ▷ Posterior part of turbinates normal on both sides.
  - ▷ *Nasopharynx (roof and posterior wall):* Normal: No adenoid hypertrophy seen
  - ▷ *Eustachian tube opening:* Normal
  - ▷ No discharge or secretions seen
  - ▷ *PNS :* No PNS tenderness
  - ▷ Tests for nasal patency

- ❖ **Cold spatula test:** Equal fogging on both sides
- ❖ **Cotton wool test:** Air blast adequate on both sides
- ❖ **Cottle's test:** No improvement in nasal airway
- ❖ **Tests for smell:** Intact

Ear

	Right	Left
Pinna	Normal in size, shape, and position	Normal in size, shape, and position
Preauricular region	Normal	Normal
Infra-auricular region	Normal	Normal
Postauricular region	Normal	Normal
External auditory canal	Normal	Normal
Tympanic membrane (TM)		
TM mobility	TM mobile	TM mobile
Tuning fork tests	Right	Left
Rinne's test 256 Hz	Positive (+)	Positive (+)
Rinne's test 512 Hz	Positive (+)	Positive (+)
Rinne's test 1024 Hz	Positive (+)	Positive (+)
Weber's test	←————————————————→	
Absolute bone conduction (ABC) test	Normal	Normal

- ❖ **Mastoid tenderness:** Not present bilaterally
- ❖ **Fistula test:** Negative bilaterally
- ❖ **Facial nerve:** Intact
- ❖ **No spontaneous:** Nystagmus
- ❖ **Gaze test:** No nystagmus
- ❖ **Otoneurological tests:** Normal

Provisional Diagnosis

Chronic palatine Grade 3 tonsillitis with bilateral jugulodiagastric lymphadenitis without any complications.

■ SHORT CASE 3: NOSE (DEVIATED NASAL SEPTUM)

"My patient Mr. XYZ, 26-year-old, male, resident of Kalyan, Mumbai, and Hindu by religion came with the **chief complaints of**......."
- ❖ Left-sided nasal obstruction since 3 years
- ❖ Headache on and off

History of Presenting Illness

❖ Patient was apparently asymptomatic 3 years ago when he had trauma to nose with cricket ball, following this patient had one episode of epistaxis and since then he has left-sided nasal obstruction.
❖ History of difficulty in breathing through left nostril
❖ History of on and off headache since then
❖ No history of anosmia, dryness of nose, recurrent epistaxis, nasal discharge, cold, cough, postnasal drip, nasal twang of voice, proptosis, and loose teeth
❖ No history of otalgia/fullness in the ear/deceased hearing/otorrhea
❖ No history of odynophagia, oral breathing, dryness in throat/nose, difficulty in swallowing
❖ No history of fever

Local Examination of Nose

Nose Examination

❖ **External nose examination**:
  ▷ No external deformity or scars/sinuses/swelling over dorsum of nose
  ▷ *Philtrum:* Normal
  ▷ *Columella:* Normal
  ▷ *Vestibule:* Normal on both sides
❖ **Anterior rhinoscopy:**
  ▷ Mucosa of nose is normal on both sides
  ▷ Mild "C" shaped deviated of nasal septum to left side with small synechiae present in the left nostril **(Fig. 5)**
  ▷ Left inferior turbinate hypertrophy present
  ▷ No discharge seen along floor of nose on both sides

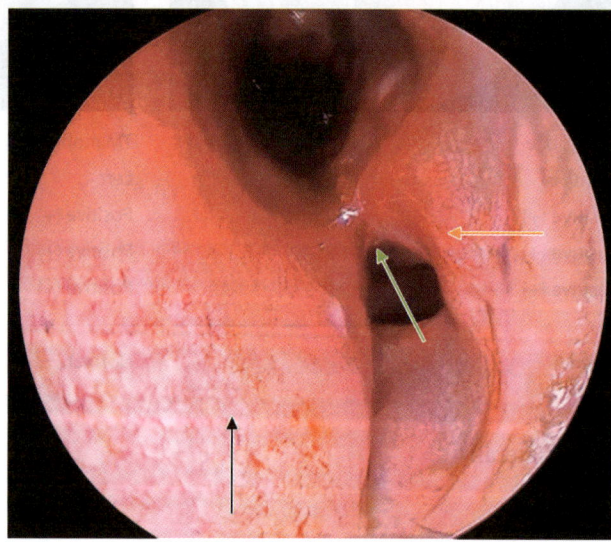

Fig. 5: Left-sided "C" shaped deviated nasal septum (DNS)(black arrow) synechiae (green arrow) inferior turbinate (yellow arrow).

❖ **Posterior rhinoscopy:**
  ▷ *Posterior part of septum:* Normal
  ▷ *Posterior part of middle and inferior turbinates*: Normal on both sides
  ▷ *Nasopharynx (roof and posterior wall):* Normal
  ▷ *Eustachian tube opening:* Normal
  ▷ No discharge or secretions (postnasal drip) seen
  ▷ *PNS:* No PNS tenderness
  Tests for nasal patency:
  ▷ *Cold spatula test:* Adequate fogging on both sides
  ▷ *Cotton wool test:* Air blast adequate on both sides
  ▷ *Cottle's test:* No improvement in nasal airway
❖ **Tests for smell:** Intact
❖ **Ear and throat examination:** Normal

Provisional Diagnosis

Left-sided "C" shaped deviated nasal septum with synechiae in left nostril without any complications

KEY POINTS

- Investigations would include hematological investigations including bleeding time, clotting time, and X-ray PNS Waters and Caldwell's view.
- Treatment in this case would be septoplasty surgery with synechiae release with nasal splint.

■ SHORT CASE 4: NOSE

"My patient Mr. ABC, 24–year-old, male, resident of Sewri, Mumbai, student, and Hindu by religion came with the chief complaints of…"

"…….**Chief complaints** of nasal obstruction right side more than left side since 5 years"

KEY POINTS

- Males: Nasopharyngeal angiofibroma
- Females: Atrophic rhinitis
- Elderly: Malignancies

History of Presenting Illness

My patient was apparently well when he complained of nasal obstruction which insidious in onset, gradually progressive, more on right side, continuous in nature, initially present with nasal discharge but now continuously present and also associated with mouth breathing. The nasal obstruction aggravates with URTIs and nasal discharge but partially relieved with medications and decongestants.

KEY POINTS

- Onset, duration, and progression of nasal obstruction should always be elicited in history.
- Sudden onset: Trauma, foreign body
- Insidious onset: Nasal polyps, DNS
- Unilateral: DNS (spur), antrochoanal polyp, malignancy
- Bilateral: DNS (S-shaped), ethmoidal polyp, chronic rhinosinusitis

❖ No history of recurrent rhinorrhea
❖ No history of excessive sneezing
❖ No history of facial heaviness
❖ No history of postnasal drip, epistaxis
❖ No history of mouth breathing, snoring
❖ No history of headache
❖ No history nasal pain, nasal swelling
❖ No history of visual disturbances, fever, vomiting, paresthesia over cheek
❖ No history of smell disturbances/altered or decreased smell/excessive lacrimation
❖ No history of trauma
❖ No history of ear pain, ear discharge
❖ No history of reduced hearing, aural fullness, tinnitus, giddiness
❖ No history of recurrent throat pain, dysphagia, odynophagia, dyspnea, cough, change in voice

KEY POINTS

- Nasal pain, nasal swelling: Seen in acute vestibulitis, septal abscess
- Fever, vomiting, headache, visual disturbances, diplopia: Orbital complications (like orbital cellulitis, cavernous sinus thrombosis)
- Associated earache and aural fullness: Eustachian tube dysfunction

Local ENT Examination

Nose

- ❖ **External nose:**
  - ➢ No external deformity or scars
  - ➢ *Philtrum:* Normal
  - ➢ *Columella:* Normal
  - ➢ *Vestibule:* Normal on both sides
- ❖ **Anterior rhinoscopy:**
  - ➢ Mucosa of nose is normal on both sides
  - ➢ Deviated nasal "C" shaped septum to right side with spur which touches the upper part of inferior turbinate **(Fig. 6A)**
  - ➢ Left inferior turbinate hypertrophy present **(Fig. 6B)**
  - ➢ No discharge seen along floor of nose on both sides

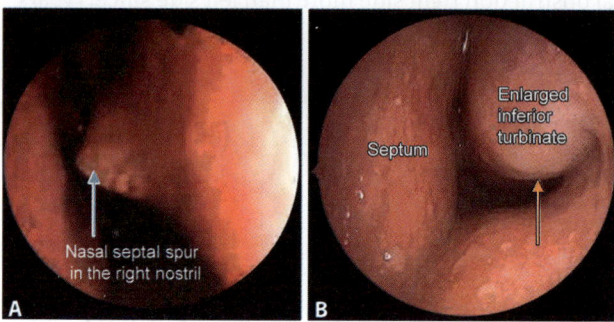

Figs. 6A and B: (A) Nasal septal spur in the right nostril; (B) Left nostril with inferior turbinate hypertrophy.

KEY POINTS

- Examine the nasal mucosa, floor of nose, septum, lateral wall, and roof of nose.
- Look for findings like nasal discharge, polyps, septal deviation, turbinate hypertrophy, foreign body.

- ❖ **Posterior rhinoscopy:**
  - ➢ *Posterior part of septum:* Normal
  - ➢ Posterior part of turbinates normal on both sides
  - ➢ *Nasopharynx (roof and posterior wall):* Normal
  - ➢ *Eustachian tube opening:* Normal
  - ➢ No discharge or secretions seen
  - ➢ *PNS:* No PNS tenderness
- ❖ **Tests for nasal patency:**
  - ➢ *Cold spatula test:* Fogging decreased on right side
  - ➢ *Cotton wool test:* Air blast decreased on right side
  - ➢ *Cottle's test:* No improvement in nasal airway
  - ➢ *Tests for smell:* Intact

> Improvement in airway if seen in Cottle's test suggests nasal valve collapse

Ear

	Right	Left
Pinna	Normal in size, shape, and position	Normal in size, shape, and position
Preauricular region	Normal	Normal
Infra-auricular region	Normal	Normal
Postauricular region	Normal	Normal
External auditory canal	Normal	Normal

Contd...

Contd...

	Right	Left
Tympanic membrane (TM)	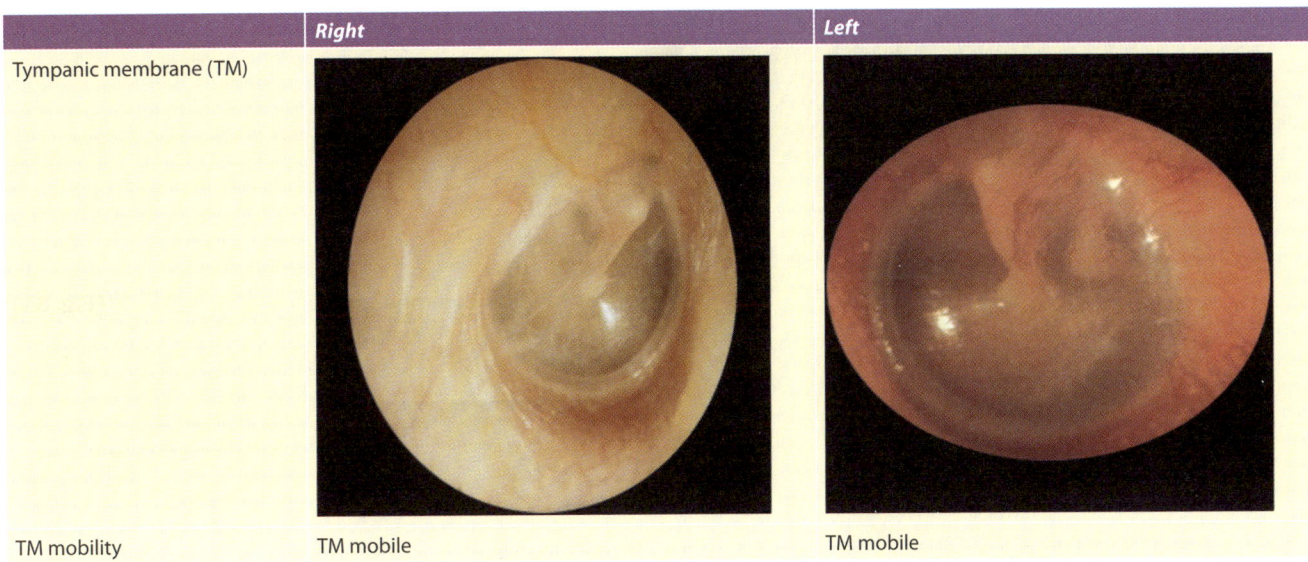	
TM mobility	TM mobile	TM mobile

Tuning Fork Tests

	Right	Left
Rinne's test 256 Hz	Positive (+)	Positive (+)
Rinne's test 512 Hz	Positive (+)	Positive (+)
Rinne's test 1024 Hz	Positive (+)	Positive (+)
Weber's test	←――――――――――→	
Absolute bone conduction (ABC) test	Normal	Normal

- **Mastoid tenderness**: Not present bilaterally
- **Fistula test**: Negative bilaterally
- **Facial nerve:** Intact
- No spontaneous nystagmus
- **Gaze test:** No nystagmus
- **Otoneurological tests:** Normal

Oral Cavity and Throat

- **Lips:** Normal
- **Teeth and gingiva:** Normal
- **Tongue (anterior two-third):** Normal; Tongue movements: Normal
- **Floor of mouth:** Normal, no bulge seen
- **Hard palate:** Normal
- **Buccal mucosa:** Mucosa normal
- **Retromolar trigone:** Normal
- **Uvula:** Normal, midline
- **Soft palate:** Normal
- **Anterior pillars:** Normal
- **Tonsils:** Not enlarged
- **Posterior pillars:** Normal
- **Base of tongue (posterior one-third of tongue):** Normal
- **PPW:** Clear, no postnasal drip
- **IDL**: Normal

Neck

- No neck nodes or swelling palpable
- Laryngeal crepitus present
- **Laryngeal framework:** Normal
- **Trachea:** Palpable in midline

Provisional Diagnosis

DNS to right side with right-sided nasal spur and left-sided turbinate hypertrophy without any complications.

Index

Page numbers followed by *f* refer to figure and *t* refer to table.

A

Abscess 151, 250
   brain 168
   cerebellar 90*f*, 493*f*, 494*f*
   cerebral 89
   chronic retropharyngeal 253
   cold 282
   cyst, septal 150
   drainage of 250, 253, 255
   epiglottic 273
   extradural 88, 166, 168
   intratonsillar 241
   mastoid 84
   orbital 167
   otogenic brain 89
   parapharyngeal 252, 254, 255*f*, 395, 498*f*
   parotid 248
   peritonsillar 251, 252
   postaural mastoid 85
   potential parapharyngeal 252
   prevertebral 253
   septal 161, 162
   subdural 88, 168
   submandibular 250*f*
   subperiosteal 167, 168
Absolute bone conduction test 50
Acellular dermal homografts 359
Achalasia cardiac 327, 329
Achlorhydria 323
Acid 322
   reflux 320
Acid-fast bacillus 195
Acidic foods 342
Acoustic canal, external 3, 4, 46, 58, 61, 110, 130, 134, 135, 361, 374, 442
Acoustic neuroma 114, 143-145, 145*f*, 491*f*, 508
Acquired immunodeficiency syndrome 335, 336
   infection, prevention of 353
Actinomyces israelii 197
Actinomycin D 431, 433
Actinomycosis 197
Acute pharyngitis 246, 246*f*
   causes of 246
   management of 246
Acute respiratory tract infection 389
Acute retropharyngeal abscess 252, 253*f*
   causes of 252
Acyclovir 340
Adenocarcinoma 62, 324.
Adenoid 31, 175, 176
   anatomy of 243
   cystic carcinoma 228, 236
   differential diagnosis of 476
   facies 244
   hypertrophy 243, 244*f*
      grading of 244
   surgery 389

Adenoidectomy 172, 389, 422, 460*f*
   complications of 390
   contraindications of 389
   surgery 389, 390
Adenoiditis 243, 244*f*
Adenolymphoma 235
Aditus 6
Adolescent transitional voice disorder 305
Adrenaline nebulization 274
Adriamycin 433
Air cell system 6, 362
Airway 502
   laser fire of 419
   maintenance 276
   obstruction 251, 277
   threatening of 250
Alae nasi movements 152
Alcohol 225
   abuse 222
Alexander's law 51
Alkaline
   douches 199
   phosphatase 194
Alkalis 322
Allergic fungal sinusitis 170, 495*f*
   fungal concretions of 495*f*
Allergic shiners 175
Allergy 166, 271, 277, 279, 385
   management of 167
Alpha-interferon 201
Alpha-tocopherol 228
Alveolar ridge carcinoma 228, 228*f*
Ameloblastoma 209
American leishmaniasis 198
Amikacin 347
Aminoglysides 347
Amoxicillin 165, 172
Amoxyclav 349
Amphotericin 198
Ampicillin 165, 273, 274
Analgesics 164, 165, 252
Anesthesia 358, 364, 377, 379, 386, 397, 407, 412, 414, 499
   complications of 415
   instruments 502
   local 358, 364, 500
   machine 502, 502*f*
   topical 416
Anesthetic drugs, local 501
Angiofibroma 258*f*, 460*f*, 494*f*
   mass 257*f*
Ankyloglossia 210
Anorexia 282
Anosmia 150, 160, 164
Anotia 55, 56*f*
Antacids 328
Anterior laryngeal web steroid therapy 286*f*
Anterior pillar
   congestion of 239*f*
   retractor 463, 464*f*
Anthracyclines 431

Antibiotics 166, 167, 172, 242
Anticancer drugs, toxicity of 432
Antifungal therapy 171
Antihistaminics 166, 376
Antimetabolites 430
Antimony compounds 198
Antireflux
   medication 280, 320
   surgery 328
Antiretroviral therapy 352
Antisyphilitic treatment 281
Antitubercular drugs 195, 508
   therapy 253, 283
Antral cell, large 482
Antral lavage 165
Antral puncture 164
Antrochoanal polyp 178, 178*f*, 213*f*, 375, 474, 475*f*, 523
Antrum 6
   exposure of 362
Aortic aneurysm 414
Aphonia 290
   functional 307
Apnea index 310
Aqueductal anomalies 121
Armstrong grommet 366*f*
Arousal
   index 309
   test 122
Arrhythmias 276
Aryepiglottic folds 520
Arytenoid
   cartilage 520
   identification of 412
Asch's forceps 458, 458*f*
Aspergillus 171
   fumigatus 349
Aspiration 210, 290, 300, 396
   pneumonia 251
   prevention of 276
Asthma 166, 271, 385
   bronchial 175
Atelectasis 67*f*, 476
Atelectatic tympanic membrane 364
Ateroids 221
Atresia 151
   acquired 63
Atrophic rhinitis 162, 168, 192
   management of 168
   primary 169
   secondary 170
Atropine 397
Attacks, acute 97
Atticoantrostomy 361*f*
Audiograms 506
Audiometry curves 506*f*
Audiometry test 114
Auditory 124
   brainstem response 122, 123, 145
   nerve transmission pathway 12
   response cradle 122
   system 10

Aural atresia 46
Aural polyp 60, 373
Aural polypectomy 374
Auricle 3, 134
   hematoma of 56
Auricular nerve, posterior 128
Autoimmune
   disease 322
   disorder 130, 221
Axonotmesis 128
Azithromycin 172

B

Bacillary angiomatosis 344
Bacterial infection, secondary 275
Bacterial sinusitis, chronic 375
Bacteriology 74, 248, 250, 251
Ballenger swivel knife 452, 453*f*
Barium swallow 264*f*, 268, 323, 323*f*, 325-327, 331*f*
Barotrauma 510
Barrett's esophagus 324, 330
   screening for 324
Basal cell 62
   carcinoma 58, 157, 157*f*, 194
Bat ear 55
Battery cell 476*f*, 489
Baxter grommet 366*f*
Beam therapy, external 435
Behcet's syndrome 220
Bell's palsy 129, 131
Bell's phenomenon 130
Benzathine penicillin 194
Beta-carotene 228
Betamethasone drops 199
Binocular vision 409, 441
Biopsy 140, 142, 193, 194, 198, 204, 283, 324
   forceps 378
Bithermal caloric test 113
Bivona cuffed flexible tube 401
Bivona hyperflex uncuffed tube 401
Blair incision, modified 234*f*
Blast injuries 506, 508
Bleeding
   diathesis 389
   intractable 149
   nose 180
   postnasal 390
   post-tonsillectomy 388
   reasons of 179
Bleomycin 431, 433
Blepharospasm 132
Blindness 166
Blood 335
   disorders 219, 220
   pressure 181
      monitor 502
   products 335
   stained nasal discharge 208
   vessels, peripheral prominent 49

Index

Bloodless surgery 422
Blurred vision 206
Bocca's sign 300
Body movements, abnormal 311
Bone
    injuries 184
    marrow transplantation 201
Bony defect, congenital 156f
Bony destruction 151, 207f, 208
Bony labyrinth 8
Bordetella pertussis 276
Boyle Devis mouth gag 386f, 461
Boyle's apparatus 414
Brachytherapy 435
Brain 156
    computed tomography scan of 131, 168f
    magnetic resonance imaging of 145f
    tissue, herniation of 156f
Brainstem evoked audiometry 114
Branchiomeric paraganglioma 138
Brandt-Daroff exercises 116
Breathing system 502
Broken metallic tracheostomy tube 483f
Bronchial obstructions, types of 316, 316f
Bronchopneumonia 198
Bronchoscope 468, 470, 413
Bronchoscopy
    contraindications of 414
    flexible 415
    precautions during 415
Bronchus 414f
Buccal carcinoma 226f
Buccal mucosa 210, 211, 223, 226
    carcinoma of 226
Bulbar polio 325
Bulging tympanic membrane 350f
Bull's eyelamp 213
Bull's lamp 441
Bullous pemphigoid 220

C

Cacosmia 150
Caldwell's view 473, 474f
Caloric test 112, 113f, 145
Canal wall mastoidectomy surgery
    down 80, 361, 361f
    up 80, 361f
Canaloplasty surgery 135
Cancer
    spread of 330
    therapy 219
Candida albicans 349
Candidiasis 219, 338f
    atrophic 338f
    chronic hypertrophic 220
Capnometer 502
Carbon dioxide laser 417
Carcinogen, inhalation of 203
Carcinoma 207f
    cheek 226f
    esophageal 411
    hypopharynx 396
    larynx 299, 396
    maxilla 495f
    maxillary sinus 208
    nasal cavity 207
    nasopharyngeal 259
    T-cell 194
Cardiac disease 385
Cardiac surgeries 396
Cardioscope 502
Cardiospasm 327
Cardiovascular accidents 325
Carotid artery, mycotic aneurysm of 255
Carotid body tumors 138
Carotid space 255
Cartilages 16
Cartilaginous enlargement 150
Caudal deviation 160
Cauliflower ear 45
Cavernous hemangioma 205
Cavernous sinus 168
    thrombosis 162, 166, 168
Cavity, obliteration of 362
Cawthorne-Cooksey exercises 117
Ceftriaxone 347
Cefuroxime 172, 349
Cell
    cycle 429, 430
    papilloma, cylindrical 204
Cellulitis 154, 250, 273
Central facial paralysis 131
Central nervous system 123
Central nystagmus 51
    causes of 51
    types of 111
Central vertigo 109
Central vestibular disorders 119
Cephalosporin 273
Cerebellar artery 128
Cerebellar hemisphere lesions 112
Cerebellar lesion 112
Cerebellar sign 53, 145
Cerebellopontine angle 144, 145
    tumors 508
Cerebellum lesions, midline disease of 112
Cerebrospinal fluid rhinorrhea repair 376
Cerumen 62
Ceruminoma 61, 137
    malignant 62
Cervical
    adenitis 273
    esophageal
        rupture 321
        web 264f
    esophagotomy 319
    fascia 395
    group, posterior 217
    lymphadenopathy 201, 275, 346
    spine 486f
    sympathectomy 169
    vertebra, dislocation of 415
Cervicofacial branches 128
Cessation reflex 122
Cheilitis, angular 339, 339f
Chemodectoma 138
Chemosis 204
Chemotherapeutic agents, classification of 430
Chemotherapy 200, 201, 206, 225, 344, 429, 432, 437
    phase-specific 430
    posterior 432
    preparation of patient before 432
    principles of 429
    role of 429
    types of 431
Chest
    auscultation 274
    examination 274
    fixation of 37
    pain 327
        substernal 326
    physiotherapy 399
    piece 409, 471
    X-ray of 195, 198, 482f, 483, 483f
Chevalier Jackson direct laryngoscope 472f
Chills 161
Chlorambucil 430
Chloramphenicol 169
Choana
    atresia 475
    posterior 151
Cholesteatoma 77, 130, 482
Cholesterol granuloma 201
Chonal atresia, unilateral 475
Chondrodermatitis nodularis chronica helicis 57
Chondroma 150, 298
Chondrosarcoma 150
Chorda tympani 7, 128, 130
Chromium 203
Chronic suppurative otitis media 73, 74, 76, 82, 83, 87
    complications of 80, 82
    etiology of 74
    management of 53
    types of 73
Cimetidine 328
Cisplatin 433
Citelli's punch forceps 458, 458f
Clarithromycin 172
Cleft palate 151, 211
    submucous 385, 389
Coablator wands 460f
Coblation method 385
Coblation technique 420
Coblation wand 421, 459
Cochlea 9
    electrical potentials of 13
Cochlear conductive 104
Cochlear duct 9
Cochlear dysplasia 123
Cochlear hypoplasia 123
Cochlear implant 123, 124, 125f
    device 125
    electrode 125
    surgery 124, 124f
    steps of 124
Cochlear otosclerosis 508
Cochlear pathology 146
Cochleopalpebral reflex 122
Cold
    air caloric test 113
    common 163
    compression 180
    dissection 386
    methods 385
    spatula test 153f
Coloboma 2
Commando operation 227
Computed tomography virtual bronchoscopy 413f
Concha 17
    bullosa 496f
Condy's gargles 387
Congenital malformation, classification of 121
Congestion 175
Conjunctiva, cobblestone appearance of 175
Conventional septoplasty 379
Cordectomy 422
Corneal ulcer 132
Coronary artery diseases 148
Cortical mastoidectomy 361, 361f, 362
Corynebacterium diphtheriae 275
Coryza 163
Cottle's line 160
Cottle's test 152, 153f, 160
Cotton wool test 152
Cough 164, 282, 396
    croupy 253, 275
    dry 280
    nocturnal 327
    painful 396
    suppressants 276
Cranial fossa approach, middle 146
Cranial nerve 144
    examination 145
    complete 204
Craniofacial resection 206
C-reactive protein 334
Cricoarytenoid joint 34
Cricoid cartilage 520
Cricoid hook 467, 467f
Cricopharyngeal spasm 325
Cricopharyngoscope 323, 468, 469, 469f
Cricothyroid joint 34, 300
Cricothyroidotomy 404
Cricothyrotomy 394
    procedure 404f
Crocodile forceps 445, 446f
Cryosurgery 385, 425
    method, disadvantages of 385
    uses of 426
Cryptococcosis 347
Cryptococcus neoformans 349
Cryptotia 56
Cuffed tracheostomy tube 516
Cutaneous horn 58, 136
Cutaneous sarcoidosis 198f
Cyberknife 435
    stereotactic radiation 435
Cyclophosphamide 430, 433
Cyst 134
    benign lymphoepithelial 348f
    bone 202
    congenital 134, 202
    dermoid 58, 134, 156
    epidermal implantation 134
    hemorrhagic 296f
    laryngeal 284, 286, 286f
    maxillary sinus 474
    mucous retention 167
    preauricular 44, 134
    sebaceous 57, 134
    thyroglossal 218f
    tonsillar 241
    vallecular 297f, 422
    vocal cord 296f
Cystic non-neoplastic lesions 297

Cystic odontomas 202
Cystic parotid swelling 235f
Cytarabine 431
Cytomegalovirus ulcers 339, 341
Cytotoxic antibiotics 431
Cytotoxics 199

D

da Vinci surgical robotic system 428, 428f
Dacarbazine 433
Dacrocystorhinostomy 375
Darwin's tubercle 56
Daunorubicin 431
Daytime sleepiness, excessive 311
Deaf, edema of 126
Deafness 99, 120
    conductive 101
    types of 99
Decompression 132
Deformity, C-shaped 159
Dehydration 249, 275
Denis Browne tonsil holding forceps 464, 465f
Denker's approach, modified 205
Dental infection 166, 250
Dental pain 164
Dental paresthesia 204
Depressors 35
Dermoid 156, 202
Deviated nasal septum 159, 160f, 475, 547
    types of 159
Dexamethasone 273
Diabetes mellitus 148, 385, 508
Diagnostic nasal endoscopy 205, 377
Didanosine 352
Diffuse esophageal spasm 326
Dingman's mouth gag 462, 462f
Diphtheria 239
Diphtheritic laryngitis 275
Diphtheroids 169
Diplopia 205, 206, 349
Discoid lupus erythematosus, chronic 220
Distraction technique 122
Dix-Hallpike maneuver 112
Donaldson grommet 366f
Doxorubicin 431, 433
Doyen's mouth gag 462
Draffin's bipod 461f
Dressing 399
Drug
    allergy 219
    antimicrobial 165
    antiretroviral 352
    chemotherapy 508
    classes of 352
    ototoxic 101, 508
    postexposure prophylaxis 353
    therapy, single 432
Dull mask-like face 476
Dull tympanic membrane 66
Dysdiadochokinesia 145
Dysphagia 210, 214, 253, 271, 282, 300, 326, 331
    chronic 334
    disorders of 320
    evaluation of 333

Dysphonia 304
    mixed 307
    plica ventricularis 305
    types of 304
Dysplasia
    high-grade 324
    low-grade 324
Dyspnea 253, 275, 280, 282, 283, 415
    worsens 290

E

Ear 254, 337, 373, 538, 541, 547, 550
    anatomy of 3
    auditory system of 10
    canal
        infections of 59
        inflammations of 59
    cup 45, 56
    development of 10
    discharge 42
        nonfoul smelling 42
    examination 41, 541, 545
    exostoses of 136
    foreign bodies of 62
    infections 4
    instruments 442
    lobule, anomalies of 56
    lop 56
    microscopy 53
    parts of 3
    physiology of 3, 10
    sarcoma of 138
    structures of 3
    surgery 360
Ear, nose, and throat (ENT)
    disorders 429
    local examination 541
    operative specimens in 518
    radiotherapy in 434
    robotics in 427
    role of radiotherapy in 434
    scopes in 468
Earache 43, 213
Eardrum 74
Edema 175
    angioneurotic 396
Efavirenz 352
Electrical impulses 12
Electrocochleography 123
Electrodiagnostic tests 129
Electron beams 434
Electronystagmography 114, 145
Emergency tracheostomy 404
Emotional rhinitis 176
Emphysema, surgical 215
Empyema 273
Encephalocele 156, 203
Endaural speculum 444, 444f
Endolymphatic duct 9
Endoneurium, injury of 129
Endoscopes
    Jackson pattern of 468t
    Negus pattern of 468t
Endoscopic enucleation 329
Endoscopic mucosal resection 329
Endoscopic septoplasty 379
    advantages of 380
    procedure of 379

Endoscopy 323, 324
    flexible 215
Endotracheal block 476
Endotracheal tubes 502
Eosinophilia, peripheral 175
Eosinophilic count, absolute 176
Eosinophilic granuloma 200, 482
Eosinophils 193, 201
    abundance of 201
    large number of 175
Epiglottis 520
    acute 272, 275, 395
    pseudoedema of 282
Epineurium, injury of 129
Epipharynx 31
Epiphora 130, 206, 208
Epirubicin 431
Epistaxis 149, 160, 179, 205
    surgery for 375
Epithelial cell granulomas 199
Epley's repositioning maneuver 115, 116f
Epstein-Barr virus 129
Epulis, congenital 225
Erythema multiforme 220, 221
Erythematous candidiasis 339
Erythrocyte sedimentation rate 198
Erythroplakia 223
Escherichia coli 250
Esomeprazole 328
Esophageal dysphagia 332
Esophageal foreign body, complication of 319
Esophageal pH monitoring 334
Esophageal spasm 326
Esophageal stents 325
Esophageal varices, injection of 411
Esophageal web 323f
Esophagitis, acute 320
Esophagogastric dysphagia 332
Esophagogastroduodenoscopy 323
Esophagoscopy 320, 323, 325, 334, 411, 489
    flexible 490f
Esophagus 39, 320, 322, 331f, 346, 485f, 489, 490, 490f
    anatomy of 33, 38, 317
    benign stricture of 324
    carcinoma of 330, 331f
    constrictor of 38
    corrosive burns of 322
    disorders of 320
    lymphatic drainage of 39f
    narrowest constriction of 484f, 485f
    neoplasms of 329
    perforation of 321, 412
    physiology of 33, 38
    reflux disorder of 328
    scleroderma of 329
Esthesioneuroblastoma 206
Estradiol 169
    sprays 169
Ethmoid
    air cells 25
    arteries 182
    carcinoma 207
    infundibulum 24
    polyp 178
    sinusitis 495f

Ethmoid sinus 25, 208, 349f, 496f
    groups of 25
    malignancy 209
    palpation 153f
Eustachian tube 68, 69, 71
    anatomy of 68
    blockage 72
    catheter 444, 444f
    disorders of 71
    examination of 70
    function 69, 70
    obstruction, causes of 71
    physiology of 69
    testing 70
Eve's tonsillar snare 463, 463f
Exanthematous fever 508
Exostoses 61, 136
External auditory canal
    benign tumors of 136
    congenital disorders of 59
    diseases of 58
    primary cholesteatoma of 60
External canal, atresia of 59
External ear 3, 133, 349
    benign tumors of 133
    diseases of 55
    malignant tumors of 133
    nerve supply of 4
    tumors of 133
External nose 150, 154
    congenital tumors of 156
    diseases of 154
Extrapulmonary tuberculosis regimen 195
Eye
    care of 130, 351
    movement 204
    sunken 476
Eyelid
    edema 175
    of upper 165

F

Face
    computed tomography scan of 235f
    fractures of
        middle third of 185
        upper third of 184
    magnetic resonance imaging of 233f
Facial asymmetry 204
Facial edema 353f
Facial expression, muscles of 128
Facial lesion, localization of 131
Facial muscles, regular massage of 130
Facial nerve 127, 127f, 129, 131, 234, 492f
    anomalies of 128
    blood supply of 128
    branches of 128
    complications of 127
    course of 127, 127f, 128f
    function tests 131
    hyperkinetic disorders of 132
    injury 128, 129
    neuroma 508
    paralysis 129
    surgery of 132
Facial pain 164, 166, 208

Index

Facial palsy 51, 52, 130f, 142, 351
Facial paralysis 87
   complications of 132
   peripheral 131
Facial paresthesia 204, 208
Facial swelling 349
Facial trauma 183
False cords, edema of 282
Famciclovir 340
Farabeuf's periosteal elevator 444, 444f
Farrier's aural speculum 443
Fat 359
Fatigue 311
Faucial arch tumors 261
Faucial diphtheria 242, 275
Faucial pillars 223
Ferrous sulfate 323
Fever 161, 164, 271, 274, 282, 347, 349
   high 272
   low-grade 163, 275
Fiberoptic bronchoscopy, flexible 215, 416
Fiberoptic endoscopes 215
Fiberoptic flexible bronchoscope 470f
Fibrosis 75
Fibrous dysplasia 209
Fine needle aspiration cytology 301
Finger
   nose test 145
   spelling method 124
Fissure 151
Fistula 110, 151
   collaural 59
   labyrinthine 508
   oroantral 204
   oronasal 211
   sign 110
   test 53, 110
Fitzgerald-Hallpike test 113
Flail chest 396
Flap over maxilla, elevation of 209f
Fluorescent treponemal antibody absorption 118
Fluticasone propionate 172
Foley's catheter 390
Folic acid 323
   antagonists 431
Follicular hyperplasia 347
Food
   allergy 221
   passage, common foreign bodies of 318
   regurgitation of 327
Foot pedal control 421
Foreign body, laryngeal 317
Foul smelling ear discharge 42
Fracture, mandibular 190
Freer's mucoperichondrial elevator 378, 451, 451f
Frey's syndrome 132, 236
   treatment for 236
Frontal bone, fractures of 185
Frontal recess 25
Frontal sinus 24, 25, 184, 205, 456f
   mucocele of 167
   palpation 153f
Frontal sinusitis 165
Frostbite 56
Fuller's bivalve metallic tube 467f
Fulminant fungal sinusitis 171
Functional endoscopic sinus surgery 167, 172, 375, 376, 454f, 502
   complications of 377
   contraindications of 375
   extended indications of 375
   indications of 375
   principle of 375
Fungal ball 170, 375
Fungal infections 170, 347
Fungal manifestations 337
Fungal otitis externa 59
Fungiform papilloma 204
Furuncle 59, 151, 154
Fusion inhibitors 352

G

Gadre's double breasting 169
Gait test 111
Gallium-67 bone scans 350
Galvanic test 114
Gamma knife surgery 146
Gardiner tuning fork 442
Gastroesophageal reflux disease 271, 328
   complications of 329
Gastrointestinal tract 142
Gelatin, absorbable 390
Gelfoam 390
Gemcitabine 431
General anesthesia 364, 414, 500
Geniculate ganglion 128
Ghosh vestibuloplasty 170
Giant cell 201
   multinucleated 199
   reparative granuloma 201
Gillette's space 30
Gingivitis, red-band 342
Glioma 157, 203
Globus hystericus 329
Globus pharyngeus 329
Glomus bodies 138
Glomus jugulare 139
Glomus tumor 138, 139f, 140
   extensive 508
Glomus tympanicum 139, 139f
Glossitis 323
Glottic carcinoma 300f
Glottis 36, 301
   carcinoma 521
Glucose 169
Glycerine 169
Goiter 218f, 391f
Goode's T tube 366f
Gradenigo's syndrome 492f
Granular cell tumor 224, 298
Granular pharyngitis 175, 385
Granulation 151
   tissues 130
Granuloma 295
   caseating 195
   necrotizing 201
   nonhealing midline 200
Granulomatosis, allergic 201
Granulomatous nodules 192
Grommet, types of 365
Growths 211
Gruber speculum 443
Guaifenesin 349
Guillain-Barre syndrome 396
Guillotine surgery 385
Gums 210, 211
Gustatory lacrimation 132
Gustatory rhinitis 176

H

H_2 blockers 328
Habilitation, aim of 123
Haemophilus influenza 250, 272
Hairy leukoplakia 340
   whitish nonremovable lesions of 341f
Halitosis 164, 210, 213
Haptoglobin-related protein report 343
Hard palate 210, 211, 262f
   carcinoma of 227, 228f
Hartmann's dressing forceps 451, 451f
Hartmann's tuning fork 442, 442f
Head and neck 210
   cancers 433
   lymph nodes of 216
Headache 149, 160, 164, 206
   causes of 149
   frontal 161, 165
Hearing
   assessment of 122
   mechanism 11
   normal 506
   physiology of 11
Hearing aid 106, 124
   augments auditory 124
Hearing loss 96, 99, 101, 120-122, 142, 213, 504, 507f-509f
   bilateral 43, 509
   noise-induced 507f
   causes of 507, 508, 510
   conductive 99, 204, 510f
   degree of 504
   diagnosis of 101
   drug related 101
   nonorganic 102
   sensorineural 100, 118, 144, 350, 509f
   sudden sensorineural 100, 103
   unilateral 43
Heart failure 277
Heartburn 327
Heath speculum 443
Heel knee test 145
Heimlich maneuver 277, 277f
Hemangioma 58, 135, 151, 158, 205, 212f, 298
   capillary 205
   types of 205
Hematoma 151, 359
Hemifacial pain 132
Hemiglossectomy
   specimen 523
   surgery 227f
Hemodynamics, maintenance of 181
Hemorrhage 387, 427
   management of 387, 388
   secondary 388
Hemotympanum 510
Hepatic toxicity 433
Herpes simplex 129
   ulcer 340, 340f
   virus lesions 340
Herpes zoster 129, 150, 339, 340
   oral ulcers of 340f
   oticus 60, 130
   vesicles of 340f
Heuwieser antral grasping forcep 455f
Hiatal hernia 323, 328
   types of 323
Higginson's rubber syringe 459, 459f
Highly active antiretroviral therapy 352
   intensification of 344
Hilar lymphadenopathy 198
Histiocytic cells, numerous 201
Histoplasmosis 347
   treatment for 348
Hodgkin's lymphoma 348
Hondusa's sign, positive 208
Honeymoon rhinitis 176
Hook retractor, double 467
Hot fomentation 165
Hot methods 385
Human immunodeficiency virus 335, 346, 349, 508
   infection, prevention of 353
   lesions, types of 336
   lymphadenopathy 346
   management of 351
   structure of 335, 335f
Human papilloma virus lesions 340, 341
Humidification 273
Hump nose 155
   deformity 155
Hutchinson's teeth 193f
Hydration, adequate 273
Hydrocortisone 273
Hyoid bone 34
Hyperdense maxillary sinus, causes of 516
Hyperemia 150
Hypermotility disorders 325
Hyperplasia 211, 278
Hyperplastic candidiasis 339, 339f
Hypertelorism 207f
Hypertension 148, 149, 385
Hypertrophic rhinitis 173
Hypertrophy 152
   bilateral tonsillar 544f, 546f
Hypnotics 313
Hypoglossal-facial anastomosis 132
Hypomotility disorders 325
Hypopharynx 32, 314
   benign lesions of 263
   malignant lesions of 263
   tumors of 256, 263
Hypophyseal diverticulum 31
Hypophysectomy 376
Hypopnea 309
Hyposmia 149, 164
Hypothyroidism 176, 279

I

Ifosfamide 430
Immune disorders 219, 220

Index

Immunoglobulin 276
  E 174
Immunotherapy 175
In vitro allergy test 176
Incision 250, 253, 392
Induction chemotherapy 431
Infection 219, 279
  bacterial 221
  ethmoid, drainage of 168
  extragenital 197
Inflammatory disorders 57
Inhalant allergen 174
Injury 150
  axonal 128
  chemical 271
  inhalational 271
  traumatic 56
Inspiratory stridor 274, 275, 277, 282
Instrumental manipulation, technique of 368
Internal acoustic meatus 127
Internal auditory canal anomalies 121
Internal ear 8
  features of 8
Internal jugular chain 217
Intracranial complications, sinusitis with 376
Intranasal mass 206
Intranasal meningoencephalocele 205
Intratympanic muscles 7
Intravenous antibiotic 273
Intubation 295
Invasive fungal sinusitis 349, 375
Ionizing radiations 434
Iron 169
  deficiency anemia 322, 323
Irrigation system 421

J

Jackhammer esophagus 326
Jackson's metallic tracheostomy tube 467f
Jening's mouth gag 462, 462f
Jobson Horne probe 444, 444f
Jugular chain, external 217
Jugular nodes
  lower 216
  middle 216
  upper 216
Jugular vein thrombophlebitis 254
Juvenile angiofibroma 524
Juvenile nasal angiofibroma excision 422
Juvenile nasopharyngeal angiofibroma 149, 256, 259
Juxtavisceral chain 217

K

Kaposi's sarcoma 225, 343, 350
  over hard palate 344f
  over lower lip 344f
Kashima's operation 422
Keloid 57, 135
Kemicetine antiozaenae solution 169
Keratitis 130
  exposure 132

Keratoacanthoma 58, 136
Keratosis 295
  obturans 63, 135
Kerrison punch 457f
Kidney, metastasis from 482
Kiesselbach's plexus 158
Killian's elevator 452, 452f
Killian's self-retaining nasal speculum 452, 452f
Killian's triangle 29
Kilovoltage machines 436
Klebsiella ozaenae 169
Kleinsasser's microlaryngoscope 471, 472f
Kobrak test, modified 112
Kocher's incision, modified 392f
Koilonychia 323
Kuhn-Bolger frontal recess giraffe forceps 456f
Kveim test 198

L

Labyrinth, blood supply of 10
Labyrinthine
  anomalies 121
  exercises 98
Labyrinthitis 86, 508
Lacerations 56
Lack's tongue depressor 460, 460f
Lacrimation 205
Lamina papyracea 25
Lamivudine 353
Language, development of 123, 124
Lansoprazole 328
Laryngeal cancer 299
  management of 302
Laryngeal cartilages 33, 33f, 34t
Laryngeal cavity 300f
Laryngeal diphtheria 275
Laryngeal edema 250, 252, 254, 408
Laryngeal electromyography 289
Laryngeal glottic hemangioma 298f
Laryngeal inlet 35, 215f
Laryngeal joints 34
Laryngeal mask airway 502
Laryngeal membranes 34
Laryngeal mirror 215
Laryngeal muscles 35, 35f
Laryngeal nerve supply 37f
Laryngeal paralysis 276, 287
  causes of 287
Laryngeal polypectomy 374
Laryngeal signs 175
Laryngeal squamous papilloma 298f
Laryngeal stridor, congenital 284
Laryngeal trauma 396
Laryngeal web 284, 285
  steroid therapy, posterior 286f
Laryngeal widening 300
Laryngectomy, total 520, 521
Laryngitis 270, 278
  acute 270
  atrophic 280
  chronic 278
  sicca 280
Laryngocele 284, 286, 297, 297f
Laryngoesophageal cleft 284, 286
Laryngomalacia 284, 285
  congenital abnormality of 284
Laryngopharyngeal reflux 279

Laryngopharynx 32, 214, 215
Laryngoscopy 295f, 406
  direct 284, 285, 301, 406, 408, 468, 472
  flexible 268, 271, 284
  indirect 214, 214f, 215, 268, 271, 323, 408
  mirror, indirect 460, 461f
Laryngospasm 408
Laryngotracheal trauma 266
  Schaefer classification of 267
Laryngotracheobronchitis, acute 273, 275, 395
Larynx 192, 214, 215, 283, 373, 422
  acute inflammation of 270
  anatomy of 33
  benign tumors of 295
  carcinoma of 521
  cavity of 36
  chronic inflammation of 270
  congenital
    abnormality of 284
    lesions of 284
  cystic non-neoplastic lesions of 297
  development of 38
  edema of 277
  embryology of 38
  examination of 271
  external 215
  functions of 37
  intrinsic muscles of 35t
  lupus of 283
  lymphatic drainage of 36
  malignant tumors of 299
  membranes of 34
  neoplastic tumors of 298
  nerve supply of 36, 287
  parts of 36
  pediatric 38
  physiology of 33, 37
  spaces of 37
  structures of 36
  widening of 215
Laser 417
  complications of 417
  machine 418f
  principle of 417
  safety precautions 419
  types of 418
Lautenslager operation 170
Law's view 479
LeFort's fracture 189f, 190f
LeForte's facial fracture, classification of 488
Legionella pneumophila 349
Leishmania
  braziliensis 198
  donovani 198
Leishmaniasis 198
Lempert's elevator 451, 451f
Lempert's endaural incision 358f
Lempert's incision scar 46
Leprosy 131, 162, 195
Leprous laryngitis 280
Lesion
  benign 422
  intratemporal 132
  malignant 224, 263
  precancerous 322
  premalignant 221, 224
  solid non-neoplastic 295

Leukemia 220
Leukoplakia 222, 295
  patch 222f
Lichen planus 220, 221
Lichtwitz antral cannula 459f
Lids, edema of 165
Ligaments, membranes of 34
Lignocaine 221, 501f
Limbs, sudden movement of 122
Lincoln highway 487
Linear accelerator 436
Linear gingival erythema 342
Lingual thyroid reduction 423
Lingual tonsillectomy 422
Lips 210
  carcinoma of 210f, 225f
Little's area 20, 20f, 158, 159
Long face syndrome 244
Lopinavir 352, 353
Lower airway, protection of 23, 37
Lower lip
  hemangioma of 212f
  ulceroproliferative growth over 210f
Lower motor neuron facial palsy, causes of 52
Lower respiratory tract infection 482
Luc's forceps 465, 465f
Ludwig's angina 249, 250f, 395, 497f, 498f
Lumboperitoneal drain 91
Lumen catheter, double 390
Lung lesions 347
Lupus pernio 198
Lupus vulgaris 194
Lymph nodes 204, 302
  submandibular 161
Lymphadenitis 275
  regional 198
Lymphadenopathy 347
  causes of 346
  persistent generalized 347
Lymphatic drainage 21, 26, 31, 32, 39
Lymphocytes 193
Lymphoid depletion 347
Lymphoma 225, 396
  disseminated 200

M

Macrotia 55
Maculopapular rash 433
Magill's forceps 502
Maguaran plate 461f
Malaise 271, 275, 282
Malignant tumors, non-squamous 225
Mandible, fractures of 190, 191, 250
Manometry 323, 334
Mantoux skin test 195, 283
Mask 502
Masking therapy 106
Mass, complete excision of 196
Mastoid 6, 141, 360
  air cells
    exenteration 362
    primary carcinoma of 141
  antrum 6, 362
  infection 84
  interpret X-ray of 477

Index

pathology 478
sclerosis of 493f, 494f
surgery 128, 363
tenderness 50
types of 6, 478
X-ray of 478f, 481f
Mastoidectomy 87, 360
operated 482
type 363
Mastoiditis 45, 89, 130
acute coalescent 83
complications of 84
differential diagnosis of 84
Maternal-fetal transmission 335
Matrix, fibrillary nature of 206
Maxilla
carcinoma of 519
fractures of 189
osteomyelitis of 165
Maxillary artery 182
Maxillary region, tumors of 202
Maxillary sinus 170, 349f, 474f, 475f, 495f
carcinoma 208
forceps 456f
functional endoscopic sinus surgery 455f
lateral wall of 205
mucosa 169
ostium 24
palpation 153
Maxillary sinusitis 474, 475f
Maxillectomy
medial 205
partial 208, 518
total 208, 519, 520
Maximal stimulation test 129
Measles 508
Meatus
middle 18, 24
stenosis of 63
Mediastinal masses 396
Melanoma 58, 225
Melkersson syndrome 130
Melphalan 430
Membrane
extrinsic 34
intrinsic 34
Membranous labyrinth 9, 121
Meniere's disease 95, 146
staging of 96
variants of 96
Meniere's syndrome 115
Meningeal signs 349
Meningitidis 88
Meningitis 156, 162, 165, 168, 273
Meningoencephalocele 156, 156f, 206f, 203, 497f
Menstruation 176
Metal tracheostomy tubes 400
Metastatic lymphadenopathy, secondary 396
Methotrexate 433
Methylene blue tests 71
Metoclopramide 328
Microdebrider angled blade 460f
Microdebrider wand 459
Microear Baluchi scissors 446f
Microear surgery instruments 445
Microlaryngoscopy 409, 468
forceps 409
surgery procedure 410f

Microsurgical baluchi scissors 446
Microtia 55
Middle ear 5, 11, 133, 350
anatomy of 5
benign neoplasm of 138
blood supply of 7
carcinoma of 141
cleft 142
diseases of 64
effusion 204
infections 160
mastoid 134
mucosa 74
nerve supply of 7
ossicles of 7
pressure value 505
structures of 6
surgery 360
tumors of 138
walls of 5
Midfacial
destruction 198
destructive lesion 200
Mikulicz cells 193, 283
Minimal nerve excitability test 129
Minor salivary glands
carcinoma of 220
pleomorphic adenoma of 233
tumors 228, 262f
Mitomycin C 431
Mitotic index 206
Molar, roots of 250
Mollison's self-retaining hemostatic mastoid retractor 445f
Mollison's tonsillar
artery forceps 463, 463f
dissector 463, 464f
Mometazone 172
Montgomery 403
Moraxella 42
Morning headaches 311
Moro's reflex 122
absence of 122
Motility disorders 325
Mouse-nibbled appearance 282
Mousseau-Barbin tube 411
Mouth
angle of 339f
carcinoma, floor of 228
drooping of angle of 130
dry 345
floor of 210, 211
Mucocele 167, 202, 225
Mucoepidermoid carcinoma 235
Mucoid 42
Mucolytics 349
Mucoperichondrium 205
Mucormycosis 131, 196, 197f
black crust of 171f
Mucositis 221
Mucous membrane pemphigoid 220
Muller's maneuver 311
Multidrug therapy 432
Multiple sleep latency test 312
Multivitamins 323
Mumps 181, 229, 508
Muscles 68
actions of 35
extrinsic 35
intrinsic 35
tension dysphonia 304, 305

Muscular dystrophy 325
Mycobacterium
leprae 280
tuberculosis 347
Mycolytics 399
Myeloma, multiple 482
Myocutaneous flap reconstruction 226f
Myringoplasty 357, 360
Myringotomy 364, 365f
Myxedema 277, 279

N

Nasal allergy, sources of 174
Nasal biopsy 201
Nasal bones 185
fracture 185f
depressed 186f, 488f
types of 488
involvement 198
undisplaced fracture of 489f
X-ray of 488f, 489f
Nasal carcinoma 207f
Nasal cartilages 16f
Nasal catheter 502
Nasal cavity 416, 475f
carcinoma of 207
examination of 150
neoplasms of 202
patency of 150
proper 17
Nasal congestion 163
Nasal decongestant drops 165
Nasal deformity, external 162
Nasal dermoid 207, 207f
Nasal diphtheria 475
Nasal discharge 149, 165, 166, 205
Nasal endoscopy 204, 422, 453, 453f
Nasal glioma 157f
Nasal implantation 198
Nasal irrigation 167, 169
Nasal lesions 201
Nasal mass 205, 207, 423, 460f
biopsy 208
Nasal mucormycosis 171f, 197
Nasal mucosa 192
edema of 166
involvement 198
over turbinates 173
Nasal muscles 16f
Nasal myiasis 162
Nasal obstruction 148, 159, 160, 164, 166, 173, 175, 205
bilateral 148, 149, 159, 161
causes of 475
differential diagnosis of 149, 178
unilateral 148, 149, 205, 206
Nasal packing 381
anterior 180, 181, 181f, 381, 381f
posterior 180, 182, 182f, 382
Nasal papilloma specimen 205
Nasal part anteriorly 524
Nasal patency 176
Nasal polyp 167, 173, 177, 373
formation of 175
Nasal polypectomy 374, 422
Nasal polyposis 375, 514
Nasal reflexes 23

Nasal septal
hematoma 161f
spur 550f
Nasal septum 19, 151, 158, 185, 205
anteroinferior part of 158
blood supply of 19, 179, 179f
hemangioma of 158
parts of 158
perforation 162
perforation of 162
smooth bilateral swelling of 161
Nasal signs 175
Nasal skin 15
involvement 198
Nasal smear 175
cytology 176
Nasal solution 169
Nasal structures 193
Nasal stuffiness 208
Nasal suction tips 455f
Nasal synechiae 372f
Nasal valve correction, collapsed 314
Nasal vestibulitis 154
Nasal wall, lateral 17
Nasolacrimal system 192
Naso-orbital fracture 186
mode of 186
Nasopharyngeal angiofibroma 257f, 258f
extensive 257f
Nasopharyngeal bursa 31
Nasopharyngeal culture and assay 276
Nasopharyngeal pathology, symptoms of 69
Nasopharyngeal tonsil 31, 243
Nasopharynx 31, 152, 192, 196f, 198, 314
tumors of 256
X-ray of 475, 475f
Nebulization 399
Neck 546, 551
computed tomography scan of 297f, 498f
cystic hygroma of 218f
dissections 428
examination 543, 544
interpret X-ray of 483
magnetic resonance imaging of 262f
mass in 214
posterior triangle of 218f
trauma 267f
triangles 216f
ultrasonography 273
X-ray of 253f, 482f, 483, 483f-490f
Neck nodes 216f, 301
classification of 216
examination of 216, 217, 217f
levels of 216
Neck swelling 300
anterior 217, 218f
differential diagnosis of 217
lateral 217
midline 218f
Neonatal screening procedure 122
Neoplasm 131, 151, 219, 474
affecting esophagus, malignant 329

Index

benign 211, 329
  intratemporal 131
  malignant 211
Neoplastic oral manifestations 343
Neoplastic tumors 298
Nephritis 277
Nerve
  graft 132
  injury, Sunderland classification of 129, 129f
Neural pathways 12
Neurapraxia 128
Neurilemmoma 143
Neurofibroma 58
Neuroma 508
Neurotmesis 128
Nevirapine 352
Nissen's fundoplication 328
Nitrogen mustards 430
Nocardia 347
Nocturia 311
Nocturnal polysomnography 312
Noise
  breathing 290
  exposure 503
  safe limits of 102
Noise-induced hearing loss 102, 506
  types of 102
Nonairflow rhinitis 176, 173, 176
  etiological classification of 176
Noncaseating granulomas 194
Non-chromaffin paraganglioma 138
Non-Hodgkin's lymphoma 220, 225, 344, 345, 345f
Nose 314, 337, 546, 549, 550
  anatomy of 15
  anterior rhinoscopy examination of 151
  computed tomography scan of 156f, 160, 208
  contrast-enhanced computed tomography scan of 258f
  cysts of 202
  examination 150, 151, 542, 545, 548
  floor of 151
  functional examination of 150, 152
  granulomatous diseases of 192, 193f
  instruments 449
  internal 17
  inverted papilloma of 204
  lateral wall of 205
  magnetic resonance imaging of 197f
  nerve supply of 21
  nonolfactory mucosa of 205
  parts of 15
  physiology of 15, 21
  rhinophyma of 157
  rhinosporidiosis of 196
  Schneiderian membrane of 205
  vestibule of 17
  X-ray of 160, 475f-477f
Nuclear polymorphism 206
Nucleotide reverse transcriptase inhibitors 352
Nutcracker esophagus 326
Nutrition 438
  deficiency 221

Nystagmus 51, 111, 144
  degree of 111
  direction of 110, 111
  Ewald's laws for 111
  generation of 14
  grading of 51
  peripheral 51
  vestibular 110

O

Obital fat, prolapse of 377f
Obstruction, level of 308
Obstructive sleep 310, 311
  apnea 310, 313, 423
  pathophysiology of 310
Occupational rhinitis 176
Ocular signs 175
Odynophagia 210, 213, 250, 271, 282, 300, 326, 331
Ohngren's line 203
Olfaction 22
  pathway of 22
Olfactory neuroblastoma 206
Olfactory pathways 22
Onodi cell 25
Operation, steps of 365
Ophthalmoplegia 204
Optic nerve decompression 376
Optokinetic test 114
Oral appliances 314
Oral candidiasis 337
Oral cavity 27, 210, 337, 338f, 339f
  anatomy of 27
  and throat 543, 545, 551
  benign conditions of 219
  carcinoma of 225
  care of 438
  common disorders of 219
  conditions of 221
  disorders of 219
  examination of 213f
  lesion 210, 423
  lymphatic drainage of 28
  parts of 27
  physiology of 27
  tumor of 224
Oral communication 124
Oral hairy leukoplakia 339
Oral hygiene 252
Oral lymphangioma 224
Oral manifestations, bacterial 342
Oral mass lesions surgeries 460f
Oral mucosa, injury of 250
Oral papilloma 224
Oral rifampicin 283
Oral steroids 376
Oral submucous fibrosis 223, 223f
Oral ulcers 219
  etiological causes of 219
Oral warts over tongue 341f
Orbit 171f
  invasion 206
Orbital apex syndrome 167, 168
Orbital cellulitis 165-168
Orbital decompression 376
Orbital floor fractures 188, 189
Orbital invasion 205
Orbital proptosis 496f
Oropharyngeal dysphagia 332
Oropharynx 32, 192, 196f, 212, 213f, 215, 314, 337

benign tumors of 260
malignancy in 260
malignant tumors of 260
tumors of 256, 260
Ossicles 74
Osteoma 61, 136, 209
Osteomeatal complex 18
Osteomyelitis 165-167
Osteotome 449
Ostmann's pad of fat 69
Otalgia 43, 476, 503
  referred 282, 300
Otic hydrocephalus 91
  bacterial 59
  hemorrhagica 59
  malignant 60
Otitis externa 59, 350
Otitis media 66, 168
  acute 74, 350, 350f, 476
    necrotizing 66
    suppurative 64, 87, 131, 364
  adhesive 67
  chronic 130, 476
    secretory 67
  secretory 476
  serous 175, 350, 364
  tubercular 81
Otoacoustic emission test 122, 123
Otolaryngological surgeries 422
Otologic signs 175
Otological examination 144
Otorrhea 42, 503
Otosclerosis 92, 509
  foci of 92
Otoscope 350, 442, 442f
Overweight 328
Oxazaphosphorines 430
Oxidized cellulose 390
Oxygen 273
  cylinder 502
  flow meter 502
  mask 502
  supplement 274
Oxymetazoline 165, 377

P

Pachydermia larynges 279
Paclitaxel 433
Pain 210, 349
  killers 376
  relief of 130
Palatal mucormycosis 171f
Palatal paralysis 276
Palatal perforation 197f, 228f
Palate, high-arched 476
Palatine tonsillar hypertrophy 240f
Palatine tonsils 239f
  anatomy of 237
Palliative chemotherapy 431
Pallor 323
Palpable cervical nodes 204
Pantoprazole 328
Papillary cystadenoma lymphomatosum 235
Papillary sinusitis 204
Papilloma 58, 135, 422
  inverted 474, 475
Paraesophageal dysphagia 332
Paralysis, pharyngeal 276

Paranasal sinuses 53, 147, 150, 202, 208, 337, 373, 494f-496f
  anatomy of 15, 23
  benign neoplasm of 209
  cysts of 202
  examination of 150, 152
  extensive mucormycosis of 171f
  functions of 26
  mucous membrane of 26
  physiology of 15, 23, 26
  X-ray of 160, 165, 198, 473, 474f
Parapharyngeal space 30, 254, 262
  tumors of 262
Parathyroid glands, inferior 393f
Parathyroidectomy 428
Paresthesias 349
Parkinson's disease 325
Parosmia 150
Parotid gland 234f, 348f
  injury 184
  pleomorphic adenoma of 233, 233f, 525
  swelling, bilateral 232, 232f
Parotid nodes 207
Parotid space 248
Parotid surgery 236
Parotid swelling 348, 348f
Parotidectomy 502
Parotitis, acute 230
  suppurative 230, 230f
Paroxysmal sneezing 173, 175
Pars flaccida perforation 79
Pars tensa 75f, 76f
Passavants ridge 31
Passing cardia 412
Paterson-Brown-Kelly syndrome 322
Patulous eustachian tube 72
Penicillin 194, 197, 276
Penicillinosis, treatment for 348
Percutaneous dilatational tracheostomy 405, 405f
  prerequisites for 405
Perennial allergy 175
Perichondritis 57, 282
Periodic acid-Schiff 194
Periodontal disease 342, 342f
Periodontal tissue 342f
Periodontitis, acute necrotizing 342
Periosteal elevator 452
Permanent tracheostomy, indications for 396
Persistent laryngitis 168
Persistent perforation, causes of 74
Pertussis 85, 276
Petrosal artery, superfiacial 128
Petrosal nerve, greater superficial 128
Petrotympanic fissure 128
pH monitoring 323, 324
Pharmacotherapy 107, 175
Pharyngeal pouch 265
  tumors of 256, 263
Pharyngeal signs 175
Pharyngeal space 30, 254
Pharyngeal wall
  outline structure of 29
  posterior 213
    carcinoma of 265
Pharyngitis 168
  acute 246, 246f
  chronic 247

Index

Pharyngomaxillary space, abscess of 254
Pharynx 29, 254
    anatomy of 27, 28
    divisions of 31
    physiology of 27, 28
Phonation 37
Photon beams 434
Physiotherapy 130
Pinna 3, 5, 45, 56, 137
    anatomy of 3
    avulsion of 56
    benign lesions of 134
    diseases of 55
    forward downward displacement of 85
Pituitary tumor excision 376
Plasma
    cells 193, 201
    effect of 420
    exchange 200
    generation, stages of 420
Plasmapheresis 351
Pleomorphic adenoma 232, 262f, 497f
Plester's side knife 448
Plummer-Vinson syndrome 264f, 322
Plunging ranula 225
Pneumatic mastoid 478f
Pneumatization, type of 477
Pneumocystis carinii 350
Pneumomediastinum 396
Pneumonia 273
Pneumothorax 275, 396
Polanyi 417
Polio epidemic 385
Politzer's aural speculum 443
Polychondritis 57
Polycyclic hydrocarbons 203
Polymerase chain reaction 195
Polyp 74, 151, 167, 373
    formation 201
    removal 314
        methods of 373
        surgeries 460f
Polypectomy 373
Polypoid mass 207f
Polyposis 166, 167
Polysomnography 312
Portex tracheostomy tube 466f, 467
Postaural incision 124f
Postauricular region 46
Postcricoid region, carcinoma of 264
Postnasal discharge 166
Postnasal drips 173
Postnasal mirror 152
Postnasal packing 390
    methods of 390
Post-tracheostomy care 399
Postural tests 144
Posturography 114
Potassium iodide tablets 169
Preauricular accessory lobule 56
Preauricular lobule 56f
Pregnancy 176
Premolar, roots of 250
Presbycusis 103
Presbylaryngis 305
Presbyosmia 150
Pretracheal fascia 395
Proptosis 205, 206, 349

Protease inhibitors 352
Proteus vulgaris 169
Proton pump inhibitors 324
Pseudocyst 134
Pseudoephedrine 349
Pseudomonas 42, 250, 349
    aeruginosa 272, 349
Pseudorosettes, formation of 206
Puberphonia 305
Puberty 176
Pulmonary tuberculosis 282
Pulse 387
    oximeter 502
    rate monitoring 181
Pure tone audiometry 53, 93, 123, 131, 145, 503
Purine analogues 431
Purulent discharge 166
Purulent rhinorrhea 164
Pyoceles 202
Pyogenic granuloma 224
Pyriform sinus, carcinoma of 263
Pyrimidine analogues 431

Q

Quinsy 241, 251

R

Rabeprazole 328
Radiation 193, 203, 436, 437
    postoperative 437
    units of 436
Radical dose radiotherapy 200
Radical mastoid cavities 141
Radical mastoidectomy 362
    modified 361f, 362
    steps in modified 362
Radioactive material 436
    types of 435
Radioallergosorbent test 175
Radiofrequency 423f
Radiofrequency assisted
    adenoidectomy surgery 424
    somnoplasty surgery 424
    tongue base reduction surgery 424
    tonsillectomy surgery 424
    uvulopalatopharyngoplasty 424
    uvulopalatoplasty 424
Radiolucent cavity, causes of 482
Radiotherapy 142, 146, 201, 434
    complications of 437
    intensity modulated 435
    modes of 435
    uses of 434
Raghav Sharan's operation 169
Rampley's sponge holding forceps 466
Ramsay-Hunt syndrome 130, 351
Ranitidine 328
Ranula 225, 225f
Rapid eye movement sleep 309
Rat tail appearance 331f
Ratkhe's pouch 31
Recurrent laryngeal nerve 287, 287f, 393f
Rehabilitation 123
    care 269
    vestibular 109
Reinke's edema 279, 295

Reinke's space 279
Renal function tests 200
Respiration 22, 37
    cessation of 309
Respiratory distress 274
Respiratory disturbance index 309
Respiratory failure 395
Respiratory gas monitor 502
Respiratory insufficiency 396
Respiratory obstruction 214, 254, 395
Respiratory paralysis 395
Respiratory rate 387
Respiratory sleep disorders 310
Resuscitation bag 502
Reticuloendothelial cells 198
Retracted tympanic membrane 175
Retromolar trigone 210, 212
    involvement of 226f
Retropharyngeal abscess 252, 253f, 395, 483, 486, 486f, 487, 487f, 488f
    management of 487
Retropharyngeal space 30
    anatomy of 252
Reuter Bobbin grommet 366f
Rhabdomyosarcoma 142
Rhinitis 201, 475
    acute 163
    allergic 173, 174
    chronic 151, 163
    drug-induced 176
    hormone-related 176
    medicamentosa 176
Rhinocerebral disease 171
Rhinolalia
    aperta 307
    clausa 307
Rhinolith 162
    removal 375
Rhinometry, acoustic 176
Rhinophyma 150, 157
    correction of 423
    excision 422
Rhinoplasty, augmentation 162
Rhinorrhea 163, 204, 476
    excessive 173
Rhinoscleroma 192
Rhinoscopy
    anterior 150, 151, 542f
    posterior 150, 151, 152f, 542f
Rhinosinusitis 163, 167, 168f
    acute 163, 172
        bacterial 164
        viral 163, 164
    allergic fungal 375
    chronic 163, 166, 167, 172
    pediatric 172
    recurrent 163
    subacute 163
Rhinosporidiosis 151, 195, 475
    removal 375
Riecker's chest holder 471
Rifampicin 169
Rigid fiberoptic endoscopy 215
Rima glottidis 36
Ringertz tumor 204
Rinne's test 49, 49f, 50
Ritonavir 352, 353
Robotic surgery
    advantages of 427
    disadvantages of 427
Rodent ulcer 150, 157, 157f
Romberg's test 111, 144

Rose's position 386f
Rosen's aural speculum 443, 443f
Rosen's circular knife 447, 448f
Rosen's endomeatal incision 359f
Rotational test 114
Russell body 193, 283
Ryle's tube feeding 320

S

Saddle nose 155
    deformity 155
Saline irrigation 166
Saliva, drooling of 130, 210, 476
Salivary gland
    disorders of 229
    granulomatous infections of 230
    malignancy
        signs of 233
        symptoms of 233
    tumors of 212, 229, 232, 262
Salivary stone, huge 231f
Salivation, disturbance of 210
Salt and pepper appearance 494f
Sarcoidosis 198
Sarcoma 138
Scars 150
Schirmer test 132
Schneiderian papilloma 204
Schwabach's test 50
Schwann cells 143
Scleroderma 328, 329
Scleroma 283, 395
    affecting larynx 283
Sclerosis, multiple 325
Scratch disease 347
Seasonal nasal allergy 175
Sebaceous adenoma 61
Sebaceous glands, retention cysts of 134
Seborrheic dermatitis 349
Selenium 228
Semicircular canal 8, 14
    fistula, lateral 87
Semicircular ducts 9
Sensorineural deafness 101
Sensorineural hearing loss, bilateral 508
Sensory 103
Septal deviation, minor degree of 160
Septal flaps, necrosis of 162
Septal hematoma 161, 162, 162f, 199f, 201
    secondary infection of 161
Septal perforation 372f
Septic shock 273
Septicemia 251, 252, 254
    signs of 272
Septoplasty 161, 314, 369-372
    complications of 371
Septum 151, 185
    blood supply of 20
    retaining mucosa 161
    submucous resection of 369
Seromucinous glands 169
Serum
    angiotensin-converting enzyme 198
    calcium 198
Shah grommet 366f
Shea's aural speculum 443, 443f
Sheehy grommet 366f

Index

Shenoid sinus 494f
Shepard grommet 366f
Sialadenitis, submandibular 250
Sialectasis 230
Sialolithiasis 230
Sickle knife 409, 447, 447f
Siegel's speculum 442
Siegelization test 442
Sigmoid sinus 90
Silicon 365
Simpson's aural syringe 442, 443f
Sinonasal
    infections 349
    lymphoma 200
    malignancy 203, 206
    mass excision 376
    type papilloma 204
Sinus 24, 156
    fungal infection of 170
    infection 181
    of Morgagni 31
    osteomyelitis of 376
    ostium 165
    plate
        complete 89
        erosion of 90f, 493f, 494f
    preauricular 44, 56, 134
    thrombophlebitis, lateral 90
    ventilation of 26, 26f
Sinusitis 149, 160, 163, 167, 173, 349, 349f
    acute
        ethmoid 165
        frontal 165
        maxillary 164, 165
    allergic fungal 170, 495f
    chronic 279
        frontal 165
        invasive 170
    complications of 167
    intracranial complications of 168
    recurrent 175, 375
Sjogren's syndrome 231
    types of 231
Skin 176
    care of 438
    disorders 219, 220
    incision 397
    lesions 347
        cosmetic removal of 423
    prick test 175
    redness of 215
Skull-base osteomyelitis 60, 350
Sleep 309
    disturbances 311
    physiology of 309
    syndrome 310
Sleep apnea 308, 310, 311
    evaluation of 311
    risk factors of 310
    surgeries 314
    treatment of 313, 314
    types of 310
Sliding hiatus hernia 328
Sluder's neuralgia 149
Small internal auditory canal 123
Small round blue cell tumors 206
Smell
    altered sense of 149
    disturbance of 166
    loss of 160
    sense of 150
Smooth muscle tumor 329
Snare method 374, 386
Sneezing 163
Snoring 213, 308
    effects of 310
    mechanism of 308
Soft cystic swelling 156f
Soft palate 213, 339f
Soft papilloma 204
Soft tissue 475f, 493f
    injuries 183
    mass 208
Sonotubometry 71
Sore throat 213, 275
Sound, conduction of 11
Spasmodic dysphonia 306
    abductor 306
    adductor 306
Spasms 132
Spatula test 152
Speech 37
    development 120, 123, 124
    discrimination 145
    disorder 304
    therapy 279, 280
Sphenoethmoid recess 152
Sphenoid sinus 25, 152, 168, 205, 473, 495f
Sphenoid sinusitis 496f
Sphenopalatine
    foramina 494f
    ganglion block 170
Spindle poisons 431
Split night polysomnography 312
Sponge holding forceps 466f
Spontaneous nystagmus 110
Squamous cell carcinoma 58, 61, 141, 150, 157, 194, 220, 25, 226
Squamous papilloma 298
S-shaped deformity 159
St. Clair Thompson
    adenoid curette 464
        with guard 464f
    nasal speculum 450, 450f
    posterior rhinoscopy mirror 152, 449, 449f
    quinsy draining forceps 468, 468f
Stahl's ear 45, 56
Stammberger straight mushroom punch 456f
Stapedial reflex 131, 132, 145
Stapedotomy surgery, steps of 94
Stapes footplate 94f
    fenestra in 94f
Stapes suprastructure, fractures of 94f
Staphylococcus aureus 248
Stavudine 352
Steam inhalation 165
Stellate ganglion block 170
Stenson's duct 249
Sterilization 468
Steroid 130, 193, 199, 276
    intranasal 164
    nasal spray 162, 167
    sprays 166, 376
Stertor 291, 294
Stomatitis, angular 323
Strap muscle 395

Streptococcus
    pneumoniae 42, 349
    pyogenes 251
Streptomycin 169, 193
    systemic use of 169
Stress 221, 342
Stridor 253, 272, 283, 292, 294, 300
Stroboscopy 215
Styloid foramen 127
Stylomastoid foramen 128
Subglottic edema 415
Subglottic hemangioma 284, 285
Subglottic stenosis 283, 285f
    congenital 284, 285
Subglottis 302, 520
Subjective tinnitus, causes of 106
Submandibular duct, opening of 212
Submandibular gland 526
    duct 231f
    normal 526
    pleomorphic adenoma of 233, 234
Submandibular salivary flow test 132
Submandibular space, infections of 249
Submucous resection 369
    surgery 161
Suction cannula 409
Sulfamethoxazole 347
Superficial parotidectomy surgery 234f
    complications of 236
Supraglottic
    cancer 300
    laryngitis 272
Supraglottis 301
Supraorbital ridge fracture 185
Surgery 146, 201, 205
    exacerbates condition 199
    steps of 358, 391
Swallowing
    phases of 331
    physiology of 40
Swelling 150, 151, 167, 210, 215
Swimmer's ear 45
Synechia 475
Synkinesis 132
Synthetic tubes 401
Syphilis 131, 151, 193, 193f, 395
    acquired 281
    congenital 281
Syphilitic laryngitis 281
Systemic antibiotics 250, 255
Systemic disorders 219
Systemic lupus erythematosus 220
Systemic steroids 167
Systemic therapy 199

T

Tachycardia 387
Tampons 182, 182f
Tandem walking 144
Tarsorrhaphy 351
Taste
    disturbance of 210
    loss of 130
    test 132
Taxoids 431
Tear
    artificial 351
    bronchial 415

Teeth 210, 211, 254
    care of 438
    crowded 476
    fall 462f
    loose 201, 204, 208
    protruding 476
    upper incisor 38
Teflon paste, submucosal injection of 170
Teflon piston 94f
Telescope forceps 469f
Teletherapy 435
Temporal bone 90f, 123, 131, 492f
    fractures of 131, 492f, 508, 510
    high-resolution computed tomography of 54, 492f, 493f
    longitudinal fracture of 492f
    malignancy of 508
Temporalis fascia 359
Temporomandibular joint 208
Tenderness 152, 165, 217
Tetanus 396
Tetracycline 221
Thermal causes 220
Thermal necrosis, middle area of 417
Thoracic esophageal rupture 321
Thornwaldt's cyst 202, 203, 203f, 476
Thready pulse 387
Three fingers test 50
Throat 210, 543, 545
    discomfort 253
    examination 544
    instruments 460
    irritation 280
Thrush 219
Thudicum's nasal speculum 450, 450f
Thumb sign 273
Thyroid
    artery, inferior 393f
    carcinomas 522
    cartilage 520
    gland 393f, 395
    malignant 334
    vessels, superior 392f
Thyroidectomy 391, 396, 422
    surgery
        complications of 393
        steps of 391
        total 393f, 522
Tics 132
Tilley's nasal packing forceps 451, 451f
Tilly Lichtwitz antral trocar and cannula 459
Tinnitus 43, 96, 105, 106, 503
    evaluation of 106
    management of 106
    pathophysiology of 106
    retraining therapy 107
    treatment options of 106
Tissue 420
    blanching of 195
    damage, zones of 417
    destruction, mechanism of 425
Titanium 365
Tongue 211, 212f
    anatomy of 27
    anterior two-third of 210
    base of 213
    carcinoma of 211f, 227, 227f, 523

Index

channeling 422
depressor 213*f*, 461
deviation of 211*f*
dry 346*f*
erythematous candidiasis of 339*f*
palpation of base of 214
protrusion of 218*f*
pseudomembranous candidiasis of 338, 338*f*
Tonsil 212
   physiology of 237
   tumors of 261
Tonsillar bed structures 237*f*
Tonsillar fossa 261
Tonsillar grading 241*f*
Tonsillar hypertrophy, Brodsky grading of 240
Tonsillar tissue 385
Tonsillectomy 384, 385, 387, 422
   surgery 386*f*
      complications of 387
      steps of 386
Tonsillitis 168, 543
   acute 237, 238, 239*f*, 385
   chronic 237, 240, 240*f*
Tonsilloadenoid resection 423
Tonsilloliths 241
Toothache 201
Tophi 57
Topical nasal spray 172
Topoisomerase inhibitors 431
Torticollis 253
Torus 224
Towne's view 480
Toxic
   myocarditis 276
   shock syndrome 181
Toynbee's aural speculum 443, 443*f*
Toynbee's test 70
Trachea 34, 192, 317, 489
   anatomy of 315, 395
   exposure 398
   incision 398
   tear 415
   transection, complete 269, 269*f*
Tracheobronchitis 168
Tracheostomy 250, 252, 272, 273, 286, 314, 394, 403
   advantages of 395
   complications of 399
   contraindications of 396
   functions of 395
   indications of 395
   preoperative 255
   procedure 397
   surgical anatomy of 395
   tube 398-400, 402, 466
      size of 402
      types of 400
   types of 397
Tragal tenderness 51
Transaxillary thyroidectomy 428
Transillumination test 165
Transitional cell papilloma 204
Transoral robotic surgery (TORS) 427*f*, 428

Transthoracic esophagotomy 319
Trauma 131, 159, 219
   acoustic 508
   external 254
Traumatic perforation 162
Treponema pallidum 281
   hemagglutination 118
Treponema pertenue 197
Treponemal infection 197
Trimethoprim 347
Tripod fracture 187
Trismus 210, 226, 414
Trosseau's tracheal dilator 468, 468*f*
True vocal cords 289*f*
   mouse nibbled appearance of 282*f*
Tubal tonsil 31
Tuberculosis 131, 162, 194, 198, 482, 487
   lymphadenopathy 347
Tuberculous laryngitis 281, 282*f*
Tumor 142, 144, 151
   benign 57, 61, 157, 204, 224, 256, 260
   congenital 156
   malignant 58, 61, 134, 137, 157, 225, 256, 260
   necrosis 206
   over hard palate 211*f*
   spread of 142
   treatment with radiation, modes of 436
Tuning fork
   tests 49, 93, 514, 541, 551
   types of 442
Turban epiglottis 282
Turbinoplasty 314
Tutopatch 359
Tympanic membrane 4, 5, 46, 47*f*, 65, 67*f*, 75*f*, 105, 442
   attic perforation 47*f*
   diseases of 63
   large sized perforation 48
   layers of 4
   marginal perforation 47*f*
   medium sized perforation 48
   multiple perforations of 44
   normal 46
      right 48*f*
   outer surface of 128
   perforation 47, 75
      small central 48*f*
      subtotal 48
      total 48
Tympanic plexus 7
Tympanic segment 128
Tympanogram, type of 505
Tympanomastoidectomy 360
Tympanoplasty 357, 359, 360
   complications of 359
   Wullstein's classification of 359
Tympanosclerosis 67, 75, 509

U

Uglydepigmented scar 385
Ulcer 150, 210, 212*f*
   aphthous 220, 342, 343*f*
   traumatic 220

Ulcerative lesion 227*f*, 344*f*
Ulcerative periodontitis, necrotizing 342, 342*f*
Uncuffed tube 401, 516
Unifocal disease 201
Unilateral vocal cord paralysis 289
   management of 288
Unterberger's test 112, 144
Upper lip, distortion of 192
Utricle 9, 14
Uvula 212, 213
Uvulopalatopharyngoplasty 422

V

Vagus nerve, course of 288*f*
Valleculae, base of 213
Valsalva test 70
Vascular ischemia 130
Vasculitis 201
Vaseline gauze packing 181, 182
Vasomotor rhinitis 173, 176
   pathogenesis of 173
Venereal disease research laboratory 118
Venous drainage 39
Ventilating rigid bronchoscopy 470*t*
Venturi bronchoscope 471*f*
Venturi rigid bronchoscopy 470*t*
Vertebral angiography 145
Vertigo 43, 96, 108, 142, 503
   benign paroxysmal positional 114, 118
   peripheral 109
   types of 108
Vessels, ligation of 182
Vestibular disorder, peripheral 118
Vestibular nerve 9
Vestibular neuritis 115
Vestibular schwannoma 143
   microscopy of 143
Vestibular system 13
   disorders of 108, 109, 114
   mechanism of 13
   physiology of 14
Vestibular testing 145
Vestibule 8, 36, 150, 151
Vestibulo-ocular reflexes 111
Vidian neurectomy 173
Vinca alkaloids 431
Vincristine 433
Vindesine 431
Vinorelbine 431
Viral infection 129, 221
Viral parotitis 229
Vision 349
Visual loss 204
Visual reinforcement audiometry 123
Vitamin
   A 169, 228
   D 169
   deficiency 169, 219, 322
   E 228
Vocal cord 35, 296*f*, 298*f*, 300*f*
   lesion 410*f*
   palsy 290*f*, 300*f*
      bilateral 288, 290
      congenital 284, 285

positions 289*f*
spreader 409
Vocal nodules 295
Vocal polyp 295, 373
Vocal trauma 271
Voice
   abuse, chronic 279
   assessment of 216
   disorders of 214, 304
   fatigue 271
   hoarseness of 275, 280, 282, 300
   hypernasality of 307
   hyponasality of 307
   rest 271, 279, 283
Vulgaris 194

W

Waldeyer's ring 29, 30
Walsham's forceps 458, 458*f*
Wart 135
Warthin's tumor 235, 235*f*
Watery nasal discharge 175
Wax
   complications of 367
   role of 367
   solvents 368
Wax removal 367
   technique of 367
Weber's test 50, 50*f*
Weber-Ferguson-Longmire incision 208, 209*f*
Wegener's granulomatosis 199, 199*f*
Wegener's triad 199
Weight loss 300, 313, 327
Weil-Blakesley straight cupped forceps 454*f*, 455*f*
White cholesteatoma matrix 79
Whooping cough 276
William Wilde's
   incision scar 46
   postaural incision 359*f*
Wison's operation 170
Wound, closure of 362

X

Xenograft-bovine pericardium 359
Xerostomia 210, 345
X-ray
   chest 273, 274, 334
   mastoid Schuller's view 54
   neck 274
Xylometazoline 165

Y

Yankauer suction tube 463, 463*f*
Yaws 197
Young's operation 169

Z

Zidovudine 352, 353
Zollner speculum 443
Zygoma, fractures of 187, 188